PIERCE COLLEGE LIBRARY
PUYALLUP WA 98374
LAKEWOOD WA 98498

Medical-Surgical Nursing

Rationales

Mary Ann Hogan, RN, CS, MSN

Clinical Assistant Professor
University of Massachusetts, Amherst
Amherst, Massachusetts

Tomas Madayag, ARNP, MEd, MSN, EdD

Associate Professor
Barry University, School of Nursing
Miami Shores, Florida

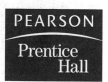

PEARSON

Prentice
Hall

Upper Saddle River, New Jersey 07458

Library of Congress Cataloging-in-Publication Data

Medical-surgical nursing : reviews & rationales / [edited by] Mary Ann Hogan, Tomas Madayag.
   p. ; cm.—(Prentice Hall nursing reviews & rationales)
Includes bibliographical references and index.
   ISBN 0-13-030457-3
   1. Nursing—Examinations, questions, etc. 2. Surgical nursing—Examinations, questions, etc.
   [DNLM: 1. Nursing Process—Examination Questions. 2. Nursing Process—Outlines. 3. Nursing Care—methods—Examination Questions. 4. Nursing Care—methods—Outlines. 5. Perioperative Nursing—methods—Examination Questions. 6. Perioperative Nursing—methods—Outlines. WY 18.2 M4896 2004] I. Hogan, Mary Ann, MSN. II. Madayag, Tomas. III. Series.
   RT41.M498 2004
   610.73—dc22

2003017414

Notice: Care has been taken to confirm the accuracy of the information presented in this book. The authors, editors, and the publisher, however, cannot accept any responsibility for errors or omissions or for the consequences for application of the information in this book and make no warranty, express or implied, with respect to its contents.

The authors and the publisher have exerted every effort to ensure that drug selections and dosages set forth in this text are in accord with current recommendations and practice at time of publication. However, in view of ongoing research, changes in government regulations, and the constant flow of information relating to drug therapy and drug reactions, the reader is urged to check the package inserts of all drugs for any change in indications of dosage and for added warnings and precautions. This is particularly important when the recommended agent is a new and/or infrequently employed drug.

The authors and publisher disclaim all responsibility for any liability, loss, injury, or damage incurred as a consequence, directly or indirectly, of the use and application of any of the contents of this volume.

Publisher: Julie Levin Alexander
Assistant to Publisher: Regina Bruno
Editor-in-Chief: Maura Connor
Executive Development Editor: Marilyn Meserve
Development Editor: Jeanne Allison
Director of Production and Manufacturing: Bruce Johnson
Managing Production Editor: Patrick Walsh
Production Liaison: Danielle Newhouse
Production Editor: Jessica Balch, Pine Tree Composition
Manufacturing Manager: Ilene Sanford
Manufacturing Buyer: Pat Brown
Design Director: Cheryl Asherman

Design Coordinator: Maria Guglielmo Walsh
Interior Designer: Jill Little
Cover Designer: Joseph DePinho
Electronic Art Creation: Precision Graphics
Marketing Manager: Nicole Benson
Assistant Editor: Sladjana Repic
Channel Marketing Manager: Rachele Strober
Manager of Media Production: Amy Peltier
New Media Project Manager: Stephen Hartner
Composition: Pine Tree Composition, Inc.
Printer/Binder: Courier/Westford
Cover Printer: Phoenix Color

Copyright © 2004 by Pearson Education, Inc., Upper Saddle River, New Jersey 07458. All rights reserved. Printed in the United States of America. This publication is protected by Copyright and permission should be obtained from the publisher prior to any prohibited reproduction, storage in a retrieval system, or transmission in any form or by any means, electronic, mechanical, photocopying, recording, or likewise. For Information regarding permission(s), write to: Rights and Permissions Department.

Pearson Prentice Hall™ is a trademark of Pearson Education, Inc.
Pearson® is a registered trademark of Pearson plc.
Prentice Hall® is a registered trademark of Pearson Education, Inc.

Pearson Education Ltd., *London*
Pearson Education Australia Pty. Limited, *Sydney*
Pearson Education Singapore, Pte. Ltd.
Pearson Education North Asia Ltd., *Hong Kong*
Pearson Education Canada, Ltd., *Toronto*
Pearson Educación de Mexico, S.A. de C.V.
Pearson Education—Japan, *Tokyo*
Pearson Education Malaysia, Pte. Ltd.
Pearson Education, Upper Saddle River, New Jersey

10 9 8 7 6 5 4 3 2 1
ISBN 0-13-030457-3

Contents

Preface

INTRODUCTION

Welcome to the new Prentice Hall Reviews and Rationales Series! This 9-book series has been specifically designed to provide a clear and concentrated review of important nursing knowledge in the following content areas:

- Child Health Nursing
- Maternal-Newborn Nursing
- Mental Health Nursing
- Medical-Surgical Nursing
- Pathophysiology
- Pharmacology
- Fundamentals and Skills
- Nutrition and Diet Therapy
- Fluids, Electrolytes, & Acid-Base Balance

The books in this series have been designed for use either by current nursing students as a study aid for nursing course work or NCLEX-RN licensing exam preparation, or by practicing nurses seeking a comprehensive yet concise review of a nursing specialty or subject area.

This series is truly unique. One of its most special features is that it has been authored by a large team of nurse educators from across the United States and Canada to ensure that each chapter is written by a nurse expert in the content area under study. Prentice Hall Health representatives from across North America submitted names of nurse educators and/or clinicians who excel in their respective fields, and these authors were then invited to write a chapter in one or more books. The consulting editor for each book, who is also an expert in that specialty area, then reviewed all chapters submitted for comprehensiveness and accuracy. The series editor designed the overall series in collaboration with a core Prentice Hall team to take full advantage of Prentice Hall's cutting edge technology, and also reviewed the chapters in each book.

All books in the series are identical in their overall design for your convenience (further details follow at the end of this section). As an added value, each book comes with a comprehensive support package, including free CD-ROM, free companion website access, and a Nursing Notes card for quick clinical reference.

STUDY TIPS

Use of this review book should help simplify your study. To make the most of your valuable study time, also follow these simple but important suggestions:

- Use a weekly calendar to schedule study sessions.
  - Outline the timeframes for all of your activities (home, school, appointments, etc.) on a weekly calendar.
  - Find the "holes" in your calendar—the times in which you can plan to study. Add study sessions to the calendar at times when you can expect to be mentally alert and follow it!
- Create the optimal study environment.
  - Eliminate external sources of distraction, such as television, telephone, etc.
  - Eliminate internal sources of distraction, such as hunger, thirst, or dwelling on items or problems that cannot be worked on at the moment.
  - Take a break for 10 minutes or so after each hour of concentrated study both as a reward and an incentive to keep studying.
- Use pre-reading strategies to increase comprehension of chapter material.
  - Skim the headings in the chapter (because they identify chapter content).
  - Read the definitions of key terms, which will help you learn new words to comprehend chapter information.
  - Review all graphic aids (figures, tables, boxes) because they are often used to explain important points in the chapter.
- Read the chapter thoroughly but at a reasonable speed.
  - Comprehension and retention are actually enhanced by not reading too slowly.
  - Do take the time to reread any section that is unclear to you.
- Summarize what you have learned.
  - Use questions supplied with this book, CD-ROM, and companion website to test your recall of chapter content.
  - Review again any sections that correspond to questions you answered incorrectly or incompletely.

TEST TAKING STRATEGIES

Use the following strategies to increase your success on multiple-choice nursing tests or examinations:

- Get sufficient sleep and have something to eat before taking a test. Take deep breaths during the test as needed. Remember, the brain requires oxygen and glucose as fuel. Avoid concentrated sweets before a test, however, to avoid rapid upward and then downward surges in blood glucose levels.
- Read each question carefully, identifying the stem, the four options, and any key words or phrases in either the stem or options.
  - Key words in the stem such as "most important" indicate the need to set priorities, since more than one option is likely to contain a statement that is technically correct.
  - Remember that the presence of absolute words such as "never" or "only" in an option is more likely to make that option incorrect.

- Determine who is the client in the question; often this is the person with the health problem, but it may also be a significant other, relative, friend, or another nurse.
- Decide whether the stem is a true response stem or a false response stem. With a true response stem, the correct answer will be a true statement, and vice-versa.
- Determine what the question is really asking, sometimes referred to as the issue of the question. Evaluate all answer options in relation to this issue, and not strictly to the "correctness" of the statement in each individual option.
- Eliminate options that are obviously incorrect, then go back and reread the stem. Evaluate the remaining options against the stem once more.
- If two answers seem similar and correct, try to decide whether one of them is more global or comprehensive. If the global option includes the alternative option within it, it is likely that the more global response is the correct answer.

THE NCLEX-RN LICENSING EXAMINATION

The NCLEX-RN licensing examination is a Computer Adaptive Test (CAT) that ranges in length from 75 to 265 individual (stand-alone) test items, depending on individual performance during the examination. Upon graduation from a nursing program, successful completion of this exam is the gateway to your professional nursing practice. The blueprint for the exam is reviewed and revised every three years by the National Council of State Boards of Nursing according to the results of a job analysis study of new graduate nurses (practicing within the first six months after graduation). Each question on the exam is coded to one *Client Need Category* and one or more *Integrated Concepts and Processes*.

Client Need Categories

There are 4 categories of client needs, and each exam will contain a minimum and maximum percent of questions from each category. Each major category has subcategories within it. The *Client Need* categories according to the NCLEX-RN Test Plan effective April 2001 are as follows:

- Safe, Effective Care Environment
  - Management of Care (7–13%)
  - Safety and Infection Control (5–11%)
- Health Promotion and Maintenance
  - Growth and Development Throughout the Lifespan (7–13%)
  - Prevention and Early Detection of Disease (5–11%)
- Psychosocial Integrity
  - Coping and Adaptation (5–11%)
  - Psychosocial Adaptation (5–11%)
- Physiological Integrity
  - Basic Care and Comfort (7–13%)
  - Pharmacological and Parenteral Therapies (5–11%)
  - Reduction of Risk Potential (12–18%)
  - Physiological Adaptation (12–18%)

Integrated Concepts and Processes

The integrated concepts and processes identified on the NCLEX-RN Test Plan effective April 2001, with condensed definitions, are as follows:

- Nursing Process: a scientific problem-solving approach used in nursing practice; consisting of assessment, analysis, planning, implementation, and evaluation.

- Caring: client-nurse interaction(s) characterized by mutual respect and trust and directed toward achieving desired client outcomes.
- Communication and Documentation: verbal and/or nonverbal interactions between nurse and others (client, family, health care team); a written or electronic recording of activities or events that occur during client care.
- Cultural Awareness: knowledge and sensitivity to the client's beliefs/values and how these might impact on the client's healthcare experience.
- Self-Care: assisting clients to meet their health care needs, which may include maintaining health or restoring function.
- Teaching/Learning: facilitating client's acquisition of knowledge, skills, and attitudes that lead to behavior change.

More detailed information about this examination may be obtained by visiting the National Council of State Boards of Nursing website at http://www.ncsbn.org and viewing the *NCLEX-RN Examination Test Plan for the National Council Licensure Examination for Registered Nurses.* *

HOW TO GET THE MOST OUT OF THIS BOOK

Chapter Organization

Each chapter has the following elements to guide you during review and study:

- Chapter Objectives: describe what you will be able to know or do after learning the material covered in the chapter.

OBJECTIVES

▌ Review basic principles of growth and development.

▌ Describe major physical expectations for each developmental age group.

▌ Identify developmental milestones for various age groups.

▌ Discuss the reactions to illness and hospitalization for children at various stages of development.

- Review at a Glance: contains a glossary of key terms used in the chapter, with definitions provided up-front and available at your fingertips, to help you stay focused and make the best use of your study time.

REVIEW AT A GLANCE

anticipatory guidance *the process of understanding upcoming developmental needs and then teaching caregivers to meet those needs*

cephalocaudal development *the process by which development proceeds from the head downward through the body and towards the feet*

chronological age *age in years*

critical periods *times when an individual is especially responsive to certain environmental effects, sometimes called sensitive periods*

development *an increase in capability or function; a more complex concept that*

is a continuous, orderly series of conditions that lead to activities, new motives for activities; and eventual patterns of behavior

developmental age *age based on functional behavior and ability to adapt to the environment; does not necessarily correspond to chronological age*

- Pretest: this 10-question multiple choice test provides a sample overview of content covered in the chapter and helps you decide what areas need the most—or the least—review.

Pretest

1 The nurse discusses dental care with the parents of a 3-year-old. The nurse explains that by the age of 3, their child should have:

(1) 5 "temporary" teeth.
(2) 10 "temporary" teeth.
(3) 15 "temporary" teeth.
(4) 20 "temporary" teeth.

2 The mother of a 6-month-old infant is concerned that the infant's anterior fontanel is still open. The nurse would inform the mother that further evaluation is needed if the anterior fontanel is open after:

(1) 6 months.
(2) 10 months.
(3) 18 months.
(4) 24 months.

- Practice to Pass questions: these are open-ended questions that stimulate critical thinking and reinforce mastery of the chapter content.

➤ Practice to Pass

What would you explain as normal motor development for a 10-month old infant?

- NCLEX Alerts: the NCLEX icon identifies information or concepts that are likely to be tested on the NCLEX licensing examination. Be sure to learn the information flagged by this type of icon.

NCLEX!

- Case Study: found at the end of the chapter, it provides an opportunity for you to use your critical thinking and clinical reasoning skills to "put it all together;" it describes a true-to-life client case situation and asks you open-ended questions about how you would provide care for that client and/or family.

Case Study

A 6-month-old female infant is brought into the pediatric clinic for a well-baby visit. You as the pediatric nurse will be assigned to care for this family.

❶ Identify the primary growth and development expectations for a 6-month-old.

❷ What type common behavior is expected of this 6-month-old towards the nurse?

❸ What immunization(s) are recommended at this age to maintain health and wellness?

For suggested responses, see page 406.

- Posttest: a 10-question multiple-choice test at the end of the chapter provides new questions that are representative of chapter content, and provide you with feedback about mastery of that content following review and study. All pretest and posttest questions contain rationales for the correct answer, and are coded according to the phase of the nursing process used and the NCLEX category of client need (called the Test Plan). The Test plan codes are PHYS (Physiological Integrity), PSYC (Psychosocial Integrity), SECE (Safe Effective Care Environment), and HPM (Health Promotion and Maintenance).

Posttest

1 **When using the otoscope to examine the ears of a 2-year-old child, the nurse should:**

(1) Pull the pinna up and back.
(2) Pull the pinna down and back.
(3) Hold the pinna gently but firmly in its normal position.
(4) Hold the pinna against the skull.

2 **To assess the height of an 18-month-old child who is brought to the clinic for routine examination, the nurse should:**

(1) Measure arm span to estimate adult height.
(2) Use a tape measure.
(3) Use a horizontal measuring board.
(4) Have the child stand on an upright scale and use the measuring arm.

CD-ROM

For those who want to practice taking tests on a computer, the CD-ROM that accompanies the book contains the pretest and posttest questions found in all chapters of the book. In addition, it contains 10 NEW questions for each chapter to help you further evaluate your knowledge base and hone your test-taking skills. In several chapters, one of the questions will have embedded art to use in answering the question. Some of the newly developed NCLEX test items are also designed in this way, so these items will give you valuable practice with this type of question.

Companion Website (CW)

The companion website is a "virtual" reference for virtually all your needs! The CW contains the following:

- 50 NCLEX-style questions: 10 pretest, 10 posttest, 10 CD-ROM, and 20 additional new questions
- Definitions of key terms: the glossary is also stored on the companion website for ease of reference
- In Depth With NCLEX: features drawings or photos that are each accompanied by a one- to two-paragraph explanation. These are especially useful when describing something that is complex, technical (such as equipment), or difficult to mentally visualize.
- Suggested Answers to Practice to Pass and Case Study Questions: easily located on the website, these allow for timely feedback for those who answer chapter questions on the web.

Nursing Notes Clinical Reference Card

This laminated card provides a reference for frequently used facts and information related to the subject matter of the book. These are designed to be useful in the clinical setting, when quick and easy access to information is so important!

ABOUT THE MEDICAL-SURGICAL NURSING BOOK

Chapters in this book cover "need-to-know" information about nursing management of a wide variety of health problems. The first chapter reviews nursing process and diagnostic and laboratory studies relevant to medical-surgical nursing. Chapters 2 through 16 explore health problems related to specific body systems. The final chapter discusses health problems commonly encountered in emergency and critical care settings. Mastery of the information in this book and effective use of the test-taking strategies described will help the student be confident and successful in testing situations, including the NCLEX-RN, and in actual clinical practice.

ACKNOWLEDGMENTS

This book is a monumental effort of collaboration. Without the contributions of many individuals, this first edition of *Medical-Surgical Nursing: Reviews and Rationales* would not have been possible. We gratefully acknowledge all the contributors who devoted their time and talents to this book. Their chapters will surely assist both students and practicing nurses alike to extend their knowledge in the area of medical-surgical nursing.

We owe a special debt of gratitude to the wonderful team at Prentice Hall Health for their enthusiasm for this project, as well as their good humor, expertise, and encouragement as the series developed. Maura Connor, Executive Editor for Nursing, was unending in her creativity, support, encouragement, and belief in the need for this series. Marilyn Meserve, Senior Managing Editor for Nursing, devoted many long hours to coordinating different facets of this project, and tirelessly and cheerfully encouraged our efforts as well. Her high standards and attention to detail contributed greatly to the final "look" of this series. Jeanne Allison, Developmental Editor, actively kept in communication with the different writers in this book and also facilitated getting the book itself into production. Editorial assistants, including Beth Ann Romph, Sladjana Repic, and others, helped to keep the project moving forward on a day-to-day basis, and we are grateful for their efforts as well. A very special thank you goes to the designers of the book and the production team, led by Danielle Newhouse, who brought our ideas and manuscript into final form.

Thank you to the team at Pine Tree Composition, led by Project Coordinator Jessica Balch, for the detail-oriented work of creating this book. We greatly appreciate their hard work, attention to detail, and spirit of collaboration. A special thanks also goes to Carlos Cooper, Lisa Donovan, and staff at the Pearson Education Development Group for designing and producing the *Nursing Notes* clinical reference card that accompanies this book.

Mary Ann Hogan acknowledges and gratefully thanks husband Michael and children Mike Jr., Katie, Kristen, and Billy, who sacrificed hours of quality time so that this book could come to publication. Your love and support kept me energized, motivated, and at times, even sane. I love you all!

Tomas Madayag dedicates this work to his parents who have instilled in him the value of education. He would also like to thank his brothers and sisters for their unending support. Lastly, to all past and present students who continue to inspire him with their questions and dialogue, a special thank you.

---

*Reference: National Council of State Boards of Nursing, Inc. *NCLEX Examination Test Plan for National Council Licensure Examination for Registered Nurses.* Effective April, 2001. Retrieved from the World Wide Web September 5, 2001 at http://www.ncsbn.org/public/resources/res/NCSBNRNTestPlan Booklet.pdf.

Contributors

Julie A. Adkins, RN, MSN, FNP
Private Practice
West Frankfort, Illinois
Chapter 10

Carol Wolfensperger Bashford, MS, RN, CS
Assistant Professor, Nursing
Miami University
Hamilton, Ohio
Chapter 13

Jill C. Cash, RN-CS, MSN, FNP
Family Nurse Practitioner
Southern Illinois OB/GYN Associates
Carbondale, Illinois
Chapter 10

Joseann Helmes DeWitt, MSN, RN, C, CLNC
Assistant Professor
Alcorn State University, School of Nursing
Natchez, Mississippi
Chapter 12

Lynn L. Fletcher, MSN, FNP, RN-CS
Veterans Administration Medical Center
West Palm Beach, Florida
Chapter 7

Mary Ann Hogan, RN, CS, MSN
Clinical Assistant Professor
University of Massachusetts, Amherst
Amherst, Massachusetts
Chapter 16

Ann Marie John, MS, RN
Nursing Department
Monroe Community College, Brighton Campus
Rochester, New York
Chapter 9

Sammie L. Justesen
Providence, Utah
Chapter 6 and 15

Susan Letvak, PhD, RN
Assistant Professor of Nursing
University of North Carolina, Greensboro
Greensboro, North Carolina
Chapter 4

Theresa Loan, PhD, RN
Associate Professor of Nursing
Eastern Kentucky University
Richmond, Kentucky
Chapter 2

Tomas M. Madayag, ARNP, MEd, MSN, EdD
Associate Professor,
Barry University, School of Nursing
Miami Shores, Florida
Chapter 14

Eileen Reilly-Mitchell, MSN, RN, BC-APN
Family Nurse Practitioner
Austin, Texas
Chapter 5

Joan Roche, APRN, MS, CCRN
Assistant Clinical Professor
University of Massachusetts, Amherst
Amherst, Massachusetts
Chapter 3

Deborah Jane Schwytzer, RN, MSN, CEN
Assistant Professor of Nursing
University of Cincinnati
Cincinnati, Ohio
Chapter 1 and 17

Debera Jane Thomas, DNS, FNP/ANP, RN-CS
Associate Professor
School of Nursing, University of Connecticut
Storrs, Connecticut
Chapter 7 and 8

Daryle Wane, APRN, BC, MSN, BSN
Assistant Professor of Nursing
Pasco Hernando Community College
New Port Richey, Florida
Chapter 11

Reviewers

Mary L. Anthony, MSN, RN
Associate Professor of Nursing
MacMurray College
Jacksonville, Illinois

Sharon Chappy, RN, PhD, CNOR
Assistant Professor
University of Wisconsin, Oshkosh
Oshkosh, Wisconsin

Martha Cobb, MS, RN, MEd, CWOCN
Clinical Associate Professor
The University of Arizona, College of Nursing
Tucson, Arizona

Deborah Conaway, RN, MSN
Assistant Professor
Samuel Merritt College/Kaiser Permanente
San Leandro, California

Kelly Jo Cone, RN, PhD
Assistant Professor
St. Francis Medical Center, College of Nursing
Peoria, Illinois

Kathy Patton Hall, RN, MSN, OCN
Assistant Professor of Nursing
Arkansas State University, Department of
    Nursing
State University, Arkansas

Mary Beth Kuehn, RN, MSN
Assistant Professor of Nursing
St. Olaf College
Northfield, MN

Mercy Mammah Popoola, RN,CNS, PhD
Assistant Professor
Georgia Southern University, School of Nursing
Statesboro, Georgia

Vincent Salyers, EdD(c), RN
Associate Professor
Palomar College
San Marcos, CA
Adjunct Professor
University of Phoenix, San Diego Campus
San Diego, California

Marian Tabi, PhD, RN
Assistant Professor
Georgia Southern University, School of Nursing
Statesboro, Georgia

Student Consultants

Alisa Beaulieu
Santa Fe Community College
Gainesville, Florida

Alison Cody
Germanna Community College
Locust Grove, Virginia

Daniel Dale
Valdosta State University
Valdosta, Georgia

Stephanie Hornby
George Mason University
Fairfax, Virgina

Amy Jeter
Ohio University-Chillicothe
Chillicothe, Ohio

Joan Lawrence
Auburn University
Auburn, Alabama

Lisa Marie Mays
Boise State University
Boise, Idaho

Shawn Shaughnessy
Santa Fe Community College
Gainesville, Florida

Phyllis Thieken
Ohio University-Chillicothe
Chillicothe, Ohio

Jenefer Thomas
Boise State University
Boise, Idaho

Gyleen Vickerman
Boise State University
Boise, Idaho

Carolyn Wilkinson
Auburn University
Auburn, Alabama

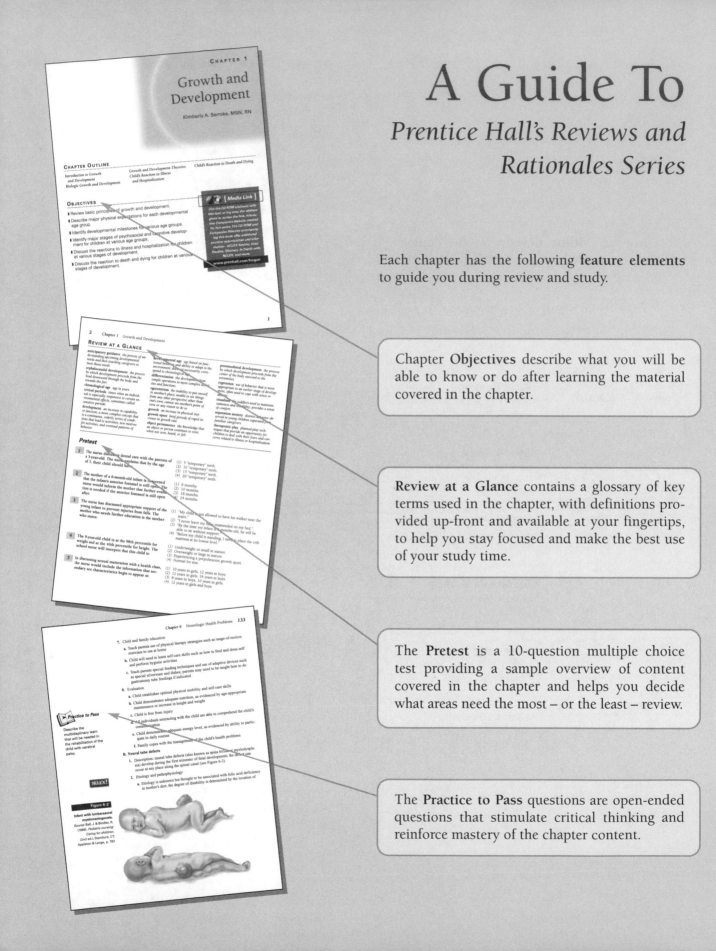

A Guide To
Prentice Hall's Reviews and Rationales Series

Each chapter has the following **feature elements** to guide you during review and study.

Chapter **Objectives** describe what you will be able to know or do after learning the material covered in the chapter.

Review at a Glance contains a glossary of key terms used in the chapter, with definitions provided up-front and available at your fingertips, to help you stay focused and make the best use of your study time.

The **Pretest** is a 10-question multiple choice test providing a sample overview of content covered in the chapter and helps you decide what areas need the most – or the least – review.

The **Practice to Pass** questions are open-ended questions that stimulate critical thinking and reinforce mastery of the chapter content.

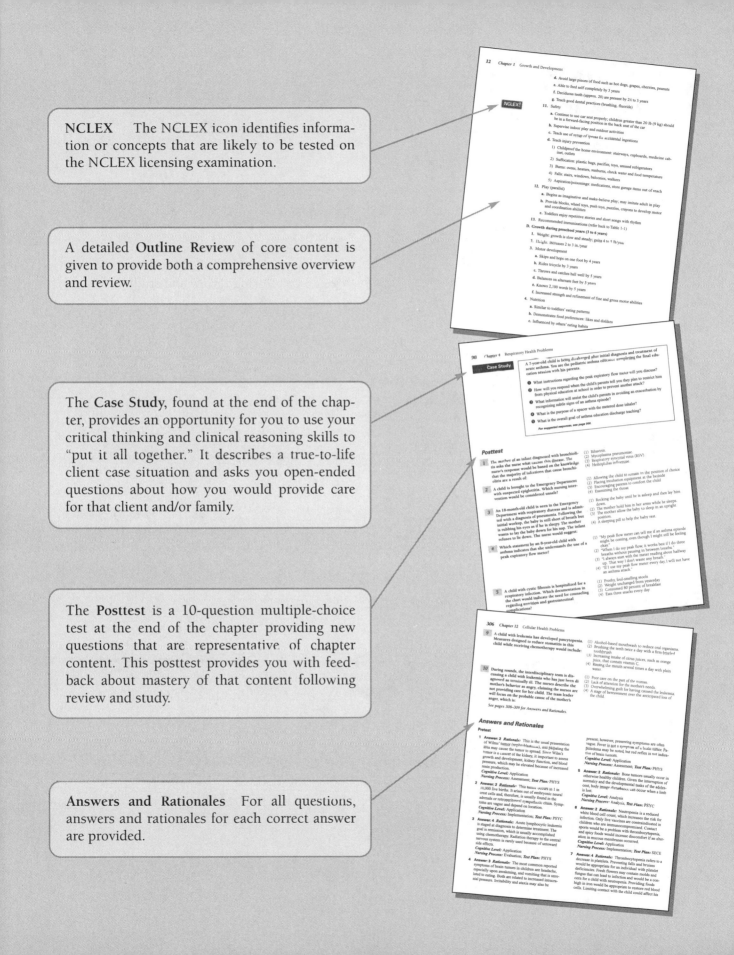

NCLEX The NCLEX icon identifies information or concepts that are likely to be tested on the NCLEX licensing examination.

A detailed **Outline Review** of core content is given to provide both a comprehensive overview and review.

The **Case Study**, found at the end of the chapter, provides an opportunity for you to use your critical thinking and clinical reasoning skills to "put it all together." It describes a true-to-life client case situation and asks you open-ended questions about how you would provide care for that client and/or family.

The **Posttest** is a 10-question multiple-choice test at the end of the chapter providing new questions that are representative of chapter content. This posttest provides you with feedback about mastery of that content following review and study.

Answers and Rationales For all questions, answers and rationales for each correct answer are provided.

Nursing Process, Physical Assessment, and Common Laboratory and Diagnostic Tests

Deborah Jane Schwytzer, RN, MSN, CEN

CHAPTER OUTLINE

OBJECTIVES

▪ Discuss the use of the nursing process as it applies to care of the adult client.

▪ Describe common physical assessment procedures used to examine the adult client.

▪ Identify laboratory tests commonly used to monitor the status of the adult client.

▪ Identify diagnostic tests commonly used to detect health problems in the adult client.

[**Media Link**]

Use the CD-ROM enclosed with this text, or log onto the address given to access the free, interactive Companion Website created for this series. The CD-ROM and Companion Website accompanying this book offer additional practice opportunities and information—NCLEX Review, Case Studies, Glossary, In Depth with NCLEX, and more.

www.prenhall.com/hogan

REVIEW AT A GLANCE

assessment *first step in the nursing process that involves the systematic gathering, sorting, and documentation of information collected*

auscultation *active listening to sounds within the body to gather information about the client's health status*

database *client-specific data collected through the client health history, physical assessment, and diagnostic test findings*

defining characteristics *signs and symptoms that support the specific nursing diagnosis*

diagnosis *application of standardized nursing labels to identified health problems or needs identified during client assessment*

etiology *identifiable causes or contributing factors defining the presence of a client need or problem*

evaluation *analysis of data gathered about the client's progress towards*

achievement of the identified goals or outcomes

implementation *operationalization of interventions assigned to achieve client-specific goals*

inspection *utilization of the senses of vision and smell to obtain information pertinent to the client's health status*

nonverbal communication *nonspoken messages conveyed through the use of body, facial expressions, or attitude*

nursing process *a systematic problem-solving approach to the collaborative identification of client health needs and the application of nursing care to effectively meet those needs*

objective data *any observable information that can be corroborated with assessment and diagnostic testing*

outcomes *measurable achievement of goals of treatment*

palpation *the touching of a client in a therapeutic manner to gain specific information pertinent to his or her health status*

percussion *the striking of one object against another to produce characteristic vibration sounds*

PES *format method for creating a client-specific nursing diagnostic statement by combining the client identified need, etiology, and signs or symptoms that identify the need*

planning *identification of achievable client goals and outcomes with the assignment of appropriate interventions to achieve these goals*

subjective data *data obtained from the client; includes feelings, perceptions and beliefs*

therapeutic communication *interaction between nurse and client aimed at gathering information and achievement of client goals*

Pretest

1 The nurse obtaining a nursing history can enhance data collection by utilizing the communication technique contained in which of the following questions?

(1) "Did your pain begin recently?"
(2) "You said the pain started yesterday?"
(3) "Can you tell me more about how the pain began?"
(4) "The pain isn't bad right now, is it?"

2 A nurse who is revising the nursing plan's goals and interventions would require which of the following?

(1) Knowledge of the hospital's standards of care
(2) Medical assessment and written orders
(3) Healthcare team conferences
(4) Validation of the effectiveness of the interventions

3 The nurse assesses for hyperkalemia in a client with which of the following problems?

(1) Renal failure
(2) Nausea and vomiting
(3) Excessive laxative use
(4) Loop diuretic use

4 Baseline arterial blood gases are drawn on a healthy adult scheduled for surgery. The nurse expects the findings to be which of the following?

(1) PO_2 30 mmHg and PCO_2 15 mmHg
(2) pH 7.32 and HCO_3 21 mEq/L
(3) PO_2 90 mmHg and pH 7.40
(4) PCO_2 49 mmHg and HCO_3 21 mEq/L

5 In assessing the laboratory findings for a client the nurse should be aware that a decrease in the serum level of which laboratory value might cause digitalis toxicity?

(1) Sodium
(2) Potassium
(3) Chloride
(4) Calcium

6 The nurse is preparing the client for an ultrasound of the gallbladder. Which of the following statements would be the most important to prepare the client for the test?

(1) "You will have food and fluids restricted for 4 to 8 hours prior to the test."
(2) "Stool in the bowel may cause a reporting of inaccurate findings."
(3) "There is no special preparation for this procedure. You may eat and drink as usual."
(4) "You will be asked to drink a solution of radionuclide 2 hours prior to the procedure."

7 Your client has recently returned to the unit following a bronchoscopy and is requesting a glass of water. Your first consideration in fulfilling the request would be which of the following?

(1) Is the client able to ambulate without assistance?
(2) Are the side rails up on the client's bed?
(3) Did the client receive a local anesthetic during the procedure?
(4) Is the call light within reach?

8 Your client is experiencing shortness of breath after oxygen that was being delivered by nasal cannula was decreased to 2 L/min. Pulse oximetry reveals an oxygen saturation reading of 71 percent. Which of the following would be the most appropriate immediate nursing action?

(1) Closely monitor the client's condition and increase the oxygen concentration to 15 L/min.
(2) Place the client in a semi-Fowler's position and continue to monitor.
(3) Do nothing; the drop in oxygen concentration is expected with the change in oxygen being delivered.
(4) Sit the client up, assess the client's status, and notify the physician immediately.

9 Which of the following steps of the nursing process would the nurse use when determining specific client needs based on the admission history database?

(1) Client teaching
(2) Team collaboration
(3) Diagnosing
(4) Developing a clinical pathway

10 The nurse is implementing a plan of care. Which of the following actions would the nurse take in this phase of the nursing process?

(1) Listen for carotid bruits
(2) Assist the client to use the incentive spirometer every 2 hours
(3) Prioritize care issues
(4) Consult the physical therapist about the client's progress

See pages 42–43 for Answers and Rationales.

I. The Nursing Process

A. Overview of the five steps (or phases) of the nursing process

1. **Assessment** is a systematic, comprehensive process of collecting, organizing, and documenting client specific data gathered from various available sources; it includes the client's medical, personal, social, and environmental status; data is also obtained from a comprehensive or system-specific physical assessment

2. Diagnosing/analysis is the interpretation of assessment data collected to identify client specific needs and strengths, and the formulation of an appropriate nursing **diagnosis;** it includes both actual and potential identified needs

3. **Planning** utilizes the assessment data and diagnoses to formulate client goals (desired outcomes), to prioritize the nursing diagnoses, and to identify the specific interventions to meet these goals

   a. It is a collaborative effort that assigns achievable and measurable, prioritized short and long-term goals and appropriate interventions to meet these goals in a specified time-frame

   NCLEX!

   b. Since it is a written plan of care, it allows for continuity and communication among the client, family, and all healthcare providers

4. **Implementation** is the actual carrying out of the client's plan of care through direct or appropriately delegated nursing orders; communication, supervision, and collaboration are essential to the successful achievement of this step

5. **Evaluation** includes an ongoing determination of the effectiveness of the implemented plan of care and the revision of the plan as needed to achieve the desired client outcomes

   a. The nurse assesses the actual outcomes and compares them with the desired outcomes

   b. If appropriate, new client goals are identified and reprioritized; appropriate interventions are prescribed; and the revised plan of care is implemented

   c. This is an ongoing process throughout the client's period of care

B. **Relationships** of the steps of the nursing process

1. The **nursing process** is a systematic, problem-solving technique

2. It is client-oriented and goal-directed to meet the identified actual and potential needs of the client and family

3. All five steps are adaptable to meet the ever-changing needs of the client and depend upon successful application of critical thinking and human caring skills during the previous step

4. It requires open communication, excellent listening skills, and the use of critical thinking

5. It promotes nurse-client-healthcare team interaction to effectively determine the appropriate means to meet the identified client needs and to achieve the desired outcomes (see Figure 1-1)

II. Assessment Phase

A. **Database collection:** client-specific data collected through the client health history, physical assessment, and diagnostic test findings

1. **Subjective data**

   a. This data is a collection of the client's symptoms, feelings, or individual perception of problems and needs

   b. It includes the health history and chief complaint in the client's own words

   c. Data can also be obtained from the client's family, friends, or other healthcare providers but is the interpretation of the perceived client needs

Figure 1-1

The nursing process is a continual process whose steps overlap to meet client's changing needs.

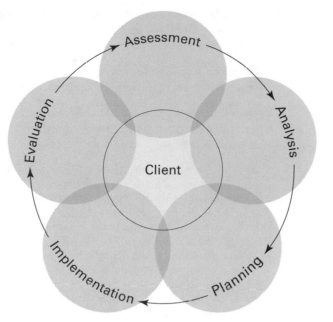

2. Objective data

    a. This is data that can be substantiated by physical examination, laboratory findings, or direct observation

    b. It is measurable against normal reference data or ranges and can be verified by more than one person

B. Nursing interview skills

    1. Establish rapport: the approach to the client is essential to the success of the nursing interview; introduce yourself, your title, and the purpose of the interview to begin the interview process; call the client by formal name to show respect and then ask how he/she wishes to be addressed during the interview; this recognition enhances the client's sense of being unique

        a. Set up the environment to have a quiet, undisturbed atmosphere and controlled lighting and temperature; this reduces distractions and enhances client comfort, which may in turn enhance data collection

        b. Good interpersonal skills demonstrated by the nurse during the interview process also affect data collection in a positive way and may increase the usefulness of the information gathered

            1) The nurse must demonstrate a nonjudgmental, accepting attitude towards the client when gathering assessment data

            2) Expressing concern, genuine caring and establishing rapport will place the client at ease and facilitate the client's comfort to provide accurate and thorough information

2. Questions are asked during the nursing interview process to gather information for use in all phases of the nursing process; a combination of types of questions should be used to elicit this information

   a. Questions should be formulated to gather information about the client's health concerns, perceived needs, chief complaint, and symptoms

   NCLEX!

   b. *Open-ended questions* are useful because they allow the client to provide general information rather than focus on facts and provide the client with a sense of control

      1) The client can decide how much information to give and how to say it

      2) Questions such as "What usually causes the onset of this pain?" or "When did these concerns begin?" can be very effective

      3) Open-ended questions require more than a one- or two-word response and are useful at the beginning of the interview process when the nurse and client are establishing a trusting relationship

      4) Disadvantages are that this type of question can be time-consuming and may cause the nurse to miss some important information; it is also not useful when interviewing a confused client or in emergent situations

   c. *Closed-ended questions* are directed towards fact-finding and are generally used to restrict the client's response to specifically focus on a certain area or concern, or to elicit information quickly and efficiently

      1) Questions such as "Are you thinking of hurting yourself or others?" or "Where is the pain now?" will encourage short and to-the-point answers

      2) Closed-ended questions, if overused, may also discourage open communication and the conveying of valuable information

3. **Therapeutic communication** (a nurse–client interaction aimed at information gathering and client goal achievement) is fundamental to developing a constructive and understanding relationship between the client and nurse that is directed toward meeting the client's identified needs; the following techniques are helpful:

   NCLEX!

   a. *Active listening* involves not only hearing the words that the client is saying but also processing this information to understand the client's feelings and unspoken concerns; it involves watching the client's body language and facial expressions as the client conveys his or her message; the use of good listening skills will convey to the client a sense that the nurse is accepting, caring, and attentive to the client's concerns

   b. *Rephrasing* information that the client has stated indicates to the client that the message has been heard by the nurse and allows for clarification (if needed), and serves to focus further discussion

   c. *Reflecting* on the information shared by the client conveys not only an understanding of the message and associated feelings, but also encourages further discussion and information sharing; remember that the use of reflection should not convey a message of being judgmental or giving advice

        d. *Summarizing* reviews the main information gathered during the interview and allows the client and nurse to identify any information that may have been omitted or to assure that the information was interpreted appropriately

    4. Compare verbal and nonverbal cues

        a. Be aware that body language and other nonverbal cues that the client expresses are frequently just as important as the client's verbal information

        b. Nonverbal communication (such as appearance, posture, gestures, or facial expressions) can often tell as much about the client's health, feelings, and self-image as the client's verbalization

        c. Take into consideration cultural differences that may affect a client's nonverbal communication

        d. Always validate interpretation of nonverbal cues with the client to ensure accuracy

    5. Terminating the interview is a necessary part of the interviewing process; it summarizes and validates the information gathered and gives the client an opportunity to share any additional information or comments about the interview process; it also allows opportunity to plan for future interactions

C. Organizing data

    1. Utilizing a nursing model: all data must be systematically collected, organized, and documented by the nurse using a consistent framework

    2. *Human Response Patterns* from the North American Nursing Diagnosis Association (NANDA) is one framework that organizes client data into nine patterns that reflect the client's interaction with the environment and provides a basis for developing nursing diagnoses

    3. Gordon's *Functional Health Patterns* is another commonly used format for organizing data into categories that can be used to develop nursing diagnoses and a plan of nursing care

III. Diagnosis Phase

A. Problem identification

    1. Involves critical analysis of assessment data gathered and compared to standards or established criteria used to recognize quality

    2. Identifies the client's strengths, actual or potential health care risks or needs, and the client's response to those identified actual or potential health care needs

    3. Identified needs must be amenable to nursing intervention

B. Selecting a diagnosis

    1. NANDA has developed a universal taxonomy of diagnostic labels that can be individualized to the identified client based upon the client's human response pattern

    2. NANDA has defined nursing diagnosis as a clinical judgment about individual, family, or community response to an actual or potential health problem or life process

3. NANDA has stated that these nursing diagnoses provide the basis for the applied interventions

C. **Writing a diagnostic statement**

1. Utilize the **PES format** (problem, etiology, signs and symptoms)

2. Problem identification is based on analysis of the assessment data to determine the client's individual health problem or response that may respond to nursing intervention

3. The problem is stated with a NANDA diagnostic label for the general area of client need; i.e., Activity intolerance, Knowledge deficit, etc.

4. **Etiology** of the problem is the probable cause or causes of the identified problem, (related to [r/t]) i.e., related to physical immobility, related to hospitalization, etc.

5. Signs and symptoms (**defining characteristics**) are the observable, measured, or reported evidence of the diagnosis (as manifested/evidenced by)

6. Sample PES format: Anxiety related to hospitalization as manifested by crying and withdrawal

IV. **Planning Phase**

A. **Priority setting** involves establishing a hierarchy of needs

1. Those needs that are life-threatening are usually given highest priority

2. Determination is based on the client's and family/significant other's input and value/belief system

3. *Maslow's Hierarchy of Needs Theory* is frequently used in priority setting

4. Prioritization will also be affected by resource availability

5. The medical plan must also be taken into consideration when prioritizing the nursing care plan

B. **Goals/outcomes** are those identifiable client responses that are the result of the prescribed nursing orders or interventions

1. Short-term goals are expected client responses and accomplishments over a brief period of time; they are goals that meet the client's immediate needs; i.e., "client will be tolerating a clear liquid diet by Monday"

2. Long-term goals focus on the client's long-term healthcare needs or condition; they may be focused on criteria for discharge, rehabilitation, or health care promotion, i.e., "Client will be able to perform self-tracheostomy suctioning"

3. Discharge planning should begin at the time of the first nurse-client encounter

4. Nursing orders or interventions that are prescribed to achieve client goals must be client-specific, congruent with approved standards and medical plan, and must be clearly communicated in writing

V. **Implementation Phase**

A. **Nursing plan** of care is carried out

B. **Daily priorities** are set based upon client status

    C. Activities may be delegated as appropriate

    D. Data is collected as interventions are completed related to client's response

    E. Continual assessment and documentation, both written and verbal, are essential

    F. Nursing care plans provide a scientific basic/rationale for client care and help to ensure optimal outcomes

VI. Evaluation Phase

    A. Determines achievement of client goals and effectiveness of the plan of care

       1. Data is collected on an ongoing basis about client's progress and achievement of desired outcomes

       2. Nursing interventions are evaluated for their effectiveness in achievement of desired outcomes

NCLEX!

    B. Nursing plan of care is modified or terminated as needed based upon results of evaluation

       1. Modification may occur in the nursing diagnoses, goals, or interventions

       2. Termination of care plan will occur if goals have been met

VII. Documentation

    A. A vehicle for communication

       1. Delineates all steps of the nursing process in a clear, concise manner

       2. Allows for feedback between or among all healthcare providers

NCLEX!

       3. Provides information for educational purposes and reimbursement issues but must assure a degree of confidentiality

       4. Must be legible and utilize standardized abbreviations and terms

       5. Provides a written record of care and its outcomes

    B. Legal implications

       1. The medical record is a legal document and can be used in court related to care provided and outcomes

NCLEX!

       2. Must adhere to professional standards and agency policies

VIII. History-Taking as Part of Physical Assessment

    A. Communicating with the adult client

       1. Prior to beginning an assessment of the adult client, it is essential to gather all necessary client information, medical records, and needed equipment

       2. An environment free of potential interruptions with good lighting and appropriate temperature setting enhances the comfort of the client

       3. When beginning the health history-taking and the physical review of systems, assure the client of the confidentiality of this process

       4. Be sure to allow enough time to complete the history and physical examination

5. Use language at a level appropriate for the client during the history and the physical examination

6. Use proper names unless otherwise agreed upon

7. Use specific medical terms only if understood by the client, and give a full explanation of what to expect during the exam

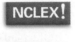

8. Be aware of any cultural influences or values that may affect the assessment process

9. Special care should be taken with the elderly or clients with special needs, such as the visually or hearing impaired, mentally or physically challenged, or those with language difficulties; in these cases, a family member or support person should be included in the process if authorized by the client

B. Health history and interview

1. The health history and interview are the initial steps in the physical assessment process and provide the subjective information needed to develop an individualized plan of nursing care

2. Information gathered will serve as the basis for an understanding of the client's expectations of this episode of health care, his/her concerns and needs, and provide a means to identify possible areas for specific physical and laboratory data collection

C. Outline of client's health history

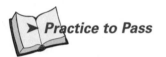

Practice to Pass

An elderly client who is hearing-impaired has been scheduled for a routine physical examination. What actions should be taken to enhance the ability to obtain an accurate health history?

1. The *chief complaint/current problem* is the reason the client seeks health care; it should be quoted in the client's own words; include documentation of the history of the chief complaint such as onset, location, duration, quality, alleviating and aggravating factors, and associated symptoms

2. The *past medical history* includes a summary of all the medical problems that the client has experienced during his/her lifetime

   a. It should include all allergies, chronic and acute illnesses, communicable diseases, blood transfusions, major injuries, accidents, or surgeries with dates and where hospitalized

   b. An immunization history should be obtained; particular attention should be paid to Hepatitis B and TB in at risk populations, flu and pneumonia vaccines in the elderly and chronically ill populations, and tetanus toxoid in the general population

   c. A list of the current and past over-the-counter (OTC) and prescription medication use is also obtained

3. The *family history* includes a record of the health status of the client's immediate blood relatives (parents, aunts, uncles, grandparents, siblings, spouse and children), including the age, current health status, and any chronic illnesses that may be known; a *genogram* (see Figure 1-2) is often used to depict this information; any genetic or familial diseases are also documented in this section

4. The *personal history* reviews aspects of the client's lifestyle that may affect current health or identify risk factors for health problems

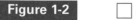

Figure 1-2

Interpreting a genogram.
A. Standard symbols; B.
Combining symbols to
provide additional
information; C. A family
genogram.

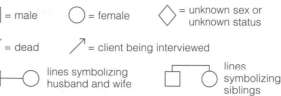

☐ = male   ◯ = female   ◇ = unknown sex or unknown status

╱ = dead   ↗ = client being interviewed

☐—◯ lines symbolizing husband and wife

☐ ◯ lines symbolizing siblings

A Genogram symbols

☐53 = 53-year-old male with diabetes
Diabetes

⊘65 = 65-year-old female dead of colon cancer
Colon cancer

↗(24) = 24-year-old female being interviewed

◇2 = two unknown individuals

B Combining symbols to provide additional information

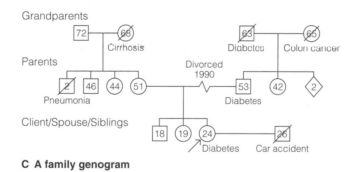

Grandparents

[72]—⊘68
      Cirrhosis

[63]—⊘65
Diabetes Colon cancer

Parents

Divorced
1990

⊘2 [46] (44) (51)
Pneumonia

[53] (42) ◇2
Diabetes

Client/Spouse/Siblings

[18] (19) (24)—[26]
      ↗Diabetes Car accident

C A family genogram

a. Note alcohol use and quantity of consumption along with timing and occasions of use

b. Note tobacco use, i.e., cigarettes, cigars, chewing tobacco, snuff, or pipe smoking; cigarettes are usually calculated in pack/year history (number of packs per day multiplied by the number of years smoked)

c. Document the use of illegal drugs or inappropriate use of drugs as well as the route of their use; although this is a sensitive issue, it is vital to appropriately assessing and diagnosing the client's needs

d. Address the client's sexual practices in order to identify areas of risk and potential educational needs

e. Obtain a personal history, including the client's education, financial status, religious and ethnic background, work and home environment, travel history, hobbies, sleep pattern, stress management activities, and date of last health check-up

5. The *review of systems* is a detailed history according to body systems

a. General: assess the client's perception of overall health at present and in the past; note presence of fatigue, malaise, fever, chills, night sweats, sensitivity to heat and cold, or recent weight or appetite changes

b. Skin: ask about changes in skin pigmentation, jaundice, rashes, moles, lumps, sores, odors, excessive sweating, changes in hair growth pattern or hair growth in unusual places, changes in skin or nail texture

c. Head and neck: ask whether the client has experienced any recent head trauma, headaches, vertigo, syncope, changes in mental status, pain, tenderness, decreased movement in the neck, difficulty swallowing, or swelling in the head or neck

d. Eyes: ask about any visual changes, pain, use of glasses, contact lenses, reading devices, double vision, night blindness, visual halos, flashing lights, blind spots, excessive tearing or drainage, glaucoma, or cataracts

e. Ears: inquire about use of hearing aids, changes in hearing acuity, discharge, pain, ringing in the ears (tinnitus), recent or chronic earaches or infections

f. Nose and sinuses: ask about recent colds, pain, stuffiness, discharge, polyps, obstructions, nosebleeds, difficulty breathing, or feeling of sinus pressure

g. Mouth and throat: ask about any dentures, toothaches, caries, abscesses, bleeding or swelling, changes in the appearance of the tongue or pain in the tongue, chewing difficulties or pain, changes in taste or salivation, hoarseness, throat pain, or enlarged thyroid

h. Breasts: ask male and female clients about any noted pain, tenderness, discharge from nipples, and changes in size or dimpling

i. Respiratory: ask about any shortness of breath, breathing pattern changes, acute or chronic cough, sputum production or change in color, bloody sputum, wheezing, and date of last chest x-ray

j. Cardiac: inquire about edema, shortness of breath at night relieved by sleeping on several pillows, chest pain, murmurs, palpitations, and date and results of last electrocardiogram (ECG)

k. Gastrointestinal: ask about any changes in appetite, nausea, vomiting, heartburn, frequent indigestion, excessive thirst, diarrhea, constipation, bowel movement frequency, change in stool color, flatulence, hemorrhoids, abdominal pain with location and intensity, or abdominal swelling

l. Urinary: inquire about any urinary burning or frequency, nocturia, decreased stream of flow, hesitancy, polyuria, bedwetting, incontinence, frequent urinary tract infection or history of kidney stones

m. Genital

1) Female client: ask about onset of menarche, date of last menstrual period, any premenstrual symptoms, intermenstrual bleeding, painful periods, vaginal discharges, pain, sexually transmitted diseases, sexual activity, use of birth control, safe sex practices, last pap smear and

mammogram, pregnancy history, hormonal replacement therapy, and regular practice of self-breast examinations

2) Male client: ask about penile discharge, testicular pain or lumps, sexually transmitted diseases, sexual activity, safe sex practices, impotence, infertility, erections, hernias, enlarged prostate, and regular practice of testicular self-examination

n. Peripheral vascular: ask client about any noted varicosities, pain in calf when walking, hand, leg, or foot cramps, blood clots in legs, ankle or hand swelling, and changes in temperature or sensation in fingers or feet

o. Musculoskeletal: inquire about joint stiffness, heat, or pain, decreased range of motion, weakness, swelling, bony deformities, bone tenderness, gout, arthritis, osteoarthritis, muscle atrophy, herniated discs, or broken bones

p. Neurological: ask about any changes in balance, coordination, sensory perception, changes in speech or thought processes, aphasia, headaches, tremors, seizures, weakness, head injuries, or fainting

q. Hematologic: inquire about bruising, bleeding, anemia, blood type, sickle cell anemia, and history of blood transfusions (and reactions)

r. Endocrine: ask about fatigue, heat or cold intolerance, bulging eyes, weight changes, changes in urine volume, changes in hair distribution, changes in the size of head, hands or feet, swelling in anterior neck, diabetes mellitus, or hormone replacement therapy

s. Psychiatric: inquire about depression, irritability, tension and feeling of excessive stress, suicidal or homicidal ideations, or disturbances in thought processes

D. Impact of cultural and religious beliefs

1. The client's cultural and religious norms and values will affect his/her view and response to illness, the need to seek care, and the care he/she believes to be appropriate

2. The nurse must recognize the importance of the individual's beliefs and values, identify the specific practices, and incorporate these into the plan of care

3. Communication style, both verbal and nonverbal, must be assessed (for example, some Asian cultures value silence and suppression of emotions, and view eye contact as disrespectful); the client may require the services of a translator or family member (if available and appropriate) to convey their needs

4. Family and social relationships must be considered

   a. Family is the center of many cultures, and as such, many decisions about healthcare are made by the family or a particular family member and not by the client

   b. Strong family values and traditions may require that a family member be present at all times while the client is receiving care; others may require privacy at all times

5. Health customs and practices such as the use of folk practitioners, ointments, heat, cold, and/or special foods, may be essential components of the client's care

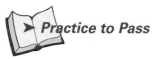

Practice to Pass

You are obtaining a health history on a client with a chief complaint of nausea. What information would be important to obtain?

      a. Make every attempt to allow the incorporation of these practices into the plan of care

      b. If serious conflicts exist, attempt to collaborate with the client

  6. Religious beliefs are essential to the well being of the client; respect and honor the client's belief systems and document any specific spiritual needs and requests of the client

IX. Physical Examination Techniques

NCLEX!

  A. Inspection: the visual observation of all parts of the body during the health assessment; involves visually comparing the size, shape, symmetry, color, position, and appearance of the client; it can also involve utilizing the sense of smell to detect unusual odors

  B. Palpation: the use of touch to determine the characteristics of exposed and underlying tissues and organs; is best performed when the client is relaxed

    1. Various parts of the hands are used to palpate certain areas of the body or gain specific information

      a. Use the dorsal surface to assess body temperature because of its increased sensitivity

      b. Use the palmar surface finger pads to assess moisture, texture, masses, pulses, crepitus, fine tactile discrimination, and organ size, shape, position, and consistency

      c. Use the ulnar surface, ball of the hand, and the palmar metacarpophalangeal joints to assess using vibrations

    2. Types of palpation

      a. Light palpation: uses superficial, gentle, delicate touch with the finger pads for surface assessments or skin and the assessment of superficial or enlarged masses, fluid, and tender or guarded areas

      b. Deep palpation: uses the fingertips and hand to assess internal organs and structures to a depth of about 2 to 3 cm or more using either one or two hands

      c. Ballottement: utilizes the fingers to tap around suspected masses floating in a fluid-filled cavity and sense the rebound of the mass as it returns to its original position

  C. Percussion: the striking of one object against another to cause vibrations that produce a sound

    1. Percussion sounds are assessed according to their location, intensity, pitch, duration, and quality; each body part or area percussed has a normal or expected sound and any deviation is further assessed

    2. Percussion produces five distinct sounds: flatness, dullness, resonance, hyperresonance, and tympany; each sound is normal in certain areas; there are two types of percussion

      a. Direct percussion utilizes the fingers or fist of the examiner's hand to tap directly on the client's skin to elicit a sound, such as when percussing the sinus region; a percussion hammer can also be utilized to assess reflexes

b. Indirect percussion involves the nurse tapping the finger or fingers of one hand with the other hand that is in contact with the client's skin, such as when assessing over the lung fields

D. Auscultation: utilizes the sense of hearing to assess sounds produced by body organs

1. Auscultated sounds are classified by presence, location, intensity, pitch quality, and duration

2. Types of auscultation

a. Direct: involves the detection of sounds with the ear alone either away from the client or with the ear in contact with the client's skin; wheezing or hyperactive bowel sounds can sometimes be heard with direct auscultation

b. Indirect or mediated: involves the detection of sound with the assistance of some type of amplified or nonamplified listening device

1) The most common device is the acoustic stethoscope, which does not amplify the sound but rather blocks out environmental noises

2) Another type of mediated auscultation device is the Doppler, which will amplify sounds to allow detection and characterization

E. Measurement of vital signs, height, and weight

1. The client's vital signs include temperature, pulse, respirations, and blood pressure; these are considered essential components of the physical assessment to obtain a baseline for the client as well as to evaluate health status changes or needs

a. Temperature: the measurement of the body's balance between heat production and heat loss to the environment

1) The usual sites of measurement are oral, rectal, axillary, or the tympanic membrane

2) Normal temperature for the adult client is 98°F (36.7°C) to 98.6°F (37°C)

3) Factors affecting temperature can include age, exercise, circadian rhythms, hormones, stress, and the environment

b. Pulse: a measurement of a wave of blood as generated by the left ventricle

1) The most common sites of measurement are the radial or apical pulse; however the pulse can also be obtained in the temporal, carotid, brachial, femoral, popliteal, posterior tibial, or dorsalis pedis areas

2) Normal pulse range is considered to be 60 to 100 beats per minute but is very client-specific

3) Factors affecting the pulse rate can include age, gender, medications, exercise, stress, temperature, hemorrhage, position change, and preexisting medical condition(s)

c. Respirations: the measurement of the act of breathing characterized by its rate, rhythm, depth, and character

1) Respirations are normally measured with the client at rest

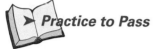
Practice to Pass

You are performing a physical examination on a client who has recently had abdominal surgery. What changes would occur in your physical assessment?

NCLEX!

NCLEX!

2) Normal respiratory rate is considered to be 12 to 20 respirations per minute

3) Factors that may affect the respiratory rate are exercise, stress, temperature, medication, altitude, and preexisting medical conditions such as asthma

   d. Blood pressure: the measurement of blood flow through the arteries; it is recorded as the systolic and the diastolic pressure

1) Blood pressure is measured in millimeters of mercury (mmHg) and is recorded as a fraction of systolic/diastolic; although usually measured indirectly at the brachial artery, it may also be obtained at the radial and popliteal arteries with a blood pressure cuff

2) Normal adult blood pressure is considered to be 120/80, however it is more accurate to compare a client's blood pressure to his or her baseline when assessing current health status

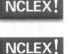

3) Age, gender, race, obesity, medications, exercise, stress, time of day, or preexisting medical condition affects blood pressure readings

4) Blood pressure cuff bladder should be 40 percent of the circumference of the extremity and its length should be two-thirds of the limb circumference; the use of an inappropriate size blood pressure cuff can cause erroneous blood pressure readings

5) Blood pressure readings may also be obtained directly and continuously through the use of a catheter inserted directly into the brachial, radial, or femoral artery, which is then connected to hemodynamic monitoring equipment and displayed on a monitor

  2. Height: the client's length; is gathered to establish a baseline upon which to compare subsequent measurements and serves as an indicator of health status; is often used to assist in identifying hormonal, genetic, or organ system dysfunction

  3. Weight: a measure of the client's body mass in pounds or kilograms; is gathered to establish a baseline for future measurements and to assist in identifying actual or potential healthcare needs; often the height and weight measurements are plotted together on a graph for comparison to establish norms of growth, development, and nutritional status

X. Common Laboratory Tests Used to Monitor the Health Status of Adults

A. Blood chemistries

  1. Albumin (serum): normal range is 3.5 to 5.0 g/dL; 52 to 68 percent of total protein

   a. Description: a component of protein that is synthesized by the liver; it is responsible for increasing osmotic pressure to maintain intravascular fluid retention and transportation of hormones, fatty acids, bilirubin, medications, and substances insoluble in water; a decrease in albumin will cause fluid shifts from the blood vessels into the tissues causing edema formation

   b. Clinical problems: *decreased levels* of albumin occur in acute liver failure, cirrhosis of the liver, malnutrition, malabsorption syndromes, ulcerative colitis, renal disorders, and preeclampsia; *increased levels* may occur in dehydration, severe diarrhea, or vomiting

c. Medications that may affect albumin levels: *decrease*: aspirin, ascorbic acid, penicillin, and sulfonamides; *increase*: heparin

NCLEX!

d. Nursing implications

1) No dietary or fluid restrictions prior to the blood being drawn

2) Assess for edema or ascites formation; prevent skin breakdown

2. Ammonia (serum): normal range is 15 to 45µg/dL

a. Description: a by-product of nitrogen breakdown in protein metabolism; it is normally converted to urea in the liver and excreted by the kidney

b. Clinical problems: *decreased levels* may occur in renal failure, and in malignant or essential hypertension; *increased levels* may occur in hepatic failure, hepatic encephalopathy, hepatic coma, cor pulmonale, Reye's syndrome, severe congestive failure, high-protein diets with liver dysfunction, acidosis, hyperalimentation, and exercise

c. Medications that may affect ammonia levels: *increase*: ammonium chloride, acetazolamide, and isoniazid (INH), diuretics such as furosemide, thiazides, and ethacrynic acid

d. Nursing implications

1) Client should fast prior to blood being drawn

NCLEX!

2) Specimen should be placed in ice and immediately transported to the laboratory for analysis since ammonia will increase over time

3) Monitor client for symptoms of hepatic failure such as confusion, lethargy, tremors, or twitching

4) Decreased ammonia levels are seen with intake of a low-protein diet, antibiotics such as neomycin that destroy ammonia-producing intestinal flora and use of lactulose that increases bowel evacuation of ammonia

3. Amylase (serum): normal range is 60 to 160 Somogyi U/dL; slightly increased in pregnancy and the elderly; urine amylase: 4 to 37 U/L over 2hr

a. Description: an enzyme produced in the pancreas, salivary glands, and liver that aids in the digestion of complex carbohydrates

b. Clinical problems: *decreased levels* of amylase can be seen in chronic pancreatitis, acute and subacute liver necrosis, chronic alcoholism, toxic hepatitis, severe burns, severe thyrotoxicosis, or hydration with D_5W IV solution; *increased levels* may occur with acute and chronic pancreatitis, acute cholecystitis, obstruction of the pancreatic duct, peptic ulcer perforation, gastric surgery, acute alcohol intoxication, diabetes mellitus, diabetic acidosis, burns, pregnancy, benign prostatic hypertrophy, and renal failure

c. Medications that may affect amylase levels: *decrease*: citrates, glucose, fluorides, oxalates; *increase*: ACTH, ethyl alcohol, narcotics, salicylates, tetracycline, and thiazide diuretics

d. Nursing implications: restrict food and narcotics for 2 hours prior to blood being drawn

NCLEX!

4. Arterial blood gases (whole blood): normal range is pH: 7.35 to 7.45; $PaCO_2$: 35 to 45 mmHg; PaO_2: 80 to 100 mgHg; HCO_3 (bicarbonate): 22 to 26 mEq/L; base excess (BE): +2 to –2 mEq/L

a. Description: arterial blood gases are utilized to assess acid-base imbalances caused by metabolic or respiratory conditions; the findings are utilized to detect metabolic acidosis or metabolic alkalosis, or respiratory acidosis or respiratory alkalosis, or a combination of both metabolic and respiratory imbalances

NCLEX!

b. Table 1-1 demonstrates the relationship among the pH, $PaCO_2$, HCO_3 and base excess with each condition

1) Respiratory acidosis is characterized by a low pH and elevated $PaCO_2$

2) Respiratory alkalosis is characterized by an elevated pH and decreased $PaCO_2$

3) Metabolic acidosis is characterized by a low pH, decreased HCO_3, and a decreased BE

4) Metabolic alkalosis is characterized by an elevated pH, increased HCO_3, and increased BE

Table 1-1

Acid-Base Disturbances

Acid-Base Imbalance	pH	$PaCO_2$	HCO_3	BE	Clinical Problems
Respiratory acidosis	↓	↑	Normal	Normal	Chronic lung diseases ARDS Anesthesia Pneumonia Pneumothorax
Respiratory alkalosis	↑	↓	Normal	Normal	Hyperventilation Anxiety Sepsis Pulmonary emboli Tetany Fever
Metabolic acidosis	↓	Normal	↓	↓	Diabetes Renal failure Burns Shock Starvation Malnutrition
Metabolic alkalosis	↑	Normal	↑	↑	Excessive bicarbonate intake Severe vomiting Hepatic failure Cushing's syndrome Hyperaldosteronism

c. Medications that may affect pH levels: *decreased*: narcotics, barbiturates, ammonium chloride, acetazolamide; *increased*: sodium bicarbonate, antacids, steroids, salicylate overdose, or diuretics

NCLEX!

d. Nursing implications

1) Monitor vital signs, level of consciousness, respiratory status, and lung sounds frequently to assess acid-base imbalance

2) Administer IV fluids, medications, and respiratory therapy as ordered

3) Advise laboratory personnel to anticipate arrival of ABG specimen for immediate processing

4) Explain procedure to the client

5. Bicarbonate (serum): normal range is 22 to 26 mEq/L

a. Description: an essential *anion* (negatively charged ion) that is a part of the renal and respiratory buffer systems; it is responsible for maintaining an appropriate acid-base environment within the body for vital biologic processes at the tissue and cellular levels; a decrease in bicarbonate will lead to an acidic environment while an excess of bicarbonate will lead to an alkaline environment within the body

b. Clinical problems: *decreased levels* of bicarbonate occur with renal failure, diarrhea, lactic acidosis, and diabetic ketoacidosis; *increased levels* may occur with excessive bicarbonate or antacid intake, excessive GI suctioning or vomiting, hyperaldosteronism, or diuretic therapy

c. Medications that affect bicarbonate levels: *increase:* diuretics, OTC antacids, or excessive administration of sodium bicarbonate

d. Nursing implications: the health history data helps determine possible causes for alterations in bicarbonate levels and assessment of respiratory and renal status is important

6. Bilirubin (serum): normal ranges are total bilirubin: 0.1 to 1.2 mg/dL; direct bilirubin: 0.0 to 0.3 mg/dL; indirect bilirubin: 0.1 to 1.0 mg/dL

a. Description: a breakdown product of hemoglobin in the reticuloendothelial system; it is transported in the plasma to the liver where it is broken down and excreted in the bile; there are two forms of bilirubin: direct or conjugated (soluble in the plasma) and indirect or unconjugated (protein-bound)

b. Clinical problems: *decreased levels* of direct bilirubin occur with iron-deficiency anemia; *Increased levels* of direct bilirubin occur with hepatic disease such as hepatitis, cirrhosis, cancer of the liver, obstructions with stones or tumors, and infectious mononucleosis; *increased levels* of indirect bilirubin can be seen with hemolytic anemias, sickle cell anemia, septicemia, transfusion reactions, congestive heart failure, and malaria

c. Medications that may affect bilirubin levels: *decrease*: aspirin, penicillin, caffeine, and barbiturates; *increase*: antibiotics, barbiturates, diuretics, isoniazid (INH), oral contraceptives, steroids, and vitamins A, C, and K

d. Nursing implications

NCLEX!

1) The client should not eat a high-fat diet or yellow vegetables immediately prior to blood being drawn

2) The specimen should be protected from light and processed immediately upon arrival in the laboratory to reduce effects of light on bilirubin

3) Monitor client for evidence of jaundice

7. Calcium (serum): normal range is 4.5 to 5.5 mEq/L or 9 to 11 mg/dL

a. Description: an essential *cation* (a positively charged ion), necessary for structure of bones and teeth, contraction of muscles and conduction of nerve impulses, secretion of hormones, blood clotting, and selective transportation across cell membranes

b. Clinical problems: *decreased levels* of calcium occur in GI malabsorption diseases, decreased calcium and vitamin D intake, hypoparathyroidism, chronic renal failure, infections, pancreatitis, alcoholism, trauma to or removal of the parathyroid glands, and pregnancy; *increased levels* may occur with hyperparathyroidism; cancers of the bone, breast, lung, kidney, or bladder; multiple fractures; immobility; or renal calculi

c. Medications that may affect calcium levels: *decrease*: antibiotics, cortisone, heparin, laxatives, insulin, and antacids high in magnesium; *increase:* calcium salts, vitamin D, estrogen preparations, and thiazide diuretics

NCLEX!

d. Nursing implications

1) No dietary limitations prior to blood being drawn

2) Assess the client for signs of tetany, positive Chvostek's or Trousseau's sign, or digoxin toxicity

3) Do not add calcium to solutions that contain bicarbonate, as they will form a precipitate

8. Carbon dioxide (serum): normal range is 22 to 30 mEq/L

a. Description: an important compound utilized in the maintenance of metabolic acid-base balance; the concentration of bicarbonate is closely linked to carbon dioxide concentration in acid-base balance

b. Clinical problems: *decreased levels*: diabetic ketoacidosis, metabolic acidosis, starvation, dehydration, shock, acute renal failure, and salicylate toxicity; *increased levels*: metabolic alkalosis, severe vomiting, and hypothyroidism

c. Medications that may affect carbon dioxide levels: *decrease*: antibiotics, diuretics, thiazides, and paraldehyde; *increase*: barbiturates, loop diuretics, and steroids

d. Nursing implications: assess for signs and symptoms of metabolic acidosis and alkalosis

9. Cholesterol/lipoproteins (serum): normal ranges see Table 1-2

a. Description: a blood lipoprotein that is synthesized in the liver

1) Cholesterol assists in formation of bile salts for fat digestion and formation of adrenal, ovarian, and testicular hormones

Table 1-2	**Type of Cholesterol**	**Value**	**Implications**
Cholesterol Levels and Implications	Total cholesterol	<200 mg/dL	Desirable
		200–240 mg/dL	Moderate risk
		>240 mg/dL	High risk
	High-density lipoproteins	29–77mg/dL	
		>60 mg/dL	Very low risk for coronary heart disease (CHD)
		46–59 mg/dL	Low risk for CHD
		35–45 mg/dL	Moderate risk for CHD
		<35 mg/dL	High risk for CHD
	Low-density lipoproteins	60–160 mg/dL	Low risk for CHD
		<130 mg/dL	Moderate risk for CHD
		130–159 mg/d	High risk for CHD
		>160 mg/dL	
	HDL: LDL ratio	3:1	

2) High-density lipoproteins (HDL) and low-density lipoproteins (LDL) are fractions of lipoproteins that contain varying amounts of cholesterol, protein, triglycerides, and phospholipids

3) HDL are primarily composed of protein and have about 20 percent cholesterol; they have been called the "good" lipids because they are believed to serve a protective function against coronary artery disease (CAD)

4) LDL are primarily composed of cholesterol and are felt to increase the risk of CAD

5) In general, the higher the ratio of HDL: LDL, the lower the risk of CAD

b. Clinical problems: *decreased levels* of cholesterol will be observed in malnutrition, starvation, and hyperthyroidism; *increased levels* of cholesterol and lipoproteins will be seen with hypercholesterolemia, hyperlipoproteinemia, acute myocardial infarction, diabetes, cirrhosis, nephrotic syndrome, hypothyroidism, pregnancy and eclampsia, and intake of high-fat diets

c. Medications that may affect lipoprotein levels: *decrease:* estrogen, aspirin, antibiotics, heparin, colchicine, thyroxine; *increase:* aspirin, oral contraceptives, steroids, phenothiazides, sulfonamides, and phenytoin

d. Nursing implications: a diet high in fat or cholesterol may cause elevated levels of lipoproteins

10. Cortisol: (plasma) normal in morning is 5 to 23 μg/dL; afternoon is 3 to 13 μg/dL

a. Description: a glucocorticoid released from the adrenal cortex in response to adrenocorticotropic hormone (ACTH) levels

b. Clinical problems: *decreased levels:* Addison's disease, decreased functioning of the anterior pituitary gland, and hypothyroidism; *increased levels:* Cushing's syndrome, adrenal gland neoplasms, pregnancy, stress, hyperthyroidism, and acute myocardial infarction

    c. Medications that may affect cortisol levels: *decrease*: androgens, phenytoin; *increase:* estrogen, oral contraceptives, and spironolactone

    d. Nursing implications: the client should be NPO and on bedrest immediately prior to the blood being drawn due to the utilization of cortisol with physical exercise

11. Creatine kinase (serum) normal range is male 5 to 35 μg/mL; female 5 to 25 μg/mL

    a. Description: an enzyme found in skeletal and heart muscle and brain tissue; has three isoenzymes that can be separated to isolate the specific location of enzyme released: CK-MM—skeletal muscle, CK-MB—heart muscle, and CK-BB—brain tissue; this differentiation can help determine the specific tissue damaged and monitor progression of the condition

    b. Clinical problems: *increased levels* of creatine kinase and its isoenzymes are observed in myocardial infarction, excessive physical activity, skeletal muscle diseases, trauma, surgery, intramuscular (IM) injections, cerebrovascular accident, head trauma, seizures, or pulmonary embolism

    c. Medications that may affect creatine kinase levels: *increase:* high-dose aspirin, ampicillin, carbenicillin, or dexamethasone

    d. Nursing implications: hold IM injections if creatine kinase levels are expected to be drawn; assess clinical signs and symptoms of diseases that may cause elevated CK or CK isoenzyme levels

12. Creatinine (serum and urine) normal range is serum 0.5 to 1.5 mg/dL; urine 1 to 2g/24h

    a. Description: a by-product of muscle catabolism that is excreted by the kidney; it is utilized to determine renal function

    b. Clinical problems: *decreased levels* of creatinine are sometimes seen in females due to their decreased muscle mass; *increased levels* occur in acute and chronic renal failure, neoplasms, congestive heart failure, acute myocardial infarction, lupus erythematosus, and a diet high in muscle meats

    c. Medications that may affect creatinine levels: *increase:* nephrotoxic antibiotics, lithium, and methyldopa

NCLEX!

    d. Nursing implications: clients suspected of having decreased serum creatinine and creatinine clearance levels should be monitored for signs and symptoms of renal disease

13. Glucose, fasting (serum): normal range is 70 to 110 mg/dL

    a. Description: test to determine the client's ability to convert glucose to glycogen

    b. Clinical problems: *decreased levels* of glucose may occur with hypoglycemia, adrenal gland dysfunction, malnutrition, alcoholism, liver disease, or malabsorption syndromes; *increased levels* of glucose occur with diabetes mellitus, Cushing's syndrome, stress, burns, infection, acute pancreatitis, and extensive trauma

    c. Medications that may affect glucose levels: *decrease:* excessive insulin intake; *increase:* anesthetic agents, steroids, ACTH, diuretics, epinephrine, or phenytoin

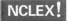

d. Nursing implications

1) Assure that the client has been NPO for at least 12 hours and all morning insulin has been held prior to blood draw

2) Observe for signs and symptoms of hypoglycemia and hyperglycemia

14. Glucose tolerance test (serum) normal range is <140 mg/dL

a. Description: test utilized to detect diabetes mellitus; client ingests a fluid containing 75 g of glucose after a fasting serum glucose level has been drawn; serum blood specimens are collected every 30 minutes for 2 hours after the ingestion

b. Clinical problems: *increased levels*: impaired glucose tolerance, diabetes mellitus

c. Medications that may affect glucose levels: *increase:* steroids, phenytoin, diuretics, nicotinic acid

d. Nursing implications: the client should be at rest for the length of the test and should receive thorough instructions about the test, purpose, and what to expect during the test

15. Iron (serum) normal range is 50 to 150 µ/dL

a. Description: iron is necessary for the synthesis of hemoglobin in the bone marrow

b. Clinical problems: *decreased levels* of iron occur with iron-deficiency anemia, malabsorption diseases, chronic bleeding disorders, pregnancy, and chronic renal failure; *increased levels* of iron occur with pernicious and hemolytic anemias, liver disease, lead toxicity, and thalassemia

c. Medications that may affect iron levels: *increase*: iron preparations and oral contraceptives

d. Nursing implications: monitor for signs and symptoms of iron-deficiency anemia and take care with the blood specimen to avoid hemolysis that may cause elevated results

16. Lactic dehydrogenase (serum) normal ranges are total LDH 100 to 190 IU/L; LDH isoenzymes: LDH^1—14 to 26%, LDH^2—27 to 37%, LDH^3—13 to 26%, LDH^4—8 to 16%, LDH^5—6 to 16%

a. Description: intracellular enzyme important for cellular metabolism; there are five isoenzymes of LDH: LDH^1 and LDH^2 are primarily found in cardiac cells, LDH^3 is primarily found in pulmonary cells; and LDH^4 and LDH^5 are primarily found in hepatic cells

b. Clinical problems: *increased levels* of total LDH and specific isoenzymes can be found in myocardial infarction, acute hepatic diseases, pulmonary embolus, pulmonary infarction, skeletal muscle diseases, cancers, cerebral vascular accident, anemia, and excessive exercise

c. Medications that may affect LDH levels: *increase:* narcotics and frequent IM injections

d. Nursing implications

1) Assess for signs and symptoms of cardiac, hepatic, musculoskeletal, and pulmonary diseases

        2) Assess the levels and trends of LDH values and report them to the physician as appropriate

        3) Minimize IM injections at least 8 hours prior to blood draw

17. Lipase (serum) normal range is 20 to 180 IU/L

    a. Description: an enzyme secreted by the pancreas that aids in fat digestion

    b. Clinical problems: *elevated levels* of lipase will occur with acute and chronic pancreatitis, pancreatic cancers, acute renal failure, and obstruction of the pancreatic duct; (because lipase remains in the blood for up to 14 days after an episode of acute pancreatitis, it is useful in the late diagnosis of this condition)

    c. Medications that may affect lipase levels: *increase:* narcotics and steroids

    d. Nursing implications: client should be NPO except water for 8 hours prior to blood draw

18. Magnesium (serum) normal range is 1.5 to 2.5 mEq/L

    a. Description: essential cation primarily stored in bones and cartilage; it facilitates muscle contraction, carbohydrate and protein metabolism, and regulation of potassium and calcium

    b. Clinical problems: *decreased levels* of magnesium occur in malabsorption syndromes, cirrhosis, alcoholism, hypokalemia, dehydration, malnutrition, and hypoparathyroidism; *increased levels* of magnesium occur in renal failure, dehydration, and diabetes mellitus

    c. Medications that may affect magnesium levels: *increase:* magnesium-rich antacids and laxatives high in magnesium such as milk of magnesia and magnesium citrate; *decrease:* diuretics, insulin, calcium gluconate, and neomycin

    d. Nursing implications

        1) Monitor for signs and symptoms of magnesium imbalance

NCLEX!

        2) Monitor ECG strips for peaked T wave or widened QRS complex that would indicate the need to evaluate serum magnesium and potassium levels

19. Osmolality normal range (serum) is 280 to 300 mOsm/kg H_2O; normal range for (urine) is 50 to 1200 mOsm/kg H_2O

    a. Description: measurement of serum and urine concentration as a result of the number of particles dissolved in solution

    b. Clinical problems

        1) *Decreased serum osmolality levels* could indicate intravascular fluid overload or syndrome of inappropriate ADH (SIADH)

        2) *Decreased urine osmolality levels* could indicate diabetes insipidus, acute renal failure, or hyponatremia

        3) *Increased serum osmolality levels* could indicate dehydration, hypernatremia, hyperglycemia, or diabetes insipidus

        4) *Increased urine osmolality* could indicate SIADH

c. Medications that affect osmolality levels: *decrease*: excessive IV fluid infusion of D_5W

d. Nursing implications

1) There are no special restrictions when preparing for serum collection

2) Urine osmolality testing requires intake of a high-protein diet for several days prior to the urine collection and fluid restriction for 8 to 12 hours prior to urine collection

3) The second specimen of the morning is sent for analysis

20. Phosphorus (serum) normal range is 1.7 to 2.6 mEq/L or 2.5 to 4.5 mg/dL

a. Description: an essential intracellular anion stored primarily in the bones; it serves to regulate energy transfer as ATP, and assist in metabolism of carbohydrate, fat, and protein

b. Clinical problems: *decreased levels* occur in malabsorption syndromes, starvation, hyperparathyroidism, hypercalcemia, chronic alcoholism, and diabetic acidosis; *increased levels* occur in hypoparathyroidism, bone tumors, renal insufficiency and failure, Cushing's syndrome, and multiple fractures

c. Medications that may affect phosphorus levels: *decrease:* antacids, insulin, mannitol; *increase*: heparin, phenytoin, and phosphate

d. Nursing implications: because phosphorus levels are the inverse of calcium levels, check calcium levels and observe for signs of tetany if phosphorus levels are elevated

21. Potassium (serum) normal range is 3.5 to 5.1 mEq/L

a. Description: an essential intracellular cation needed for protein synthesis, glucose storage and use, and electrical activity of excitable membranes such as cardiac muscle

b. Clinical problems: *decreased levels* of potassium occur in dehydration, excessive vomiting and diarrhea, starvation, stress, trauma, burns, metabolic alkalosis, diabetic acidosis, and gastric suctioning; *increased levels* of potassium occur in acute renal failure, excessive use of salt substitutes, metabolic acidosis, oliguria, and anuria

c. Medications that may affect potassium levels: *decrease*: diuretics (potassium-wasting), sodium polystyrene (Kayexalate), lactulose, insulin, aspirin, and laxatives; *increase*: potassium-sparing diuretics, heparin, histamine, antibiotics, and epinephrine

NCLEX!

d. Nursing implications

1) Closely monitor serum potassium levels and signs and symptoms of potassium imbalance

2) Decreased potassium levels can cause ECG changes such as AV conduction defects, depressed S-T segments and inverted or flat T waves

3) Increased potassium levels can cause widened QRS complexes and peaked T waves

4) Clients with hypokalemia are predisposed to the development of digitalis toxicity

22. Prostate-specific antigen (PSA) (serum) normal ranges are 1 to 4 ng/mL; benign prostatic hypertrophy 4 to 19 ng/mL; prostate cancer 10 to 120 ng/mL

    a. Description: glycoprotein present in prostate tissue; PSA is a highly sensitive indicator of prostatic cancer and is used to diagnose and monitor treatment effectiveness and prognosis

    b. Clinical problems: *increased levels* of prostate-specific antigen occur in prostatic cancer and benign prostatic hypertrophy

    c. Nursing implications: a thorough client genitourinary history and health assessment will help determine the need for this test and monitor progression of the disease process

23. Protein (serum and urine) normal ranges are *serum*—total protein = 6.0 to 8.0 g/dL, albumin = 52 to 68% of total protein, globulin = 32 to 48% of total protein; *urine:* normal range is 0 to 5mg/dL (random); 24-hour specimen, is 25 to 150 mg

    a. Protein and its components (albumin and globulin) are essential for maintenance of colloid osmotic pressure, supply of amino acids, and for immunity to diseases

    b. Clinical problems

        1) *Decreased levels of serum proteins* occur in malnutrition, starvation, malabsorption syndromes, severe burns, chronic renal failure, toxemia, and nephrotic syndromes

        2) *Increased levels of serum proteins* occur with dehydration, nausea, vomiting, diarrhea, and excessive exercise

        3) *Increased levels of urine proteins* occur with glomerulonephritis, nephrotic syndrome, systemic lupus, erythematosus drug toxicities, renal infections, and toxemia of pregnancy

    c. Medications that may affect protein levels: *increased*: supplemental infusions of protein-rich solutions; increased urine proteins may occur with the use of contrast media, nephrotoxic antibiotics, and tolbutamide

    d. Nursing implications: monitor the client's nutritional status and start replacement therapies as ordered; continually monitor I & O

24. Sodium (serum) normal range is 135 to 145 mEq/L

    a. Description: major cation in the extracellular fluid responsible for maintaining extracellular volume, osmolality, urine concentration, and cardiac and skeletal muscle contraction through the sodium-potassium pump

    b. Clinical problems: *decreased levels* of sodium occur in vomiting, diarrhea, gastric suctioning, SIADH, burn injury, and renal failure; *increased levels* occur in diabetes insipidus, congestive heart failure, hepatic failure, severe vomiting, and diarrhea

    c. Medications that may affect sodium levels: *decrease:* diuretics including mannitol and thiazides; *increase:* laxatives, steroids, antibiotics

d. Nursing implications: closely monitor for signs and symptoms of sodium imbalance (high sodium intake immediately prior to blood draw will affect results)

25. Thyroid hormones: thyroid-stimulating hormone (TSH)(serum) normal range is 0.35 to 5.5 μIU/mL; triiodothyronine (T^3)(serum) normal range is 80 to 200 ng/dL; thyroxine (T^4)(serum) normal range is 4.6 to 11 μg/dL

    a. Description: thyroid-stimulating hormone is secreted by the anterior pituitary gland, which stimulates the release of T^3 and T^4 through a negative feedback mechanism; thyroid hormones are responsible for controlling the rate of metabolic processes, normal growth and development, and nervous system maturation

    b. Clinical problems: *decreased levels* of thyroid hormones occur in hypothyroidism caused by pituitary malfunction, myxedema, cretinism, renal failure, strenuous exercise, and trauma; *increased levels* of thyroid hormones occur in hyperthyroidism caused by thyroid malfunction, goiter, Graves' disease, thyroiditis, and thyrotoxic crisis

    c. Medications that may affect thyroid hormone levels: *decrease:* aspirin, steroids, dopamine, phenytoin, lithium, and testosterone; *increase:* oral contraceptive, estrogen, lithium, potassium iodide, and perphenazine

    d. Nursing implications: closely monitor client for signs and symptoms of thyroid hormone imbalances, particularly tachycardia and cardiovascular changes

26. Triglycerides (serum) normal ranges: 12 to 29 yr–10 to 140 mg/dL; 30 to 39 yr–20 to 150 mg/dL; 40 to 49 yr–30 to 160 mg dL; >50 yr–40 to 190 mg/dL

    a. Description: the most common blood lipid in the body involved in energy production, storage, and insulation; this lipid is a major contributor to the development of coronary artery disease and other arterial diseases

    b. Clinical problems: *decreased levels* of triglycerides occur in hyperthyroidism, protein malnutrition, congenital lipoproteinemia, and excessive exercise; *increased levels* of triglycerides occur in hyperlipoproteinemia, hypertension, acute myocardial infarction, nephrotic syndrome, alcoholic cirrhosis, Down syndrome, high-carbohydrate diet, and pregnancy

    c. Medications that may affect triglyceride levels: *decrease:* clofibrate, phenformin, metformin, and ascorbic acid; *increase:* oral contraceptives and estrogen

    d. Nursing implications: client should be NPO for at least 12 hours prior to blood draw; recent alcohol or high-carbohydrate diet intake will elevate the triglyceride level

27. Troponin I (serum) normal level is < 1.0 ng/mL; diagnostic for MI > 2.2 ng/mL

    a. Description: a cardiac-specific protein marker for myocardial injury; elevation begins 4 to 6 hours after the onset of chest pain and peaks at approximately 12 to 24 hours making it a very useful diagnostic tool for determining myocardial injury

b. Clinical problems: *increased levels* of Troponin I occur with myocardial injury and infarction

c. Medication that may affect the Troponin I levels: none known at the present

d. Nursing implications

1) A thorough and serial cardiac assessment is essential in monitoring clients with suspected or diagnosed myocardial injury

2) A screening test for Troponin I is performed at the bedside

3) The nurse must be aware of the correct test procedures and interpretation of the test results

28. Urea nitrogen (serum) normal range is 5 to 25 mg/dL; also known as BUN

a. Description: urea is an end product of protein metabolism formed in the liver and excreted by the kidneys

b. Clinical problems: *decreased levels* of BUN occur with severe liver disease, malnutrition, overhydration, low protein intake, and pregnancy; *increased levels* of BUN occur with dehydration, renal insufficiency or failure, other kidney diseases, diabetes mellitus, sepsis, GI bleeding, and high protein diet

c. Medications that may affect urea nitrogen levels: *decrease:* phenothiazines; *increase:* diuretics, antibiotics, lithium, morphine, propranolol, and methyldopa

NCLEX!

d. Nursing implications: assess for adequate hydration status and monitor intake and output (I & O) if renal disease is suspected

29. Uric acid (serum) normal range is 3.5 to 8.0 mg/dL (male); 2.8 to 6.8 mg/dL (female)

a. Description: a by-product of purine metabolism that is normally excreted by the kidneys

b. Clinical problems: *decreased levels* of uric acid occur in acidosis, folic acid anemia, and pregnancy; *increased levels* of uric acid occur with gout, alcoholism, renal failure, leukemias and metastatic carcinomas, hyperlipoproteinemia, diabetes mellitus, stress, and polycythemia

c. Medications that may affect uric acid levels: *decrease:* allopurinol, warfarin, probenecid, and sulfinpyrazone; *increase:* acetaminophen, ascorbic acid, diuretics, levodopa, methyldopa, aspirin, and theophylline

NCLEX!

d. Nursing implications: monitor urinary output and assess for signs of gout and kidney stones

B. Hematology

1. Activated partial thromboplastin time (APTT) (serum) normal range is 20 to 35 seconds; for anticoagulation therapy it is 1.5 to 2.5 times normal

a. Description: screening test utilized to detect clotting deficiencies and to monitor effectiveness of heparin therapy

b. Clinical problems: *increased levels* occur with clotting factor V, VIII, IX, X, XI, and XII deficiencies, cirrhosis of the liver, disseminated intravascular coagulopathy (DIC), leukemia, and Hodgkin's disease

c. Medications that may affect the APPT: *increase:* heparin, salicylates, and enoxaparin

    d. Nursing implications: assess for signs and symptoms of bleeding and report APPT results to physician

2. Prothrombin time (PT) (plasma) normal range is 10 to 13 seconds; anticoagulation therapy range is 1.5 to 2.0 times control

    a. Description: measures the clotting abilities of fibrinogen, prothrombin, and factors V, VII, and X; the PT is used to monitor the effectiveness of oral anticoagulation therapy with warfarin

    b. Clinical problems: *decreased levels* occur in pulmonary embolism, acute myocardial infarction, and thrombophlebitis; *increased levels* may occur with alcohol ingestion, liver disease, clotting factor deficiencies, congestive heart failure, erythroblastosis fetalis, and leukemias

    c. Medications that may affect the PT: *decrease:* oral contraceptives, vitamin K, digitalis, diuretics, rifampin, and metaproterenol; *increase:* oral anticoagulants, salicylates, phenytoin, methyldopa, and chlordiazepoxide

    d. Nursing implications

      1) Monitor the plasma PT level and report to physician

      2) Monitor for signs and symptoms of bleeding

      3) Vitamin K is the antidote for elevated PT levels

    e. The international normalized ratio (INR) may be used instead of PT; therapeutic level is commonly 2.0 to 3.0

3. Erythrocyte sedimentation rate (ESR) normal range: < 20 mm/hr

    a. Description: measures the rate at which red blood cells settle out of unclotted blood; primary influence on the ESR is the presence of acute phase reactants in the presence of inflammation

    b. Clinical problems: *decreased rate* will occur with sickle cell anemia, degenerative arthritis, angina pectoris, and factor V deficiency; *increased rate* will occur with acute infections, inflammatory conditions, systemic lupus erythematosus (SLE), pregnancy, cancers, burns, rheumatoid arthritis, and rheumatic fever

    c. Medications that may affect the ESR: *decrease the rate:* aspirin, quinine, and steroids; *increase the rate:* oral contraceptives, dextran, methyldopa, theophylline, and procainamide

    d. Nursing implications: withhold any medications that can affect the ESR 4 hours prior to blood draw

4. Hematocrit (HCT) normal range: male—40 to 54%; female—36 to 46%

    a. Description: the percent of packed red blood cells per 100 mL of blood

    b. Clinical problems: *decreased levels* may occur with acute blood loss, chronic liver failure, anemias, chronic renal failure, malnutrition, bone marrow deficiencies, SLE, rheumatoid arthritis, and vitamin B and C deficiencies; *increased levels* may occur with hypovolemia, severe diarrhea, burns, trauma, eclampsia, chronic anoxia, and diabetic acidosis

c. Medications that may *decrease levels:* penicillin and chloramphenicol

d. Nursing implications: assess change in vital signs; monitor signs and symptoms of anemia, fluid volume status, and output

5. Hemoglobin (Hgb) normal range is male: 13.5 to 17 g/dL; female: 12 to 15 g/dL

a. Description: oxygen carrying component of the red blood cell

b. Clinical problems: *decreased levels* may occur in anemias, renal disease, and overhydration; *increased levels* may occur in dehydration, chronic pulmonary disease, severe burns, polycythemia, and high altitudes

c. Medications that may affect hemoglobin levels: *decrease:* antibiotics, aspirin, indomethacin, rifampin, and antineoplastic medications; *increase:* gentamicin and methyldopa

d. Nursing implications: assess for signs and symptoms of dehydration and anemia

6. Platelet count normal range is 150,000 to 400,000/μL

a. Description: basic blood element primarily responsible for clotting

b. Clinical problems: *decreased levels* of platelets may occur in cancer, leukemias, liver disease, kidney disease, DIC, and SLE; *increased levels* of platelets may occur in polycythemia, acute blood loss, splenectomy, and infections

c. Medications that may affect platelet levels: *decrease:* aspirin, chloromycetin, chemotherapeutic agents, thiazide diuretics, and quinidine

d. Nursing implications: assess for signs and symptoms of bleeding disorders and monitor platelet levels in clients undergoing chemotherapy and radiation therapy

7. Reticulocyte count normal level is 0.5 to 1.5 percent of all red blood cells

a. Description: immature red blood cells released by the bone marrow that become mature red blood cells in 1 to 2 days

b. Clinical problems that may affect the reticulocyte count: *decreased levels* may occur in anemias, radiation therapy, hypopituitary and hypoadrenal functioning, and excessive alcohol intake; *increased levels* may occur with chronic blood loss, anemias, thalassemia, leukemias, and as an effect of treatment of iron, vitamin B_{12}, and folic acid deficiencies

c. Nursing implications: monitor effectiveness of anemia therapy

8. White blood cell count (WBC) normal range is 4500 to 11,000 cells/μL

a. Description: component of the body's defense system; an increase indicates the presence of infection

b. Clinical problems: *decreased levels* may occur in anemias, viral infections, malaria, alcoholism, SLE, and rheumatoid arthritis; *increased levels* may occur in acute infections, tissue injury and necrosis, stress, sickle cell anemia, and hemolytic anemia

NCLEX !

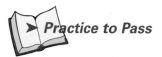

Practice to Pass

Your client who was recently started on daily warfarin sodium (Coumadin) therapy has just received an order from the physician to have biweekly prothrombin times (PT) drawn. The client asks you why. What would your response be?

      c. Medications that may affect the WBC: *decrease:* antibiotics, acetaminophen, chemotherapeutic agents, chlordiazepoxide, oral hypoglycemics, indomethacin, rifampin, and phenothiazide; *increase:* aspirin, antibiotics, allopurinol, heparin, digitalis, lithium, and epinephrine

NCLEX!

      d. Nursing implications: monitor for signs and symptoms of inflammation and infection

  9. White blood cell differential

      a. Description: there are five types of white blood cells with each having a specific function in the body's defense systems; the differential provides specific information about infection and disease process based upon WBC cell type

      b. Clinical problems: see Table 1-3

NCLEX!

      c. Nursing implications: assess for signs and symptoms of infection, allergic reaction, and wound healing process

C. Serology and immunology

  1. Antinuclear antibody (ANA) (serum): normal finding is negative

      a. Description: measures presence of antibodies that destroy the nucleus of cells and cause tissue death; is a screening test for collagen diseases and is specific for systemic lupus erythematosus (SLE)

      b. Clinical problems: *positive or increased levels* occur in SLE, scleroderma, rheumatoid arthritis, leukemia, systemic sclerosis, infectious mononucleosis, and myasthenia gravis

Table 1-3	Type	Normal Value	Function	Clinical Problems
White Blood Cell Differential	Neutrophils	50–70%	First response to tissue injury and inflammation	*Decreased:* viral diseases, anemias, leukemias, and agranulocytosis *Increased:* acute infections, acute appendicitis, inflammation, acute pancreatitis
	Eosinophils	1–3%	Response to allergic and parasite conditions	*Decreased:* burns, shock *Increased:* allergies, cancer, phlebitis
	Basophils	0.4–1.0%	Promote healing	*Decreased:* hypersensitivity reaction, stress, pregnancy *Increased:* inflammatory process, wound healing, leukemia
	Monocytes	4–6%	Second response to infection	*Decreased:* aplastic anemia *Increased:* viral diseases, cancer, collagen diseases
	Lymphocytes	25–35%	Assist in immune response (B and T lymphocytes)	*Decreased:* cancer, leukemia, aplastic anemia, multiple sclerosis, renal failure, nephrotic syndrome, SLE

    c. Medications that affect ANA value: *increase:* antibiotics, antihypertensives, isoniazid, thiazides, diuretics, oral contraceptives, antiarrhythmics, and chlorpromazine

    d. Nursing implications: monitor for signs and symptoms of collagen diseases

2. C-reactive protein (serum): normal finding is negative

    a. Description: elevated levels of C-reactive protein occur with an acute bacterial inflammatory process approximately 6 to 10 hours after tissue damage has begun and begins to decline approximately 48 to 72 hours after

    b. Clinical problems: *increased levels* may occur with acute myocardial infarction, rheumatoid arthritis, rheumatic fever, pyelonephritis, metastatic cancer, inflammatory bowel syndromes, and bacterial infections

    c. Medications that may affect C-reactive protein levels: *increase:* oral contraceptives

    d. Nursing implications: client should be NPO except for water for 8 to 12 hours prior to blood draw; assess the client for signs and symptoms of acute inflammatory responses

3. Carcinoembryonic antigen (CEA) (serum): normal in nonsmokers is < 2.5 ng/dL; in smokers is < 5.0 ng/dL

    a. Description: utilized to detect colon and pancreatic carcinoma and monitor the effectiveness of treatment

    b. Clinical problems: *increased levels* of CEA occur with carcinomas of the GI tract, pancreatic, liver, lung, breast, cervical, prostate, bladder, testes, and kidney; leukemia; inflammatory bowel disease; chronic smoking; ulcerative colitis; acute renal failure; acute pancreatitis; and chronic ischemic cardiac disease

    c. Nursing implications: heparin should be withheld for 2 days prior to blood draw; since results are not absolute, give support to client and family while awaiting results

4. Immunoglobulins (Ig)(serum): normal ranges are total Ig = 900 to 2200 mg/dL; IgG = 650 to 1700 mg/dL; IgA = 70 to 400 mg/dL; IgM = 40 to 350 mg/dL; IgD = 0 to 8 mg/dL; IgE = < 40 U/mL

    a. Description: specific blood proteins involved in the antibody-antigen immune response

        1) IgG: provides early immunity in the newborn and results from exposure to antiviral and antibody activity

        2) IgA: protects mucous membranes from bacterial and viral infections

        3) IgM: is responsible for primary immunity from antigen exposure

        4) IgD: unknown

        5) IgE: response to allergic and anaphylactic reactions

    b. Nursing implications: assess a client's immunization and vaccination status, infectious disease exposure history, and blood transfusion history

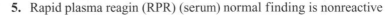

5. Rapid plasma reagin (RPR) (serum) normal finding is nonreactive

   a. Description: The RPR test is used to diagnose syphilis

   b. Clinical problems that may affect a false-positive RPR include TB, pneumonia, chickenpox, mononucleosis, rheumatoid arthritis, SLE, hepatitis, and pregnancy

   c. Nursing implications: assessment of the client's sexual history is necessary to ensure notification of possible contacts if testing proves positive for syphilis

6. Venereal disease research laboratory (VDRL) (serum) normal findings is nonreactive

   a. Description: the VDRL test is used to detect the presence of syphilis

   b. Clinical problems that may cause a false positive VDRL include tuberculosis, rheumatoid arthritis, SLE, hepatitis, infectious mononucleosis, or recent smallpox vaccine

   c. Nursing implications: assess client's sexual history and obtain a thorough client history to rule out any possible causes of false positive results

D. Urinalysis: normal findings see Table 1-4

1. Description: the urinalysis is utilized to determine the presence of renal or urinary tract disorders; it can also be used to determine metabolic dysfunctions

2. Clinical problems that may affect the results of the urinalysis can include: contaminated specimen, fluid balance, pregnancy, liver disease, renal disease, presence of bacteria or infection, ingestion of certain foods and medications, trauma, diabetes, or pituitary gland disorders

3. Medications that may affect the urinalysis include: antibiotics, phenytoin, methylene blue, sulfisoxazole-phenazopyridine (Azo-Gantrisin), methacarbanol, iron injections, contrast media, steroids, epinephrine, and anticoagulants

4. Nursing implications

   a. Assist client in obtaining a clean specimen or obtain a catheterized specimen

Practice to Pass

Your client has told you that he is very concerned that his RPR has been reported as reactant. How would you respond to this client?

Table 1-4		
Normal Urinalysis Results	Color	pale yellow
	Protein	1–14 mg/dL
	Odor	aromatic similar to ammonia
	Bilirubin	negative
	Turbidity	clear
	RBCs	1–2 per high-power field
	Specific gravity	1.005–1.030
	WBCs	0–5 per high-power field
	PH	4.5–8
	Casts	none–few
	Glucose	<15 mg/dL
	Bacteria	<1000
	Ketones	negative
	Nitrates	negative

    b. Send specimen to the laboratory ASAP

    c. Assess the client's fluid status, medications, and foods taken recently

E. Fecal analysis: normal findings for occult blood–negative; ova and parasites–negative; fecal fat < 7 g/24 hr

  1. Description: fecal analysis is usually performed to diagnose diseases of the GI tract

  2. Clinical problems

    a. Positive stool occult blood can occur with cancer, peptic ulcer disease, ulcerative colitis, or diverticulitis

    b. The presence of ova and parasites indicates infection

    c. Increased findings of fecal fat can occur with malabsorption syndrome, pancreatic diseases, or Crohn's disease

  3. Nursing implications: assist client to obtain a fresh specimen; send specimen to the laboratory as soon as possible (ASAP) for analysis

F. Cerebrospinal fluid analysis: normal findings are color = clear; WBCs = 0 to 8 mm^3; protein = 15 to 45 mg/dL; chloride = 118 to 132 mEq/L; glucose = 40 to 80 mg/dL

  1. Description: CSF is obtained by lumbar puncture and fluid analysis is done to diagnose spinal and cerebral diseases and infections

  2. Clinical problems

    a. Color may change because of the presence of red blood cells or an elevated cell count

    b. Increased cell count may be caused by infection, tumor, or presence of blood

    c. Elevated protein levels may indicate tumor, viral or bacterial infection, or Guillain-Barré syndrome

    d. Elevated glucose levels may occur with some types of meningitis, brain cancer, or leukemia

  3. Nursing implications

    a. Assist with the lumbar puncture to obtain specimen

    b. Explain procedure to the client, provide comfort during positioning, and answer questions as needed

    c. Ensure that specimens are placed in sterile containers and sent to the laboratory for analysis ASAP

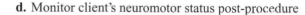

    d. Monitor client's neuromotor status post-procedure

XI. Diagnostic Tests Commonly Used to Detect Health Problems in Adults

A. Computed tomography (CT) scan

  1. General description

    a. A noninvasive, diagnostic radiographic procedure that provides cross-sectional images of the body to differentiate subtle changes in the tissue density of the selected structure

    b. CT scans are performed to rule out the presence of or evaluate enlarged nodes, lesions, abscesses, hemorrhage, and the extent of cancer metastases

    c. The x-ray beam scans a thin layer of the client's body and transmits that information to a computer that constructs images on a screen for interpretation

    d. The client will lie on a moveable scanning table and pass through the opening in the scanner; the client should be reassured that he or she will be visible to the radiology staff during the procedure

  2. CT of the head

    a. The client lies on the CT scanner table in a supine position with tape or Velcro straps across the forehead to prevent any motion

    b. Depending on the client's history and physician request, contrast media may be administered intravenously

    c. Sedation is given occasionally for restlessness, if necessary

    d. This test can be utilized to detect aneurysms, the presence of blood, fluid, tumors, or structural abnormalities

  3. CT of the abdomen

    a. The client is required to drink approximately 42 ounces of contrast media prior to the test and will also require intravenous (IV) access for the administration of contrast media

    b. The contrast media may cause the client to become flushed or nauseated, but this reaction is usually transient

    c. This test can be utilized to determine the presence of fluid, lesions, structural malformations, the presence of foreign bodies, or hemorrhage

B. Doppler studies

  1. General information: a diagnostic, noninvasive examination that utilizes the echoes of an ultrasonic beam to create three-dimensional oscilloscope pictures or waveform diagrams on a computer screen as the beam is "bounced back" to the Doppler probe

  2. Cardiac (called echocardiogram): a diagnostic test to evaluate cardiac structures and valves; an image is produced on a screen as the ultrasound waves emitted from the Doppler probe are reflected back to a transducer from the cardiac structures; this test is utilized to evaluate or diagnose cardiac tamponade, heart valve malformation or malfunctioning, left ventricular function, and septal defects; a conductive gel is utilized to enhance the transmission of the emitted waves

  3. Vascular studies: upper- and lower-extremity venous and arterial evaluations can be done to detect the presence of thrombus, structural malformation, claudication, and the effectiveness of surgical revascularization; a conductive gel is used to enhance the transmission of the emitted waves

C. Electrocardiography

  1. General description: a noninvasive diagnostic examination utilized to record the electrical activity of the heart

2. Twelve-lead electrocardiogram (ECG): involves the placement of electrodes, usually on the limbs and anterior chest, to detect electrical impulses that are transposed as waveforms to the graphic recorder or monitor screen; it is done to evaluate the configuration, duration, rate, and rhythm of these waveforms to detect dysrhythmias or conduction defects that may indicate myocardial abnormality

3. Ambulatory ECG: the monitoring of the client's cardiac electrical activity while the client is engaged in normal or diagnostic activities

   a. Holter monitor: used to record the client's ECG (2-leads) over a 24-hour period while performing normal daily activities; is used to correlate the client's symptoms to cardiac activity, and to provide information on heart rate, type, and frequency of any arrhythmias; the client is asked to keep a log of activities and any symptoms that develop during the 24-hour period

   b. Graded exercise treadmill test (GXT): a noninvasive test performed on a treadmill to evaluate chest pain, other symptoms of coronary artery disease, cardiac functional capacity, or cardiac arrhythmias that may develop during stress

      1) Electrodes are placed on the client's chest and a continuous 12-lead ECG is performed

      2) The client's blood pressure is also continuously monitored throughout the testing procedure

      3) During the procedure, the client is asked to walk on the treadmill as the speed and elevation of the grade is gradually increased until a target heart rate is reached (which is 80–90 percent of a maximum heart rate based on client's age and level of physical activity)

      4) Certain medications (such as propranolol, a beta adrenergic blocker) and conditions such as chest pain, fatigue, or peripheral vascular disease may preclude the client from reaching his or her target heart rate

D. Endoscopy

1. General description: an invasive diagnostic procedure during which a long flexible fiberoptic tube is introduced into the GI or respiratory tract to visualize the tissues; this test aids in the diagnosis of disease, bleeding, or masses

2. Bronchoscopy: an invasive procedure performed to directly visualize the bronchi for abnormal color, strictures, abscesses, masses, foreign bodies, and to obtain sputum specimens and tissue biopsies

   a. The procedure requires that the client receive a local anesthetic to enhance comfort and to inhibit the cough reflex as the tube is passed through the nasopharynx and oropharynx into the trachea

   b. During and immediately postprocedure, the client must be monitored for impaired respirations, laryngospasm, and bleeding

   c. Because of the impaired gag reflex caused by the local anesthetic and sedation caused by medications given during the procedure, the client should be carefully monitored until awake and the gag reflex has returned

3. Colonoscopy: an invasive procedure performed for direct visualization of the large intestine for abnormal color, inflammation, strictures, masses, foreign

bodies, or bleeding; biopsy and removal of tumors and polyps can also be performed; since the client will probably receive mild sedation during the procedure, it is important to carefully monitor vital signs during and after the procedure until the client is fully awake

E. Magnetic resonance imaging (MRI)

1. A noninvasive diagnostic tool utilized to create images of multiple body planes through the use of a magnetic field and radiofrequency waves

2. Its purpose is to detect tissue structures and tears, fluid accumulations, abnormal masses, and neurological and vascular disorders

3. It is particularly useful in visualizing soft tissue and fluid collections in the areas scanned throughout the body

NCLEX!

4. Because a magnetic field is utilized for the testing, all metal items must be removed prior to placing the client in the MRI cylinder

5. If the client requires emergency care, he or she must be removed from the vicinity of the MRI scanner for care

6. The client should be advised that the MRI cylinder is narrow and that various noises will be heard while the scanner is in use

7. The client should also be advised that although they are in the narrow cylinder, they are able to communicate with the technician via an intercom system within the cylinder

NCLEX!

8. Mild sedation, relaxation techniques, and earplugs may be useful for the client who is anxious about lying in a confined area

9. Advances in the MRI technology have allowed for the creation of a less confining open chamber for those clients with severe claustrophobia

F. Ophthalmoscopy: a noninvasive procedure utilized to examine the inner eye structures of the retina, optic disc, blood vessels, fundus, and macula; an ophthalmoscope is used to allow for magnification and directed lighting so the examiner can assess for any abnormalities in these structures

G. Otoscopic exam: A noninvasive procedure utilized to examine the external auditory canal and tympanic membrane

1. An otoscope is used to allow magnification, directed lighting, and access through the external auditory canal to visualize the canal and tympanic membrane

2. This allows the examiner to assess for lesions, obstructions, inflammation, and to visualize foreign bodies within the auditory canal

3. The tympanic membrane is assessed for color and evaluated for lesions or perforations

H. Pulse oximetry: a noninvasive, intermittent or continuous monitor utilized to trend a client's arterial oxygen saturation

1. A probe, usually attached to the client's finger, toe, earlobe, or bridge of nose, passes an infrared light through the tissue and measures the oxygen saturation of the blood

2. Be aware that this measurement maybe affected by abnormal hemoglobin levels and vascular insufficiencies so results should be compared to the client's ABGs initially

3. This is often measured at the time of respiratory assessment; normal is considered to be > 90% or 95%, depending on source used

I. **Radiography:** diagnostic procedures that utilize radiation exposure to visualize underlying structures

1. Chest x-ray: a noninvasive diagnostic procedure utilized for general screening and diagnosis of lung and bone abnormalities; the procedure can be performed in the radiology department or at the client's bedside; precautions to prevent excessive radiation exposure should be taken by the staff during the procedure and shielding should be provided for clients who are pregnant or of childbearing age

2. Skull x-ray: a non-invasive, diagnostic radiographic procedure utilized to examine the skull for fractures or abnormalities

   a. Skull fractures, if present, are classified by location and type, i.e., depressed, linear, or penetrating

   b. The orbit area is examined for the presence of free air indicating sinus bone fracture or fractures of the orbits that may indicate potential damage to the eyes or extensive brain damage

   c. The client should be advised to lie very still during the procedure

3. Upper GI series (barium swallow): a radiographic and fluoroscopic examination of the pharynx and esophagus as the client swallows a barium sulfate mixture

   a. The results of this procedure are utilized with other information to diagnose hiatal hernia, esophageal varices or diverticuli, head, neck, or stomach cancer, polyps, strictures, or pharyngeal muscle dysfunctions

   b. The client will be asked to be NPO for 8 hours prior to the procedure

   c. During the procedure, the client will swallow quantities of the barium mixture as a radiographic recording of its movement is made

   d. After the procedure, it is important that the client eliminates the barium from the GI tract; additional fluids or a mild cathartic may be ordered to aid in its elimination

4. Lower GI series (barium enema): a radiographic and fluoroscopic examination of the large intestine to detect structure abnormalities of the large intestine such as tumor, diverticuli, or polyps

   a. It is essential that the client's large intestine be free of stool at the time of the examination

   b. The client will be NPO for 18 hours prior to examination after a clear liquid diet

   c. Enemas or laxative suppositories will be ordered for the evening before and the morning of the examination to ensure the absence of stool

   d. After the procedure, it is important that the client eliminate the barium from the GI tract; additional fluids, a laxative, or an enema may be ordered

5. Ventilation perfusion (VQ) scan

    a. A lung perfusion scan is performed to diagnose possible pulmonary thrombosis or embolism; it involves injecting a radionuclide intravenously and obtaining a series of images to detect areas of decreased radionuclide uptake in the lung tissue, indicating decreased blood flow

    b. The ventilation scan involves the inhalation of a mixture of air and radioactive gas; a nuclear scan is performed to measure the amount of gas exchange

    c. In pulmonary embolism, indications of decreased blood flow will be noted in the area but no ventilation abnormality will be noted

    d. During the procedure, it is necessary that the client have IV access and the client is monitored postprocedure for any possible anaphylactic reaction to the radionuclide

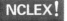

    e. Because of the excretion of the radionuclide in the urine, use of gloves and thorough handwashing should be performed for 24 hours postprocedure

J. Skin testing: a skin test is the intradermal (ID) injection or cutaneous scratch of a substance to assess for hypersensitivity to that substance

    1. Allergic reactions: this type of test involves multiple intradermal injections or cutaneous scratches applied to the client's back or forearm and subsequent monitoring for a local or systemic reaction of hypersensitivity

        a. It is necessary to have immediate access to emergency equipment because of the potential for an anaphylactic reaction whenever allergy testing is performed

        b. The client should be advised to report any symptoms of drowsiness, skin rash, or palpitations during or following testing

        c. The client should also be advised of the possibility of repeat or further testing

    2. Purified protein derivative (PPD): this skin test is administered ID to detect the presence of tuberculosis infection or exposure

        a. A 0.1 mg dose of PPD is planted on the inner aspect of the forearm using a tuberculin syringe with a 25- to 27-gauge needle

        b. The site of injection is usually observed 48 to 72 hours after administration and the result is interpreted based on the size of the induration

        c. A positive result usually indicates active TB or exposure to someone with TB and requires further testing with a chest x-ray and possible sputum culture

    3. Fungi test: a skin test to detect the presence of a fungal infection such as coccidioidomycosis or histoplasmosis

        a. The test involves the intradermal injection of fungal material

        b. Positive reactions of erythema and induration will be noted when results are read in 24 to 48 hours

        c. If positive, blood titers will usually be drawn at 1- to 2-week intervals to monitor titers

     d. A negative blood titer result does not rule out infection, however; the client should be advised that repeat testing might be necessary

K. Ultrasound: a noninvasive diagnostic procedure that passes high-frequency sound waves through the body that are then reflected by underlying body structures to a transducer; recorded images are created on a computer screen to detect abnormalities or contents of structure; a conductive gel is used to enhance the transmission of the waves

  1. Abdominal: noninvasive procedure performed to detect the presence of masses, abnormal structural changes, or the presence of ascites; the client should be instructed that he or she may be given enemas or be NPO for a period of time prior to testing because the presence of stool, gas, or air can alter the recorded images

  2. Gallbladder: a noninvasive procedure utilized to detect the presence of gallstones and detect abnormalities of the gallbladder; client teaching will include taking a clear liquid diet 24 hours prior to testing, and using laxatives the evening before and an enema on the morning of testing; the client will be NPO for 8 hours prior to the examination

  3. Hepatobiliary: a noninvasive procedure utilized to detect cirrhosis, cysts, subphrenic abscesses, tumors, and to visualize the biliary ducts; client teaching will include the need for bowel cleansing and NPO status prior to the procedure

L. Visual acuity

  1. A noninvasive test that utilizes the Snellen chart, a chart with letters of varying sizes and standardized numbers at the end of each line

  2. The top number (20) indicates the distance, measured in feet, between the client and the chart

  3. The bottom number is the distance, measured in feet, at which a person with normal vision can read the line

  4. Each eye is tested individually while covering the opposite eye with an occluder

  5. The client should be tested with and without corrective lenses as appropriate

  6. Documentation of the reading for each eye should be made

  7. Normal findings are considered to be 20/20

  8. Abnormal findings will include: absent acuity in an eye, uncorrected acuity of 20/30 or greater in one eye, or that the vision in both eyes is different by two lines or more

  9. Alternatives to Snellen chart: an "E" Snellen chart and one with pictures have been developed for use with clients who are unable to read

  10. Near vision is tested with a pocket Snellen chart, Rosenbaum card, or any printed material held approximately 14 inches from the face; inability to read comfortably at this distance without moving the card is considered abnormal and may possibly be caused by aging

Case Study

A. S., a 50-year-old male client, has been admitted for a chief complaint of upper abdominal pain, nausea, and vomiting. His primary care physician is ruling out a medical diagnosis of acute pancreatitis.

❶ What questions would you ask during the collection of his health history database pertaining to the chief complaint?

❷ What laboratory tests would you anticipate to be ordered?

❸ Which diagnostic procedures would you expect to be ordered?

❹ What is the client teaching related to these procedures?

❺ Identify three possible nursing diagnoses that would be appropriate for this client.

For suggested responses, see pages 734–735.

Posttest

1 A client has been admitted to your unit this afternoon for treatment of dehydration. The discharge planning for this client should begin:

(1) When the client is ready to discuss discharge.
(2) The morning prior to discharge.
(3) After the physician writes the discharge order.
(4) During the initial contact between the client and nurse.

2 The evaluation process of your nursing plan of care would include which of the following?

(1) Ambulating your client 20 feet down the hallway
(2) Questioning your client about his family medical history
(3) Assessing your client's progress toward a desired outcome
(4) Assigning a nursing diagnosis to an identified need

3 You would anticipate that a client with liver failure would have an elevated serum blood level of which of the following?

(1) Glucose
(2) Ammonia
(3) Albumin
(4) Platelet count

4 Which of the following should be removed from the client in preparation for an MRI procedure?

(1) Urinary catheter
(2) Plastic name band
(3) Partial dental plate
(4) Foam slippers

5 Which of the following isoenzymes of lactic dehydrogenase (LDH) would you expect to be elevated in a client with a diagnosis of acute myocardial infarction (MI)?

(1) LDH^1
(2) LDH^3
(3) LDH^5
(4) LDH^4

6 Which of the following would indicate that your client is in metabolic acidosis?

(1) High pH, high HCO_3
(2) Low pH, low pCO_2
(3) Low pH, low HCO_3
(4) High pH, low pCO_2

7   Your client has been diagnosed with renal failure. What serum laboratory value would be the best indicator of renal function?

(1) Potassium level
(2) Blood urea nitrogen (BUN)
(3) Creatinine level
(4) Specific gravity

8   A client is scheduled for a colonoscopy and asks you what will be determined from the test. Your response is that a colonoscopy would:

(1) Evaluate whether there is a tumor or other problem in the large intestine.
(2) Determine the presence of blood in the abdominal cavity.
(3) Evaluate the presence of and possibly sclerose esophageal varices.
(4) Assess the effectiveness of treatment of a peptic ulcer.

9   A client is admitted with a diagnosis of diabetic ketoacidosis (DKA). The nurse expects the ABGs to reflect which of the following?

(1) Metabolic alkalosis
(2) Respiratory acidosis
(3) Normal findings
(4) Metabolic acidosis

10 A client presents to the Emergency Department with a complaint of left arm pain following a fall. The first physical examination technique the nurse utilizes would be:

(1) Palpation for any deformities or areas of tenderness.
(2) Inspection for any deformities, discoloration, or obvious bone protrusion.
(3) Palpation of distal pulses.
(4) Information gathering about the circumstances of the injury.

See pages 43–44 for Answers and Rationales.

Answers and Rationales

Pretest

1   **Answer: 3** *Rationale:* Open-ended questions encourage the client to speak freely and to elaborate and clarify answers as needed. Restrictive questions that only require a "yes" or "no" answer (option 1) do not encourage free exchange of information nor does frequent rephrasing of the client's answer (as in option 2). Leading questions (option 4) tend to elicit the answer that the nurse anticipated.
Cognitive Level: Application
Nursing Process: Assessment; *Test Plan:* PSYC

2   **Answer: 4** *Rationale:* Validation of the effectiveness of the interventions to achieve the client-specific goals encompasses input from the healthcare team members and knowledge of hospital standards of care. Medical assessment and written orders are components of client care but not the focus of the nursing plan of care.
Cognitive Level: Application
Nursing Process: Evaluation; *Test Plan:* PHYS

3   **Answer: 1** *Rationale:* Renal failure results in the inability of the kidneys to excrete potassium and that leads to hyperkalemia. Nausea, vomiting, excessive laxative use, and loop diuretic use will cause hypokalemia.
Cognitive Level: Application
Nursing Process: Assessment; *Test Plan:* PHYS

4   **Answer: 3** *Rationale:* Arterial blood gas findings of PO_2 90 mmHg (80–100 mmHg normal) and pH 7.40 (7.35–7.45 normal) would be within the normal range for an adult. All the other options list abnormal findings.
Cognitive Level: Analysis
Nursing Process: Assessment; *Test Plan:* PHYS

5   **Answer: 2** *Rationale:* A low-serum potassium level enhances the action of digitalis and predisposes the client receiving digitalis to develop toxicity. The other lab values do not contribute to digitalis toxicity.
Cognitive Level: Application
Nursing Process: Assessment; *Test Plan:* PHYS

6 **Answer: 1** *Rationale:* The client will be required to have an empty stomach for the procedure to allow visualization of the gallbladder and adjacent structures to accurately rule out tumors, structural abnormalities, or the presence of stones. Since the lower GI tract is not visualized during this procedure, there is no need for the bowel to be empty. Also, ultrasound does not require the use of radioactive isotopes.
Cognitive Level: Application
Nursing Process: Implementation; *Test Plan:* PHYS

7 **Answer: 3** *Rationale:* The administration of a local anesthetic is possible during the procedure to decrease the gag reflex and increase comfort. The nurse should check for the return of the gag reflex to prevent the potential for aspiration. The position of the side rails, availability of the call light, and the ability to ambulate without assistance are safety concerns but are not related to the specific client request.
Cognitive Level: Analysis
Nursing Process: Assessment; *Test Plan:* PHYS

8 **Answer: 4** *Rationale:* An oxygen saturation of < 80 percent with observable signs of shortness of breath indicate respiratory distress and require immediate intervention. A full respiratory assessment should be performed and the physician advised of the findings immediately. Symptomatic respiratory distress should not be ignored. The repositioning of the client and the receiving of a physician's order to increase the oxygen being delivered would be helpful. The client should be continually monitored but 15L/min flow rate of oxygen may be excessive.
Cognitive Level: Analysis
Nursing Process: Assessment; *Test Plan:* PHYS

9 **Answer: 3** *Rationale:* Diagnosing is a specific step of the nursing process that utilizes the information collected during the client-specific database collection. Client teaching is a nursing intervention. Team collaboration is important in the intervention and evaluation phases of the nursing process. The utilization of a previously developed clinical pathway includes components of all steps of the nursing process.
Cognitive Level: Application
Nursing Process: Analysis; *Test Plan:* SECE

10 **Answer: 2** *Rationale:* Assisting the client to use the incentive spirometer actively operationalizes the client's plan of care to maintain optimal oxygenation status. Auscultation of carotid bruits would be a part of the assessment process from which a care need may be identified. Prioritization of care issues is part of the planning stage of the nursing process from

which nursing interventions are determined. Consultation with other care providers is used in evaluating the effectiveness of the planning of care and gathering information for possible revision.
Cognitive Level: Application
Nursing Process: Implementation; *Test Plan:* SECE

Posttest

1 **Answer: 4** *Rationale:* Discharge planning should begin on admission to the unit and should be an ongoing process. As a rule, clients are not ready to discuss discharge plans on the day of admission; however, planning for appropriate followup and coordination of care cannot frequently be achieved on the morning of discharge.
Cognitive Level: Application
Nursing Process: Planning; *Test Plan:* SECE

2 **Answer: 3** *Rationale:* The evaluation step of the client's plan of care includes the assessment of their progress toward a previously identified desired outcome. The desired outcome would have been the result of gathering the client's health history, identifying a nursing diagnosis, goal formulation, and implementing the assigned plan of care such as ambulation.
Cognitive Level: Application
Nursing Process: Evaluation; *Test Plan:* SECE

3 **Answer: 2** *Rationale:* In liver failure, an excess of serum ammonia results from the liver's inability to convert ammonia to urea for excretion. Because of the liver's inability to perform it's normal functions, glucose, albumin, and the client's platelet count may be decreased rather than increased.
Cognitive Level: Application
Nursing Process: Assessment; *Test Plan:* PHYS

4 **Answer: 3** *Rationale:* MRI testing involves the use of a magnetic field and radiofrequency waves. Any object that contains metal of any kind will be attracted to the magnetic field, affect the diagnostic ability of the test, and can potentially harm the client. Foam, plastic, and the urinary catheter are not attracted to the magnetic field.
Cognitive Level: Application
Nursing Process: Planning; *Test Plan:* SECE

5 **Answer: 1** *Rationale:* LDH[1] and LDH[2] are the primary isoenzymes for cardiac muscle and are utilized to diagnose an acute MI. LDH[3] is the primary pulmonary isoenzyme, and LDH[4] and LDH[5] are indicators of hepatic dysfunction.
Cognitive Level: Application
Nursing Process: Assessment; *Test Plan:* PHYS

6 Answer: 3 *Rationale:* Normal ABG pH is 7.35 to 7.45 and a normal bicarbonate level is 22 to 26 mEq/L. A low pH would indicate a client is in an acidotic state and the low bicarbonate would indicate a metabolic cause for the acidosis. The pCO_2 level is an indicator of the respiratory component of the client's acid-base balance.
Cognitive Level: Application
Nursing Process: Analysis; *Test Plan:* PHYS

7 Answer: 3 *Rationale:* Creatinine levels are more sensitive and specific for renal disease. Although the BUN level is used to assess renal function, it can also be affected by diet and fluid status. The potassium level can be affected by many factors as well. Specific gravity is not a blood test, but rather is performed on the urine itself.
Cognitive Level: Application
Nursing Process: Assessment; *Test Plan:* PHYS

8 Answer: 1 *Rationale:* A colonoscopy is the insertion of a flexible tube into the lower GI tract for evaluation and treatment of conditions of the lower bowel. An evaluation of the esophagus and stomach would require an approach from the upper GI tract such as an esophagogastroduodenoscopy (EGD). The presence of blood in the abdominal cavity would require an abdominal ultrasound or other x-ray procedure.
Cognitive Level: Application
Nursing Process: Implementation; *Test Plan:* PHYS

9 Answer: 4 *Rationale:* DKA produces an excess release of hydrogen ions into the serum that cannot be buffered by the already depleted bicarbonate level due to an osmotic diuresis that occurs. Therefore the client is in metabolic acidosis. There is no essential respiratory cause for this metabolic condition and the results will not be within normal limits due to the pathophysiology of the disease process.
Cognitive Level: Application
Nursing Process: Assessment; *Test Plan:* PHYS

10 Answer: 2 *Rationale:* The first nursing assessment technique utilized to gather data is inspection of the area. Palpation of any of the area would be attempted after the inspection. Obtaining the client history is not a component of the physical examination.
Cognitive Level: Application
Nursing Process: Assessment; *Test Plan:* PHYS

References

Berger, K. J. & Williams, M. B. (1999). *Fundamentals of nursing: Collaborating for optimal health.* Stamford, CT: Appleton & Lange, pp. 348–382.

Doenges, M. E., Moorhouse, M. F., Burley, J. T. (2000). *Application of nursing process and nursing diagnosis: An interactive text for diagnostic reasoning.* (3rd ed.). Philadelphia: F.A. Davis Company, pp. 2–4.

Estes, M .E. (2002). *Health assessment & physical examination* (2nd ed.). Albany, NY: Delmar Publishers, pp. 18–58, 505–510.

Huether, S. E. (2002). Structure and function of the digestive tract. In: K. L. McCance & S. E. Huether. *Pathophysiology: The biologic basis for disease in adults and children* (4th ed.). St. Louis, MO: Mosby, pp. 1314–1317.

Ignatavicius, D. D. & Workman, M. L. *Medical-surgical nursing: Critical thinking for collaborative care* (4th ed.) Philadelphia: W. B. Saunders Company, pp. 946–947, 1329–1330, 1505–1510, 1803.

Kee, J. F. (2001). *Handbook of laboratory and diagnostic tests with nursing implications.* Upper Saddle River, NJ: Prentice Hall.

Kozier, B., Erb, G., Berman, A., & Burke, K. (2004). *Fundamentals of nursing: Concepts, process, and practice* (7th ed.). Upper Saddle River, NJ: Prentice Hall, Inc., pp. 266–267, 501–503, 508–510, 518–520, 556.

Lehne, R. A. (2002). *Pharmacology for nursing care* (4th ed). Philadelphia: W. B. Saunders, pp. 393–401, 539.

LeMone, P. & Burke, K. M. (2004). *Medical surgical nursing: Critical thinking in client care* (3rd ed.). Upper Saddle River, NJ: Prentice Hall, Inc., pp. 119–160, 542–549.

Lewis, S. M., Heitkemper, M. M., & Dirksen, S. R. (2000). *Medical-surgical nursing: Assessment and management of clinical problems* (5th ed.). St. Louis, MO: Mosby, Inc., pp 4–13, 225, 809.

McCance, K. L. & Huether, S. E. (2002), *Pathophysiology: The biologic basis for disease in adults and children* (4th ed.). St. Louis, MO: Mosby, Inc., pp. 86–97, 1011–1013, 1363.

Wilkinson, J. M. (2001). *Nursing process and critical thinking* (3rd ed.). Upper Saddle River, NJ: Prentice Hall.

CHAPTER 2

Respiratory Disorders

Theresa Loan, PhD, RN

CHAPTER OUTLINE

OBJECTIVES

▊ Identify basic structures and functions of the respiratory system.

▊ Describe the pathophysiology and etiology of common respiratory disorders.

▊ Discuss expected assessment data and diagnostic test findings for selected respiratory disorders.

▊ Identify priority nursing diagnoses for selected respiratory disorders.

▊ Discuss therapeutic management of a client experiencing a respiratory disorder.

▊ Discuss nursing management of a client experiencing a respiratory disorder.

▊ Identify expected outcomes for the client experiencing a respiratory disorder.

[*Media Link*]

Use the CD-ROM enclosed with this text, or log onto the address given to access the free, interactive Companion Website created for this series. The CD-ROM and Companion Website accompanying this book offer additional practice opportunities and information—NCLEX Review, Case Studies, Glossary, In Depth with NCLEX, and more.

www.prenhall.com/hogan

REVIEW AT A GLANCE

acid *a substance that is capable of losing hydrogen ions*

acidosis *the condition of increased hydrogen ion concentration in the blood*

alkalosis *the condition of decreased hydrogen ion concentration in the blood*

alveolar ventilation *volume of air that undergoes gas exchange*

anatomic dead space *the portion of the respiratory system from the nose to the respiratory bronchioles that functions only as an air passageway; about 25 percent of air inhaled with each breath remains in the anatomic dead space and is therefore unavailable for gas exchange*

base *a substance that is capable of accepting hydrogen ions*

buffer *a weak acid or a weak base that transfers hydrogen ions between solutions to maintain acid-base balance; the respiratory system plays a vital role in maintenance of acid-base balance; carbon dioxide combined with water forms car-*

bonic acid and is eliminated from the body during exhalation

compliance *elastic property of the lungs and thorax; also referred to as distensibility*

diffusion *movement of gas from an area of greater pressure to an area of lower pressure*

expiration *movement of gas from the respiratory system into the atmospheric air; process is generally passive, but may become more conscious and forced with obstructive lung disease*

inspiration *movement of air from the atmosphere into the respiratory system; process is generally passive but may be voluntary*

oxygen saturation *the percentage of oxygen bound to hemoglobin compared to the volume that the hemoglobin is capable of binding*

perfusion *circulation of blood into the tissues and cells*

pH *refers to the hydrogen ion concentration of a solution; indicator of the ratio of acid and base in the blood; a lower pH value indicates greater hydrogen ion concentration and greater acidity; a higher pH value indicates lower hydrogen ion concentration and higher alkalinity*

pulmonary ventilation *total volume of gas exchange between the atmosphere and the lungs*

respiration *the mechanical and metabolic processes involved with oxygen transport from the atmospheric air into the blood and carbon dioxide transport from the blood back into the atmospheric air*

ventilation–perfusion mismatch *clinically significant imbalance between volume of air and volume of blood circulating to the gas exchange area of the lungs; average ratio is 4 L of air passing into the alveoli for every 5 L of blood that flows into the alveoli (ratio of 0.8); also commonly known as VQ (ventilation quotient) mismatch*

Pretest

1 A client underwent bronchoscopy using conscious sedation. Which of the following outcomes is most important to be met prior to discharging the client?

(1) The client verbalizes symptoms to report to the physician following discharge.
(2) The client has an intact gag reflex.
(3) The client is afebrile.
(4) The client is taking oral fluids.

2 A client is admitted to the hospital with the medical diagnosis of traumatic brain injury. From the assessment finding of slow, shallow respirations, the nurse concludes that which area of the brain is affected by the injury?

(1) Anterior pituitary
(2) Hypothalamus
(3) Medulla
(4) Cerebral cortex

3 In the client with right lung pneumonia, the nurse should encourage which position to facilitate optimal oxygenation?

(1) Prone position
(2) Supine position with head elevated 30 degrees
(3) Positioned with the right side dependent
(4) Positioned with the left side dependent

4 The nurse is making a home visit to a 70-year-old client with emphysema. Which assessment finding has the most serious implication for this client's nursing care?

(1) Increased anterior-posterior diameter of the chest
(2) Bilateral crackles throughout the lung fields
(3) Pursed-lip breathing
(4) Circumoral cyanosis

5 A postoperative client with emphysema is receiving oxygen at 2 L/min via nasal cannula when he/she complains of feeling dyspneic. The spouse asks the nurse to increase the oxygen intake to help him/her breathe easier. Which response by the nurse is appropriate?

(1) Switch the oxygen to a 100% non-rebreathing mask
(2) Explain to the spouse that high concentration of oxygen may depress breathing
(3) Ask the spouse to leave the room to let the client get some sleep
(4) Administer pain medication

6 For the client with bacterial pneumonia, the nurse assesses for which of the following findings?

(1) Normal white blood cell count
(2) Atelectasis
(3) Productive cough
(4) Unremarkable chest x-ray

7 The occupational health nurse teaches a group of employees to follow all safety policies because irreversible lung damage can result from occupational exposure to substances such as coal, asbestos, or glass, because of:

(1) Chronic inflammation of lung tissue.
(2) Frequent antigen-antibody reaction to foreign substances.
(3) Chronic air trapping.
(4) Surfactant deficiency.

8 In developing the care plan for a client with pulmonary mycobacterium tuberculosis, what primary precaution should be included?

(1) Contact skin precautions
(2) Use of special mask to avoid inhaling infected airborne droplets
(3) Avoidance of blood contamination
(4) Containment of draining wounds

9 The family of a client with emphysema asks the nurse about the disease process. The nurse explains that the disorder results from a decreased oxygen supply because of:

(1) Paralysis of respiratory muscles.
(2) Infectious obstructions.
(3) Pleural effusion.
(4) Loss of surface area for gas exchange.

10 In the client with new rib fractures, which assessment finding would best alert the nurse to the possible development of a pneumothorax?

(1) Pink, frothy sputum
(2) Hoarseness
(3) Decreased breath sounds on affected side
(4) Dullness to percussion on the unaffected side

See pages 93–94 for Answers and Rationales.

I. Overview of Anatomy and Physiology

A. Respiratory system structures: anatomic areas include upper and lower respiratory tract, accessory structures, and blood supply; functional areas include conducting airways (**anatomic dead space**) from the nose to the terminal bronchioles, and gas exchange airways, from the respiratory bronchioles to the alveoli and alveolar ducts

1. Upper respiratory tract (conducting airways)

   a. Nose: passageway for air exchange between atmospheric air and the respiratory tract; filters, humidifies [requires about 250 milliliters (mL) of fluid daily], and heats inspired air; nasal hairs trap airborne particles in mucus and cilia propel them into the nasopharynx, where they are expelled by coughing or diverted into the gastrointestinal (GI) tract; olfactory nerve receptors are responsible for the sense of smell

    b. Paranasal sinuses: air-filled cavities in frontal, maxillary, ethmoid, and sphenoid bones that contribute to mucus production and voice resonance

    c. Pharynx: nasopharynx, laryngopharynx (passageway for air), and oropharynx (passageway for food); adenoids in the nasopharynx and tonsils in the oropharynx contain lymphatic tissue that contributes to immune function

    d. Larynx: vibration of vocal cords within the larynx produces the voice; remains open only when air is passing through; epiglottis closes during swallowing to prevent passage of food into the trachea

    e. Trachea: passageway between the upper and lower respiratory tract; divides into the right and left mainstem bronchus

2. Lower respiratory tract (conducting airways and gas exchange airways)

    a. Bronchi: passageway for air from trachea, through the right mainstem bronchus and left mainstem bronchus (conducting airways) into the lungs; mainstem bronchi branch into smaller bronchioles that eventually terminate in the alveoli; right mainstem bronchus is more evenly aligned with the trachea, making it a more common passage for aspirated gastric contents and dislocated endotracheal tubes; terminal bronchioles (gas exchange airways) have a semi-permeable membrane and participate in gas exchange

    b. Alveoli: air-filled sacs in the lungs; oxygen diffuses from alveoli (gas exchange airways) into the blood across the alveolar-capillary membrane (primary site of gas exchange); carbon dioxide diffuses across the pulmonary capillary membrane into the alveoli; spherical shape of the alveoli provides greater surface area for gas exchange

        1) Type I alveolar cells: squamous epithelium cells that participate in gas exchange

        2) Type II alveolar cells: manufacture Type I alveolar cells and surfactant, a lipoprotein substance that decreases alveolar surface tension, an essential element in gas exchange

    c. Lungs: function is air exchange; store blood and neutralize some vasoactive substances; right lung is divided into three lobes—upper, middle, and lower; left lung is divided into 2 lobes—upper and lower; upper area is called the apex; lower area is called the base

    d. Pleura: two-layer membrane covering the lungs and thoracic cavity; visceral pleura attaches to the external lung surface; parietal pleura lines the thoracic cavity; pleural fluid lubricates pleural layers and holds them together during inspiration and expiration

    e. Pleural cavity: air-filled space of the thoracic cavity housing the lower respiratory tract

3. Accessory structures: contribute to the mechanics of breathing

    a. Rib cage: 12 pairs of ribs and the sternum provide skeletal support and protection for the heart and lungs

    b. Intercostal muscles: located between the ribs, contraction facilitates chest expansion during inspiration by increasing the anterior-posterior and lateral diameter of the chest

    c. Diaphragm: separates the thoracic cavity from the abdominal cavity; brain's respiratory center controls contraction of diaphragm via the phrenic nerve;

flattens during inspiration to allow greater chest expansion during inspiration; an intact nervous system is essential to proper functioning of the diaphragm

B. Respiratory system functions: primary function of the respiratory system is the exchange of gases between the external environment and the blood; process of respiration involves ventilation, perfusion, diffusion, and nervous system control; **respiration** refers to the mechanical and metabolic processes involved with oxygen (O_2) transport from the atmospheric air into the blood and carbon dioxide (CO_2) transport from the blood back to the atmospheric air

 1. Ventilation: passage of gases between the atmosphere and the lungs; ventilation phases include inspiration and expiration; adequacy of ventilation is influenced by respiratory system pressures, respiratory tissue properties, airway resistance, lung volumes and capacities, body position, and disease processes

     a. **Pulmonary ventilation**: total volume of gas exchange between the atmosphere and the lungs

     b. **Alveolar ventilation**: volume of air that undergoes gas exchange

     c. Ventilation phases

         1) **Inspiration**: nerve impulses travel from brain via phrenic nerve to contract the diaphragm, increasing the diameter of the thoracic cavity; intrapleural pressure increases, becoming more negative compared to atmospheric air; air moves from area of higher pressure (atmosphere) to lower pressure (respiratory system); air moves through structures of the respiratory system to alveoli and pulmonary capillaries where gas exchange occurs

         2) **Expiration**: diaphragm relaxes and pushes upward, decreasing thoracic cavity diameter; intrapleural pressure remains negative compared to atmospheric air, but becomes less negative than during inspiration; intrapulmonic pressure becomes higher than atmospheric pressure allowing passive air flow from lung through respiratory structures into the atmosphere; smaller airways may collapse during expiration, particularly in the supine position

     d. Respiratory system pressures: atmospheric pressure of 760 mmHg serves as reference point for comparison to respiratory pressures

         1) Intrapulmonary pressure: also called intra-alveolar pressure; equals atmospheric pressure when glottis is open and there is no air movement

         2) Intrapleural pressure: negative pressure produced by opposite forces of elastic recoil between the lungs and chest wall; with glottis open and alveolar air in communication with the atmosphere, it measures negative compared to intrapulmonary pressure; with glottis closed, during coughing or with forced expiration, it measures positive compared to atmospheric air; normally negative intrapleural pressure prevents lung collapse

         3) Intrathoracic pressure: compared to atmospheric air, negative pressure inside the thoracic cavity equals intrapleural pressure; with forced expiration against a closed glottis, intrathoracic pressure becomes positive

e. Respiratory tissue properties: respiratory vessels and airways are implanted in elastic tissues

1) **Compliance**: elastic property of lung related to elastic and collagen fibers; compliance changes with change in respiratory system pressures and/or change in lung fluid content; higher compliance occurs in lung that is more easily distended; lower compliance occurs in lung that is not easily distended

2) Elastic recoil: ability of lungs to return to original shape after air is expelled; recoil is present because of opposing forces created by movement of lungs and chest wall

3) Distensibility: ease of lung inflation made more difficult by increased volume of lung fluid content or consolidation of lung tissue

4) Stiffness: resistance of lungs to stretch to accommodate air volume; increasing lung stiffness lowers compliance

f. Airway resistance: obstruction to airflow caused by conditions of respiratory system tissues (elastic recoil, compliance), changes in airway diameter (bronchoconstriction, mucus obstruction), and/or pressure differences between atmospheric air and intrapulmonary air

g. Lung volumes and capacities: lung volumes describe normal individual quantities of air exchanged during specific times of the breathing cycle; lung capacities describe combined quantities of lung volumes during specific periods of the breathing cycle (see Box 2-1)

NCLEX!

h. Body position: gravity accounts for greater ventilation in dependent areas of lung; with inspiration and body upright, sitting, or standing, airway opening allows for airflow to follow the path of least resistance into the more compliant lung bases

---

Box 2-1

Lung Volumes and Capacities

- Tidal volume (V_T): total air volume inspired and expired during one breathing cycle.
- Inspiratory reserve volume (IRV): maximum air volume inspired with forced **inspiration** (i.e., movement of air from the atmosphere into the respiratory system) following normal inspiration.
- Expiratory reserve volume (ERV): air volume that can be expired with force following normal expiration.
- Residual volume (RV): air volume remaining in lungs following forced expiration.
- Total lung capacity (TLC): maximum capacity of air volume of the lungs.
  $TLC = IRV + V_T + ERV + RV$
- Inspiratory capacity (IC): maximum air volume that can be inhaled following a normal exhalation.
  $IC = V_T + IRV$
- Vital capacity (VC): maximum air volume that can be exhaled after a maximum inhalation.
  $VC = IRV + V_T + ERV$
- Functional residual capacity (FRC): residual air volume in lungs after a normal exhalation.
  $FRC = ERV + RV$

2. **Perfusion:** blood flow through the pulmonary capillary bed and to the respiratory system structures; respiratory system circulation includes the pulmonary circulation and bronchial circulation

   a. Pulmonary circulation: pulmonary artery carries deoxygenated (venous) blood from the right ventricle, branches into pulmonary capillaries, and connects to alveoli; CO_2 is exchanged for O_2 at the pulmonary capillary membranes; capillary membranes merge into pulmonary venules and pulmonary veins that carry oxygenated blood back to the left atrium of the heart

   b. Bronchial circulation: bronchial arteries branching from the thoracic aorta circulate blood to the conducting airways and other respiratory tract tissues; bronchial blood does not circulate to the alveoli and is not included in gas exchange; deoxygenated bronchial blood drains through bronchial capillaries and veins into the vena cava and the right side of the heart; deoxygenated blood from small bronchial veins drains into azygos and pulmonary veins into the left side of the heart then combines with oxygenated blood from the pulmonary circulation

   c. Characteristics of respiratory system circulation: blood pressure and resistance to blood flow are lower in pulmonary blood vessels compared to systemic blood vessels; adequacy of pulmonary capillary blood flow depends upon a mean pulmonary arterial pressure (MPAP) that is greater than mean pulmonary venous pressure (MPVP); blood volume in pulmonary capillary bed increases when MPVP exceeds MPAP, causing pulmonary edema; pulmonary blood vessels constrict in response to hypoxia

3. **Diffusion:** movement of gas from an area of higher pressure to lower pressure; O_2 diffuses from the atmosphere into the alveoli, across the pulmonary capillary membrane and into the pulmonary capillaries for circulation throughout the body; CO_2 diffuses out of the pulmonary capillaries across the capillary membrane and into the alveoli to be exhaled; diffusion continues until pressure differences become equal between the two areas

   a. Fick's Law: describes the process of gas diffusion

   Gas volume = Partial pressure of gas 1 – Partial pressure of gas 2 × Surface area of membrane × Diffusion coefficient / Membrane thickness

   b. Variables that influence gas exchange (see Table 2-1)

Table 2-1	Variable	Example
Variables that Influence Gas Exchange	Partial pressure of the gas	Supplemental oxygen increases partial pressure of inspired air
	Surface area	Loss of lung tissue by surgery or disease decreases surface area available for gas exchange
	Molecular weight and gas solubility	CO_2 is more soluble in the membranes and diffuses more quickly than oxygen
	Thickness of membrane	Membrane is thickened by some disease processes such as pneumonia, pulmonary edema; a thicker membrane impedes effective air exchange

c. Ventilation-perfusion relationship: adequate gas exchange requires alveolar ventilation of about 4 L/min balanced with alveolar capillary perfusion of about 5 L/min (see Figure 2-1)

1) Normal ventilation-perfusion (V/Q) ratio: 4:5

2) V/Q ratio is influenced by partial pressure of O_2 and partial pressure of CO_2

3) Average normal PaO_2 = 100 mmHg; average normal $PaCO_2$ = 40 mmHg

4) Partial pressure of gases varies in different lung areas

5) Under normal conditions and in the upright position, ventilation is greater than perfusion in the lung apices; ventilation greater than perfusion yields a V/Q ratio greater than 4:5; perfusion greater than ventilation yields a V/Q ratio less than 4:5

6) Under normal conditions and in the upright position, perfusion and ventilation are greater in the lung bases

Figure 2-1   Ventilation-perfusion relationships. A. Normal alveolar-capillary unit with an ideal match of ventilation and blood flow. Maximum gas exchange occurs between alveolar wall and blood. B. Physiologic shunting: A unit with adequate perfusion but inadequate ventilation. C. Dead space: A unit with adequate ventilation but inadequate perfusion. In the latter two cases, gas exchange is impaired.

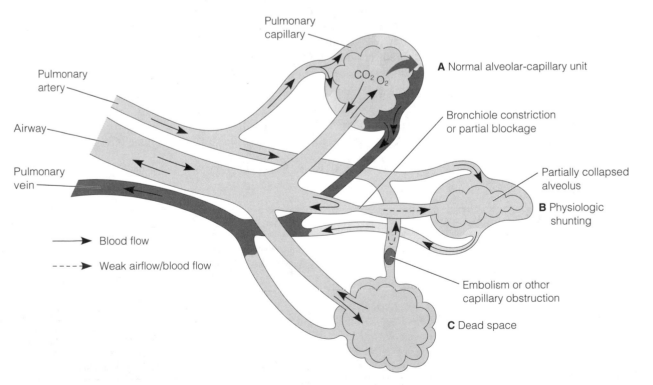

4. Nervous system control of breathing: initiates within the medulla oblongata and pons of the brainstem

   a. Medulla oblongata: controls inspiration, expiration, and breathing pattern

   b. Pons: controls rate and depth of respiration

   c. Sensory input to brainstem: impulses that influence breathing and respiration are transmitted to the brainstem from chemoreceptors, stretch receptors, proprioceptors, baroreceptors, and the external environment

   1) Central chemoreceptors in medulla: increased PCO_2 and/or decreased blood pH causes increased alveolar ventilation as a compensatory mechanism to maintain PCO_2 and pH at normal levels

   2) Peripheral chemoreceptors in the aortic arch and carotid bodies: increased PCO_2 and/or decreased pH, and/or decreased partial pressure of arterial oxygen (PO_2) causes increased alveolar ventilation

   3) Stretch receptors in the alveolar septa, bronchi, and bronchioles: prevent overdistention of the lungs when they are inflated

   4) Proprioceptors in muscles and tendons of moveable joints: stimulate ventilation with exercise to increase oxygen supply during increased oxygen demand

   5) Baroreceptors in the aortic arch and carotid sinus: alter respiration relative to changes in arterial blood pressure; elevated arterial blood pressure lowers respiration; blood pressure below 80 mmHg increases respiration

   6) External environment: factors such as cold, physical stress, air pollution, smoking, and pain alter respiration; infection and fever increase respiration caused by increased oxygen demand

   d. Nerve impulses travel from brain stem via phrenic nerve to diaphragm and stimulate muscle contraction for breathing

II. Diagnostic Tests and Assessments

A. Radiological studies

1. Chest x-ray: performed to visualize structures, fluid, and air in the thoracic cavity; anterior-posterior and lateral views are the most common; appropriate use of lead shielding reduces overall exposure to x-rays

2. Computed tomography (CT): provides a cross-sectional visualization of examined tissue; identifies slight variations in tissue thickness so it may detect lesions not identified by x-ray; performed with or without contrast (check allergies to iodine or seafood if contrast used); computerized images are greatly enhanced compared to traditional x-rays

3. Magnetic resonance imaging (MRI): computerized images similar to CT identify subtle changes in tissue structure; utilizes the body's natural radio frequency impulses; assess client to ensure metal sources are removed; clients with metal implants may be ineligible for MRI

4. Pulmonary angiogram: provides visualization of the pulmonary vasculature; radioactive contrast medium injected is injected through a central venous catheter into the right side of the heart and pulmonary artery for visualization of the pulmonary circulation pathway; identifies circulation alterations (congenital abnormalities, thromboembolism) and tumor demarcation; assess for iodine and/or seafood allergies

5. Ventilation-perfusion scan: radioactive isotope injected to identify areas of ventilation and perfusion within the lungs

B. Pulse oximetry

1. Continuously monitors arterial or venous **oxygen saturation,** the percentage of oxygen bound to hemoglobin compared to the volume that the hemoglobin is capable of binding

2. Uses a light spectroscopy probe attached to a local tissue site such as the finger, earlobe, or nose

NCLEX!

3. Lowered accuracy occurs with diminished peripheral perfusion, brightly-lit environment, acrylic fingernails, and dark skin color

C. Pulmonary function test

1. Uses a spirometer to measure lung volumes and capacities during forced breathing techniques

2. Identifies normal or abnormal pulmonary functions

3. Differentiates restrictive versus obstructive alterations of pulmonary function

4. Assesses effects of bronchodilator therapy

D. Bronchoscopy

1. Visualizes the bronchi and branches using a fiberoptic scope

2. Is performed for diagnostic and/or therapeutic reasons

3. Obtains tissue and/or fluid specimens from the lung

4. Removes foreign bodies from lungs

5. May be performed on individuals breathing room air, supplemental oxygen, or receiving mechanical ventilation

NCLEX!

6. Preprocedure care

    a. Client NPO 6 to 12 hours before procedure

    b. Requires informed consent

    c. Administer analgesia/sedation as ordered

    d. Local/topical anesthesia applied to nasal, pharyngeal areas

7. Postprocedure care

    a. Priority is airway maintenance

NCLEX!

    b. Assess for return of gag reflex and symptoms of laryngeal edema—hoarseness, stridor, dyspnea, vital signs, and chest pain

E. Thoracentesis

1. Is the introduction of a needle into the thoracic cavity for diagnostic and/or therapeutic reasons

2. Allows withdrawal of pleural fluid for laboratory analysis—microbiology, cytology

3. Permits drainage of pleural effusion

F. Laboratory

1. Arterial blood gases: blood specimen obtained by arterial puncture or drawn from arterial line; identifies acid-base status and compensatory mechanisms

Parameter	Normal Value
pH	7.35 – 7.45
PCO_2	35 – 45 mm Hg
HCO_3^-	22 – 26 mEq/ L
PO_2	80 – 100 mm Hg

   a. Identification of acid-base status

   1) **Acid:** donates hydrogen ions

   2) **Base:** accepts hydrogen ions

   3) Acid-base balance is classified as normal, acidotic, or alkalotic; acid-base balance can be altered by the respiratory or metabolic components, either individually or in combination

   b. Check **pH** (first step): reflects concentration of hydrogen ions in the blood; pH is an overall indicator of acid-base balance or buffering; a **buffer** is a weak acid or a weak base that transfers hydrogen ions between solutions to maintain acid-base balance

   1) pH value < 7.35 indicates **acidosis** (the condition of increased hydrogen ion concentration in the blood)

   2) pH value > 7.45 indicates **alkalosis** (the condition of decreased hydrogen ion concentration in the blood)

   c. Check PCO_2 (second step): is an indicator of respiratory buffering

   1) PCO_2 < 35 mmHg indicates alkalosis

   2) PCO_2 > 45 mmHg indicates acidosis

   Examples: pH < 7.35 + PCO_2 > 45 mmHg = respiratory acidosis

   pH > 7.45 + PCO_2 < 35 mm Hg = respiratory alkalosis

   d. Check HCO_3 (third step): is an indicator of metabolic buffering

   1) HCO_3^- < 22 mEq/L indicates acidosis

   2) HCO_3^- > 26 mEq/L indicates alkalosis

   Examples: pH < 7.35 + HCO_3^- < 22 mEq/L = metabolic acidosis

   pH > 7.45 + HCO_3^- > 26 mEq/L = metabolic alkalosis

  e. After interpreting the pH value as normal, acidotic, or alkalotic, determine whether the respiratory or the metabolic buffering component matches the acid-base component identified by the pH

Example 1:   pH of 7.2 = Acidosis

  PCO_2 of 50 mm Hg = Acidosis

  HCO_3^- of 24 mEq/L = Normal

  Interpretation: respiratory acidosis

Example 2:   pH of 7.5 = Alkalosis

  PCO_2 of 30 mm Hg = Alkalosis

  HCO_3^- of 23 mEq/L = Normal

  Interpretation: respiratory alkalosis

Example 3:   pH of 7.25 = Acidosis

  PCO_2 of 42 mmHg = Normal

  HCO_3^- of 20 mEq/L = Acidosis

  Interpretation: metabolic acidosis

Example 4:   pH of 7.55 = Alkalosis

  PCO_2 of 38 mmHg = Normal

  HCO_3^- of 30 mEq/L = Alkalosis

  Interpretation: metabolic alkalosis

Example 5:   pH of 7.2 = Acidosis

  PCO_2 of 50 mm Hg = Acidosis

  HCO_3^- of 20 mEq/L = Acidosis

  Interpretation: combined respiratory and metabolic acidosis

Example 6:   pH of 7.5 = Alkalosis

  PCO_2 of 30 mm Hg = Alkalosis

  HCO_3^- of 30 mEq/L = Alkalosis

  Interpretation: combined respiratory and metabolic alkalosis

  f. Identification of acid-base compensation: acid-base balance can be normal, uncompensated, partially compensated, or compensated (see Table 2-2)

2. Sputum analysis: specimen obtained for microbiology (gram stain, culture and sensitivity) or cytology; performed to identify infectious organisms and appropriate antimicrobial therapy

  a. Sputum collection procedure: sputum obtained by expectoration, suctioning, saline-induced from the airways, thoracentesis, lung needle biopsy, or transtracheal aspiration; for sputum collection from individuals who can cooperate, have client to rinse mouth prior to attempting to obtain expectorated specimen

Table 2-2	**Acid-Base Compensation**	**Arterial Blood Gas Analysis**
Determining Acid-Base Compensation in Arterial Blood Gases	Normal	Normal pH, normal PCO_2, and normal HCO_3^-
	Uncompensated	Abnormal pH, abnormal PCO_2 or abnormal HCO_3^-
	Partially compensated	Abnormal pH, abnormal PCO_2 or HCO_3^-
		pH condition (acidosis or alkalosis) matches either PCO_2 or HCO_3^-, but not both
	Compensated	Normal pH, abnormal PCO_2 or abnormal HCO_3^-

NCLEX!

1) Specimens for acid-fast bacilli (mycobacterium tuberculosis) may be collected on three different days; specimen collection following a long sleep period (early morning) is desirable because of greater concentration; if unable to obtain a sputum specimen for acid-fast bacilli, gastric specimen may be obtained because mycobacterium tuberculosis is not altered by the acidic gastric contents

2) Specimens for cytology require collection container with a fixative agent

b. Specimen processing: specimens should be collected in the appropriate type of container and sent to the laboratory promptly

3. Skin testing: performed to assess for allergic reactions to specified antigens (Type I hypersensitivity), exposure to tuberculosis-causing organisms (Type IV hypersensitivity), or fungi

a. Skin test administration: injection must be intradermal

1) Circle the injection site with a long-lasting marker

2) Diagram the forearm injection site on chart

b. Skin test interpretation

NCLEX!

1) Measure area of induration (if present) not reddened areas; size of induration is related to positive result with tuberculin testing; result should be read 48 to 72 hours after placement

NCLEX!

2) Positive result: individual has been exposed to the antigen; positive result from tuberculin testing does not mean that the individual has active disease, only that there has been exposure

a) Induration of 5 mm or greater: indicates recent exposure to infectious tuberculosis, or possible human immunodeficiency virus infection; chest x-ray findings with characteristic Ghon tubercles are likely healed and not active infection sites

b) Induration of 10 mm or greater: indicates typical finding of active tuberculosis infection in populations with chronic, complicating diseases such as diabetes, end-stage renal disease, gastrointestinal cancer; finding is compatible in high risk populations such as intravenous drug users, homeless, and residents of high infection incidence areas

3) Negative result: indicates no exposure to the antigen or tuberculosis; false-negative findings occur with suppression of cell-mediated immunity such as occurs with human immunodeficiency virus

III. Common Nursing Techniques and Procedures

A. Airway management: goal is to maintain patent airway

1. Head and jaw position

   a. Upper airway obstruction is often caused by loss of local muscle tone or a foreign object

   b. Open airway by head tilt and anterior chin lift maneuver

   c. In individuals with suspected neck injury, open airway by anterior chin displacement and/or jaw thrust; do *not* perform head tilt

   d. Perform Heimlich maneuver in individuals who are conscious with suspected foreign body obstruction of airway

2. Artificial airways

   a. Oropharyngeal airway: maintains airway patency by preventing posterior tongue displacement

      1) Oropharyngeal airway is intended only for unconscious individuals due to possible vomiting or laryngeal spasms

      2) Airway must be sized for the individual

      3) Assess oral cavity for possible foreign body or vomitus

      4) Tongue blade may be needed to temporarily displace tongue during insertion

      5) Head and jaw position must be maintained independent of airway placement

   b. Nasopharyngeal airway: maintains airway patency via nasal route in individual who is semi-conscious or in whom placement of oropharyngeal airway is not feasible

      1) Airway must be sized for individual; a tube that is longer than appropriate may pass into the esophagus, causing stomach distention and inadequate ventilation

      2) Head and jaw position must be maintained independent of airway placement

   c. Endotracheal intubation: a long, cuffed endotracheal tube is inserted with a laryngoscope by specially trained personnel for long-term airway management or for connection to a mechanical ventilator

      1) Endotracheal tube must be sized for individual

      2) Lung auscultation immediately following placement should yield bilaterally equal breath sounds

      3) Proper placement is confirmed by chest x-ray as soon as feasible relative to individual's location and condition

4) Endotracheal tube tip must be located above the carina to facilitate ventilation of both lungs

d. Tracheostomy: surgical placement of cuffed airway into the trachea by specially trained personnel

1) Ventilation may be voluntary or via mechanical ventilation

2) Supplemental oxygen can be delivered via a trach collar or mechanical ventilator

e. Cricothyrotomy: emergency surgical opening of the cricothyroid membrane to maintain patent airway when other methods fail or are not feasible

3. Techniques for airway clearance

a. Oropharyngeal suctioning: non-sterile procedure to remove secretions from upper airway; alert individuals may be taught to do self-suctioning

b. Nasotracheal suctioning: sterile procedure to remove secretions from tracheal area; may be performed to obtain a sterile sputum specimen

c. Tracheobronchial suctioning: sterile procedure using individual suction catheters or in-line suction catheter for clearing secretions via endotracheal tube

B. Body positioning

1. Physiology: fluid shift theory

a. Lung ventilation and perfusion are gravity-dependent

b. Changes in body position from supine (0 degrees) to varying degrees of head elevation or lateral positioning activates reflexive cardiovascular changes that produce fluid shifts in lungs and chest vessels

2. Specific conditions

a. Acute respiratory failure

1) Elevate head at least 45 degrees

2) Position increases chest expansion

3) Elevation mobilizes fluid from the chest into more dependent areas

b. Unilateral lung disease

1) Place individual with unaffected lung in dependent position ("good lung down")

2) Position by using gravity to promote ventilation-perfusion matching

c. Acute respiratory distress syndrome (ARDS)

1) Prone positioning may be attempted in individuals on maximal mechanical ventilation with unresponsive hypoxemia

2) With position change from supine to prone, previously nondependent air-filled alveoli become dependent, perfusion becomes greater to air-filled alveoli opposed to previously fluid-filled dependent alveoli, thereby possibly improving ventilation—perfusion matching

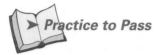

Practice to Pass

How should the client with unilateral lung disease be positioned to achieve optimal oxygenation and why?

3) Oxygenation improves in some individuals with ARDS placed into prone position

4) Caution should be used to avoid unintentional dislodgment of endotracheal tube during positioning

C. Oxygen administration

1. Nasal cannula

   a. Oxygen dose delivered is related to individual's tidal volume and the amount of oxygen flow

   b. Typical oxygen flow of 1 to 6 L/min will provide oxygen concentrations of 24 to 44 percent

   c. Oxygen concentration increases by about 4 percent for each 1 L of oxygen flow (room air oxygen concentration is about 21 percent)

   d. Individuals with chronic obstructive pulmonary disease (COPD) should receive low dose of oxygen flow, about 1 to 2 L/min to prevent respiratory depression; these clients are used to high CO_2 levels and low O_2 levels, so increased O_2 can cause a loss of respiratory drive

2. Face mask

   a. Similar to nasal cannula oxygen administration, oxygen dose delivered is diluted by room air

   b. Exhaled carbon dioxide trapped by mask can be re-breathed

   c. Oxygen flow should be greater than 5 L/min to minimize re-breathing carbon dioxide

   d. Provides oxygen concentration of 40 to 60 percent

3. Face mask with oxygen reservoir

   a. Constant flow of oxygen into attached reservoir bag attached to mask minimizes re-breathing of exhaled carbon dioxide

   b. Typical oxygen dose of 6 to 10 /min provides 60 to 100 percent oxygen concentration

   c. Delivery system used for individuals who require higher oxygen concentrations, but in whom endotracheal intubation is not yet feasible

4. Venturi mask

   a. Utilizes oxygen delivery device that provides more control over oxygen concentration than previously described delivery systems

   b. Delivers oxygen in concentrations of 24, 28, 35, and 40 percent

   c. Used in individuals with COPD and chronic carbon dioxide retention

5. Continuous positive airway pressure (CPAP): discussed in chapter 17

6. Mechanical ventilation: discussed in chapter 17

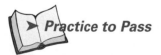

Practice to Pass

Why should individuals with chronic lung disease initially be given low concentration (1 to 2 L/min) of supplemental oxygen?

D. Pulmonary hygiene

    1. Pursed lip breathing

        a. Client exhales through pursed lips

        b. Slows down speed of exhalation and reduces airway collapse, thus enhancing respiration

    2. Coughing

        a. Coughing adequate for airway clearance requires higher airway pressures

        b. Augmented coughing: caregiver places hand below xiphoid process and thrusts downward on abdomen as client ends inspiration

        c. Huff coughing: client attempts sequential coughing while saying "huff"; maneuver keeps glottis open during coughing; beneficial in clients with COPD

    3. Chest physical therapy

        a. Purpose: to mobilize bronchial secretions into larger airways for removal by coughing or suctioning

        b. Indications: greater than 30 mL secretions per day, secretions with artificial airway, and/or atelectasis

        c. Percussion

            1) Client positioned for maximal drainage from appropriate area

            2) Technique involves use of cupped hands alternately percussing indicated area

            3) Contraindications: lung cancer, hemoptysis, and bronchospasm

        d. Vibration

            1) Pressure is applied with palm of hand or electrical vibrator over appropriate area of chest

            2) Vibration may be used in some clients when percussion is contraindicated

        e. Postural drainage

            1) Uses gravity to mobilize bronchial secretions

            2) Nebulized bronchodilators may be administered prior to postural drainage

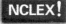

            3) Contraindicated about 1 hour before and within 3 hours after a meal to reduce risk of vomiting and/or aspiration

E. Tracheostomy care

    1. Purpose: temporary or permanent artificial airway

        a. Temporary

            1) Maintains airway when endotracheal intubation is not feasible or possible

2) Facilitates ventilator management and/or weaning

   b. Permanent

     1) Maintains airway following surgical alteration of head/neck

     2) Tracheostomy tube may be temporary or permanent; stoma may not require tracheostomy tube for long-term patency after surgical tracheostomy tract is healed

2. Maintain aseptic conditions when suctioning or cleaning tracheostomy

3. Safety precautions

   a. Keep tracheostomy tube obturator at head of bed for reinsertion in case of accidental dislodgment

   b. Keep manual ventilation bag connected to oxygen source at bedside

   c. Keep a spare unused tracheostomy tube at bedside for emergency use

F. Laryngectomy care

1. Purpose: excision of larynx as treatment for cancer

2. Preoperative teaching: client/family must be educated about the long-term implications including loss of voice, swallowing difficulties, altered route for nutrition intake, and permanent tracheostomy

3. Postoperative care

   a. Maintain patent airway

   b. Provide pain management

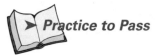

Practice to Pass

What are the key safety measures the nurse must maintain for the client with a tracheostomy?

   c. Provide appropriate nutritional support

   d. Teach client/family how to care for tracheostomy and feeding tube (if applicable)

   e. Provide access to communication devices, such as writing supplies, picture or word board, speaking tracheostomy valve, etc.

   f. Provide emotional support to client and family; make appropriate referrals

G. Respiratory isolation

1. The Occupational Safety and Health Administration (OSHA) mandates that employers provide protective materials to caregivers at risk for exposure to infectious substances

2. OSHA isolation categories were last revised in 1996

   a. Standard precautions

     1) Includes handwashing, gloves, and protective face gear utilized for all clients independent of actual or potential risk for infection

     2) Recommends universal precautions for all clients when handling or coming in possible contact with blood, mucous membranes, non-intact skin, or parenteral devices

   b. Transmission-based precautions: airborne, droplet, and/or contact precautions

1) Methods utilized for clients with known or suspected infectious processes that require isolation measures beyond those of Standard Precautions

2) Airborne and droplet precautions

a) In addition to Standard Precautions, persons around client with known or suspected pathogen transmitted by airborne or droplet method should wear mask

b) Limit client transport within facility; when transport necessary, place mask on client

c) Limit contamination of equipment and/or environment

d) Client should have private (single) room or be placed with a cohort (a client with the same diagnosis)

IV. Nursing Management of the Client Having Thoracic Surgery

A. Preoperative period

1. Reduce anxiety through preoperative teaching about procedure and postoperative course and care

2. Assess client's support systems and ability to care for self after surgery

3. Administer preoperative medications, such as antibiotics, opioid analgesics, and anti-anxiety agents, as ordered

4. Obtain baseline vital signs, oxygenation status, and cognitive status for comparison postoperatively

B. Postoperative period

1. Perform baseline assessments for vital signs, oxygenation status, and cognitive status as for all postoperative clients

2. Maintain patent airway

3. Position client for optimal ventilation and perfusion; note any specific surgeon's orders for positioning; be prepared to initiate respiratory support (intubation, emergency tracheostomy, mechanical ventilation) as needed

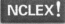

4. Maintain water seal drainage if chest tube present

5. Maintain sterility of operative dressing

6. Maintain client safety

7. Administer antibiotics, bronchodilators, corticosteroids, inhalation agents, or other medications as ordered

8. Administer analgesics as ordered; adequate pain management facilitates chest expansion and optimal ventilation

9. Assess for possible surgical complications that should be reported immediately to maintain oxygenation

a. Change in level of consciousness ranging from restlessness and agitation to lethargy or unresponsiveness

    b. Increase in respiratory rate, unequal chest expansion, decreased breath sounds, and/or use of accessory muscles for breathing

    c. Loss of water seal drainage in closed chest drainage system

    d. Greater than desired volume of chest drainage (75 mL to 100 mL drainage over 1 hour is an average acceptable upper limit); orders should specify volume of acceptable chest tube drainage

  10. Teach the client and family about post-discharge home care and follow-up

  11. Refer to community health resources for assistance with post-discharge care if needed

C. Care of the client with a chest tube

  1. Purpose of chest tube: to reestablish negative intrathoracic pressure following equalization of pressure between chest and atmosphere due to surgery, trauma, or pneumothorax

  2. Routine postprocedural care

    a. Maintain occlusive dressing at chest tube insertion site

    b. Secure chest tube to chest with heavy tape

    c. Secure all chest tube and suction tubing connections with tape

    d. Keep collection apparatus below the level of the chest to allow gravity to promote chest drainage

    e. Milk the chest tube to maintain tube patency *only if ordered*; milking chest tube can cause tissue damage

    f. Chest tube is not clamped when client is mobile and is never clamped without a physician order and/or according to agency policy

    g. In some types of disposable drainage apparatus and with use of glass bottles (rare), the water column fluctuates with breathing; check manufacturer's product description to verify

    h. Maintain indicated amount of water in water seal chamber; below normal water volume creates higher suction than may be desired, contributing to pleural tissue damage

    i. Monitor level of fluid in the suction control chamber (if fluid is used to maintain suction) to ensure it is at the proper level; fluid level in this chamber directly corresponds to the amount of suction pressure

    j. Monitor hourly chest tube drainage output (physician usually specifies hourly volume of chest tube drainage that is acceptable)

    k. Monitor respiratory status: pneumothorax can enlarge or reoccur even in the presence of a patent chest tube drainage system

  3. Types of chest tube drainage collection systems (Figure 2-2)

    a. Sterile plastic disposable collection units or sterile glass bottles (rarely) are used to apply intrathoracic suction and to collect chest tube drainage; disposable collection units are used most frequently

Figure 2-2

**Water-seal drainage system for chest tubes.
A. One-bottle system;
B. Two-bottle system;
C. Three-bottle system.**

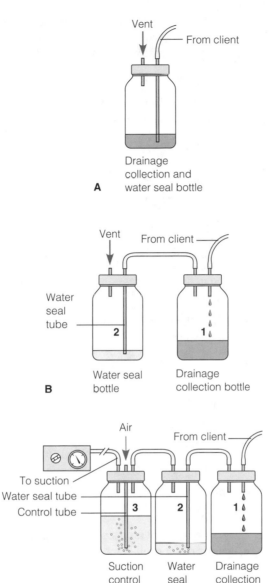

NCLEX!

b. Typically plastic chest tube drainage collection systems (also called closed chest drainage systems) have three chambers:

1) Drainage chamber: collects drainage and can be marked once per shift or more frequently to track amounts of drainage over time

2) Water seal chamber: prevents air in drainage tubing and collection container from flowing back into chest; chamber is filled to the 2-cm mark with sterile water to maintain underwater seal; it is imperative that this seal not be interrupted

3) Suction control chamber: helps to reestablish negative intrathoracic pressure; chamber can be filled with water to the proper level to regulate the amount of suction- most commonly 20 cm (e.g., Pleurevac

4000); some systems use "dry" suction (e.g., Pleurevac 6000) in which a knob is turned to the appropriate level; both types are connected to low wall suction with a connecting tube

c. One-way valve (Heimlich valve)

1) Purpose: performed for emergency treatment of tension pneumothorax during conditions of life-threatening cardiovascular collapse

2) Catheter-over-needle is inserted in the 2nd intercostal space, midclavicular line to relieve a tension pneumothorax

3) Catheter remains in chest after needle removal; audible hissing sound confirms presence of tension pneumothorax

4) Intrathoracic air escapes into the atmosphere via the chest catheter; procedure actually creates a simple pneumothorax

5) Further treatment includes placement of thoracostomy tube and connection to negative pressure drainage collection apparatus as soon as feasible

D. Positioning the client after lung surgery: orders should specify turning parameters for specific client

1. Lobectomy: positioning includes lying on back or turned to either side

2. Segmental resection: positioning includes lying on back and turned onto the non-operative side; positioning on the operative side may place tension on sutures and promote bleeding

3. Pneumonectomy

a. Positioning includes lying on back and turned toward the operative side

b. Client may be turned temporarily slightly toward the non-operative side, but should not remain in this position

c. Turning the client with the operative side in the dependent position promotes desired consolidation of fluid in the pleural space previously occupied by the removed lung and prevents the heart and remaining lung from shifting into the operative side

d. Positioning the client with the operative side dependent facilitates ventilation and perfusion

e. Avoid complete lateral turning to either side, which will change the pressure dynamics within the chest and could lead to mediastinal shift

VI. Disorders of the Respiratory System

A. Obstructive pulmonary diseases

1. Emphysema

a. Description

1) Progressive destruction of alveoli related to chronic inflammation

2) Decreased surface area of respiratory bronchioles, alveoli, and alveolar ducts available for gas exchange

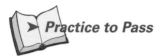

Practice to Pass

What nursing measures are used to prevent recurrence of pneumothorax?

NCLEX!

NCLEX!

NCLEX!

NCLEX!

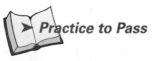

Practice to Pass

How should the nurse position the client who had a pneumonectomy in the postoperative phase and why?

   3) Airway collapse due to loss of elasticity in respiratory system tissues

   4) A chronic form of obstructive pulmonary disease (COPD)

      a) Group of diseases with the major characteristic of airflow restriction

      b) Common symptom includes difficulty with exhalation caused by airways obstructed by edema or excessive mucus production

      c) Lung hyperinflation causes alveolar air trapping and leads to frequent pulmonary infections

      d) Symptoms may be reversible in asthma, but are typically progressive with emphysema, chronic bronchitis, and cystic fibrosis

b. Etiology and pathophysiology

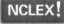

   1) Cigarette smoking is the primary etiology associated with emphysema

   2) Contributing factors include chronic respiratory inflammation from air pollution or occupational substances such as coal, glass, and asbestos

   3) Diagnosis in young and middle-aged adults may be associated with hereditary deficiency of alpha1–antitrypsin, an enzyme that prevents breakdown of lung tissue protein

   4) Air trapping in respiratory bronchioles, alveoli, and alveolar ducts leads to repeated infections and characteristic barrel chest appearance

   5) Work of breathing requires more energy and greater use of accessory muscles

c. Assessment

   1) Clinical manifestations

      a) "Pink puffer" is a classic clinical description characterized by barrel chest, pursed-lip breathing (caused by forced exhalation), obvious use of accessory muscles when breathing, and underweight appearance

      b) Exertional dyspnea progresses with advancing disease

      c) Persistent tachycardia is related to inadequate oxygenation

      d) Lung auscultation yields overall diminished breath sounds, and wheezes or crackles may be present

   2) Diagnostic and laboratory test findings

      a) Arterial blood gas analysis reveals slightly decreased PO_2; PCO_2 is not elevated until later stages

      b) Chest x-ray indicates hyperinflated lungs with a flattened diaphragm; heart size is normal or small

      c) Pulmonary function tests demonstrate low vital capacity and forced expiratory volume (FEV_1)

d. Therapeutic management

   1) Goals of therapy are to improve ventilation and promote patent airway by removal of secretions

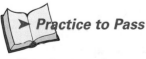

Practice to Pass

How does emphysema alter gas exchange?

2) Remove environmental pollutants and encourage smoking cessation

3) Bronchodilator therapy

4) Beta adrenergic agonists

5) Corticosteroid therapy

6) Oxygen therapy and nebulization therapy

7) Chest physiotherapy

8) Intermittent positive pressure breathing (IPPB)

9) Mechanical ventilation

10) Surgical procedures include bullectomy, lung volume reduction surgery, and lung transplantation

e. Priority nursing diagnoses: Impaired gas exchange; Dyspnea; Risk for infection; Imbalanced nutrition: less than body requirements; Activity intolerance; Deficient knowledge; Noncompliance (regarding smoking cessation)

f. Planning and implementation

1) Provide education and referrals for clients with behaviors that increase the risk for development of emphysema and other chronic obstructive pulmonary diseases

2) Refer clients to a structured pulmonary conditioning program and provide reinforcement as appropriate

3) Teach clients to avoid pulmonary irritants

4) Assist clients to develop appropriate nutritional plans to provide adequate calories

5) Administer supplemental low-flow oxygen as necessary; be prepared to initiate mechanical ventilatory support

6) Administer and teach clients about antibiotic therapy

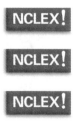

7) Administer and teach clients about bronchodilator therapy and use of measured-dose (metered dose) inhalants

8) Position clients to optimize and maintain airway and effective breathing patterns, usually with head elevated according to comfort

g. Medication therapy

1) Immunization against pneumonia and influenza

2) Antibiotics as needed for concurrent respiratory infection

3) Bronchodilators: controversial use in COPD, but maintenance therapy may be used to reduce dyspnea and attempt to increase FEV_1

4) Beta-adrenergic agonists: used as bronchodilators in COPD and administered by nebulizer or metered dose inhaler (MDI)

5) Anticholinergics: ipratropium (Atrovent) administered as maintenance therapy by inhaler; considered one of the most effective bronchodilators for COPD

6) Long-acting theophylline: controversial use in COPD but may be beneficial to strengthen diaphragm contractility and decrease work of breathing

7) Corticosteroids: controversial use in COPD but may be beneficial for clients with asthma history or with frequent exacerbations unresponsive to therapy with beta-agonists

h. Client education

1) Smoking cessation

2) Teach clients how to avoid occupational or environmental pollutants

3) Maintain adequate nutrition with emphasis on higher calorie intake

4) Teach energy conservation techniques

i. Expected outcomes/evaluation

1) Activity tolerance is optimized

2) Pulmonary irritants such as smoking, air pollution, or occupational exposure are avoided

3) Pulmonary infections are reduced in number and severity

4) Nutritional intake is adequate but not excessive for individual energy needs

2. Chronic bronchitis

a. Description

1) A disorder of chronic airway inflammation

2) Chronic productive cough lasting at least 3 months during 2 years

3) A form of chronic obstructive pulmonary disease

b. Etiology and pathophysiology

1) Cigarette smoking is the primary etiology of chronic bronchitis

2) Contributing factors include chronic respiratory inflammation from air pollution or occupational substances such as coal, glass, and asbestos

3) Chronic inflammation of airways produces hyperplasia of mucous glands, resulting in excessive sputum production

4) Cilia disappear, and their airway clearance function is lost

5) Goblet cells develop in abnormal sites of the terminal bronchioles, also increasing sputum production

6) Mucosal edema and increased production of thick mucus progressively obstructs airflow

7) Work of breathing increases with progressive airway obstruction

8) Repeated pulmonary infections result from increased sputum production with ineffective airway clearance

9) Polycythemia develops as a compensatory response to chronic hypoxemia

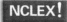

c. Assessment

1) Clinical manifestations

a) Frequent cough, occurring during the winter season, with foul-smelling sputum

b) Frequent pulmonary infections

c) Classic appearance of "blue bloater" includes tendency for obesity and bluish-red skin discoloration from cyanosis and polycythemia

d) Dyspnea and activity intolerance occurs as disease progresses

e) Increased anterior-posterior chest diameter

2) Diagnostic and laboratory test findings

a) Elevated red blood cell count; hemoglobin and hematocrit elevated in later stages

b) Chest x-ray reveals enlarged heart, congested lung fields and normal or flattened diaphragm

c) Pulmonary function indicates increased residual volume, decreased vital capacity, FEV_1, and FEV_1/FVC ratio

d. Therapeutic management

1) Includes measures previously described in section on emphysema

2) Antimicrobials

e. Priority nursing diagnoses: Impaired gas exchange; Dyspnea; Ineffective airway clearance; Risk for infection; Imbalanced nutrition: more than body requirements; Activity intolerance; and Knowledge deficit

f. Planning and implementation

1) Provide education or referrals to clients with behaviors that increase the risk of developing emphysema and other chronic obstructive pulmonary diseases

2) Refer clients to a structured pulmonary conditioning program and provide reinforcement as appropriate

3) Teach clients how to avoid pulmonary irritants

4) Assist clients to develop appropriate nutritional plans that provide adequate calories but maintain ideal weight

5) Administer supplemental low-flow oxygen as necessary; be prepared to initiate mechanical ventilation

6) Administer and teach clients about antibiotic therapy

7) Surgical interventions include bullectomy, lung volume reduction surgery, and lung transplantation

g. Medication therapy

1) Immunization against pneumonia and influenza

2) Antibiotics

3) Bronchodilators: controversial use in COPD, but maintenance therapy may be used to reduce dyspnea and attempt to increase FEV_1

4) Beta-adrenergic agonists: used as bronchodilators in COPD and administered by nebulizer or MDI

5) Anticholinergics: ipratropium (Atrovent) administered as maintenance therapy by inhaler considered one of the most effective bronchodilators for COPD

6) Long-acting theophylline: controversial use in COPD but may be beneficial to strengthen diaphragm contractility and decrease work of breathing

7) Corticosteroids: controversial use in COPD but may be beneficial for clients with history of asthma or with frequent exacerbations unresponsive to beta-agonist medications

h. Client education

1) Smoking cessation

2) Avoiding occupational or environmental pollutants

3) Nutritional therapies for adequate energy needs and weight management

i. Expected outcomes/evaluation

1) Activity tolerance is optimized

2) Avoids pulmonary irritants, such as smoking, air pollution, and occupational exposure

3) Client has reduced incidence and frequency of pulmonary infections

4) Weight reduction if needed

5) Client/family describe appropriate lifestyle changes to optimize health

3. Asthma

a. Description

1) Chronic inflammation of airways leads to intermittent obstruction

2) Severity and duration of symptoms are unpredictable

3) The progressive airway obstruction unresponsive to treatment leads to status asthmaticus, an emergency condition

4) Is a form of chronic obstructive pulmonary disease

b. Etiology and pathophysiology

1) Intrinsic etiologies: uncertain causes; physical or psychological stress; exercise-induced

2) Extrinsic etiologies: antigen-antibody (allergic) reaction to specific irritants; common triggers include air pollutants, sinusitis, cold and dry air, medications, food additives, hormonal influences, and gastroesophageal reflux

3) Characterized by widespread spasms of bronchiole smooth muscle with airway edema

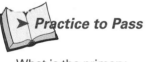

Practice to Pass

What is the primary lifestyle change that the nurse should teach the client with chronic bronchitis?

    4) Excessive secretion of thick mucus contributes to airway obstruction

    5) Lungs become hyperinflated and alveolar air trapping occurs

    6) Gas exchange becomes impaired as ventilation-perfusion mismatching occurs

  c. Assessment

    1) Clinical manifestations

      a) Severe dyspnea

      b) Wheezing with expiration; intensity of wheezing is not related to severity of airway obstruction; clients with severe airway obstruction may not be able to move enough air to produce wheezing sound

      c) Cough

      d) Feelings of chest tightness

      e) Prolonged expiration is noted

      f) Mild to greatly diminished breath sounds upon auscultation; diminished or absent breath sounds may be related to atelectasis or pneumothorax

      g) Hyperresonant sound on percussion

      h) Increased heart rate and blood pressure

      i) Extreme restlessness, anxiety, agitation

      j) Tachypnea with use of accessory muscles

    2) Diagnostic and laboratory test findings (during an episode or "attack")

      a) Decreased PO_2, mild respiratory alkalosis

      b) Elevated eosinophil count

      c) Increased residual volume, decreased vital capacity, decreased forced expiratory volume and peak expiratory flow rate

  d. Therapeutic management

    1) Acute episodes are managed with inhaled beta agonists, bronchodilators, anti-inflammatory agents, corticosteroids, and oxygen therapy; in severe cases, mechanical ventilation may be instituted

    2) Chronic management includes administration of drugs described in the medication section

  e. Priority nursing diagnoses: Ineffective breathing pattern, Ineffective airway clearance, Risk for infection, and Anxiety

  f. Planning and implementation

    1) Assess respiratory and oxygenation status

    2) Administer supplemental oxygen as needed

    3) Administer bronchodilators as prescribed

NCLEX!

    4) Observe characteristics of sputum

    5) Identify/avoid/remove precipitating factors

    6) Teach client relaxation techniques during non-acute periods

    7) Allergy desensitization therapy if appropriate

    8) Be prepared to establish IV access

    9) Be prepared to initiate mechanical ventilation if indicated

   10) Diagnostic testing during non-acute period includes chest x-ray, pulmonary function studies, allergy skin testing, serum eosinophils, and IgE

   11) Provide emotional support to client and family

g. Medication therapy

    1) Short-acting beta-agonist inhaler: used for mild symptoms occurring twice weekly or less; also used for intermittent symptomatic relief and may be combined with long-acting medications

    2) Anti-inflammatory inhaler: used for mild symptoms occurring daily

    3) Anti-inflammatory inhaler plus medium-dose corticosteroid inhaler: used for moderate symptoms occurring daily or more often

    4) Anti-inflammatory inhaler plus long-acting bronchodilator plus oral corticosteroid: used for severe symptoms occurring daily or more often

    5) If appropriate, allergy desensitization therapy

h. Client education

    1) Identify asthma triggers

    2) Teach client/family proper use of metered-dose inhaler

    3) Instruct client regarding the use of peak flow meter for self-assessment of asthma status

    4) Asthma symptoms requiring emergency intervention

i. Expected outcomes/evaluation

    1) Absence of dyspnea, chest tightness, wheezing

    2) Respiratory rate 12 to 24 breaths per minute

    3) Pulse oximetry/arterial blood gas values within normal range

    4) Bilaterally clear and equal breath sounds

    5) Afebrile

    6) Adequate airway clearance of clear, thin secretions

    7) Absence/resolution of anxiety

    8) Clear chest x-ray or return to client's usual baseline

    9) Normal or improved pulmonary function tests

B. Restrictive pulmonary diseases

1. Pleural effusion

   a. Description

      1) Accumulation of fluid in the pleural space

      2) Indicates underlying pulmonary disease/abnormality

      3) A form of restrictive lung disease

   b. Etiology and pathophysiology

      1) Transudative pleural effusion

         a) Pleural fluid contains a small quantity of protein

         b) Fluid moves from capillaries into pleural space

         c) Most common cause is increased hydrostatic pressure, such as what occurs with heart failure

         d) Decreased oncotic pressure caused by an inadequate albumin level occurs more frequently with chronic renal and liver disease

      2) Exudative pleural effusion

         a) Pleural fluid contains a large quantity of protein

         b) Inflammatory response causes increased capillary permeability with fluid shift out of capillaries

         c) Exudation is associated with pulmonary tumors, pulmonary infections, pulmonary emboli, pancreatitis, and ruptured esophagus

      3) Empyema

         a) Pleural fluid containing pus

         b) Empyema is associated with infectious processes such as pneumonia, lung abscess, and tuberculosis

      4) Chylothorax

         a) Disruption of pulmonary lymph vessels caused by surgery or trauma can lead to abnormal accumulation of lymph fluid in pleural space

         b) Produces fat malabsorption from GI tract

   c. Assessment

NCLEX!

      1) Clinical manifestations

         a) Worsening dyspnea

         b) Diminished or absent breath sounds on affected side

         c) Dullness to percussion on affected side

         d) Chest wall pain

         e) Fever, persistent cough, night sweats, and weight loss with empyema

2) Diagnostic and laboratory test findings

    a) Visible on chest x-ray if greater than 250 mL fluid accumulates

    b) Diagnostic thoracentesis: differentiates source of pleural fluid

d. Therapeutic management

    1) Goal is to treat the underlying cause

    2) Thoracentesis for drainage of the pleural cavity

    3) Antibiotic therapy

    4) Surgical procedure may include decortication, or the separation of the pleural membranes

e. Priority nursing diagnoses: Ineffective breathing pattern; Pain; Risk for infection; Hyperthermia; Impaired gas exchange

f. Planning and implementation

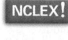

    1) Monitor respiratory and oxygenation status

    2) Physician performs thoracentesis; thoracostomy if indicated

    3) Treatment of the underlying cause

    4) Provide supplemental oxygen if indicated

    5) Provide adequate nutrition with focus on adequate protein intake

g. Medication therapy

    1) Analgesics

    2) Antipyretics

    3) Intravenous lipids, if chylothorax present

h. Client education

    1) Explain underlying cause of pleural effusion

    2) Teach client/family to monitor for changes in respiratory and oxygenation status

    3) Instruct about purpose of thoracentesis/thoracostomy

i. Expected outcomes/evaluation

    1) Resolution or reduction of accumulated pleural fluid

    2) Afebrile

    3) Control of chest wall pain

    4) Adequate protein intake

    5) Respiratory rate 12 to 24 breaths per minute

C. Pneumothorax/hemothorax

  1. Description

    a. Pneumothorax: air accumulation in the pleural space

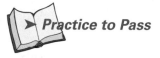

Practice to Pass

What nutritional alterations are necessary for the client with pleural effusion caused by chylothorax?

NCLEX!

1) Spontaneous: rupture of air-filled bleb allows pathway for air movement between respiratory system and pleural space; collapse of involved tissue may seal leak with minimal client symptoms; air leak may progress until pressure between thoracic cavity and atmosphere equalizes and client is symptomatic

   a) Primary: spontaneous rupture of bleb in otherwise healthy individual; occurs more often in tall, slender males aged 20 to 40

   b) Secondary: rupture of overly distended alveolus/alveoli; occurs in individuals with known COPD; severity of symptoms varies with size of pneumothorax

NCLEX!

2) Tension: disruption of the chest wall or lungs causes air accumulation in the pleural space; pressure on the mediastinum causes pressure on the other lung and interrupts venous return to the heart; is a medical emergency that requires emergency placement of chest tube to relieve increasing pressure in the thoracic cavity to restore adequate cardiac output

3) Traumatic: disruption of the pleura, bronchi, or lung tissue caused by blunt or penetrating trauma with air accumulation in the pleural space

4) Iatrogenic: disruption of the pleura, bronchi, or lung tissue during instrumentation for central venous line placement, lung biopsy, or thoracentesis produces unintentional air leak within the respiratory system; clinical manifestations and treatment are the same as for spontaneous pneumothorax

   b. Hemothorax: blood accumulation in the pleural space; clinical manifestations and treatment are the same as for pneumothorax

2. Etiology and pathophysiology

   a. Normal intrapleural pressure is negative compared to atmospheric air pressure

   b. Pressure difference between the thoracic cavity and the atmosphere is one of the stimuli for breathing

   c. Disruption of the pleura causes air accumulation within the pleural space

   d. Intrapleural pressure equalizes with atmospheric air, removing one of the stimuli for breathing

   e. The lung collapses as pressure increases in the thoracic cavity

   f. Excessive pressure is placed on the chest organs and great vessels

   g. Preload decreases and cardiac output is compromised

3. Assessment

NCLEX!

   a. Clinical manifestations

   1) Dyspnea

   2) Tracheal deviation toward the unaffected side

   3) Diminished breath sounds on affected side

   4) Percussion dullness on affected side

      5) Unequal chest expansion (reduced on affected side)

      6) Crepitus over the chest

   b. Diagnostic and laboratory test findings

      1) Chest x-ray reveals pneumothorax

      2) ABG shows decreased PO_2

4. Therapeutic management

NCLEX!

   a. In mild cases, no chest tube is required; if the pneumothorax is significant, a chest tube is inserted

   b. Placement of chest tube with water seal drainage

   c. Spontaneous pneumothorax: in otherwise healthy client may resolve without invasive treatment

   d. If spontaneous pneumothorax occurs repeatedly, may require pleurodesis, an instillation of an agent (such as tetracycline) in the pleural spaces to allow the pleura to adhere together; other procedures include partial pleurectomy, stapling, or laser pleurodesis for pleural sealing

5. Priority nursing diagnoses: Impaired gas exchange; Risk for injury; Ineffective breathing pattern; Decreased cardiac output; Risk for infection; Pain, Anxiety

6. Planning and implementation

   a. Care of the client with a chest tube: previously discussed in this chapter (see section IV C)

   b. Monitor respiratory and oxygenation status

   c. Provide supplemental oxygen as indicated

   d. Maintain infection control practices

7. Medication therapy: analgesics and antibiotics

NCLEX!

8. Client education

   a. Purpose of chest tube

   b. Activity limitations

   c. Pain management

9. Expected outcomes/evaluation

   a. Absence/resolution of dyspnea

   b. Afebrile

   c. Pulse oximetry or arterial blood gas results within normal range

   d. Control of pain

   e. Bilaterally clear and equal breath sounds

   f. Client is able to participate in activities of daily living

D. Atelectasis

1. Description

   a. Collapsed alveoli

   b. Common complication among postoperative or immobilized clients

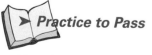

Practice to Pass

How does tension pneumothorax cause life-threatening cardiovascular collapse?

PIERCE COLLEGE LIBRARY

2. Etiology and pathophysiology

   a. Pulmonary secretions and/or exudates contribute to airway obstruction

   b. Airway obstruction increases intra-alveolar pressure causing alveolar collapse

   c. Surface area available for gas exchange is decreased

3. Assessment

   NCLEX!

   a. Clinical manifestations

      1) Low-grade fever

      2) Breath sounds diminished or absent in affected area

      3) Diminished rate and depth of respiration

      4) Physical inactivity caused by immobility or pain

   b. Diagnostic and laboratory test findings: chest x-ray reveals area of collapse

4. Therapeutic management

   NCLEX!

   a. The primary goal is the prevention of atelectasis

   b. Chest physical therapy and general pulmonary hygiene measures

   c. Intermittent positive pressure breathing treatments

   d. Supplemental oxygen as indicated

5. Priority nursing diagnoses: Ineffective airway clearance; Ineffective breathing pattern; Impaired gas exchange

6. Planning and implementation

   NCLEX!

   a. Monitor respiratory and oxygenation status

   b. Deep breathing and coughing exercises

   c. Incentive spirometry

   d. Frequent position change

   e. Ambulation as soon as feasible with client condition

   f. Maintain adequate hydration and nutrition

7. Medication therapy: analgesics and antipyretics

8. Client education

   a. Diaphragmatic and abdominal breathing techniques

   b. Nonpharmacologic pain control measures

9. Expected outcomes/evaluation

   a. Maintenance of airway

   b. Effective cough with clear, thin secretions

   c. Afebrile

   d. Absence/resolution of dyspnea

MERCE COLLEGE LIBRARY

    e. Respiratory rate 12 to 24 breaths per minute

    f. Pulse oximetry and/or arterial blood gas results return to normal range or client's baseline

    g. Bilaterally clear and equal breath sounds

    h. Client participates in activities of daily living

E. Pneumonia

  1. Description

    a. Acute inflammation of lung parenchyma (alveoli and respiratory bronchioles)

    b. Classified as viral versus bacterial, community-acquired versus hospital-acquired, atypical, or pneumocystis

  2. Etiology and pathophysiology

    a. Causative agent can be infectious (bacteria, viruses, fungi, and other microbes) or non-infectious (aspirated or inhaled substances)

    b. Most common organism for both community-acquired and hospital-acquired is the Gram-positive bacteria, *Streptococcus pneumoniae*

    c. Other common organisms associated with community-acquired pneumonia include *Klebsiella pneumoniae, Pseudomonas aeruginosa, Escherichia coli, haemophilus influenzae,* and other influenzae viruses

    d. Spread of microbes in alveoli activates the inflammatory and immune response

    e. Antigen-antibody response damages mucous membranes of bronchioles and alveoli resulting in edema

    f. Microbe cellular debris and exudate fill alveoli and can impair gas exchange

  3. Assessment

    a. Viral

      1) Fever: low-grade

      2) Cough: non-productive

      3) White blood cell count: normal to low elevation

      4) Chest x-ray: minimal changes evident

      5) Clinical course: less severe than pneumonia of bacterial origin

    b. Bacterial

      1) Fever: high

      2) Cough: productive

      3) White blood cell count: high elevation

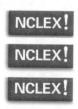

► Practice to Pass

What nursing measures are utilized to prevent atelectasis?

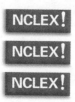

NCLEX**!**

NCLEX**!**

NCLEX**!**

NCLEX**!**

NCLEX**!**

NCLEX**!**

4) Chest x-ray: obvious infiltrates

5) Clinical course: more severe than pneumonia of viral origin

4. Therapeutic management

a. Antibiotic therapy, analgesics, antipyretics

d. Oxygen therapy to treat hypoxemia

5. Priority nursing diagnoses: Impaired gas exchange; Ineffective airway clearance; Ineffective breathing pattern; Imbalanced nutrition: less than body requirements; Activity intolerance; Anxiety; Pain; Hyperthermia

6. Planning and implementation

a. Maintain patent airway

b. Monitor respiratory and oxygenation status

c. Provide supplemental oxygen as indicated

d. Be prepared to initiate mechanical ventilatory support

e. Administer antimicrobials as prescribed

f. Provide pain management

g. Provide nutritional support and fluids via appropriate route

h. Provide adequate opportunities for physical rest

i. For all hospitalized clients, take measures to prevent pneumonia

1) Identify clients at high risk for pneumonia

2) Maintain appropriate infection control measures

3) Maintain adequate nutrition

4) Activate aspiration precautions

5) Encourage activity and mobility as soon as feasible

7. Medication therapy

a. Antibiotics as indicated

b. Other antimicrobials as indicated

c. Analgesics

d. Antipyretics

8. Client education

a. Immunization against influenza and pneumococcal pneumonia

b. Activity limitations and importance of rest

c. Effects and dosages of medications

d. Avoid pollutants and irritants such as smoke

e. Symptoms to report to health care provider (return of fever, worsening respiratory status)

> Practice to Pass

How do assessment findings differ among clients with viral versus bacterial origin of pneumonia?

9. Expected outcomes/evaluation

   a. Absence of respiratory distress

   b. Breath sounds clear to auscultation

   c. Effective coughing with expectoration of sputum if indicated

   d. Decreased or absent chest pain

   e. Resolution of fever

   f. Maintenance of normal body weight

   g. Client participates in care with decreased or no activity intolerance

F. **Pulmonary tuberculosis**

   1. Description

      a. Lung infection caused by *Mycobacterium tuberculosis*

      b. Any tissue can be infected, but tuberculosis is often found in the lung

   2. Etiology and pathophysiology

      a. *Mycobacterium tuberculosis* is an acid-fast, Gram-positive bacillus with transmission via airborne droplets

      b. Infection usually results from frequent close contact with an infected individual

      c. Inhaled bacilli inhabit the respiratory bronchioles and alveoli

      d. Bacilli travel through the lymph circulation and may spread throughout the body before cell-mediated immunity can contain its movement

      e. Eventual activation of cell-mediated immunity produces a granuloma lesion

      f. Liquified necrotic material from the Ghon tubercle portion of the granuloma lesion results in passage of infectious particles into the major airways where they can be exhaled into the air

   3. Assessment

      a. Clinical manifestations

         1) Frequent cough with copious frothy pink sputum; nonproductive cough develops first as an early symptom

         2) Night sweats

         3) Anorexia

         4) Weight loss

         5) History may indicate recent exposure to infected individual(s)

      b. Laboratory and diagnostic test findings

         1) Positive tuberculin skin test (indicated exposure)

         2) Appearance of characteristic Ghon tubercle on chest x-ray

         3) Positive acid-fast bacillus sputum cultures (provides definitive diagnosis of infection)

4. Therapeutic management: see medication therapy below

5. Priority nursing diagnoses: Ineffective breathing pattern; Ineffective health maintenance; Imbalanced nutrition: less than body requirements; Hyperthermia; Pain; Activity intolerance

6. Planning and implementation

   a. Monitor respiratory and oxygenation status

   b. Provide adequate nutrition and hydration

   NCLEX!

   c. Institute standard precautions (Center for Disease Control Tier 1) and airborne precautions (Tier 2, transmission-based precautions)

      1) Use a private room with negative air pressure that has 6 to 12 full air exchanges per hour and is vented to the outside or has its own air filtration system

      2) Wear specially fitted mask (N95 respirator) whenever entering client's room; fit-test the mask with each use

      3) Provide visitors with appropriate masks

      4) Wear gown and masks if client does not reliably cover mouth during coughing or sneezing to reduce risk of transmission to others

      5) Provide client with a surgical mask if it is necessary to bring client to another department; choose shortest and least busy route and alert that department ahead of time about client's status; schedule tests for less busy times of day

   d. Administer antimicrobial therapy as prescribed

   e. Provide supplemental oxygen as indicated

   f. Obtain periodic sputum cultures following onset of antimicrobial therapy

7. Medication therapy

   a. Antibiotic prophylaxis: for individuals exposed to clients with active disease

   NCLEX!

   b. Isoniazid (INH) drug of choice for 6 months if no clinical evidence of disease

   c. INH drug of choice for 12 months if abnormal chest x-ray or high-risk population such as with human immunodeficiency virus (HIV) or drug-induced immunosuppression

   d. Active disease: treatment options prescribed by Centers for Disease Control (CDC)

   NCLEX!

      1) Option 1: INH, rifampin (Rifadin), pyrazinamide (Tebrazid), and ethambutol (Myambutol) or streptomycin given daily or 2 to 3 times weekly (if therapy verified); if cultures report sensitivity to rifampin or isoniazid, ethambutol or streptomycin can be stopped; minimal 6 months drug therapy; drug therapy continues for at least 3 months after first negative sputum culture obtained

      2) Option 2: INH, rifampin, pyrazinamide, and ethambutol or streptomycin given daily for 2 weeks, then 2 times weekly for 6 weeks, then 2 times weekly isoniazid and rifampin for 16 weeks

3) Option 3: INH, rifampin, pyrazinamide, and ethambutol or strepto-mycin 3 times weekly for 6 months

4) Option 4: active TB with HIV; option 1, 2, or 3 for minimum of 9 months and to continue for at least 6 months after first negative sputum culture

8. Client education

a. Infection control measures, including handwashing, coughing into tissues and disposing of them in a closed bag

b. No special precautions need to be taken with clothing, books, personal objects or eating utensils because inanimate objects do not easily spread the bacteria

c. Teach client/family/close contacts about mechanisms of transmission and antimicrobial therapy, including the need to take medication for the full course of therapy to prevent recurrence and/or development of drug-resistant organisms

d. Teach client about adverse effects of medications, including but not limited to the following:

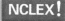

1) INH: hepatotoxicity that requires assessment of onset of jaundice, periodic monitoring of liver function tests, peripheral neuritis (numbness and tingling) that can be minimized with intake of vitamin B_6, hematologic effects (anemia, agranulocytosis, bleeding), or hypersensitivity

2) Rifampin: relatively low toxicity, but monitor CBC, liver function tests, and renal status; medication causes orange discoloration of body fluids

3) Pyrazinamide: primarily causes hepatotoxicity and elevates uric acid levels; periodic monitoring of blood levels is indicated and assessment of jaundice and symptoms of gout (joint pain)

4) Ethambutol: causes optic neuritis; obtain baseline vision screening and periodic eye exams (changes can include loss of visual acuity and red/green color discrimination)

5) Streptomycin: primarily causes ototoxicity and nephrotoxicity (similar to other aminoglycoside antibiotics); monitor hearing ability and renal function; maintain fluid intake of 2.5 to 3 liters of fluid per day

e. Maintain good nutrition and provide adequate rest periods for healing and to minimize fatigue

9. Expected outcomes/evaluation

a. Adherence to prescribed medication therapy

b. Resolution of productive cough

c. Afebrile

d. Respiratory rate 12 to 24 breaths per minute

e. Pulse oximetry or arterial blood gases within normal range or client's baseline

f. Maintenance of appropriate body weight

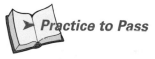

Practice to Pass

What therapies are used as tuberculosis prophylaxis for individuals who have been exposed to an individual with active disease?

      g. Resolution of active infectious phase

      h. Prevention of spread to contacts

G. Pulmonary embolism

  1. Description

      a. Emboli lodge in pulmonary vasculature and obstruct adequate blood flow through pulmonary capillaries

      b. **Ventilation-perfusion mismatch**: a clinically significant imbalance between volume of air and volume of blood circulating to the gas exchange area of the lungs; causes impaired gas exchange

      c. Pulmonary embolism is a frequent complication of hospitalized clients

  2. Etiology and pathophysiology

      a. Most common sites for origin of emboli include venous thromboses in the deep veins of lower extremities, pelvis, or right side of the heart

      b. Risk factors for pulmonary embolism include immobility, hypercoagulability, trauma to endothelial layer of blood vessels, and long bone fractures

      c. Dislodgment of venous thromboses occurs with movement into pulmonary vasculature; fat emboli travel from site of long bone fractures and traumatized vessels

      d. Emboli obstruct small to large areas of the pulmonary vasculature, preventing adequate perfusion and gas exchange

      e. A massive area of obstructed tissue leads to pulmonary infarction

      f. Severe impairment of gas exchange can be rapidly fatal

  3. Assessment

      a. Clinical manifestations

        1) Restlessness, anxiety, agitation

        2) Vital signs: tachycardia, tachypnea, hypotension, fever

        3) Chest pain

        4) Hemoptysis

        5) Mental status changes

        6) Decreasing level of consciousness

        7) Cyanosis

        8) Recent history of thromboembolism and/or long bone fractures

        9) Lung crackles upon auscultation

      b. Diagnostic and laboratory test findings

        1) Atrial fibrillation

        2) Chest x-ray may be normal

        3) Pulmonary angiogram reveals pulmonary embolism

NCLEX!

      4) Ventilation-perfusion scan indicates areas of mismatch

      5) Abnormal arterial blood gases

  4. Therapeutic management

    a. Oxygen therapy

    b. Anticoagulant therapy

    c. Embolectomy

    d. Thrombolytic therapy

    e. To prevent future pulmonary emboli, an intracaval filter may be inserted into the inferior vena cava to trap emboli from a known source

  5. Priority nursing diagnoses: Ineffective breathing pattern; Impaired gas exchange; Anxiety; Pain; Impaired physical mobility

  6. Planning and implementation

    a. Maintain patent airway

    b. Supplemental oxygen

    c. Be prepared to initiate mechanical ventilation

    d. Maintain IV access

    e. Circulatory support as indicated

    f. Placement of vena cava filter

    g. Pain management

    h. Pulmonary embolectomy

  7. Medication therapy

    a. Thrombolytic therapy

    b. Anticoagulant therapy

    c. Opioid analgesics

    d. Anti-anxiety agents

  8. Client education

    a. Prevention of thromboembolism

    b. Avoid immobility as much as feasible

    c. Teach signs/symptoms of venous occlusion

    d. Instruct client/family regarding anticoagulant therapy as indicated

  9. Expected outcomes/evaluation

    a. Respiratory rate 12 to 24 breaths per minute

    b. Pulse oximetry, arterial blood gas results within normal range or client's baseline

    c. Alert and oriented mental status

    d. Absence/resolution of chest pain

► *Practice to Pass*

What nursing measures are indicated for prevention of pulmonary emboli?

NCLEX!

NCLEX!

e. Absence/resolution of anxiety

f. Prevention of further thromboembolic phenomena

H. Bronchogenic carcinoma

1. Description

   a. Lung cancer is the leading cause of death resulting from malignancy

   b. Five-year survival rate is less than 15 percent

   c. Greater than 90 percent of lung cancers originate in the bronchus epithelium

2. Etiology and pathophysiology

   a. Cigarette smoking is the leading cause; cancer risk increases with length of smoking exposure

   b. Contributing factors include inhaled environmental substances such as air pollution, arsenic, asbestos, iron, radon, and aromatic hydrocarbons

   c. Some individuals have a genetic predisposition to bronchogenic carcinoma

   d. Tumor growth commonly begins in bronchus then migrates to upper lobes of the lungs

   e. Nonspecific inflammatory cellular changes lead to excessive mucus production, desquamation, metaplasia of epithelium, and slow-growing bronchogenic carcinoma

   f. Tumor types include small cell and non-small cell

   g. Metastasis occurs by direct contact and transport in the blood and lymph

3. Assessment

   a. Clinical manifestations

      1) Symptom onset is often late in course of disease

      2) Persistent cough with or without hemoptysis

      3) Localized chest pain

      4) Dyspnea

      5) Unilateral wheeze upon auscultation

      6) Swallowing difficulty

      7) Anorexia

      8) Weight loss

      9) Enlarged neck lymph nodes

   b. Diagnostic and laboratory test findings

      1) Mass visible on chest x-ray

      2) CT scan or MRI of chest may better differentiate mass

      3) Sputum for cytology reveals tumor cells

      4) Bronchoscopy for direct biopsy or washings for cytology reveal tumor cells

NCLEX!

4. Therapeutic management

   a. Surgical resection

      1) Pneumonectomy: removal of an entire lung

      2) Lobectomy: removal of a lobe of the lung

      3) Segmentectomy (segmental resection): removal of a segment or segments of a lung

      4) Wedge resection: dissection and removal of a defined area in the lung

   b. Chemotherapy: see chapter 12 for overview

   c. Radiation therapy: see chapter 12 for overview

   d. Laser therapy

   e. Immunotherapy

5. Priority nursing diagnoses: Anticipatory grieving; Anxiety; Pain; Knowledge deficit; Ineffective airway clearance; Ineffective breathing pattern; Impaired gas exchange; Powerlessness; Hopelessness

6. Planning and implementation

   a. Provide psychological support for client/family

   b. Provide preoperative and postoperative care for the client having surgery

   c. Administer oxygen therapy as prescribed

   d. Assist the client with pain management

   e. Position to optimize oxygenation

   f. Provide care of chest tubes as previously discussed

7. Medication therapy

   a. Opioid analgesics

   b. Chemotherapy

   c. Immunotherapy

   d. Antiemetics

8. Client education

   a. Treatment plan

   b. Assistance with coping skills

   c. Pain management

9. Expected outcomes/evaluation

   a. Pain control

   b. Effective airway clearance

   c. Effective breathing pattern

   d. Coping skills, realistic personal goals

I. Cancer of the larynx

1. Description

    a. Most laryngeal tumors are benign

    b. Most common form of malignant laryngeal cancer is squamous cell carcinoma

2. Etiology and pathophysiology

    a. Primary etiologies for laryngeal cancer include long-term cigarette smoking and alcohol ingestion

    b. Contributing factors include chronic laryngeal irritation caused by singing, air pollution, and environmental hazards

    c. Tumor growth occurs in glottis, supraglottis, and subglottis; symptoms are specific to site of tumor

    d. Chronic laryngeal irritation leads to precancerous lesions, leukoplakia and erythroplakia

    e. Carcinoma may develop at site of precancerous lesions

    f. Most common site for laryngeal metastasis is the lungs; larynx is however a rare site for metastasis

3. Assessment

    a. Clinical manifestations

        1) Hoarseness

        2) Palpable jugular nodes

        3) Change in voice characteristics

        4) Pain when swallowing

        5) Unexplained earache

    b. Diagnostic and laboratory test findings

        1) Biopsy finding

        2) X-ray visualization

        3) MRI, CT findings

        4) Barium swallow visualization

4. Therapeutic management

    a. The choice of treatment depends on the stage of the disease and the general condition of the client

    b. Radiation therapy or brachytherapy; brachytherapy is the placement of a radioactive source next to the tumor site

    c. Chemotherapy

    d. Laryngectomy

    e. Radical neck dissection

5. Priority nursing diagnoses: Impaired verbal communication; Ineffective airway clearance; Impaired swallowing; Pain; Anxiety; Deficient knowledge; Imbalanced nutrition: less than body requirements

6. Planning and implementation

a. Biopsy of laryngeal lesions and other diagnostic tests, such as CT scan, MRI of head and neck, chest x-ray

NCLEX!

b. Maintain patent airway (tracheostomy performed with laryngectomy)

c. Pain management

d. Provide adequate hydration and nutrition (temporary or permanent altered route for nutrition)

NCLEX!

e. Provide alternate means for communication as previously discussed and plan for permanent means of communication (artificial larynx or esophageal speech)

f. Monitor respiratory and oxygenation status

g. Provide oxygen supplementation as indicated

7. Medication therapy: opioid analgesics and antipyretics

8. Client education

a. Smoking cessation

b. Changes in body image

c. Care of tracheostomy

d. Use of artificial larynx

e. Supraglottic swallowing for voice production (esophageal speech)

f. Nutritional access device if indicated

g. Pain management

h. Signs of tumor spread

9. Expected outcomes/evaluation

a. Absence of cancer spread

b. Effective communication

c. Appropriate body weight maintained

d. Absence/resolution of pain

e. Demonstration of self-care

f. Psychological adjustment to permanent loss of natural means of communication

J. Thoracic trauma

1. Description: alteration of breathing mechanics and/or gas exchange caused by respiratory system trauma

a. Blunt trauma: injury to chest wall without disruption of pleura

1) Rib fractures

2) Flail chest

3) Soft tissue rupture: diaphragm, trachea, bronchi, and major blood vessels

4) Tension pneumothorax

5) Contusion: lungs, heart

b. Penetrating trauma: injury involves disruption of pleura

1) Internal wounds communicate with external atmosphere

2) Open air-sucking wounds

3) Pneumothorax/hemothorax

4) Tissue wounds: heart, lungs, major blood vessels

2. Etiology and pathophysiology

a. Blunt trauma: mechanism of injury commonly involves motor vehicle collisions, falls, and assaults

b. Penetrating trauma: mechanism of injury commonly involves firearms, motor vehicle collisions, falls, or assaults

c. Pathophysiology varies related to the specific injury: rib fracture is most common type of chest trauma

1) Flail chest

a) Multiple rib fractures in 2 places (separated from bony skeleton)

b) Chest wall unstable with paradoxical chest expansion (flail segment moves inward with inhalation and outward with exhalation)

c) Ventilation-perfusion mismatch

d) Possible underlying lung injury

2) Rupture of diaphragm

a) Abdominal contents dislocate upward into thoracic cavity

b) Decrease in diaphragmatic control of breathing

3. Assessment

NCLEX!

a. Clinical manifestations

1) Chest pain, may be severe such as with flail chest

2) Shallow breathing with splinting

3) Possible unequal chest expansion

4) Tachycardia, tachypnea, hypotension

5) Crepitus over the chest

b. Diagnostic and laboratory test findings

1) Chest x-ray findings show white opacifications

2) ABGs reveal hypoxemia

4. Therapeutic management: same as pneumothorax and hemothorax (see section IV C, 4)

5. Priority nursing diagnoses: Pain; Ineffective breathing pattern; Ineffective airway clearance; Impaired gas exchange; Decreased cardiac output; Anxiety

6. Planning and implementation

NCLEX!

   a. Ventilation support

   b. Be prepared to initiate mechanical ventilation

   c. Maintain IV access

   d. Placement of chest tube with water seal drainage may be indicated

NCLEX!

   e. Provide pain management

7. Medication therapy: opioid analgesics, epidural analgesia may be appropriate

8. Client education

NCLEX!

   a. Techniques for pulmonary hygiene

   b. Pain management: patient-controlled analgesia may be appropriate

   c. Prevention of thromboembolic phenomena

   d. Measures to decrease anxiety

9. Expected outcomes/evaluation

   a. Adequate ventilation and perfusion

   b. Control/relief of pain

   c. Pulse oximetry, arterial blood gas results within normal range

   d. Respiratory rate 12 to 24 breaths per minute with normal depth

---

Case Study

A 62-year-old female client with a history of COPD is admitted to the hospital with an acute exacerbation and left-sided pneumonia. The nurse observes increased anterior-posterior diameter of the chest, reddish-blue skin tone, and prolonged expiratory phase when breathing. Admission vital signs: temperature 101.5°F (oral), blood pressure 154/92, heart rate 110, and respiratory rate 26 breaths/minute.

❶ What nursing diagnosis is the priority for this client?

❷ During the initial physical assessment of the client, the client exhibits a frequent cough with copious purulent secretions expectorated. This assessment finding is compatible with which etiology of pneumonia?

❸ What should the nutritional plan for this client include?

❹ To optimize oxygenation for this client with left-side pneumonia, what body position should be encouraged?

❺ The client says that she is beginning to feel slightly "short of breath." What is the appropriate choice in initiating supplemental oxygen in this client?

For suggested responses, see page 735.

Posttest

1   A client comes to the clinic with an acute asthma episode. Which breath sound characteristic does the nurse expect to find upon auscultation?

(1) Bilateral crackles
(2) Wheezing
(3) Diminished breath sounds in the upper lobes
(4) Rhonchi

2   Which of the following blood gas reports would the nurse expect in a client with progressive chronic obstructive pulmonary disease (COPD)?

(1) pH 7.55, $PaCO_2$ 30 mmHg, PaO_2 80 mmHg, HCO_3^- 24 mEq/L
(2) pH 7.40, $PaCO_2$ 40 mmHg, PaO_2 94 mmHg, HCO_3^- 22 mEq/L
(3) pH 7. 38, $PaCO_2$ 45 mmHg, PaO_2 88 mmHg, HCO_3^- 26 mEq/L
(4) pH 7.30, $PaCO_2$ 60 mmHg, PaO_2 70 mmHg, HCO_3^- 30 mEq/L

3   What is the priority item in discharge teaching for the client with chronic bronchitis?

(1) Fluid restriction
(2) Smoking cessation
(3) Avoidance of crowds
(4) Side effects of drug therapy

4   A client has returned to the clinic 72 hours following a tuberculin skin test with an induration of about 5 to 6 mm at the administration site. The client is visibly upset and states: "I can't believe I have TB!" Which statement by the nurse is appropriate?

(1) "You'll need to put on a mask and wear it whenever you are around other people."
(2) "The doctor will prescribe Isoniazid for you to take for the next 3 months."
(3) "This finding does not confirm TB; it may indicate a recent exposure to tuberculosis."
(4) "We'll need to do a chest x-ray. This may be falsely positive because of your history of diabetes."

5   What instruction is most important for the nurse to provide during discharge teaching of a client who underwent a laryngectomy?

(1) Operation of feeding pump
(2) Use of Passy Muir (speaking tracheostomy) valve
(3) Tracheostomy care
(4) Wound care

6   A postoperative client has a sudden onset of shortness of breath. What initial action by the nurse is indicated?

(1) Notify the physician
(2) Assess oxygen saturation using pulse oximetry
(3) Assist the client to a high Fowler's position
(4) Auscultate the heart and lungs

7   A client has a right chest tube following a thoracotomy. When assisting the client to ambulate what measure is appropriate to maintain the water seal?

(1) Keep the collection device below the level of the chest.
(2) Clamp the chest tube before assisting the client out of bed.
(3) Milk the chest tube when the client returns to bed to assess patency.
(4) Connect the collection device to a portable suction machine.

8   A client is brought to the Emergency Department following a motor vehicle collision with a tree. Which finding is suggestive of a tension pneumothorax?

(1) Tachypnea
(2) Hypotension
(3) Tracheal deviation
(4) Unilateral wheezing

9 What is the priority nursing diagnosis for the finding of secondary polycythemia in a client with chronic obstructive pulmonary disease?

(1) Risk for injury related to venous thrombi
(2) Risk for injury related to use of oxygen
(3) Impaired tissue perfusion related to chronic hypoxemia
(4) Impaired gas exchange related to factors other than hypoxia

10 When auscultating breath sounds in the client with an acute asthma episode, the nurse uses which of the following to guide interpretation of severity of findings?

(1) Severity of airway obstruction is associated with intensity of wheezing.
(2) Wheezing may be absent with severe airway obstruction.
(3) Unilateral wheezing indicates an origin for respiratory distress other than asthma.
(4) Breath sounds are prolonged on expiration.

See pages 94–95 for Answers and Rationales.

Answers and Rationales

Pretest

1 **Answer: 2** *Rationale:* An intact gag reflex indicates that topical sedation has lost its effect and the client is able to swallow, a major safety consideration prior to discharging the client from the healthcare facility. The ability to swallow would precede consumption of oral intake. Knowing symptoms to report to the physician following discharge is important, but the physiological condition takes priority in this case. The client's ability to verbalize discharge instructions prior to discharge is not a good predictor of post-discharge memory; therefore it is essential that written instructions be sent home with the client. Fever, if present, may take hours to days to resolve; the client may have been febrile at the onset of the procedure.
Cognitive Level: Analysis
Nursing Process: Evaluation; *Test Plan:* SECE

2 **Answer: 3** *Rationale:* The medulla and pons are the areas of brain tissue that control breathing. Injury to these tissues would produce alterations in the client's breathing rate and pattern. The other options are incorrect areas of the brain.
Cognitive Level: Application
Nursing Process: Analysis; *Test Plan:* PHYS

3 **Answer: 4** *Rationale:* With unilateral lung disease, the example to remember is "good lung down." Since ventilation and perfusion are gravity dependent, enhancing ventilation and perfusion to healthy lung

tissue and alveoli will enhance oxygenation. Perfusion refers to the circulation of blood into the tissues and cells. Supine positioning would provide near equal ventilation and perfusion to both lungs. In the diseased lung, excess fluid and fibrosis inhibit gas exchange at the pulmonary capillary membrane, thereby diminishing oxygenation.
Cognitive Level: Application
Nursing Process: Implementation; *Test Plan:* PHYS

4 **Answer: 2** *Rationale:* Increased anterior-posterior diameter of the chest, pursed-lip breathing, and circumoral cyanosis are chronic findings in clients with emphysema. They do not indicate acute changes in the client's condition. Bilateral crackles throughout the lung fields indicate excessive pulmonary fluid requiring acute intervention. The etiology of the fluid excess in the lungs needs to be explored in-depth.
Cognitive Level: Analysis
Nursing Process: Assessment; *Test Plan:* SECE

5 **Answer: 2** *Rationale:* Carbon dioxide level is one of the primary stimuli for breathing in clients with chronic obstructive lung disease, who adjust to higher than normal carbon dioxide levels. Abrupt elevation of the level will depress the stimulus oxygen for breathing and can even produce respiratory arrest. Administering 100 percent oxygen to the client with COPD who is not receiving mechanical ventilation is highly likely to lead to depressed breathing and respi-

ratory arrest. The spouse's presence may be providing comfort and support for the client. Psychological distress caused by her absence may worsen the dyspnea. Pain medication may depress breathing.
Cognitive Level: Analysis
Nursing Process: Implementation; *Test Plan:* PHYS

6 **Answer: 3** *Rationale:* Productive cough is compatible with bacterial pneumonia and differentiates it from viral pneumonia. Excessive sputum is produced as pulmonary bacteria die. White blood cell count is elevated in bacterial pneumonia compared to viral pneumonia. Chest x-ray findings with bacterial pneumonia usually show consolidation whereas the chest x-ray is often normal with viral pneumonia.
Cognitive Level: Application
Nursing Process: Assessment; *Test Plan:* PHYS

7 **Answer: 1** *Rationale:* Many foreign particles inhaled from the environment are non-biodegradable and cause chronic inflammation of lung tissue. The chronic inflammation leads to progressive scarring and fibrosis of lung tissue, thereby impairing the gas diffusion capabilities of the lungs. Antigen-antibody reactions are related to exposure to protein substances.
Cognitive Level: Compehension
Nursing Process: Implementation; *Test Plan:* PHYS

8 **Answer: 2** *Rationale:* Mycobacterium tuberculosis is transmitted via airborne droplets so use of a properly fitted particulate filter mask is indicated to prevent its spread. The other options do not represent methods of preventing airborne transmission.
Cognitive Level: Application
Nursing Process: Planning; *Test Plan:* SECE

9 **Answer: 4** *Rationale:* Emphysema is a chronic disease with progressive destruction of alveoli and loss of alveolar area available for gas exchange. Paralysis of respiratory muscles, airway obstructions, and pleural effusion would diminish ventilatory capacity that could ultimately lead to decreased oxygen supply.
Cognitive Level: Application
Nursing Process: Implementation; *Test Plan:* PHYS

10 **Answer: 3** *Rationale:* Clients with rib fractures should be assessed periodically for the possible complication of pneumothorax. Decreased or absent breath sounds are related to pneumothorax because pneumothorax compresses functional lung tissue. Pink, frothy sputum is a possible (but unlikely) finding in clients with pneumothorax. Hoarseness is in-

dicative of an airway obstruction or laryngeal nerve paralysis. Percussion sounds are hyperresonant in the area of a pneumothorax caused by the collection of air in the pleural space.
Cognitive Level: Application
Nursing Process: Assessment; *Test Plan:* PHYS

Posttest

1 **Answer: 2** *Rationale:* Expiratory wheezing is a characteristic finding in acute asthma due to airway constriction. Crackles are indicative of excess pulmonary fluid, which is not a typical finding with acute asthma. Rhonchi are related to mucus obstruction of large airways and are a common finding in chronic obstructive pulmonary disease processes.
Cognitive Level: Application
Nursing Process: Assessment; *Test Plan:* PHYS

2 **Answer: 4** *Rationale:* During the later stages of COPD, arterial blood gas findings indicate low pH, elevated pCO_2, low pO_2, and elevated HCO_3^-, which indicate the body's attempt to compensate for chronically low pH. Option 1 is indicative of respiratory alkalosis; options 2 and 3 are variations of normal ABG results.
Cognitive Level: Analysis
Nursing Process: Assessment; *Test Plan:* PHYS

3 **Answer: 2** *Rationale:* Cigarette smoking is the primary etiology of chronic bronchitis so cessation is the priority for the client. Teaching the client about potential side effects of any prescribed medications should be included in all discharge teaching. Avoidance of crowds to lower the risk of pulmonary infections is a recommendation that is more individualized and less common than the need for smoking cessation. Fluids are often increased.
Cognitive Level: Analysis
Nursing Process: Planning; *Test Plan:* HPM

4 **Answer: 3** *Rationale:* An induration of 5 to 9 mm resulting from a tuberculin skin test is indicative of close contact with an individual infected with mycobacterium tuberculosis. The client with this finding will be prescribed isoniazid for 6 to 12 months as prophylaxis against development of active TB. History of diabetes is not related to false positive tuberculin skin test. The nurse should demonstrate a calm, supportive, and informing manner with this client.
Cognitive Level: Application
Nursing Process: Implementation; *Test Plan:* PSYC

5 Answer: 3 *Rationale:* For any client with a tracheostomy, maintenance of the airway is clearly the priority. Clients are taught to perform routine tracheostomy care to prevent airway obstruction. Only those clients discharged with a feeding tube will need instruction about operation of a feeding pump. Wound care and use of a Passy Muir valve for communication are important factors to include in discharge teaching, but the airway is the clear priority.
Cognitive Level: Analysis
Nursing Process: Planning; *Test Plan:* SECE

6 Answer: 3 *Rationale:* With sudden onset of shortness of breath, the priority is for the nurse to maintain airway patency and gas exchange. Positioning the client supine with a high degree of head elevation will assist with airway maintenance and ventilation. The nurse should then rapidly assess the client's heart and lung status before notifying the physician.
Cognitive Level: Analysis
Nursing Process: Implementation; *Test Plan:* SECE

7 Answer: 1 *Rationale:* Gravity helps maintain the water seal thereby preventing backflow of air and fluid into the chest. The chest tube should never be clamped as this may cause pneumothorax. The chest tube should not be milked unless ordered by the physician for clients with visible clots in the chest drainage tubing. Milking the chest tube creates suction within the tubing and can cause pleural tissue damage.
Cognitive Level: Application
Nursing Process: Implementation; *Test Plan:* SECE

8 Answer: 3 *Rationale:* Tension pneumothorax is a life-threatening condition so the nurse must recognize potential indicators. Deviation of the trachea toward the unaffected side occurs due to increased pressure within the pleural cavity. Increasing pressure on the great vessels in the chest causes decreased cardiac output, which can be fatal. Hypotension and tachypnea occur with pneumothorax but are also related to numerous other conditions. Unilateral wheezing is indicative of narrowing of the airways.
Cognitive Level: Application
Nursing Process: Assessment; *Test Plan:* SECE

9 Answer: 3 *Rationale:* Secondary polycythemia, or increased red blood cell count, develops as chronic obstructive pulmonary disease occurs, in response to chronic hypoxemia. Of the possible options, impaired tissue perfusion related to chronic hypoxemia is the only factor related to development of secondary polycythemia. Risk for injury in these clients related to venous thrombi or use of oxygen may or may not be present. Impaired gas exchange may also be a factor; however, it is related to hypoxia.
Cognitive Level: Analysis
Nursing Process: Analysis; *Test Plan:* PHYS

10 Answer: 2 *Rationale:* Wheezing is a common finding during an acute asthma episode, however; the wheezing is not a consistent predictor of the severity of the attack. Airway obstruction may be so severe that the client is moving little or no air and is experiencing severe respiratory distress. Breath sounds are prolonged in expiration with asthma, but this factor does not alter the plan of care in any way.
Cognitive Level: Application
Nursing Process: Analysis; *Test Plan:* PHYS

References

Anonymous. (2002). Understanding pneumothorax. *Nursing 32*(11), 74, 76.

Brashers, V. L. (2000). Alterations of pulmonary function. In S. E. Huether & K. L. McCance (Eds.), *Understanding pathophysiology.* St. Louis, MO: Mosby, pp. 740–774.

Brashers, V. L. & Huether, S. E. (2000). Structure and function of the pulmonary system. In S. E. Huether & K. L. McCance (Eds.), *Understanding pathophysiology.* St. Louis, MO: Mosby, pp. 718–739.

Corbett, J. V. (2000). *Laboratory tests and diagnostic procedures with nursing diagnoses.* Upper Saddle River, NJ: Prentice Hall Health.

Corwin, E. J. (2000). *Handbook of pathophysiology* (2nd ed.). Philadelphia: Lippincott.

Harkness, G. A. & Dincher, J. R. (1999). Respiratory problems. In G. Harkness (Ed.), *Medical-surgical nursing: Total patient care.* St. Louis, MO: Mosby, pp. 557–624.

Hickey, M. M. & Hoffman, L. A. (2000). Upper respiratory problems. In S. M. Lewis, M. M. Heitkemper, & S. R. Dirksen (Eds.), *Medical-surgical nursing: Assessment and management of clinical problems.* St. Louis, MO: Mosby, pp. 579–610.

Lemone, P. & Burke, K. M. (2000). *Medical-surgical nursing: Critical thinking in client care* (2nd ed). Upper Saddle

River, NJ: Prentice Hall, Inc., pp. 1326–1340, 1341–1389, 1390–1507.

Lewis, S. M. (2000). Lower respiratory problems. In S. M. Lewis, M. M. Heitkemper, & S. R. Dirksen (Eds.), *Medical-surgical nursing: Assessment and management of clinical problems* (5th ed.). St. Louis, MO: Mosby, pp. 611–659.

Lindell, K. O. & Va Sciver, T. (2000). Obstructive pulmonary diseases. In S. M. Lewis, M. M. Heitkemper, & S. R. Dirksen (Eds.), *Medical-surgical nursing: Assessment and management of clinical problems* (5th ed.). St. Louis, MO: Mosby, pp. 660–715.

Mackin, L. & Bullock, B. L. (2000). Altered pulmonary function. In B. A. Bullock & R. L. Henze (Eds.). *Focus on pathophysiology.* Philadelphia: Lippincott, Williams & Wilkins, pp.549–586.

Mackin, L. & Bullock, B. L. (2000). Pulmonary function. In B. A. Bullock & R. L. Henze (Eds.). *Focus on pathophysiology.* Philadelphia: Lippincott, Williams & Wilkins, pp. 527–548.

Mehta, M. (2003). Assessing respiratory status. *Nursing 33*(2), 54–56.

Porth, C. M. (2000). *Pathophysiology: Concepts of altered health states:* Philadephia: Lippincott, pp. 473–500, 501–528, 529–564, 625–642.

Reinke, L. F. & Hoffman, L. A. (2000). Respiratory system. In S. M. Lewis, M. M. Heitkemper, & S. R. Dirksen (Eds.), *Medical-surgical nursing: Assessment and management of clinical problems* (5th ed.). St. Louis, MO: Mosby, pp. 553–578.

Schumann, L. (2000). Obstructive pulmonary disorders. In L. C. Copstead & J. L. Banasik (Eds.), *Pathophysiology: Biological and behavioral perspectives* (2nd ed.). Philadelphia: W. B. Saunders, pp. 534–560.

Schumann, L. (2000). Respiratory function and alterations in gas exchange. In L. C. Copstead & J. L. Banasik (Eds.). *Pathophysiology: Biological and behavioral perspectives* (2nd ed.). Philadelphia: W. B. Saunders, pp. 504–532.

Schumann, L. (2000). Restrictive pulmonary disorders. In L. C. Copstead & J. L. Banasik (Eds.). *Pathophysiology: Biological and behavioral perspectives* (2nd ed.). Philadelphia: W. B. Saunders, pp. 562–586.

Wagner, K. D. (2001). Arterial blood gas analysis. In P. S. Kidd & K. D. Wagner (Eds.), *High acuity nursing.* Upper Saddle River, NJ: Prentice Hall, pp. 143–164.

Wagner, K. D. (2001). Respiratory process. In P. S. Kidd & K. D. Wagner (Eds.), *High acuity nursing.* Upper Saddle River, NJ: Prentice Hall, pp. 107–142.

CHAPTER 3

Cardiac Disorders

Joan Roche, APRN, MS, CCRN

CHAPTER OUTLINE

OBJECTIVES

▌ Identify basic structures and function of the heart.

▌ Describe the pathophysiology and etiology of common cardiac disorders.

▌ Describe expected assessment data and diagnostic test findings for selected cardiac disorders.

▌ Identify priority nursing diagnoses for selected cardiac disorders.

▌ Discuss therapeutic management of selected cardiac disorders.

▌ Discuss nursing management of a client experiencing a cardiac disorder.

▌ Identify expected outcomes for the client experiencing a cardiac disorder.

[*Media Link*]

Use the CD-ROM enclosed with this text, or log onto the address given to access the free, interactive Companion Website created for this series. The CD-ROM and Companion Website accompanying this book offer additional practice opportunities and information—NCLEX Review, Case Studies, Glossary, In Depth with NCLEX, and more.

www.prenhall.com/hogan

Review at a Glance with definitions

afterload *resistance that the ventricles must overcome to eject blood into the systemic circulation; directly related to arterial blood pressure*

angina pectoris *chest pain resulting from restricted blood flow to the myocardium*

cardiac cycle *one complete heartbeat; includes two phases: systole (ventricular contraction) and diastole (relaxation and ventricular refilling)*

cardiac output (CO) *volume of blood in liters ejected by the heart each minute; indicator of pump function of the heart; normal adult CO is 4 to 8 L/min; CO = HR × SV*

contractility *strength of contraction regardless of preload; decreased by hypoxia and some drugs (beta blockers and calcium channel blockers); increased by drugs (digoxin and dopamine)*

coronary artery disease (CAD) *refers to the build up of atherosclerotic plaque in the coronary arteries that restricts the blood flow to heart muscle*

cor pulmonale *right-sided failure and enlarged right atrium caused by chronic pulmonary hypertension*

ejection fraction (EF) *portion of the blood ejected during systole, compared with the total ventricular filling volume, normal EF is 55 to 65 percent*

ischemia *decreased supply of oxygenated blood to heart muscle*

infarction *myocardial tissue injury from lack of oxygenation*

jugular venous distention (JVD) *increased pressure in the jugular veins, visible more than a few millimeters above the clavicle with the client supine at a 45-degree angle*

preload *degree of myocardial fiber stretch at the end of ventricular diastole;*

influenced by ventricular filling volume and myocardial compliance

pulmonary edema *significant fluid overload in the lungs with acute exacerbation of left heart failure*

regurgitation *improper or incomplete closure of heart valves, resulting in back flow of blood*

stenosis *condition in which heart valve leaflets are fused together, have a narrow opening, or are stiff, unable to open or close properly*

stroke volume (SV) *volume of blood ejected from the left ventricle each cardiac cycle*

tamponade *life-threatening medical emergency resulting from excess fluid collection in the pericardial sac; interferes with heart filling and severely decreases cardiac output; if left untreated will lead to cardiac arrest and possible death*

Pretest

1. The nurse is monitoring a client who has recently undergone pericardiocentesis. The nurse suspects cardiac tamponade after observing which of the following?

(1) A rapid increase in blood pressure and flushing
(2) Jugular vein distention (JVD) and narrowing pulse pressure
(3) Bradycardia and bilateral crackles
(4) Louder and harsher heart sounds

2. A 54-year-old male client was recently diagnosed with subacute bacterial endocarditis (SBE). The nurse determines that the client understands the discharge teaching when he does which of the following?

(1) Asks for a referral to a dietician for a low-sodium diet
(2) Explains to his wife why he needs antibiotics before seeing the dentist
(3) Asks when he can start to take his antibiotics in pill form
(4) Explains his plans to quit smoking

3. The nurse on a cardiac unit is caring for a client admitted with an acute exacerbation of heart failure. The nurse concludes that the client is developing pulmonary edema after observing which change in the client?

(1) Bradycardia
(2) Increased urination
(3) Cough with pink frothy sputum
(4) Increased sleepiness

4. A client is scheduled for a cardiac angiography. In reviewing the client's record what significant finding needs to be reported to the physician before the exam?

(1) The client reported an allergy to shrimp.
(2) The client 's ECG shows atrial fibrillation.
(3) The potassium level is 5.0 mEq/L.
(4) The client has a history of chronic renal failure.

5 The nurse is developing a plan for a client who is going home with a new diagnosis of heart failure. The nurse is teaching the client to monitor fluid status. The best instruction is to teach the client to do which of the following?

(1) Restrict fluid intake to 800 mL per day
(2) Increase the dose of diuretics if there is decreased urination
(3) Record body weight every day before breakfast and report a weight gain of 3 or more pounds in a week
(4) Keep track of daily output and call the doctor for if it is less than 1 L on any day

6 The nurse is caring for a client who has just had a cardiac catheterization. The client insists on getting up to go to the bathroom to urinate immediately when he is brought back to his room. Which of the following would be the nurse's best response?

(1) "You can't walk yet. You may be too weak after the procedure and may fall."
(2) "If you bend your leg, you will risk bleeding from the insertion site. It is an artery, and it could lead to complications."
(3) "If you get out of bed, you may have an arrhythmia from the catheterization. Your heart has to rest after this procedure."
(4) "The doctor has ordered that you stay on bedrest for the next 6 hours. It is important that you follow these orders."

7 A client is getting ready to go home after a myocardial infarction (MI). The client is asking questions about his medications, and wants to know why metoprolol (Lopressor) was prescribed. The nurse's best response would be which of the following?

(1) "Your heart was beating too slowly, and Lopressor increases your heart rate."
(2) "Lopressor helps to increase the blood supply to the heart by dilating your coronary arteries."
(3) "This medication helps make your heart beat stronger to supply more blood to your body."
(4) "It slows your heart rate and decreases the amount of work it has to do so it can heal."

8 A client is taking digoxin (Lanoxin) and furosemide (Lasix) for heart failure. Which of the following would be the best menu choices for this client?

(1) Chicken with baked potato and cantaloupe
(2) Eggs and ham
(3) Grilled cheese sandwich and French fried potatoes
(4) Pizza with pepperoni

9 A nurse is preparing to admit a client with restrictive cardiomyopathy to the hospital for management of worsening heart failure. Which of the following would be the most appropriate nursing diagnosis for this client?

(1) Fear related to new onset of symptoms
(2) Hopelessness related to lack of cure and debilitating symptoms
(3) Knowledge deficit related to medication regime
(4) Activity intolerance related to decreased cardiac output

10 The nurse is preparing to utilize an external pacemaker for a client with a dysrhythmia. The nurse knows that this pacemaker is often necessary when a client is in which of the following cardiac rhythms?

(1) Ventricular fibrillation
(2) Atrial fibrillation
(3) Ventricular tachycardia
(4) Second-degree heart block

See pages 130–131 for Answers and Rationales.

I. Overview of Anatomy and Physiology of the Heart

A. Structures of the heart

1. The heart is a hollow muscular organ enclosed in a protective sac, divided into four chambers

2. The heart wall has three layers: *epicardium,* fibrous outside protective layer; *myocardium,* middle layer of specialized cardiac muscle; *endocardium,* endothelial lining of the chambers

3. *Pericardium:* protective sac encasing the heart; two fibrous layers with small amount of serous fluid separating the layers for lubrication

4. Chambers

   a. Heart has four hollow chambers, divided by a septum into a right side and a left side

   b. Each side has an upper chamber (*atrium*) and a lower chamber (*ventricle*)

      1) The atria are smaller than the ventricles

      2) Blood flows from the body into the right atrium and from the lungs into the left atrium

      3) With atrial contraction, the blood is pumped from the atria into the ventricles

      4) With ventricular contraction, the blood is pumped from the right ventricle into the pulmonary artery and lungs, and from the left ventricle into the aorta and the arterial circulation

5. Valves of the heart

   a. Atrioventricular (A-V) valves separate the atria from the ventricles; they control the blood flow between the atria and the ventricles

      1) Tricuspid valve, between the right atrium and the right ventricle, has three flaps

      2) Mitral valve, between the left atrium and the left ventricle, has two flaps

      3) Flaps of the A-V valves are connected to the papillary muscles by the chordae tendinae to prevent backflow

      4) S_1, the first heart sound ("lub"), is heard when the A-V valves close

   b. Semilunar valves separate the cardiac chambers from the great vessels and control blood flow out of the cardiac chambers

      1) Pulmonic valve is between the right ventricle and the pulmonic artery, and unoxygenated blood flows through this valve to the lungs

      2) Aortic valve is between the left ventricle and the aorta, and oxygenated blood is pumped from the heart through this valve into systemic circulation

      3) Each of the semilunar valves has three cusps that prevent backflow

      4) S_2, the second heart sound ("dub"), is heard when the semilunar valves close

B. Function of the Heart

1. Circulation (see Figure 3-1): each side of the heart acts as a pump to circulate the blood through the lungs to be oxygenated, and through the body to perfuse the tissues

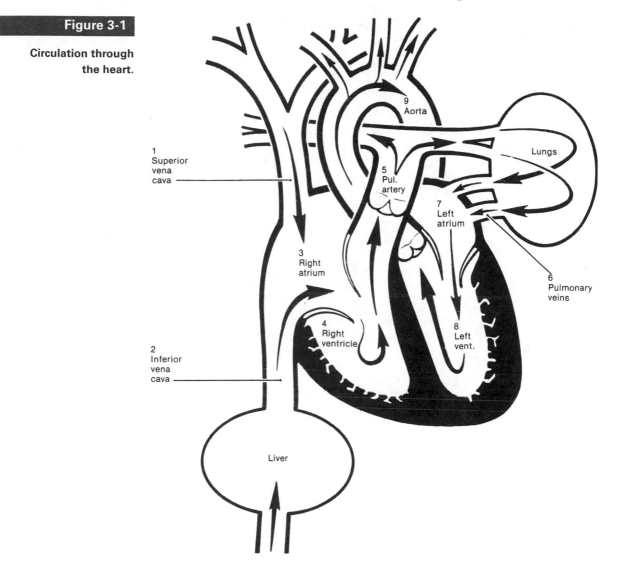

Figure 3-1

Circulation through the heart.

1 Superior vena cava

2 Inferior vena cava

3 Right atrium

4 Right ventricle

5 Pul. artery

6 Pulmonary veins

7 Left atrium

8 Left vent.

9 Aorta

Lungs

Liver

a. Double pump: right side responsible for pulmonary circulation; left side responsible for systemic circulation

b. Right heart circulation—deoxygenated blood:

Venous system ⇒ right atrium ⇒ right ventricle ⇒ lungs for oxygenation

c. Left heart circulation—oxygenated blood:

Lungs ⇒ left atrium ⇒ left ventricle ⇒ aorta ⇒ systemic circulation for tissue perfusion

d. Coronary arteries branch off the aorta to supply oxygenated blood to the heart

2. Cardiac conduction system (see Figure 3-2) is a series of pathways that conduct electrical impulses through the heart, stimulate depolarization and result-

| Figure 3-2 | The normal conduction system of the heart. |

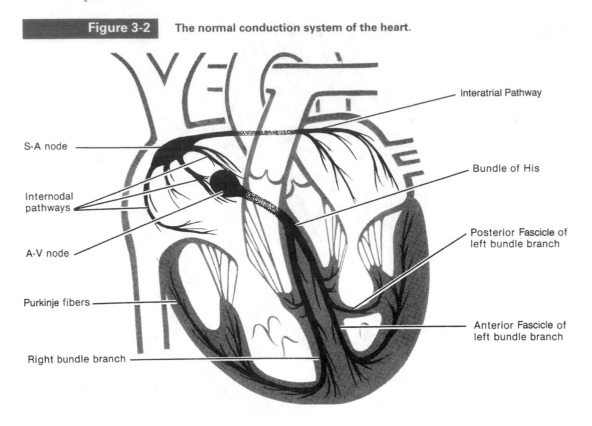

ing muscle contraction of the chambers in a specific sequence, and initiate the pumping action of the heart

a. This conduction takes place because of the special electrophysiologic properties of the specialized cells in the conduction system

b. These properties include *automaticity,* the ability to initiate an electrical impulse; *excitability,* the ability of a cell to respond to a stimulus, and *conductivity,* the ability to transmit impulses from one cell to another

c. The components of the cardiac conduction system are as follows:

1) Sinoatrial (SA) node: natural pacemaker; concentration of cells responsible for initiating the conduction impulse in the healthy heart; located in right atrium at juncture with superior vena cava; rate 60 to 100 beats per minute (bpm)

2) Internodal pathways: carry impulse from SA node to AV node through both right and left atria; impulse initiates process of depolarization in both atria; depolarization results in myocardial contraction of both atria

3) Atrioventricular (AV) node: located at the base of the atrial septum; slows the impulse; allows atria to fully empty before initiating depolarization of ventricles; when SA node is not functioning, can initiate an impulse at the rate of 40 to 60 beats per minute

4) Bundle of His: short branch of conductive cells connecting the AV node to the bundle branches at the intraventricular septum

5) Bundle branches: right (RBB) and left (LBB) split off on either side of intraventricular septum; carry impulse to purkinje fibers

6) Purkinje fibers: diffuse network of conduction pathways; are the terminal branches of the conduction system; conduct impulses rapidly throughout the ventricles; initiate rapid depolarization wave throughout the myocardium and resulting ventricular contraction; when the SA and AV nodes fail, can initiate impulses at the rate of 20 to 40 beats per minute

3. **Cardiac cycle:** each cardiac cycle is one complete heartbeat; includes two parts—systole (ventricular contraction) and diastole (relaxation and ventricular refilling):

   a. Systole: portion of the cardiac cycle when ventricles depolarize and contract to pump blood into pulmonary and systemic circulation; begins with closure of the AV valves; ends with closure of the semilunar valves

   b. Diastole: portion of the cardiac cycle when the ventricles repolarize and refill with blood; begins with closure of the semilunar valves; ends with closure of the AV valves

   c. Atrial systole (depolarization and contraction) is part of late ventricular diastole and atrial diastole occurs during ventricular systole

4. **Cardiac output (CO):** volume of blood in liters ejected by the heart each minute; indicator of pump function of the heart; normal adult CO is 4 to 8 L/min; CO is measured directly by pulmonary artery catheter (e.g., Swan-Ganz) in a critical care setting; clinical indicators of decreased CO include signs of decreased tissue perfusion including change in level of consciousness (early), decreased blood pressure (late)

$$CO = HR \times SV$$

   a. **Heart rate (HR):** number of complete cardiac cycles per minute

   b. **Stroke volume (SV):** volume of blood ejected from the left ventricle each cardiac cycle; stroke volume and ultimately cardiac output influenced by preload, afterload and contractility

   c. **Preload:** degree of myocardial fiber stretch at the end of ventricular diastole; influenced by ventricular filling volume and myocardial compliance

   d. **Afterload:** resistance that the ventricles must overcome to eject blood into the systemic circulation; directly related to arterial blood pressure

   e. **Contractility:** strength of contraction regardless of preload; decreased by hypoxia and some drugs (e.g., beta blockers and calcium channel blockers); increased by drugs (e.g., digoxin and dopamine)

5. Autonomic nervous system: regulates cardiac function and blood pressure; balance exists between sympathetic and parasympathetic branches

   a. Sympathetic nerve stimulation produces norepinephrine; results in increased heart rate, increased myocardial contractility and increased peripheral vasoconstriction; results in increased arterial blood pressure

   b. Parasympathetic nerve stimulation produces acetylcholine, results in lowered heart rate and decreased contractility; is the opposite effect of sympathetic stimulation

c. Changes in sympathetic and parasympathetic activity occur in response to sensory receptors in the body, chemoreceptors, baroreceptors, and stretch receptors

   1) Chemoreceptors: located in the aortic arch and carotid bodies; sense chemical changes in the blood, primarily hypoxia and to a lesser degree hypercapnia; respond by inducing vasoconstriction

   2) Baroreceptors: provide a rapid response to changes in pressure; sensation of low pressure initiates sympathetic stimulation resulting in increased heart rate, vasoconstricton, and consequently increased pressure; sensation of increased pressure sends impulses to medulla, decreasing heart rate and blood pressure (vagal response)

II. Diagnostic Tests and Assessments

A. Laboratory tests

1. Client preparation: the following blood tests involve simple phlebotomy, following agency procedure

2. Postprocedure nursing care: apply pressure and small dressing to site; assess for bleeding

3. Serum enzymes: increased in blood with heart damage; measurement of serum enzyme levels evaluates myocardial tissue **infarction** (injury to myocardium from decreased oxygenation); serial testing over time detects trend and determines peak time and extent of injury

   a. Creatine kinase (CK): formerly known as creatine phosphokinase (CPK), elevation indicates muscle injury; CK-MB is specific to myocardial muscle; rises within 6 hours of injury, peaks at 18 hours postinjury and returns to normal in 2 to 3 days; is useful for early diagnosis of myocardial infarction (MI)

   b. Lactic dehydrogenase (LDH): is found in many body tissues; cardiac origin is confirmed with analysis of isoenzymes (L_1 is greater than L_2; "flipped" from normal levels); elevation is detected within 24 to 72 hours after MI, peaks in 3 to 4 days and returns to normal around 2 weeks; is useful in delayed diagnosis of MI

   c. Troponin: onset is before CK-MB in MI, peaks at 24 hours and returns to normal around 2 weeks; provides early sensitivity, extended blood levels, and is more specific to cardiac injury for diagnosis of MI with an uncertain timeframe

4. Drug levels: blood tests to detect toxic levels of cardiac medications

   a. Digitoxin: therapeutic range is 0.5 to 2.0 ng/mL; early signs of toxicity include nausea, vomiting, anorexia; abdominal pain, bradycardia, other dysrhythmias, and visual disturbances (yellow/green halos) may occur

   b. Quinidine: therapeutic range is 2 to 6 mcg/mL; signs of toxicity include tinnitus, hearing loss, visual disturbances, nausea, dizziness, widened QRS, ventricular dysrhythmias

5. Electrolytes: normal levels of electrolytes are essential for proper cardiac function; cardiac disorders and medications can alter electrolyte balance

   a. Potassium (K^+)

1) Hypokalemia can occur with diuretic therapy (especially loop diuretics such as furosemide); cardiac effects include increased risk of digitalis toxicity, ventricular dysrhythmias, flattening and inversion of T wave or presence of U wave

2) Hyperkalemia is usually related to renal dysfunction or consumption of excess potassium dietary supplements; cardiac effects include ventricular dysrhythmias and asystole

3) Normal potassium level: 3.5 to 5.1 mEq/L

b. Sodium (Na^+)

1) Hyponatremia with long term diuretic therapy

2) Normal sodium level: 135 to 145 mEq/L

c. Calcium: blood levels are affected by hormonal imbalances, renal failure, and several medications

1) Cardiac effects of hypocalcemia include ventricular dysrhythmias, prolonged QT interval and cardiac arrest

2) Hypercalcemia shortens the QT interval and causes AV block, digitalis hypersensitivity, and cardiac arrest

3) Normal calcium level: 8.6 to 10.2 mg/dL

d. Magnesium

1) Cardiac effects of decreased magnesium include ventricular tachycardia and fibrillation

2) Cardiac effects of increased magnesium include bradycardia, hypotension, prolonged PR and QRS intervals

3) Normal magnesium level: 1.8 to 2.6 mg/dL

6. Serum lipid profile: a measurement used to determine risk of developing atherosclerosis

a. Total serum lipids normal value: 400 to 800 mg/dL

b. Triglycerides: lipids stored in fat tissue, readily available for energy production; normal serum value is generally accepted at 10 to 190 mg/dL, (without elevated cholesterol, up to 250 mg/dL may be acceptable)

c. Cholesterol: the main lipid associated with atherosclerotic disease; normal serum value generally accepted is < 200 mg/dL in adults

d. Lipoproteins: proteins in the blood to transport cholesterol, triglycerides, and other fats

1) High-density lipoproteins (HDL): transport cholesterol to liver for excretion; HDL/total cholesterol ratio should be at least 1:5, 1:3 more ideal

2) Low-density lipoproteins (LDL): transport cholesterol to peripheral tissues, associated with increased risk of coronary artery disease

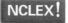

e. Pre-procedure nursing care: instruct client to fast for 12 to 14 hours before testing to ensure accurate results

B. Electrocardiography

1. Is a graphic recording of electrical activity of the heart

2. Resting electrocardiogram (ECG): represents a single recorded picture of the electrical activity of the heart

   a. Client preparation: secure electrodes to appropriate locations on chest and extremities; instruct client to remain still during test; reassure client that he or she will not receive any electrical shock or impulses

   b. No postprocedure nursing care

3. Holter monitoring: continuous ambulatory ECG monitoring over time (usual 24 hours) with small, timed, portable ECG recording device

   a. Client preparation: secure electrodes to appropriate locations on the chest; instruct client to continue normal activity and maintain a log of activities and any symptoms

   b. No postprocedure nursing care

4. Stress test: continuous multi-lead ECG monitoring during controlled and supervised exercise, usually on treadmill

   NCLEX!

   a. Client preparation: obtained written consent; explain procedure, instruct client to eat a light meal 1 to 2 hours before the exam (no caffeine, alcohol, or smoking), wear comfortable clothing and rubber-soled walking shoes

   b. Nursing care during procedure: secure electrodes to appropriate locations on chest, obtain and record baseline BP and ECG tracing; instruct client to exercise as instructed and report any pain, weakness, shortness of breath, or other symptoms immediately; monitor BP and ECG continuously, record at frequent intervals and with any symptoms or changes in vital signs, ST segments, or cardiac rhythm

   NCLEX!

   c. Postprocedure nursing care: continue to monitor ECG and BP until client returns completely to baseline and is symptom-free

C. Echocardiography

1. Is an ultrasound of the heart to evaluate structure and function of the heart chambers and valves

2. Client preparation: instruct client to remain still during test; secure electrodes for simultaneous ECG tracing; explain that there will be no pain or electrical shocks, however, the lubricant placed on skin will be cool

3. Postprocedure nursing care: cleanse lubricant from client's chest wall

D. Phonocardiography

1. Is a graphic recording of heart sounds with simultaneous ECG

2. Client preparation: instruct client to remain quiet and still during test; secure electrodes for simultaneous ECG tracing; explain that there will be no pain or electrical shocks

3. No postprocedure nursing care

E. Coronary angiography/arteriography

   1. Is an invasive procedure during which physician injects dye into coronary arteries and immediately takes a series of x-ray films to assess the structure of the arteries

NCLEX!

   2. Client preparation: obtain written consent; explain procedure, assess client for history of allergies to dye or shellfish; initiate IV site with fluids as ordered

   3. Postprocedure nursing care: same as postprocedure care for cardiac catheterization (see section below)

F. Cardiac catheterization

   1. Is the insertion of a catheter into the heart and surrounding vessels to obtain diagnostic information about the structure and function of the heart

   2. Can be performed on right or left side of the heart

NCLEX!

   3. Client preparation, nursing care during procedure, and postprocedure nursing care are outlined in Box 3-1

G. Radionuclide tests

   1. Are safe methods of evaluating left ventricular muscle function and coronary artery blood distribution; can provide some of the same information as radiographic angiography with less risk to client

      a. Client preparation: obtain written consent if required; explain procedure, instruct client that fasting may be required for a short period before the exam; contrast material will be injected through a venipuncture; it will be necessary to alternately change position and remain still during the exam; there is no associated pain or discomfort

      b. Nursing care during procedure: none, procedure is performed in nuclear medicine

      c. Postprocedure nursing care: encourage client to drink fluids to facilitate the excretion of the contrast material; assess venipuncture site for bleeding or hematoma; if stress testing was performed, assess client's BP and pulse at frequent intervals and maintain continuous ECG monitoring as indicated

   2. Allows visualization of ventricles through several cardiac cycles; calculates **ejection fraction** (EF), the portion of the blood ejected during systole, compared with the total ventricular filling volume, (normal EF = 55 to 65 percent)

   3. MUGA (gated pool imaging or multigated acquisition) scan

   4. Thallium imaging: used to assess myocardial **ischemia** (decreased supply of oxygenated blood) during stress testing

   5. PET (positron emission tomography) scan: evaluates cardiac metabolism and assesses tissue perfusion

H. Hemodynamic monitoring

   1. Is the measurement of pressures of the heart and calculation of hemodynamic parameters

Box 3-1

**Care of the Client
Undergoing Cardiac
Catheterization**

Client Preparation

- Obtain written consent
- Assess client history of allergies to iodine, dye or shellfish
- Explain that client will be awake and may experience various sensations during the procedure, including flushing sensation as dye is injected, or fluttering feeling as the catheter passes through the heart
- Explain the postprocedure routine (see postprocedure nursing care)
- Prepare insertion site by shaving and cleansing with antiseptic
- Nothing by mouth (NPO) except sips of water with cardiac medications as indicated for 6 to 8 hours
- Initiate IV site with fluids as ordered
- Administer preprocedure medications as ordered

Nursing Care During Procedure

- Procedure is performed in catheterization lab by cardiologist; nurse monitors ECG and vital signs continuously, administers conscious sedation as ordered, and provides emotional support

Postprocedure Nursing Care

- Maintain client on bedrest for 4 to 6 hours
- Keep affected extremity straight; after 1 to 2 hours head may be elevated < 30° for those who had the femoral artery as the insertion site
- Maintain pressure dressing at insertion site
- Monitor BP, HR, distal pulses, color and temperature of extremity, and assess for signs of bleeding at the site (with leg site, check under client for bleeding) according to agency schedule, (routinely q 15 minutes for 1 hour, q 30 minutes for 2 hours, q hour for 4 hours, or q 8 hours for associated procedure of percutaneous transluminal coronary angioplasty [PTCA])
- Report signs of chest pain, dysrhythmias, bleeding, hematoma formation or other changes; significant changes in vital signs, pulses, color or temperature of extremity should be reported immediately to the physician. Bleeding may be reported by the client as a feeling of warmth in the insertion area
- If bleeding occurs, restore manual pressure to site
- Maintain IV and encourage oral fluids as ordered to eliminate dye as soon as possible; the contrast medium can be nephrotoxic
- Monitor I & O to determine whether client is becoming dehydrated from increased urine output because of dye excretion

2. Central venous pressure (CVP) monitoring: appropriate for clients who require accurate monitoring of fluid volume status but are not candidates for the more invasive pulmonary artery pressure monitoring

   a. CVP monitoring is done by central catheter with the tip lying in the superior vena cava at the juncture with the right atrium

   b. Measures pressure that indicates the right heart filling pressure; is not a satisfactory method of determining left heart pressures

c. Normal CVP is 2 to 8 cm H_2O or 2 to 6 mm Hg; decreased CVP indicates decreased circulating volume; increased CVP indicates increased blood volume or right heart failure

3. Pulmonary artery pressure (PAP) monitoring: appropriate for critically ill clients requiring more accurate assessments of left heart pressures, including clients undergoing open heart surgery, clients in shock or with serious MIs

a. Pulmonary artery (Swan-Ganz) catheter has the tip in the pulmonary artery

b. Pressure measurement from this catheter is obtained after catheter tip is wedged in a pulmonary capillary, and is called the pulmonary capillary wedge pressure or PCWP; is a good indicator of left ventricular end diastolic pressure (LVEDP)

c. Allows calculation of actual cardiac output and other hemodynamic parameters at frequent intervals in critically ill clients

1) Client preparation: obtain consent according to policy; insertion is under strict sterile technique, usually at the bedside; explain to client that sterile drapes may cover the face (with an internal jugular or subclavian insertion site); assist to position client flat or slight Trendelenburg as tolerated and instruct client to remain still during the procedure

2) Nursing care during insertion procedure: assist physician in maintaining a sterile field; administer medications as ordered; monitor and document HR, BP, and ECG during procedure; reassure client through procedure

3) Postprocedure nursing care: monitor vital signs (VS), ECG at frequent intervals postinsertion; maintain client on bedrest and avoid unnecessary movements; follow policy to maintain patency and sterility of catheter

NCLEX!

4) Nursing responsibilities in hemodynamic monitoring: position the transducer at the level of the right atrium (left midaxillary line, fourth intercostal space—this point is known as the phlebostatic axis): level the CVP or pulmonary artery catheter (Swan-Ganz) transducer to this point at regular intervals according to policy (usually each shift) and before each measurement; maintain patency of catheter with a constant small amount of fluid delivered under pressure

III. Common Nursing Techniques and Procedures

A. Dysrhythmia monitoring

1. Continuous ECG monitoring in one lead with portable telemetry unit; indicated for clients undergoing surgery at risk for life-threatening conditions, with cardiac and non-cardiac diseases, and those undergoing procedures and pharmacological therapies affecting the heart

2. Lead placements (ECG continuous monitors have three leads or five leads)

a. Placement of leads with three-lead monitor

1) Below the right clavicle (right arm)

2) Below the left clavicle (left arm)

3) Lowest rib, left midclavicular line (left leg)

    b. Placement of leads with 5-lead monitor include same as three-lead (above) with the additional placements:

        1) Lowest rib, right midclavicular line (right leg)

        2) Fifth lead on one of six chest leads (V leads)

3. Preparation of client: explain procedure and reassure client that he or she will not receive electrical impulses or shocks; identify proper placement, cleanse skin with soap and water, shave hairy areas, use alcohol or skin prep according to agency policy, dry with cloth or gauze, and apply fresh electrodes

4. Interpretations of ECG patterns originating in the sinus node (see Table 3-1)

    a. Sinus rhythm

    b. Sinus tachycardia

    c. Sinus bradycardia

    d. Sinus arrhythmia

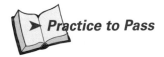

    e. Nursing and therapeutic interventions: with sinus arrest, tachycardia, or bradycardia, assess for signs of inadequate cardiac output and tissue perfusion, including changes in blood pressure, activity tolerance, and level of consciousness; the cause of sinus tachycardia should be identified and treated; medical treatment is appropriate for the symptomatic client or with long-term high rates (> 150) or extreme low rates (< 50)

5. ECG patterns originating in the atria (refer again to Table 3-1)

    a. Premature atrial contraction (PAC)

    b. Atrial tachycardia

    c. Atrial flutter

    d. Atrial fibrillation

    e. Nursing and therapeutic interventions: carotid massage, synchronized cardioversion, anti-dysrhythmia medications including beta blockers and calcium channel blockers (cardizem), and digoxin; anticoagulant therapy to reduce the risk of thrombus development

6. ECG patterns originating from the AV node (refer again to Table 3-1)

    a. Junctional (nodal) tachycardia

    b. First-degree heart block

    c. Second-degree heart block, Mobitz type I (Wenckebach)

    d. Second-degree heart block, Mobitz type II

    e. Third-degree (complete) heart block

    f. Nursing and therapeutic interventions

        1) Monitoring and observation

        2) Atropine or isoproterenol or pacemakers for symptomatic heart block

        3) *Pacemakers:* permanent pacemakers are inserted in the operating room to treat permanent conduction deficits

► *Practice to Pass*

The nurse is discharging a client from the hospital with a new diagnosis of atrial fibrillation. What would the nurse include in the client and family teaching?

Table 3-1	ECG Characteristics of Selected Cardiac Rhythms and Dysrhythmias

Rhythm/ECG Appearance	ECG Characteristics	Management

Supraventricular Rhythms

Normal sinus rhythm (NSR)

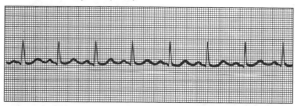

Rate: 60 to 100 bpm
Rhythm: Regular
P:QRS: 1:1
PR interval: 0.12 to 0.20 sec
QRS complex: 0.06 to 0.10 sec

None; normal heart rhythm.

Sinus arrhythmia

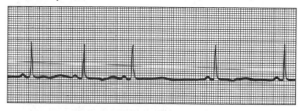

Rate: 60 to 100 bpm
Rhythm: Irregular, varying with respirations
P:QRS: 1:1
PR interval: 0.12 to 0.20 sec
QRS complex: 0.06 to 0.10 sec

Generally none; considered a normal rhythm in the very young and very old.

Sinus tachycardia

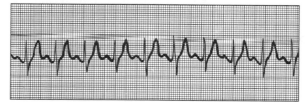

Rate: 101 to 150 bpm
Rhythm: Regular
P:QRS: 1:1 (With very fast rates, P wave may be hidden in preceding T wave)
PR interval: 0.12 to 0.20 sec
QRS complex: 0.06 to 0.10 sec

Treated only if the client is experiencing symptoms or is at risk for myocardial damage.
Treat underlying cause (e.g., hypovolemia, fever, pain).
Beta blockers or verapamil may be used.

Sinus bradycardia

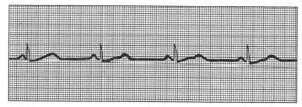

Rate:< 60 bpm
Rhythm: Regular
P:QRS: 1:1
PR interval: 0.12 to 0.20 sec
QRS complex: 0.06 to 0.10 sec

Treated only if the client is experiencing symptoms. Intravenous atropine and/or pacemaker therapy may be used.

Premature atrial contractions (PAC)

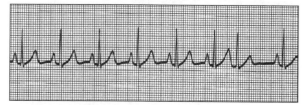

Rate: Variable
Rhythm: Irregular, with normal rhythm interrrupted by early beats arising in the atria
P:QRS: 1:1
PR interval: 0.12 to 0.20 sec, but may be prolonged
QRS complex: 0.6 to 0.10 sec

Usually require no treatment. Advise client to reduce alcohol and caffeine intake, to reduce stress, and to stop smoking.

Paroxysmal supraventricular tachycardia (PSVT)

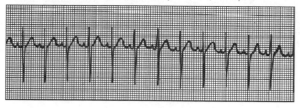

Rate: 100 to 280 bpm (usually 150 to 200 bpm)
Rhythm: Regular
P:QRS: P waves often not identifiable
PR interval: Not measured
QRS complex: 0.06 to 0.10 sec

Treat if client is experiencing symptoms. Treatment may include vagal manuevers (Valsalva, carotid sinus massage); oxygen therapy; adenosine, verapamil, procainamide, propranolol, and esmolol; and synchronized cardioversion.

Table 3-1 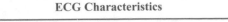 **ECG Characteristics of Selected Cardiac Rhythms and Dysrhythmias (*cont.*)**

Rhythm/ECG Appearance	ECG Characteristics	Management
Atrial flutter 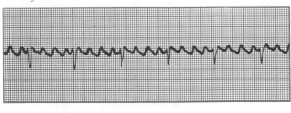	Rate: Atrial 240 to 360 bpm; ventricular rate depends on degree of AV block and usually is < 150 bpm Rhythm: Atrial regular, ventricular usually regular P:QRS: 2:1, 4:1, 6:1; may vary PR interval: Not measured QRS complex: 0.06 to 0.10 sec	Synchronized cardioversion; medications to slow ventricular response such as a beta blocker or calcium channel blocker (verapamil), followed by quinidine, procainamide, flecainide, or amiodarone.
Atrial fibrillation 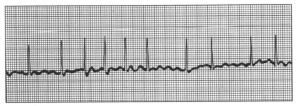	Rate: Atrial 300 to 600 bpm (too rapid to count); ventricular 100 to 180 bpm in untreated clients Rhythm: Irregularly irregular P:QRS: Variable PR interval: Not measured QRS complex: 0.06 to 0.10 sec	Synchronized cardioversion; medications to reduce ventricular response rate: verapamil, propranolol, digoxin, anticoagulant therapy to reduce risk of clot formation and stroke.
Junctional escape rhythm 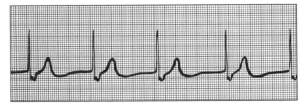	Rate: 40 to 60 bpm; junctional tachycardia 60 to 140 bpm Rhythm: Regular P:QRS: P waves may be absent, inverted and immediately preceding or succeeding QRS complex, or hidden in QRS complex PR interval: < 0.10 sec if P wave is prior to QRS complex QRS complex: 0.06 to 0.10 sec	Treat cause if client is experiencing symptoms.
Ventricular Rhythms *Premature ventricular contractions (PVC)* 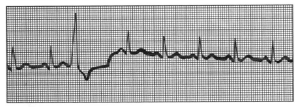	Rate: Variable Rhythm: Irregular, with PVC interrupting underlying rhythm and followed by a compensatory pause P:QRS: No P wave noted before PVC PR interval: Absent with PVC QRS complex: Wide (> 0.12 sec) and bizarre in appearance; differs from normal QRS complex	Treat if client is experiencing symptoms. Advise against stimulant use (caffeine, nicotine). Drug therapy includes intravenous lidocaine, procainamide, quinidine, propranolol, phenytoin, bretylium.
Ventricular tachycardia (VT or V tach) 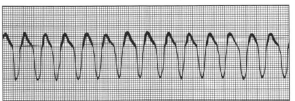	Rate: 100 to 250 bpm Rhythm: Regular P:QRS: P waves usually not identifiable PR interval: Not measured QRS complex: 0.12 sec or greater; bizarre shape	Treat if VT is sustained or if the client is experiencing symptoms. Treatment includes intravenous procainamide or lidocaine and/or immediate defibrillation if the client is unconscious or unstable.

Table 3-1	ECG Characteristics of Selected Cardiac Rhythms and Dysrhythmias *(cont.)*

Rhythm/ECG Appearance	ECG Characteristics	Management
Ventricular fibrillation (VF, V fib) 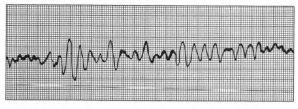	Rate: Too rapid to count Rhythm: Grossly irregular P:QRS: No identifiable P waves PR interval: None QRS: Bizarre, varying in shape and direction	Immediate defibrillation.
Atrioventricular Conduction Blocks *First-degree AV block* 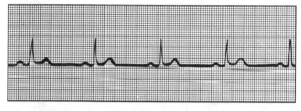	Rate: Usually 60 to 100 bpm Rhythm: Regular P:QRS: 1:1 PR interval: > 0.20 sec QRS complex: 0.06 to 0.10 sec	None required.
Second-degree AV block, type I (Mobitz I, Wenckebach) 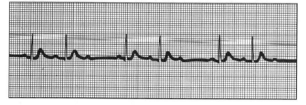	Rate: 60 to 100 bpm Rhythm: Atrial regular; ventricular irregular P:QRS: 1:1 until P wave blocked with no subsequent QRS complex PR interval: Progressively lengthens in a regular pattern QRS complex: 0.06 to 0.10 sec; sudden absence of QRS complex	Monitoring and observation; atropine or isoproterenol if client is experiencing symptoms.
Second-degree AV block, type II (Mobitz II) 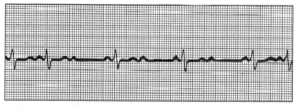	Rate: Atrial 60 to 100 bpm; ventricular < 60 bpm Rhythm: Atrial regular; ventricular irregular P:QRS: Typically 2:1, may vary PR interval: Constant PR interval for each conducted QRS complex QRS complex: 0.06 to 0.10 sec	Atropine or isoproterenol; pacemaker therapy.
Third-degree AV block (Complete heart block) 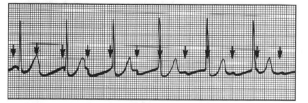	Rate: Atrial 60 to 100 bpm; ventricular 15 to 60 bpm Rhythm: Atrial regular; ventricular regular P:QRS: No relationship between P waves and QRS complexes; independent rhythms PR interval: Not measured QRS complex: 0.06 to 0.10 sec if junctional escape rhythm; > 0.12 sec if ventricular escape rhythm	Immediate pacemaker therapy.

4) For temporary conduction deficits, physicians insert temporary pacemakers in a critical care unit through a catheter or nurses may apply an external (transthoracic) pacemaker to stimulate the heart with an electrical impulse through the chest wall

7. ECG patterns originating from the ventricles (refer again to Table 3-1)

   a. Premature ventricular contraction (PVC)

   b. Ventricular tachycardia (VT)

   c. Ventricular fibrillation (VF)

   NCLEX!

   d. Nursing and therapeutic interventions: for PVCs monitor for symptoms of decreased cardiac output; instruct client to avoid caffeine or nicotine; with VT, assess immediately to determine level of consciousness (LOC) and if client has stable BP and pulse; if stable, treat with lidocaine, procainamide, and finally defibrillation if client becomes unconscious or unstable; pulseless VT and VF both require immediate defibrillation

B. Cardiac surgery or endovascular interventions

1. Percutaneous transluminal coronary angioplasty (PTCA): procedure to increase blood flow to coronary arteries by inserting a catheter with a balloon tip into the narrowed segment of an affected artery, inflating the balloon to expand the opening of the vessel and removing the catheter; may also include the insertion of an expandable intracoronary stent, which is inserted over the balloon and remains in place after the balloon is removed

   NCLEX!

   a. Client preparation, nursing care during procedure, and postprocedure nursing care are as outlined previously in Box 3-1

   NCLEX!

   b. In addition, administer anticoagulants as ordered to prevent thrombus formation, and monitor coagulation studies as indicated

   c. Because of the anticoagulants used during the procedure, the site may have a vice-type pressure device requiring a longer period of hourly site checks; monitor closely for any changes in ECG or signs of chest pain (even minor changes may be indicators of ischemia); obtain a 12-lead ECG and notify physician of any complications

2. Coronary artery bypass grafting (CABG): surgical treatment of coronary artery disease for clients with more than 50 percent occlusion in the left main coronary artery or severe blockage in several vessels; the diseased arteries are "bypassed" with saphenous veins, mammary arteries, or less frequently, artificial grafts; indicated for myocardial ischemia that cannot be managed by medical treatment; the client is maintained on cardiopulmonary bypass machine during surgery

   NCLEX!

   a. Client preparation

      1) Ensure that all consents are signed

      2) Instruct client in routine preoperative teaching, including turning and deep breathing (vigorous coughing is discouraged because it may increase intrathoracic pressure and cause instability in the sternal area), incentive spirometry to prevent respiratory complications, and leg exercises to prevent emboli formation

3) Explain the client status immediately postoperatively, including respiratory support on a ventilator with an endotracheal tube; suctioning; surgical incisions, chest tubes, multiple intravenous lines, tubes, drains, and monitors with alarms and noises; pain management, communication techniques, visiting policies, and expected length of hospitalization and recovery period

NCLEX!

b. Postprocedure nursing care: critical care nurses manage the complex nursing care of the cardiac surgical client (CABG and valvular repair/replacement) in the immediate postoperative period in special cardiac surgical units; tamponade is a life-threatening complication that may occur in the postoperative period; within 1 to 2 days client is transferred to a step-down/telemetry unit where care includes the following:

1) Monitor client for signs of decreased cardiac output, continuous ECG monitoring; I and O; full assessments with lung sounds and heart sounds at regular intervals (every 4 hours initially, then at least every 8 hours)

2) Assess and treat postoperative pain

3) Monitor indicators of cardiac output with client's increasing activity

4) Monitor respiratory status and encouraging deep-breathing and incentive spirometry

5) Monitor surgical wounds and treating as needed

NCLEX!

6) Instruct client about new medication regime, activity plan for home, cardiac rehabilitation, resumption of sexual activity (client may resume sexual activity when he or she can walk up two full flights of stairs without shortness of breath or chest pain; client should be rested, not after a heavy meal or alcohol consumption)

NCLEX!

7) Instruct client about symptoms to report to MD upon discharge, including chest pain, shortness of breath, decrease in activity tolerance, fever, redness, swelling or drainage from surgical incisions

8) Instruct client that clinical depression occurs in about 20 percent of clients up to 6 months after cardiac surgery, and client should notify physician because antidepressants are very effective; include family in teaching and planning for discharge

3. Valvular surgery repair or replacement of dysfunctional valve

a. Repair

1) *Valvuloplasty:* reconstruction including repair or removal of calcification or vegetation

2) *Annuloplasty:* narrowing a dilated valve with a prosthetic ring or purse-string sutures, or enlarging a stenosed valve with a balloon

3) Repair is the preferred option, because of the lower incidence of post-surgical complications or mortality than valve replacement

b. Replacement: valve is completely replaced

1) Mechanical valves: more durable and longer lasting; subject to mechanical failure; require lifetime anticoagulation with warfarin (coumadin)

and infections are harder to treat; an example is the St. Jude Medical valve

2) Tissue valves: may deteriorate; frequent replacement is required; not associated with thrombus formation, no long-term anticoagulation; infections are easier to treat

NCLEX!

c. Client preparation and postprocedure nursing care: (same as for cardiac surgery, see above); include instructions about preventing infection including prophylactic antibiotic therapy prior to invasive procedures including dental care, gentle oral care to prevent bacteria from entering the bloodstream through the gums; and management of anticoagulation therapy if appropriate

4. Pacemakers: permanent pacemakers are inserted in the operating room to treat permanent cardiac conduction defects

NCLEX!

a. Client preparation: obtain consent; instruct client that bedrest is required for 24 hours and activity will gradually be increased to prevent dislodging of the leads

NCLEX!

b. Postprocedure nursing care: monitor ECG continuously to ensure that pacing beats are being captured and that intrinsic heartbeats are sensed; monitor the pacemaker site for signs of bleeding or infection; dressing should remain clean and dry with no temperature elevation, swelling, redness, or tenderness; right arm and shoulder movements may be minimized immediately post-procedure to ensure that pacemaker wire remains in contact with ventricular wall

IV. Myocardial Infarction (MI)

A. Description

1. Myocardial injury from sudden restriction of blood supply to a portion of the heart

2. Is a life threatening condition

B. Etiology and pathophysiology

NCLEX!

1. Main cause is **coronary artery disease** (CAD), the build up of atherosclerotic plaque in coronary arteries that restricts blood flow to the heart

a. Nonmodifiable risk factors include age, gender, family history, diabetes, and ethnic background

b. Modifiable risk factors include smoking, obesity, stress, elevated cholesterol, and hypertension

2. Coronary artery blood flow is blocked by atherosclerotic narrowing, thrombus formation or (less frequently) persistent vasospasm; myocardium supplied by the arteries is deprived of oxygen; persistent ischemia may rapidly lead to tissue death

3. **Angina pectoris** is chest pain resulting from this restricted blood flow; it may occur in the following forms:

a. *Stable angina,* a predictable response to increased activity

b. *Unstable angina* with unpredictability and increasing severity

        c. *Prinzmetal's angina,* caused by arterial spasm often awaking the client from sleep

        d. Angina pectoris may change in character and may progress to MI

C. Assessment

    1. Chest pain unrelieved by nitroglycerine or rest; may be crushing substernal pain; may radiate to jaw, neck, back, or left arm (some clients report no pain—especially diabetics)

    2. Other symptoms may include diaphoresis, nausea, fear, anxiety, dyspnea, dysrhythmias

    3. ECG (12-lead): ST elevation, accompanied by T-wave inversion; and later new pathologic Q wave

    4. Lab findings: elevated CK with MB isoenzymes > 5 percent (early diagnosis); elevated troponin (early to late diagnosis); or elevated LDH with "flipped" isoenzymes (late diagnosis)

D. Priority nursing diagnoses: Pain; Ineffective tissue perfusion: cardiac; Decreased cardiac output; Anxiety; Fear

E. Planning and implementation

    1. Assess pain status frequently with pain scale or appropriate tool to estimate changes in pain level; pain is usually the first presenting sign of new or extended MI

    2. Assess hemodynamic status including BP, HR, LOC, skin color, and temperature frequently (every 5 minutes during episodes of pain; every 15 minutes post-pain) during the acute phase to evaluate CO; continue to monitor frequently (every 1 to 2 hours) for the first 24 hours post-MI

    3. Monitor continuous ECG to detect dysrhythmias (PVCs and tachycardia common)

    4. Perform 12-lead ECG immediately with new pain or changes in level or character of pain to identify ischemia and injury

    5. Monitor respirations, breath sounds, and input and output to detect early signs of heart failure

    6. Monitor O_2 saturation and administer O_2 (usually via nasal cannula at 2 to 4 L/min) as prescribed to increase oxygenation to heart

    7. Provide for physiological rest to decrease oxygen demands on heart

    8. Keep client NPO or progress to liquid diet as ordered; maintain IV access for medications as needed

    9. Provide a calm environment and reassure client and family to decrease stress, fear, and anxiety

    10. Report significant changes immediately to physician to ensure rapid treatment of complications

    11. Interventions in the recovery phase: maintain bedrest (with commode) for 24 to 36 hours and gradually increase activity as ordered while closely monitoring CO, ECG, and pain status; reinforce to client the importance of reporting any new pain immediately; progress diet from NPO or liquids to soft diet as ordered

NCLEX!

NCLEX!

NCLEX!

NCLEX!

NCLEX!

F. Medication therapy

NCLEX!

1. Administer nitroglycerine as prescribed to dilate coronary vessels and increase blood flow; sublingual nitroglycerine may be given 1 tab every 5 minutes for 3 times to relieve chest pain; IV nitroglycerine is administered to dilate coronary arteries and increase blood flow to the heart; do not expose nitroglycerine to heat or light; keep sublingual nitroglycerine in a dark glass container, away from heat and discard tablets that are not used in 6 months; tablets should tingle under the tongue if potent

2. Administer morphine sulfate as ordered to relieve chest pain

NCLEX!

3. Administer anticoagulants (IV heparin) and aspirin (antiplatelet) as ordered to prevent additional clot formation, monitor PTT to maintain heparin at therapeutic level

4. Administer thrombolytic therapy (alteplase recombinant [Activase], tissue plasminogen activator [t-PA] or streptokinase [Streptase]) as ordered to dissolve clot, stop progress of MI and decrease myocardial damage; monitor frequently for signs of bleeding

NCLEX!

5. Monitor neurological status frequently for changes; alteplase recombinant and streptokinase are not clot-specific and will dissolve other clots—can cause thrombolytic (hemorrhagic) CVA, a life-threatening complication

6. Administer beta-blockers post-MI as ordered to decrease cardiac work and decrease oxygen demands on the heart

7. Administer anti-dysrhythmic drugs as prescribed or by emergency protocol for dysrhythmias

G. Surgical interventions: PTCA, CABG (see previous discussion)

H. Client education

1. Include appropriate family members whenever possible

2. Explain cardiac rehabilitation program if ordered

3. Explain modifiable risk factors and develop a plan with client including supportive resources to change lifestyle to decrease these factors

4. Explain medication regime as prescribed; identify side effects to report (provide written instructions for later reference)

NCLEX!

5. Stress the importance of immediate reporting of chest pain or signs of decreased CO

NCLEX!

6. Instruct about bleeding precautions if client is on anticoagulant therapy: use soft toothbrush, electric razor, avoid trauma or injury; wear or carry medical alert identification

I. Expected outcomes/evaluation

1. Client reports decrease in pain

2. Indicators of cardiac output within client's normal range

3. No serious dysrhythmias

4. Client reports decreased anxiety or fear

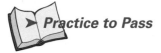

Practice to Pass

A client is admitted to the emergency room with chest pain and is being evaluated for a possible MI. What assessments would the nurse make?

5. No occurrence of complications

6. Client identifies modifiable risk factors and develops a plan including family and community supports to decrease risk

V. Heart Failure

A. Description

1. Inability of the heart to pump adequate blood to meet the metabolic needs of the body

2. Formerly called congestive heart failure

B. Etiology and pathophysiology

1. Multiple causes include myocardial damage from MI, incompetent valves, inflammatory conditions of the heart, cardiomyopathy, pulmonary hypertension (right-sided failure, called **cor pulmonale**)

2. Compensatory phase (early): CO falls $\Rightarrow$ sensed by baroreceptors $\Rightarrow$ stimulate sympathetic nervous system $\Rightarrow$ release norepinephrine $\Rightarrow$ increase in HR and vasoconstriction $\Rightarrow$ increased in filling pressures $\Rightarrow$ increase in SV and CO, (because $CO = HR \times SV$, CO is increased); compensatory mechanisms increase cardiac metabolic demands and in time decrease cardiac function and the ability to compensate

3. Depending upon the cause, heart failure presents initially as right-sided failure or left-sided failure; as it progresses the other side becomes affected

   a. Left heart failure: the left ventricle has reduced capacity to pump blood into systemic circulation causing decreased CO and stasis or "backup" of fluid into the pulmonary circulation

   b. Right heart failure: the right ventricle has reduced capacity to pump blood into pulmonary circulation causing stasis or "backup" of fluid into the venous circulation

4. Onset of heart failure

   a. Acute, with significant overload in the lungs (**pulmonary edema,** characterized by acute restlessness, anxiety, increased crackles, tachypnea, tachycardia, pink frothy sputum, decreased SO_2 and PO_2)

   b. Chronic, with fatigue and activity intolerance as the main features; clients with advanced chronic heart failure require careful management to prevent acute exacerbations

C. Assessment

1. Presenting symptoms

   a. Left failure: dyspnea on exertion (often first clinical sign), orthopnea, paroxysmal nocturnal dyspnea, new S_3 (ventricular gallop) as early sign; pulmonary edema is acute life-threatening left heart failure, as previously described

   b. Right failure: lower extremity edema; **jugular venous distention (JVD)** is visible more than a few millimeters above the clavicle with the client supine at a 45-degree angle, abdominal discomfort and nausea occur from fluid congestion in the abdominal organs

   c. Both sides: unexplained fatigue, decreased exercise tolerance, unexplained altered mental status

2. Diagnostic findings

   a. Chest x-ray may show cardiomegaly or vascular congestion

   b. Echocardiogram shows decreased ventricular function and decreased ejection fraction

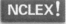

   c. CVP elevated in right-sided failure

   d. Pulmonary artery pressure monitoring may be used to guide treatment in serious case of pulmonary edema

D. **Priority nursing diagnoses:** Decreased cardiac output, Excess fluid volume, Impaired gas exchange, Activity intolerance, Deficient knowledge: diet and medication regime

E. **Planning and implementation**

   1. Acute phase

      a. Monitor and record BP, pulse, respirations, ECG, and CVP or PCWP (if appropriate) to detect changes in cardiac output

      b. Maintain client in sitting position to decrease pulmonary congestion and facilitate improved gas exchange

      c. Auscultate heart and lung sounds frequently: increasing crackles, increasing dyspnea, decreasing lungs sounds or new S_3 heart sound indicate worsening failure

      d. Administer O_2 as ordered to improve gas exchange and increase oxygenation of blood; monitor SO_2 and arterial blood gases (ABG) as ordered to assess oxygenation

      e. Administer prescribed medications on accurate schedule

      f. Monitor serum electrolytes to detect hypokalemia secondary to diuretic therapy

      g. Monitor accurate input and output (may require Foley catheter to allow for accurate measurement of urine output) to evaluate fluid status

      h. If fluid restriction is prescribed, spread the fluid throughout the day to reduce thirst

      i. Encourage physical rest and organized activities with frequent rest periods to reduce the work of the heart

      j. Provide a calm reassuring environment to decrease anxiety; this decreases oxygen consumption and decreases demands on the heart

   2. Chronic heart failure

      a. Educate client and family (see client education) about the rationale for the therapeutic regime

      b. Establish baseline assessment for fluid status and functional abilities: it is baseline "normal" for some clients with heart failure to have bilateral crackles in the bases, or some level of peripheral edema, or to be unable to walk more than a specific number of feet before tiring

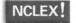

      c. Monitor daily weights to evaluate changes in fluid status

     d. Assess at regular intervals for changes in fluid status or functional activity level

F. Medication therapy

    1. Angiotensin converting enzyme (ACE) inhibitors to reduce afterload and consequently increase cardiac output (primarily used in ongoing management); monitor for hypotension, especially orthostatic

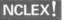

    2. Diuretics (often loop diuretics such as furosemide/Lasix) to decrease preload and pulmonary congestion, which decreases cardiac work and increases cardiac output; carefully monitor potassium levels with diuretic therapy except for potassium-sparing diuretics (important in the acute and chronic treatment of heart failure)

    3. Vasodilators including nitroglycerine to reduce preload; monitor for hypotension

    4. Morphine to sedate and vasodilate, decreasing the work of the heart; monitor for hypotension or respiratory depression (acute pulmonary edema)

    5. Digoxin (Lanoxin) to improve contractility and correspondingly increase stroke volume and cardiac output; take apical pulse for 1 full minute and withhold if heart rate is less than 60

    6. Other inotropic agents, dopamine (Intropin) and dobutamine (Dobutrex), are used in critical care cases when decompensation of cardiac output includes hypotension; monitor BP and IV site frequently

G. Client education

    1. Include family members or others in teaching as appropriate

    2. Weight monitoring: teach client the importance of measuring and recording daily weights (with same amount of clothing at the same time of day) and report unexplained increase of 3 to 5 pounds—most sensitive indicator of increased fluid overload

    3. Diet: sodium restriction to decrease fluid overload and potassium-rich foods to replenish loss from medications; do not restrict water intake unless directed (this will not decrease fluid retention)

    4. Medication regime: explain the importance of following all medication instructions; remind client that although frequent urination is bothersome, regular diuretic therapy prevents fluid overload and acute exacerbation; instruct client how to take radial pulse for one full minute before taking digoxin, and to withhold dose and call prescriber if <60 or >120

    5. Activity: help client plan paced activity to maximize available cardiac output

    6. Symptoms: report to MD promptly any of the following: chest pain, new onset of dyspnea on exertion, paroxysmal nocturnal dyspnea

    7. Other: report even minor changes to MD or homecare nurse, as they may be an early sign of decompensation

H. Expected outcomes/evaluation

    1. Cardiac output, BP within client's normal limits

    2. Minimal edema

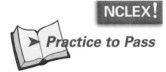

Practice to Pass

The homecare nurse is caring for a client with heart failure who reports that she skips her diuretics several times a week because she can't go out of the house after she has taken them. What should the nurse explain to this client?

3. Client weight at optimal level

4. Client maintains optimal level of function and activity

5. Client maintains medication schedule, diet, and monitors daily weight

VI. Endocarditis (Infective, Subacute Bacterial)

A. Description

1. Inflammation of the inner layer of the heart

2. Usually involves the cardiac valves

B. Etiology and pathophysiology

1. Caused by microorganisms in the blood: risk factors include IV drug use, structural defects in the heart or valves (which increase the number of platelet and fibrin strands in the endothelium)

   a. Acute endocarditis: sudden onset with *Staphylococcus aureus* the most common organism

   b. Subacute endocarditis: gradual onset with *Streptococcus viridans* or other less virulent bacteria

2. Microorganisms in the bloodstream colonize on fibrin and platelet strands in the endothelium, multiply and develop new strands; seen as "vegetation" attached to the endothelium, particularly the valves, causing valve damage; segments of vegetation may break off and travel to the extremities manifested as petechiae

C. Assessment

1. Acute: spiking fever and chills; signs of heart failure; WBC elevation

2. Subacute: fever of unknown origin; cough; dyspnea; anorexia; malaise; normal WBC; anemia; and elevated erythrocyte sedimentation rate (ESR)

3. Both: positive blood cultures; new cardiac murmurs or change in existing murmur; embolic complications from segments of vegetation circulating to the organs and the extremities including petechiae, splinter hemorrhages in the nail beds, Roth's spots

D. Priority nursing diagnoses: Risk for injury: thrombus formation; Deficient knowledge: prevention of repeated infection

E. Planning and implementation

1. Manage IV therapy; assess for any signs of infection

2. Assess the appropriateness of home infusion therapy; client may require inpatient treatment in a subacute care facility if home infusion therapy is contraindicated (as with an IV drug abuser)

3. Provide for periods of rest and moderate periods of exercise to prevent venous stasis

4. Use anti-embolism stockings to prevent thrombus formation

5. Provide for diversional activity; client is restricted from resuming normal activity for 4 to 6 weeks

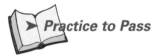

Practice to Pass

A client is completing her antibiotic treatment for subacute bacterial endocarditis (SBE). The client tells the nurse that she is so happy because now she can "finally go on with her life and forget that this ever happened." What should the nurse include in a response?

NCLEX!

F. Medication therapy

1. Consists of antibiotics given by the IV route

2. Must be given for 6 weeks

G. Client education

1. Instruct client and family about their role in home infusion therapy

NCLEX!

2. Explain that after one episode of endocarditis, client is susceptible to repeated infections because of lesions on the endocardium

NCLEX!

3. Instruct client and family about symptoms to report to physician, such as fever, anorexia, malaise

4. Instruct client about gentle, thorough oral care because infectious organisms can easily enter the bloodstream through the gums with vigorous brushing or oral treatments

NCLEX!

5. Explain the importance of prophylactic antibiotics prior to invasive procedures and routine dental care

H. Expected outcomes/evaluation

1. The client is free from signs of infection

2. The client maintains IV therapy at home (if appropriate)

3. The client describes signs and symptoms to report to MD

4. The client obtains prophylactic antibiotic therapy before invasive procedures

VII. Valvular Disorders

A. Description

1. Defects in structure or function of valves that interfere with proper cardiac circulation

2. Two major categories

   a. **Stenosis:** heart valve leaflets are fused together, opening is narrow, stiff, and unable to open or close properly

   b. **Regurgitation:** there is improper or incomplete closure of heart valves, resulting in back flow of blood

B. Etiology and pathophysiology

NCLEX!

1. Multiple causes including: rheumatic heart disease (most common), congenital, MI, endocarditis

2. Calcium deposits or scar tissue from endocarditis or MI may cause stiffening of valves in stenosis

3. Congenital malformations, scar tissue from MI, or fibrin strands from endocarditis may cause regurgitation

4. Right heart valve dysfunction usually develops in relation to other structural problems in the heart, and pulmonic defects are primarily congenital

C. Assessment

1. Heart sounds: valve dysfunctions each have characteristic changes in heart sounds (see Table 3-2)

2. Symptoms and severity depends on the extent of the valve dysfunction; from asymptomatic to signs of severe heart failure

3. Symptoms vary depending on the type of valve dysfunction (see Table 3-2)

D. Priority nursing diagnoses: Decreased cardiac output, Risk for injury: thrombus formation, Risk for infection, Deficient knowledge, Activity intolerance (late stage dysfunction)

E. Planning and implementation

1. Interventions depend upon the severity of the symptoms and type of dysfunction (refer again to Table 3-2)

2. Monitor heart sounds to assess for changes

3. With signs of decreased cardiac output, manage or restrict activity to decrease demands on the heart

4. Monitor for signs of endocarditis

5. Report changes to MD

Table 3-2

Valve Disorder	Specific Assessment	Planning and Implementation
Mitral Stenosis	Murmur: low pitched rumbling diastolic Common in young women Atrial dysrhythmias, especially atrial fibrillation (A-fib)	Monitor closely during pregnancy Administer diuretics and digitalis as prescribed Maintain sodium restricted diet Anticoagulant therapy if A-fib present Prepare for surgery
Mitral Regurgitation (Insufficiency)	Murmur: high-pitched blowing systolic Clients generally asymptomatic A-fib common with low incidence of embolization	Administer diuretics, nitrates and ACE inhibitors as prescribed Maintain sodium restricted diet
Mitral Prolapse	Murmur: systolic click Most clients asymptomatic May have PVCs and palpitations, syncope, weakness and anxiety	Administer beta blockers as prescribed for syncopy and palpitations Monitor for signs of infective endocarditis Administer prophylactic antibiotics with invasive procedures
Aortic Stenosis	Murmur: harsh systolic Late course symptoms: angina; S_3 and S_4; syncope	In symptomatic client, restrict activity to decrease myocardial oxygen consumption Monitor for signs of infective endocarditis Administer prophylactic antibiotics with invasive procedures Prepare for surgery: symptomatic aortic stenosis has poor prognosis without surgical intervention
Aortic Regurgitation (Insufficiency)	Murmur: blowing diastolic Widened pulse pressure Palpitations; tachycardia and PVCs	Medical management same as aortic stenosis Prepare for surgery which is the only effective long term therapy for aortic regurgitation

F. **Medication therapy**

   1. Is determined by symptoms

   2. Antidysrhythmic and anticoagulant therapy if atrial fibrillation present

   3. Antibiotic therapy if appropriate for endocarditis

   4. Medication regime to treat heart failure if appropriate

G. **Surgical interventions:** valve replacement

H. **Client education**

   1. Explain the importance of anticoagulant therapy to prevent thrombus formation

   2. Instruct client and family in the management of anticoagulation therapy with warfarin (Coumadin) if appropriate

      a. Monitor PT/INR values regularly because the effects of warfarin are influenced by physiological changes in the body, diet changes, or changes in medication

      b. Maintain consistent amount of food containing vitamin K in the diet including green leafy vegetables; variations may alter the effects of warfarin (Coumadin)

   3. Explain the connections among valve disorders, surgical valves, and increased risk for bacterial endocarditis

   4. Instruct client and family about methods to prevent endocarditis

I. **Expected outcomes/evaluation**

   1. The client reports no signs of endocarditis

   2. The client describes signs and symptoms to report to MD

   3. The client obtains prophylactic antibiotic therapy before invasive procedures

   4. The client with more advanced valve disorder maintains optimal level of function

VIII. **Cardiomyopathy**

A. **Description**

   1. Is an abnormality of the heart muscle

   2. Leads to functional changes in the heart

B. **Etiology and pathophysiology**

   1. Cause is unknown; however, in some cases is associated with viral infections, chronic alcohol abuse, or pregnancy

   2. Three types: dilated, hypertrophic, and restrictive

      a. Dilated cardiomyopathy (most common): enlargement of all four chambers, starting with enlarged ventricles, followed by decreased contractility; cardiac output progressively decreases

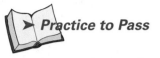

Practice to Pass

A client has had a valve repair surgery and has a new prescription for warfarin (Coumadin). What would the nurse include in the client teaching?

NCLEX!

NCLEX!

NCLEX!

b. Hypertrophic cardiomyopathy: unexplained progressive thickening of ventricular muscle mass causing increased pulmonary and venous pressures; cardiac output progressively decreases

c. Restrictive cardiomyopathy (least common): excessively rigid ventricular walls do not stretch during diastolic filling, creating back pressure and right heart failure, as well as reduced stroke volume and consequently, lowered cardiac output

C. Assessment

NCLEX!

1. Fatigue with all types

2. Dilated: weakness, signs of left heart failure, S_3 and S_4

3. Hypertrophic: exertional dyspnea, syncope, angina, signs of heart failure, S_4, sudden death often the first sign in asymptomatic individuals

4. Restrictive: dyspnea, right-sided heart failure, S_3 and S_4, emboli formation

D. Priority nursing diagnoses: Decreased cardiac output, Activity intolerance, Hopelessness

E. Planning and implementation

NCLEX!

NCLEX!

1. Monitor indicators of level of heart failure (vital signs, lung sounds, edema, dyspnea, activity tolerance)

2. Encourage rest and minimize stressful situations to reduce the workload on the heart

3. Provide counseling and psychological support because of poor prognosis

F. Medication therapy

1. There is no medical therapy to cure or prevent cardiomyopathy; medical regime is intended to treat symptoms

2. Medications are used to treat signs of heart failure (see section V F)

3. Anticoagulation therapy is used with restrictive cardiomyopathy to prevent emboli

G. Client education

1. Instruct client to avoid alcohol consumption because of its cardiac depressant effects

2. Assist clients in planning to pace their activities to reduce cardiac workload

3. Instruct client in medication and dietary for the management of heart failure

4. Explain anticoagulation therapy and monitoring if appropriate to prevent emboli formation

H. Expected outcomes/evaluation

1. The client maintains optimal level of activity

2. The client has clear lung sounds

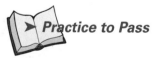

Practice to Pass

The nurse has a new admission with a diagnosis of restrictive cardiomyopathy. What signs of heart failure would the nurse expect to observe in this client?

3. The client has vital signs within normal limits (WNL)

4. The client shows decreased peripheral edema

5. The client follows medication regime

6. The client observes low-sodium, potassium-rich diet

IX. Pericarditis

A. Description: inflammation of the pericardium

B. Etiology and pathophysiology

NCLEX!

1. Acute pericarditis: may have multiple causes including infectious processes (viral the most common organism), post-MI (*Dressler's syndrome*) status, neoplasms, trauma, uremia, connective tissue diseases, or endocrine diseases

2. Chronic pericarditis: chronic pericardial inflammation causes fibrous thickening of the pericardium, constricting movement of the myocardium and restricting diastolic filling

C. Assessment

1. Acute: substernal pain, radiating to the neck, aggravated by breathing (particularly during inspiration) or coughing; friction rub (scratchy high-pitched sound on auscultation); elevated WBC; fever; malaise ECG changes including ST and T wave elevations followed by inverted T waves when ST returns to baseline

2. Chronic restrictive pericarditis: increasing dyspnea, fatigue leading to progressive signs of heart failure

D. Priority nursing diagnoses: Pain, Risk for decreased cardiac output; Risk for ineffective breathing pattern related to pain

E. Planning and implementation

1. Assess and manage pain

2. Administer oxygen as ordered and monitor SO_2

NCLEX!

3. Monitor for complications, especially cardiac **tamponade** (medical emergency resulting from excess fluid collection in the pericardial sac which interferes with heart filling and function); signs include:

   a. Jugular venous distention (JVD) with clear lungs

   b. Elevated CVP

   c. Narrowing pulse pressure

   d. Decreased cardiac output

NCLEX!

   e. Muffled heart sounds

4. Report significant changes to physician immediately

5. Position client for comfort: high Fowler's, sitting, or side-lying

6. Provide for periods of rest and limit activity to decrease cardiac workload

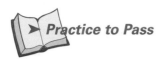

Practice to Pass

The nurse is caring for a client with pericarditis. What is a serious complication of this diagnosis, and what would the nurse recognize as signs of this complication?

NCLEX!

NCLEX!

F. Medication therapy

1. Analgesics for pain

2. Nonsteroidal anti-inflammatory medications (NSAIDs) initially, followed by steroids if inflammation doesn't respond to NSAIDs

3. Avoid anticoagulants because of risk of tamponade

4. Antibiotic therapy if inflammation is caused by bacterial microbes

G. Other medical interventions

1. Pericardiocentesis: procedure to remove fluid from the pericardial sac, performed for diagnostic analysis of the fluid to determine cause or as emergency treatment for tamponade

2. Dialysis for inflammation caused by uremia

3. Radiation to treat neoplasms

H. Client education

1. Explain inflammatory process to reduce anxiety

2. Stress medication management, especially the course of inflammatory medications, dosages, side effects

3. Instruct client to take food, milk, or antacids with anti-inflammatory medications to reduce gastric distress

4. Explain the risk for repeated episodes of pericarditis; emphasize symptoms to report (similar pain or dyspnea) promptly to physician

I. Expected outcomes/evaluation

1. The client reports no pain

2. The client describes signs and symptoms to report to physician

3. The client follows medication regime

Case Study

J. L. is a 62-year-old male who is scheduled to have coronary artery bypass surgery. His father died of a myocardial infarction(MI) at 65 years of age. J. L. has recently quit smoking. His cholesterol is 220 mg/dL with an HDL of 40 mg/dL. You are the nurse caring for J. L.

❶ What will you do to prepare J. L. for surgery?

❷ What assessments will you perform for J. L. when he is awaiting surgery?

❸ What will be your nursing diagnoses in the postoperative period?

❹ When he is transferred out of critical care, for what complications will you monitor J. L.?

❺ What discharge teaching do you plan for J. L. when he is ready to go home after his surgery?

For suggested responses, see page 735.

Posttest

1. A client is prescribed sublingual nitroglycerine for the treatment of angina pectoris. What response from the client indicates that the client understands this medication?

   (1) "Will the physician give me a year's supply of nitroglycerine tablets?"
   (2) "I will carry my nitroglycerine tablets in the inside pocket of my jacket, so they are always close."
   (3) "I usually take three of my nitroglycerine tablets at the same time. I find that they work better that way."
   (4) "I have a small labeled case for a few nitroglycerine tablets that I carry with me when I go out."

2. A client is being evaluated for a possible myocardial infarction. The nurse performs a 12-lead ECG for an episode of new chest pain. The nurse will monitor for which sign of acute myocardial injury?

   (1) ST depressions
   (2) ST elevations
   (3) New Q wave
   (4) New U wave

3. The nurse is caring for a client who underwent a percutaneous transluminal coronary angioplasty (PTCA) 4 hours previously. The client has no change in the catheter site or vital signs since returning from the procedure. The nurse obtains a 12-lead ECG and notes that the client has ST depressions. The client denies any chest pain. Which of the following is the next action that the nurse should take?

   (1) Notify the MD.
   (2) Continue to assess the client for chest pain.
   (3) Administer nitroglycerine.
   (4) Apply pressure to the catheter site.

4. The nurse is caring for a client who is being discharged after valve replacement surgery. The client has a new St. Jude Medical valve, and the nurse is reviewing the instructions for the client's follow-up care. The nurse determines that the client understands an important aspect of responsibility in the care of this valve when the client makes which of the following statements?

   (1) "I will take warfarin (Coumadin) for 2 months and get my blood drawn every week until I stop taking them."
   (2) "I will remind the doctor to give me a prescription for anticoagulant medication every time I go to the dentist."
   (3) "I will need to take anticoagulant medication for the rest of my life."
   (4) "I won't take any anticoagulant medication or blood thinners because they may cause a problem with my new valve."

5. The nurse is caring for a client on the 3rd postoperative day after coronary artery bypass (CABG) surgery. Because an important nursing diagnosis for post-CABG clients is Ineffective breathing pattern, what is the best plan by the nurse?

   (1) Ensure that the client performs deep breathing and vigorous coughing every hour
   (2) Ensure that the client uses the incentive spirometer every hour
   (3) Premedicate the client before ambulation
   (4) Auscultate lungs once a shift

6. The nurse is caring for a client with angina pectoris who was ruled out for a myocardial infarction. The nurse reviews the client's laboratory results and plans to include dietary teaching after noting that the client's lipid profile shows which of the following sets of values?

   (1) Cholesterol: 180, HDL: 40, triglycerides: 220
   (2) Cholesterol: 190, HDL: 40, triglycerides: 160
   (3) Cholesterol: 120, HDL: 25, triglycerides: 220
   (4) Cholesterol: 220, HDL: 40, triglycerides: 190

7 The nurse is caring for a client with new onset atrial fibrillation. The nurse anticipates that which of the following is a possible treatment for this dysrhythmia when it first develops?

(1) External pacemaker application
(2) Insertion of automatic internal cardiac defibrillator (AICD)
(3) Synchronized cardioversion
(4) Defibrillation

8 The nurse is assessing a client the morning of a scheduled cardiac stress test. The client reports that no breakfast was delivered this morning and the client is hungry. Which of the following is the nurse's best action?

(1) Bring the client coffee and toast.
(2) Explain that a client should have no food the morning of a cardiac stress test.
(3) Call the nutrition department and get the client's regular full breakfast.
(4) Have the nursing assistant get the client cereal with milk and orange juice.

9 A hospitalized client has continuous ECG monitoring, and the monitor shows that the rhythm has changed to ventricular tachycardia. Which of the following is the first action that the nurse should take?

(1) Administer intravenous lidocaine according to emergency protocol.
(2) Obtain the defbrillator and defribillate the client.
(3) Quickly assess the client's level of consciousness, blood pressure, and pulse.
(4) Administer a precordial thump.

10 The physician has diagnosed a myocardial infarction on the basis of ECG changes for a client in the emergency room. The nurse is assessing the client frequently, and notes that the client seems forgetful, making the nurse repeat the explanations about the ECG and non-invasive blood pressure monitors. The nurse concludes that the client's response is most likely due to which of the following reasons?

(1) The client is showing signs of Alzheimer's disease.
(2) The client is showing signs of fear and anxiety.
(3) Nurses in the emergency room are too busy to properly explain the purpose of equipment.
(4) Memory lapses are common with clients experiencing myocardial infarctions.

See pages 131–132 for Answers and Rationales.

Answers and Rationales

Pretest

1 Answer: 2 *Rationale:* When cardiac tamponade occurs, the restriction reduces stroke volume, cardiac output, and blood pressure. The right atrium is restricted causing JVD and increasing pressure during diastole. While the decreased stroke volume decreases the pressure during systole, the client compensates for decreased stroke volume and cardiac output by increasing heart rate. Because of decreased filling pressure, cardiac output drops and blood pumped from the right heart is reduced. Lung sounds are usually clear; heart sounds become more distant and muffled because they are heard through the fluid collection in the pericardium.
Cognitive Level: Analysis
Nursing Process: Assessment; *Test Plan:* SECE

2 Answer: 2 *Rationale:* Once a client is diagnosed with SBE, he or she is at risk for repeated episodes. Taking prophylactic antibiotics prior to dental care is an important activity to prevent further infections. There is no routine sodium restriction with SBE. Antibiotic treatment for SBE is given by the IV route for the entire course. Although stopping smoking will decrease his risk factor for coronary artery disease, it does not affect the SBE.
Cognitive Level: Application
Nursing Process: Evaluation; *Test Plan:* HPM

3 Answer: 3 *Rationale:* Pulmonary edema in a client with heart failure is the accumulation of fluid in the alveoli characterized by increased rales, tachypnea, tachycardia, pink frothy sputum, decreased SO_2 and PO_2. The client presents with acute restlessness and

anxiety. Urine output is generally decreased in heart failure clients; increased urinary output is usually caused by diuretic therapy.
Cognitive Level: Application
Nursing Process: Analysis; *Test Plan:* PHYS

4 **Answer: 1** *Rationale:* The dye typically used for cardiac angiography is iodine based. The client with known allergy to seafood is at risk for anaphylaxis and requires alternate media; atrial fibrillation and chronic renal failure are not contraindications to cardiac angiography; 5.0 mEq/L is a normal value for potassium.
Cognitive Level: Application
Nursing Process: Implementation; *Test Plan:* PHYS

5 **Answer: 3** *Rationale:* Daily weight is the most sensitive indicator of changes in fluid status. It is more accurate for a client at home than urine output. A fluid restriction may be recommended for a client with advanced heart failure, but it is not a method of monitoring fluid status. The client should never adjust the dose of his or her medications.
Cognitive Level: Analysis
Nursing Process: Planning; *Test Plan:* HPM

6 **Answer: 2** *Rationale:* Bedrest is prescribed to allow the arterial puncture to seal and reduce the risk of bleeding. Explaining the rationale to the client is the best way to facilitate the client's cooperation. Although the factual information in the other options may be true, it does not assist the client to understand the basis for care restrictions.
Cognitive Level: Analysis
Nursing Process: Implementation; *Test Plan:* PSYC

7 **Answer: 4** *Rationale:* Metoprolol (Lopressor) is a beta blocker, and it slows heart rate; the main therapeutic effect after a MI is to reduce cardiac workload. It does not dilate the coronary arteries, and it actually decreases the contractility (strength of the heartbeat).
Cognitive Level: Analysis
Nursing Process: Implementation; *Test Plan:* PHYS

8 **Answer: 1** *Rationale:* A prudent diet would be high in potassium because digoxin and furosemide can both deplete potassium. The diet needs to be low in sodium to prevent additional fluid overload with heart failure. Chicken, potato, and cantaloupe are all potassium-rich foods; options 2, 3, and 4 are higher in sodium.
Cognitive Level: Analysis
Nursing Process: Evaluation; *Test Plan:* PHYS

9 **Answer: 4** *Rationale:* Although some clients may have fear, hopelessness, or knowledge deficit related to their disease progression, most clients with cardiomyopathy are likely to have decreased cardiac output and corresponding activity intolerance. More data would be needed to determine whether the other nursing diagnoses apply.
Cognitive Level: Analysis
Nursing Process: Planning; *Test Plan:* PHYS

10 **Answer: 4** *Rationale:* A client who is in ventricular fibrillation requires immediate defibrillation; a client with atrial fibrillation may require synchronized cardioversion; a client with ventricular tachycardia may require defibrillation. The client with second-degree heart block is the client in this group who would most likely need a pacemaker.
Cognitive Level: Comprehension
Nursing Process: Planning; *Test Plan:* SECE

Posttest

1 **Answer: 4** *Rationale:* Nitroglycerine loses potency over time when exposed to light and heat. They should be kept cool, dry, and in a dark container. Clients should get a new bottle every 6 months, and store them in a cool place; tablets should be taken 5 minutes apart, taking more that one tablet at a time can actually decrease the effectiveness of the drug and may cause severe hypotension.
Cognitive Level: Application
Nursing Process: Evaluation; *Test Plan:* HPM

2 **Answer: 2** *Rationale:* ST elevations indicate immediate myocardial injury; ST depressions indicate myocardial ischemia; a Q wave forms several days after a myocardial infarction; a U wave is a sign of hypokalemia.
Cognitive Level: Application
Nursing Process: Assessment; *Test Plan:* PHYS

3 **Answer: 1** *Rationale:* ST depressions are a sign of ischemia. The physician should be notified immediately of any signs of ischemia after PTCA. This is the best first action, after which the nurse should continue to assess the client for chest pain. Administration of nitroglycerine without an order is not an appropriate nursing action. There is no sign of bleeding at the site; therefore, there is no indication to apply pressure.
Cognitive Level: Analysis
Nursing Process: Implementation; *Test Plan:* PHYS

4 **Answer: 3** *Rationale:* St. Jude Medical is a mechanical valve. Life-long anticoagulation therapy is required with this mechanical valve because there is a risk of thrombus formation. If a valve is replaced with a tissue valve, anticoagulation may be required during the immediate postoperative period but is not necessarily lifelong. It is recommended to take antibiotics prior to dental care.
Cognitive Level: Analysis
Nursing Process: Evaluation; *Test Plan:* HPM

5 **Answer: 2** *Rationale:* Vigorous coughing is discouraged for post-CABG clients because it may increase intrathoracic pressure and cause instability in the sternal area. Incentive spirometry and deep-breathing are the preferred techniques for lung expansion with these clients. Premedication before ambulation will facilitate activity tolerance; auscultating lungs will detect adventitious lung souds resulting from the ineffective breathing pattern, but it is not an action to encourage effective breathing patterns.
Cognitive Level: Analysis
Nursing Process: Planning; *Test Plan:* PHYS

6 **Answer: 4** *Rationale:* A cholesterol level > 200 indicates elevated cholesterol; the ratio of HDL to total cholesterol of less than 1:5 indicates increased cardiovascular risk; triglycerides > 190 indicate increased risk, (exception: triglycerides >190 without elevated cholesterol do not indicate increased cardiac risk until they reach 250).
Cognitive Level: Analysis
Nursing Process: Assessment; *Test Plan:* HPM

7 **Answer: 3** *Rationale:* Synchronized cardioversion is most effective with new-onset atrial fibrillation. Pacemakers are indicted for heart block, AICDs are used for ventricular dysrhythmias, and defibrillation is indicated for ventricular fibrillation and pulseless ventricular tachycardia.
Cognitive Level: Application
Nursing Process: Planning; *Test Plan:* PHYS

8 **Answer: 4** *Rationale:* The client should have a light meal with no caffeine before a cardiac stress test. Options 1, 2, and 3 are incorrect because they do not follow this guideline.
Cognitive Level: Application
Nursing Process: Implementation; *Test Plan:* PHYS

9 **Answer: 3** *Rationale:* The best first action is to assess the client's level of consciousness and assess if the ventricular tachycardia is perfusing the body (BP, pulse). With pulseless ventricular tachycardia, immediate defibrillation is performed by an ACLS certified nurse. If the client has a good BP and pulse, is awake and alert, the nurse may administer lidocaine as prescribed or, in some cases, administer a precordial thump.
Cognitive Level: Analysis
Nursing Process: Implementation; *Test Plan:* SECE

10 **Answer: 2** *Rationale:* Anxiety and fear are common responses to a diagnosis of myocardial infarction because of the possibility of death. This prevents the client and family from absorbing the detailed explanations about the care being provided. Memory lapses are not a common symptom of myocardial infarction, and there is not adequate information to determine that this memory lapse is associated with Alzheimer's disease. Nurses in the emergency room are able to explain procedures well to their clients.
Cognitive Level: Analysis
Nursing Process: Analysis; *Test Plan:* PSYC

References

AHCPR (1994). *Heart failure: Evaluation and care of patients with left-ventricular systolic dysfunction.* Rockville, MD: AHCRP Publication No. 94-0612, Clinical Practice Guideline Number 11.

Corbett, J. (2003). *Laboratory tests and diagnostic procedures with nursing diagoses* (6th ed). Upper Saddle River, NJ: Prentice-Hall, Inc. p. 287.

Craven, R. & Hirnle, C. (2003). *Fundamentals of nursing: Human health and function* (4th ed.). Philadelphia: Lippincott, pp. 884–889, 897.

Deglin, J. & Vallerand, A. (2003). *Davis's drug guide for nurses* (8th ed.). Philadelphia: F. A. Davis Co., pp. 287–291, 868–871.

Dudek, S. (2000). *Nutrition handbook for nursing practice* (4th ed.). Philadelphia: Lippincott, pp. 59–83, 544–599.

Gerard. P. & Tazbir, J. (2001). Management of clients with functional cardiac disorders. In J. Black, J. Hawks, & A. Keene (Eds.), *Medical-surgical nursing: Clinical management for positive outcomes* (6th ed.). Philadelphia: W. B. Saunders, pp. 1515–1550.

Grajeda-Higley, L. (2000). *Understanding pharmacology: A physiological approach.* Stamford, CT: Appleton & Lange.

Kozier, B., Erb, G., Berman, A., & Burke, K. (2004). *Fundamentals of nursing: Concepts, process and practice* (4th ed.). Upper Saddle River, NJ: Prentice Hall, Inc. p. 325.

LeMone, P. & Burke, K. (2004). *Medical-surgical nursing: Critical thinking in client care* (3rd ed.). Upper Saddle River, NJ: Prentice Hall, Inc. pp. 1015–1029, 1030–1174.

Lutz, C. & Przytulski, K. (2001). *Nutrition and diet therapy* (3rd ed.). Philadelphia: F.A. Davis, pp. 361–383.

Murphy, M. & Bending, C. (1999). Use of measurements of myoglobin and cardiac troponins in the diagnosis of acute myocardial infarction. *Critical care nurse 19,* 1:58–66.

Ochs, G. & Ochs, M. (1997). *Recognition & interpretation of ECG rhythms.* Stamford, CT: Appleton & Lange, pp. 1–66.

Ott, B. (2001). Management of clients with structural cardiac disorders. In J. Black, J. Hawks, & A. Keene (Eds.), *Medical-surgical nursing: Clinical management for positive outcomes* (6th ed.). Philadelphia: W. B. Saunders, pp. 1481–1514.

Pagana, K. & Pagana, T. (2001). *Mosby's diagnostic and laboratory test reference.* (5th ed.). St. Louis: Mosby, Inc. pp. 183, 207–210, 293–296, 332, 501–503, 514–515.

Perrin, K. (2002). Assessment of the cardiovascular system. In. D. Ignatavicius, & M. Workman (Eds.), *Medical-surgical nursing: Critical thinking for collaborative care* (4th ed.). Philadelphia: W.B. Saunders, pp. 619–652.

Perrin, K. (2002). Interventions for clients with cardiac problems. In D. Ignatavicius & M. Workman (Eds.), *Medical-surgical nursing: Critical thinking for collaborative care* (4th ed.). Philadelphia: W. B. Saunders. pp. 698–726.

Perrin, K. (2002). Interventions for critically ill clients with coronary artery disease. In D. Ignatavicius & M. Workman (Eds.), *Medical-surgical nursing: Critical thinking for collaborative care* (4th ed.). Philadelphia: W. B. Saunders, pp. 789–817.

Perrin, C. (2002). Interventions with clients with dysrhythmias. In D. Ignatavicius & M. Workman (Eds.), *Medical-surgical nursing: Critical thinking for collaborative care* (4th cd.). Philadelphia: W. B. Saunders, pp. 654–696.

Puetz, B. (1998). Nursing practice guidelines for the cardiac home care patient. Pensacola, FL: Home Healthcare Nurses Association, pp. 15–33.

Shumate, P. (2001). Assessment of the cardiac system. In J. Black, J. Hawks, & A. Keene (Eds.), *Medical-surgical nursing: Clinical management for positive outcomes* (6th ed.). Philadelphia: W. B. Saunders, pp. 1447–1480.

Vaughn, G. (1999). *Understanding and evaluating commonly requested laboratory tests.* Stamford, CT: Appleton & Lange, pp. 229–246.

Wilson, B., Shannon, M., & Stang, C. (2003). *Prentice Hall nursing drug guide 2003.* Upper Saddle River, New Jersey: Prentice Hall Health, pp. 230–237, 453–454, 910–911, 999–1002.

Peripheral Vascular Health Problems

Susan Letvak, PhD, RN

CHAPTER OUTLINE

OBJECTIVES

- Identify basic structures and functions of the peripheral vascular system.

- Describe the pathophysiology and etiology of common peripheral vascular disorders.

- Discuss expected assessment data and diagnostic findings for selected peripheral vascular disorders.

- Identify priority nursing diagnoses for selected peripheral vascular disorders.

- Discuss therapeutic management of selected vascular disorders.

- Discuss nursing management of a client experiencing a peripheral vascular disorder.

- Identify expected outcomes for the client experiencing a peripheral vascular disorder.

[*Media Link*]

Use the CD-ROM enclosed with this text, or log onto the address given to access the free, interactive Companion Website created for this series. The CD-ROM and Companion Website accompanying this book offer additional practice opportunities and information—NCLEX Review, Case Studies, Glossary, In Depth with NCLEX, and more.

www.prenhall.com/hogan

REVIEW AT A GLANCE

atherosclerosis *local accumulation of lipid and fibrous tissue along the intimal layer of an artery*

endarterectomy *opening of artery and removal of obstructing plaque*

Homan's sign *pain on dorsiflexion of the foot when the leg is raised*

intermittent claudication *ischemic muscle pain precipitated by a predictable amount of exercise and relieved by rest*

Korotkoff sounds *sounds heard in auscultation of blood pressure*

neurovascular status *color, motion, sensation, temperature, and presence of distal peripheral pulses*

orthostatic hypotension *a drop in blood pressure of 10 to 20 mmHg with upright posture*

poikilothermia *body temperature that varies with environment*

rest pain *pain while resting that may even awaken the client at night; pain is usually in the distal portion of the extremity (toes, arch, forefoot, heel) and is relieved when foot is placed in the dependent position*

sympathectomy *surgical dissection of the nerve fibers that allows vasoconstriction to occur*

vasodilation *widening of the blood vessel*

Pretest

1 A client with hypertension has a blood pressure of 170/96 after 6 months of intensive exercise and diet modifications. The nurse advises the client:

(1) To continue current treatment plan as blood pressure is being adequately controlled.
(2) To discontinue current treatment plan as it has not been effective and medications will be required.
(3) To increase his exercise by two-fold and continue dietary modifications to attempt to lower blood pressure further.
(4) That medication therapy will likely need to be started along with the exercise and diet program.

2 Evidence that the outcome of increased arterial blood supply to the extremity has been met in a client with peripheral arterial disease includes:

(1) Reduced muscle pain.
(2) Reduced sensation to touch.
(3) Increased rubor.
(4) Decreased hair on the extremity.

3 In teaching a hypertensive client about the side effects of propranolol (Inderal) the nurse plans to include which side effect of this medication therapy?

(1) Hypokalemia
(2) Constipation
(3) Heart failure
(4) Tachycardia

4 A client is at high risk for developing deep vein thrombosis. Which of the following manifestations does the nurse assess for?

(1) Absent pulse and pale extremity
(2) Ulcerated toes and rubor
(3) Cyanotic extremity and numbness
(4) Leg swelling and calf pain

5 Your client on furosemide (Lasix) therapy demonstrates understanding of how to increase potassium in his diet when he states he will add which of the following beverages to his diet?

(1) Milk
(2) Cranberry juice
(3) Coffee
(4) Orange juice

6 Which of the following findings in a client awaiting abdominal aortic aneurysm repair would you report immediately to the physician?

(1) Severe back pain
(2) Swelling of the arms and face
(3) Increased blue areas of the feet
(4) Hoarseness or difficulty swallowing

7 Which of the following laboratory values is most important for the nurse to assess to monitor therapeutic levels of heparin therapy?

(1) Prothrombin time (PT)
(2) Partial thromboplastin time (PTT)
(3) Clotting time
(4) Bleeding time

8 A client complains of pain and cramping after short periods of walking that stop when he rests. The nurse concludes he is describing which of the following symptoms of peripheral arterial disease?

(1) Arterial-venous shunting
(2) Phlebitis
(3) Intermittent claudication
(4) Raynaud's phenomenon

9 Which nursing activity would be important to add to the plan of care for an older adult suspected of having orthostatic hypotension?

(1) Teaching the client to get out of bed slowly
(2) Monitoring all blood pressure readings when the client is lying down
(3) Taking blood pressure readings in both arms
(4) Teaching the client about the use of sublingual nitroglycerin

10 When educating the client with primary hypertension, the nurse instructs the client to:

(1) Take anti-hypertensive medications when blood pressure is elevated.
(2) Monitor blood pressure annually.
(3) Avoid foods with concentrated sugars.
(4) Have regular eye exams.

See pages 163–164 for Answers and Rationales.

I. Overview of Anatomy and Physiology

A. Structure and function of blood vessels

1. Blood vessels are channels through which blood is distributed to body tissues

2. Walls of an artery or vein consist of three layers: tunica intima, tunica media, and tunica adventitia; the thickness of the walls and amount of connective tissue and smooth muscle depends upon the amount of pressure the vessel must endure

3. They are divided into the arterial system and the venous system

   a. Arterial system (Figure 4-1): consists of high-pressure vessels, the largest of which is the aorta; some branch into arterioles, which measure less than 0.5 mm in diameter; functions to deliver blood to various tissues for nourishment and contribute to tissue temperature regulation

   b. Venous system (Figure 4-2): consists of large diameter, thin-walled vessels that are under much less pressure; some veins, most commonly in the legs, contain valves to regulate one-way flow; functions to return blood from the capillaries to the right atrium for circulation and acts as a reservoir for blood volume

B. Circulation and dynamics of blood flow

1. Blood flow is the amount of fluid moved per unit of time through a vessel, organ, or throughout the entire circulatory system; regulated by:

   a. Pressure: there is a pressure differential between the arterial and venous vessels, with blood flowing from the arterial "side" of the capillaries to the lower pressured venous side

Figure 4-1 **Major arteries of the systemic circulation.**

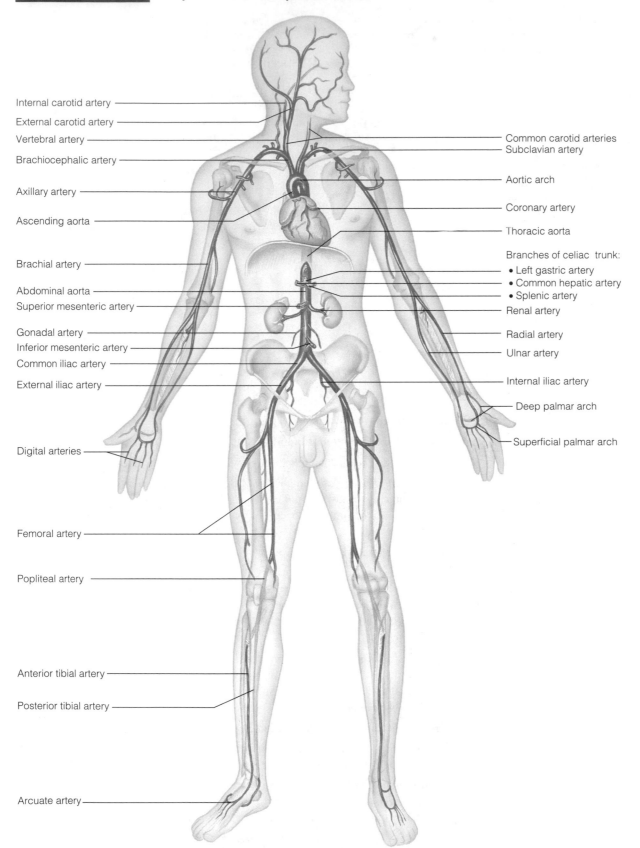

Internal carotid artery

External carotid artery

Vertebral artery

Brachiocephalic artery

Axillary artery

Ascending aorta

Brachial artery

Abdominal aorta

Superior mesenteric artery

Gonadal artery

Inferior mesenteric artery

Common iliac artery

External iliac artery

Digital arteries

Femoral artery

Popliteal artery

Anterior tibial artery

Posterior tibial artery

Arcuate artery

Common carotid arteries

Subclavian artery

Aortic arch

Coronary artery

Thoracic aorta

Branches of celiac trunk:
• Left gastric artery
• Common hepatic artery
• Splenic artery

Renal artery

Radial artery

Ulnar artery

Internal iliac artery

Deep palmar arch

Superficial palmar arch

Figure 4-2 Major veins of the systemic circulation.

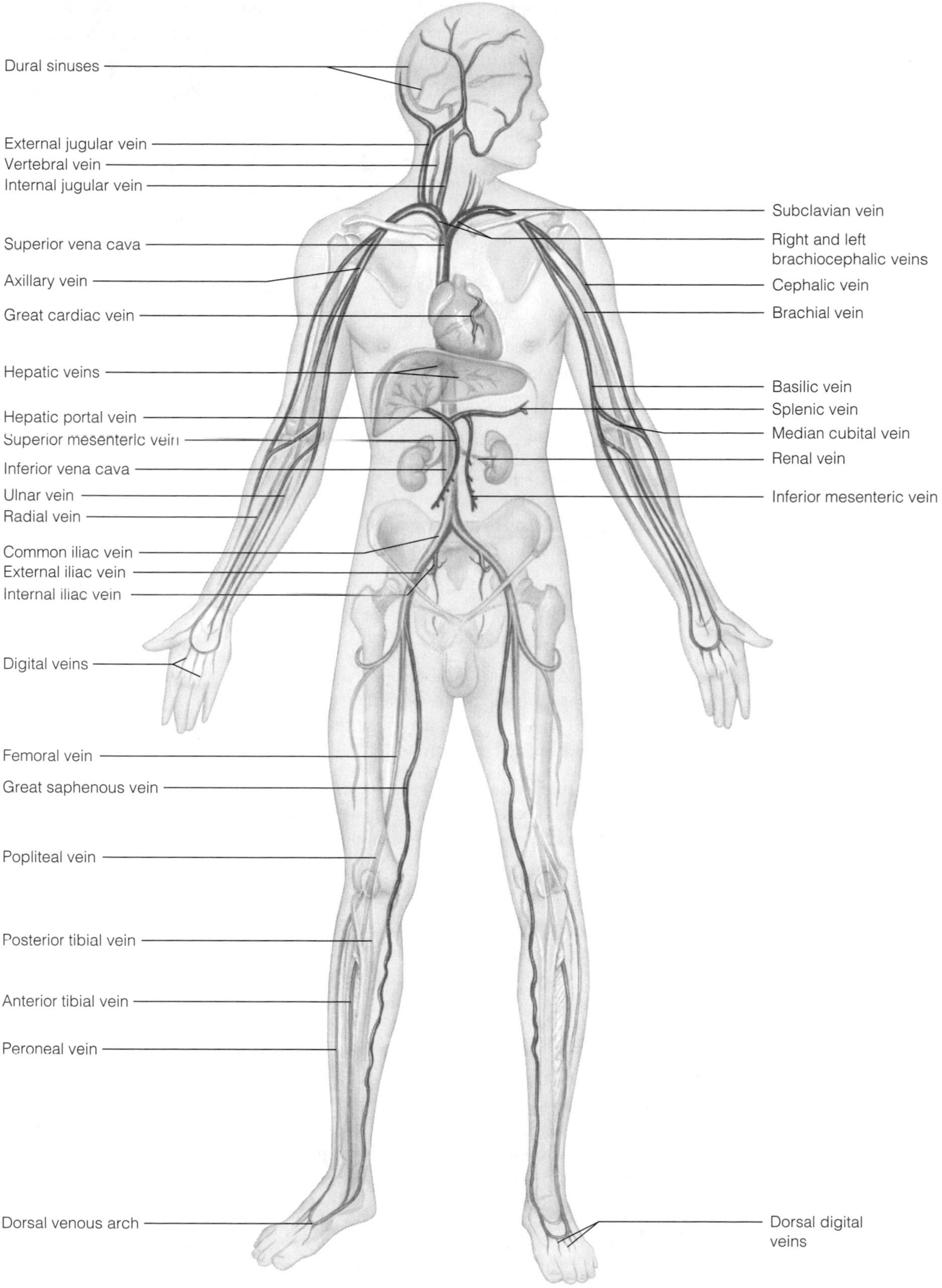

Dural sinuses

External jugular vein
Vertebral vein
Internal jugular vein

Superior vena cava

Axillary vein

Great cardiac vein

Hepatic veins

Hepatic portal vein
Superior mesenteric vein
Inferior vena cava

Ulnar vein
Radial vein

Common iliac vein
External iliac vein
Internal iliac vein

Digital veins

Femoral vein

Great saphenous vein

Popliteal vein

Posterior tibial vein

Anterior tibial vein

Peroneal vein

Dorsal venous arch

Subclavian vein
Right and left
brachiocephalic veins
Cephalic vein
Brachial vein

Basilic vein
Splenic vein
Median cubital vein
Renal vein

Inferior mesenteric vein

Dorsal digital
veins

139

    b. Resistance: opposition to blood flow; increased resistance leads to decreased blood flow; peripheral vascular resistance is determined by blood viscosity, length of vessel, and diameter of the vessel

    c. Velocity: the distance blood must travel in the unit of time

    d. Compliance: the increase in volume a vessel can accommodate for a given increase in pressure; veins are much more compliant than arteries and thus can serve as storage areas in the circulatory system

C. Blood pressure control: blood pressure is the pressure of blood against vessel walls; it is controlled by several factors

  1. Autonomic nervous system:

    a. Sympathetic nervous system: increases the heart rate (HR), the speed of impulse conduction through the atrioventricular (AV) node, and the force of atrial and ventricular contractions

    b. Parasympathetic nervous system: causes a decrease in HR by the action of the sinoatrial (SA) node and slows conduction through the AV node

  2. Baroreceptors: stimulation of these receptors located in the aortic arch and carotid sinus causes information to be sent to the vasomotor center in the brain stem to enhance the parasympathetic system, causing a decrease in HR and peripheral **vasodilation,** or widening of the blood vessel

  3. Chemoreceptors: areas stimulated by decreased arterial oxygen pressure, increased carbon dioxide pressure, and decreased plasma pH to stimulate the vasomotor center and increase cardiac activity

  4. Antidiuretic hormone (ADH): a decrease in total blood volume in the circulatory system leads the posterior pituitary gland to release ADH, causing reabsorption of water by the kidney, resulting in increased blood plasma volume and increased blood pressure

  5. Renin-angiotensin-aldosterone system: in response to sympathetic stimulation or decreased blood flow through the kidneys, the kidneys produce renin that generates angiotensin I and then angiotensin II; these are powerful vasoconstrictors that stimulate the release of aldosterone from the adrenal gland, allowing for sodium retention in the kidneys and then suppression of renin

  6. Other factors: other factors which may affect blood pressure control include temperature (cold = vasoconstriction), substances such as nicotine (vasoconstrictor) or alcohol (vasodilation), diet (sodium and fat intake), and factors such as age, gender, weight, physical health, and emotional state

II. Diagnostic Tests and Assessments

NCLEX!

A. Doppler ultrasound: measures the velocity of blood flow through a vessel and emits an audible signal; when arterial palpation is difficult or impossible because of occlusive disease, a Doppler can be useful in determining blood flow; a palpable pulse and a Doppler pulse are not equivalent and should not be used interchangeably

B. Plethysmography: records biologic changes in volume in a portion of the body associated with cardiac contractions or in response to pneumatic venous occlusion; can detect and quantify vascular disease on the basis of changes in pulse contour, blood pressure, or arterial/venous blood flow

C. Digital intravenous angiography: utilizing computer technology, visualization of blood vessels occurs after IV injection of contrast material; allows for small peripheral venous injections of contrast medium, compared with large doses that must be injected via arterial cannulation

D. Venography: injection of radiopaque dye into veins; serial x-rays are taken to detect deep vein thrombosis and incompetent valves

E. Angiography: injection of radiopaque dye into arteries to detect plaques, occlusions, injury, etc.

F. Ankle-brachial index: most commonly used parameter for overall evaluation of extremity status; ankle pressure normally is the same or higher than brachial systolic pressure

G. Computed tomography: allows for visualization of the arterial wall and its structures; used in the diagnosis of abdominal aortic aneurysm (AAA) and postoperative vascular complications such as graft occlusion and hemorrhage

H. Magnetic resonance imaging (MRI): uses magnetic fields rather than radiation; used with angiography to detect abnormalities, especially in people who are unable to have dye injected

III. Common Nursing Techniques and Procedures

A. Blood pressure measurement

1. Blood pressure (BP) is primarily a function of cardiac output and systemic vascular resistance

2. Arterial blood pressure = cardiac output × systemic vascular resistance

3. Proper technique

   a. Client should be seated with arm bared, supported, and at heart level

   b. Client should not have smoked or ingested caffeine 30 minutes prior

   c. BP should be taken in both arms initially

   d. Appropriate sized cuff must be used: rubber bladder should at least encircle the arm by 80 percent

   e. After palpating the brachial or radial pulse, inflate the cuff 30 mmHg above the level at which the pulse disappears

   f. Record systolic and diastolic sounds—known as **Korotkoff sounds** (the disappearance of sound is the diastolic reading)

   g. Two or more readings separated by 2 minutes should be averaged

   h. If the client's arms are inaccessible, you can obtain readings from the thigh or calf, auscultating the popliteal or posterior tibial arteries, respectively

IV. Primary Hypertension

A. Description: a disorder characterized by blood pressure that consistently exceeds 140/90, confirmed on at least two visits several weeks apart; onset is primarily in people 25 to 55; greatest occurrence is in African-Americans

B. Etiology and pathophysiology

    1. Hypertension can be primary (essential) or secondary; primary hypertension accounts for 90 to 95 percent of all cases; there is no known cause but risk factors include:

        a. Positive family history

        b. High sodium intake

        c. Obesity

        d. Inactivity

        e. Excessive alcohol intake

    2. Pathophysiology

        a. For arterial pressure to rise, there must be an increase in either cardiac output or systemic vascular resistance; later in the course of the disease systemic vascular resistance continues to rise as the cardiac output stabilizes

        b. There is no single cause for primary hypertension

C. Assessment

    1. Subjective data

        a. Past history of cardiovascular, cerebrovascular, renal, or thyroid diseases, diabetes, smoking, or alcohol use

        b. Family history of hypertension or cardiovascular disease

        c. Possible absence of symptoms

        d. Reports of fatigue, nocturia, dyspnea on exertion, palpitations, angina, headaches, weight gain, edema, muscle cramps, or blurred vision; symptoms may be caused by target organ damage rather than the high blood pressure itself

    2. Objective data

        a. BP consistently over 140 mmHg systolic and 90 mmHg diastolic

        b. Peripheral edema, retinal vessel changes, diminished/absent peripheral pulses, bruits, murmurs, and S_3 and S_4 heart sounds

    3. Diagnostic tests

        a. Abnormal potassium level (may be low if taking loop diuretics or high if taking potassium-sparing diuretics)

        b. Elevated blood urea nitrogen (BUN), creatinine, glucose, cholesterol and triglycerides

        c. Abnormal urinalysis

        d. Cardiomegaly on x-ray

        e. Abnormal ECG showing left ventricular hypertrophy

D. Priority nursing diagnoses: Ineffective health maintenance, Risk for noncompliance, Decreased cardiac output

E. Planning and implementation

1. Tell client the numeric blood pressure readings so he or she can keep an ongoing record

NCLEX!

2. Inform client that hypertension is usually asymptomatic, and symptoms will not reliably indicate BP levels

3. Explain that long-term followup and therapy will be necessary

4. Accurately record intake and output and daily weights of hospitalized clients

F. Medication therapy

1. No one primary drug is used; a combination of drugs are used until desired blood pressure is achieved with the least side effects

NCLEX!

2. Medications used include diuretics, beta-blockers, calcium channel blockers, angiotensin converting enzyme inhibitors (ACE) inhibitors and vasodilators (see Table 4-1)

3. The stepped care approach is often used to guide treatment; this protocol begins with lifestyle changes and adds medications based on response to previous therapy

G. Client education

NCLEX!

1. Teach lifestyle modification

   a. Sodium restriction

   b. Weight reduction

   c. DASH (dietary approaches to stop hypertension) diet: includes prescribed number of servings of food in the following categories: grains and grain products; vegetables; fruits; low-fat or nonfat dairy foods; meats, poultry, and fish; nuts, seeds, and legumes; fats and oils; and sweets

   d. Moderation of alcohol intake

   e. Exercise

   f. Relaxation techniques

   g. No smoking

2. Teach general medication therapy and potential side effects

NCLEX!

   a. Supplement potassium if taking loop diuretics

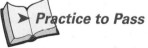

Practice to Pass

Your client with newly diagnosed hypertension has been told to follow a DASH diet by the physician. What teaching will you include when explaining the DASH diet to the client?

   b. Prevent **orthostatic hypotension** (a drop in blood pressure of 10 to 20 mmHg with upright posture) by rising out of the bed or chair slowly

   c. Avoid hot baths and strenuous exercise within 3 hours of taking vasodilators

3. Reinforce importance of adhering to treatment plan; compliance may be an issue if client does not understand that treatment can reduce risk of target organ damage or if the disorder is not taken seriously because there are no symptoms

H. Expected outcomes/evaluation

1. A decrease in blood pressure to less than 140/90

Table 4-1	Medications Commonly Used to Treat Peripheral Vascular Diseases		
Drug Class and Name: **Generic (Trade)**	**Therapeutic Use(s)**	**Mechanism of Action**	**Nursing Responsibilities**
Alpha-Adrenergic Blockers: Prazosin hydrochloride (Minipress) Doxazosin (Cardura) Terazosin (Hytrin)	Hypertension	Act by blocking the alpha$_1$ receptors on arterioles and veins to cause vasodilation	Minipress may cause a "first dose" effect: may result in syncope 30 to 60 min after first dose: • give first dose at bed time • remain in bed at least 3 hours after first dose • avoid driving for at least 24 hours. Assess BP regularly—monitor BP in lying, standing, and sitting positions to detect orthostatic hypotension. Orthostatic hypotension most common side effect; teach client to: • change positions slowly • take med at bedtime when possible • avoid hazardous activities. Other side effects include light-headedness, impotence in men, reflex tachycardia, and nasal congestion.
Angiotensin-Converting Enzyme (ACE) Inhibitors Benazepril (Lotensin) Captopril (Capoten) Enalapril (Vasotec) Lisinopril (Zestril, Prinivil) Ramipril (Altace) Quinapril (Accupril)	Hypertension Raynaud's disease Congestive heart failure	Inhibits conversation of Angiotensin I to Angiotensin II (a potent vasoconstrictor). Reduces peripheral resistance without changing cardiac output.	Monitor vital signs and compare with baseline. Teach side effects: • loss of taste • dry cough • orthostatic hypotension (especially after first dose). Teach adverse reactions: • aspirin and NSAIDs may impair hypotensive effects • take one hour before meals • always consult MD before discontinuing • can cause fetal morbidity or mortality in pregnant women.
Beta-Adrenergic Blockers Acebutolol (Sectral) Atenolol (Tenormin) Betaxolol (Kerlone) Metoprolol (Lopressor) Nadolol (Corgard)	Hypertension Myocardial infarction Arrhythmias	Decrease BP by decreasing cardiac output, response to sympathetic nerve impulses and renin secretion by the kidneys; reduces systemic vascular resistance.	Monitor vital signs and compare with baseline. Assess client for heart failure and heart block by checking pulse regularly. Avoid in clients with COPD.

(continued)

Table 4-1	Medications Commonly Used to Treat Peripheral Vascular Diseases (continued)		
Drug Class and Name: Generic (Trade)	**Therapeutic Use(s)**	**Mechanism of Action**	**Nursing Responsibilities**
Propranolol (Inderal)			Teach client: • always consult MD before discontinuing • adverse side effects: orthostatic hypotension, bronchospasm, nightmares, hallucinations.
Calcium Channel Blockers Amlodipine (Norvasc) Diltiazem (Cardizem) Felodipine (Plendil) Isradipine (Dynacirc) Nifedipine (Procardia) Verapamil (Isoptin)	Hypertension	Decrease BP by blocking the movement of calcium in the cells of smooth muscles, which decreases peripheral resistance.	Teach client side effects: • nausea • headaches • orthostatic hypotension • edema. Avoid use in clients with CHF. Procardia is given sublingually except when rapid drop in BP is required and then it is chewed.
Centrally Acting Adrenergic Blockers Clonidine (Catapres) Methyldopa (Aldomet)	Hypertension	Act within the CNS to reduce the flow of impulses through the sympathetic nerves to the blood vessels and heart resulting in dilation of arteries and veins.	Teach side effects: • dry mouth • sedation • impotence • constipation • severe rebound hypertension if stopped quickly. Teach client: • to use sugarless gum or hard candy for dry mouth • that alcohol will increase CNS depression.
Diuretics *Thiazides* Chlorothiazide (Diuril) Chlorthalidone (Hygroton) Hydrochlorothiazide (HydroDiuril) Indapamide (Lozol) Metolazone (Zaroxolyn)	Edema Hypertension	Depress the ability of the convoluted tubules to reabsorb sodium and chloride. "Where water goes, so goes sodium."	Teach client: • side effects of electrolyte imbalance: • muscle weakness • dizziness • to take diuretic in the morning • to take with food if GI upset occurs • to weigh self every morning—report weight gain of more than 2 to 3 lb • to eat foods high in potassium (oranges, bananas, broccoli, tomato juice, apricots, etc.) • to avoid alcohol • to avoid black licorice—may precipitate hypokalemia • drug increases lithium toxicity.

(continued)

Table 4-1	Medications Commonly Used to Treat Peripheral Vascular Diseases (continued)		
Drug Class and Name: Generic (Trade)	**Therapeutic Use(s)**	**Mechanism of Action**	**Nursing Responsibilities**
Loop Bumetanide (Bumex) Furosemide (Lasix)	Potent diuretic for significant diuresis with edema.	Inhibit reabsorption of sodium and chloride in the proximal and distal tubules and loop of Henle.	Explain that this type of drug is very fast acting. Teach client to: • take diuretic in the morning • take with food or milk • avoid orthostasis • use sunscreen as increased photosensitivity may occur • take potassium supplement as ordered • weigh self daily and report increases of 2 to 3 lb.
Potassium-Sparing Amiloride (Midamor) Spironolactone (Aldactone)	Used with thiazide diuretics to prevent/correct hypokalemia.	Block sodium-potassium exchange mechanism in the distal portion of the tubule; prevent sodium reabsorption and retain potassium.	Teach client to: • take with food or milk • weigh self several times a week and report a gain of over 3 lb • avoid salt substitutes and foods high in potassium. Adverse side effects include: • gynecomastia • decreased libido.
Vasodilators Hydralazine (Apresoline) Sodium nitroprusside (Nipride) Nitroglycerin (Tridil)	Apresoline: arterial vasodilation. Nipride: Direct action in hypertensive emergencies. Tridil: venous vasodilation	All will work to lower BP by acting on the smooth muscle of the vascular system to cause vasodilation.	Apresoline: • Administer IV or IM for hypertensive crisis • Take p. o. medication with food • Monitor daily weights. Nipride: • Protect drug from light, heat, and moisture • Cover IV bag and tubing with foil • Discard any solution that is not light brown in color • Administer with sodium thio-sulfate to reduce the risk of cyanide toxicity. Tridil: • IV infusion only • Use only glass bottle and ad-ministration set provided • Gradually wean off IV dose.
Other Cilostazol (Pletal)	Intermittent claudication	Not fully understood; inhibits platelet aggregation and allows for vasodilation.	Minimal side effects. Take with meals. Do not use in clients with CHF. Do not take with grapefruit juice.
Pentoxifylline (Trental)	Intermittent claudication	Decreases the viscosity of blood resulting in increased blood flow to the microcirculation.	Take with meals. Initial effects may not be noticed for 6 to 8 weeks. Minimal side effects.

2. No target organ damage (kidneys, heart, nervous system, eyes)

3. Client voices understanding of the management of hypertension

V. Peripheral Arterial Disease

A. Description: disorders that interrupt or impede arterial peripheral blood flow due to vessel compression, vasospasm, and/or structural defects in the vessel wall

B. Etiology and pathophysiology

1. Peripheral arterial occlusive disease is primarily caused by **atherosclerosis** (local accumulation of lipid and fibrous tissue along the intimal layer of an artery), but also may be caused by trauma, embolism, thrombosis, vasospasm, inflammation or autoimmunity

2. By the time symptoms appear, the vessel is about 75 percent narrowed

3. The femoral-popliteal area is the site most commonly affected in non-diabetics; diabetic clients most often develop disease in the arteries below the knees

4. Chronic arterial obstruction leads to inadequate oxygenation of the tissues causing **intermittent claudication,** which is ischemic muscle pain precipitated by a predictable amount of exercise and relieved by rest

C. Assessment

1. Subjective

   a. Client reports aching, cramping, fatigue or weakness in the legs that is relieved by rest (claudication); this is an early indication of disease

   b. Client reports **rest pain,** which is pain that occurs while resting that may even awaken the client at night; pain is usually in the distal portion of the extremity (toes, arch, forefoot, heel) and is relieved when foot is placed in the dependent position; this indicates more advanced disease

   c. Client complains of coldness or numbness in the lower extremities

2. Objective

   a. Extremities may be cool and pale with a cyanotic color on elevation

   b. Bruits may be auscultated

   c. Peripheral pulses may be diminished or absent

   d. Nails may be thickened and opaque (trophic change)

   e. Skin on the legs may be shiny and atrophic with sparse hair growth (trophic change)

   f. Ulcers may be present on the lower extremities in areas affected by reduced circulation

3. Diagnostic testing

   a. Digital subtraction angiography (DSA)

   b. Angiography

   c. Doppler ultrasound

   d. Plethysmography

D. Priority nursing diagnoses: Ineffective tissue perfusion, Impaired skin integrity, Pain

E. Planning and implementation

1. Goal: adequate tissue perfusion

   a. Assess and record strength of pulses

   b. Encourage client to stop smoking as nicotine causes vasoconstriction and hypercoagulability of blood

   c. Teach client to change position at least hourly and avoid crossing the legs

   d. Encourage client to exercise and walk to the point of pain as this decreases claudication; explain to stop walking when pain occurs to decrease oxygen needs to affected area and to resume when pain has stopped in order to build tolerance to exercise and stimulate growth of collateral circulation

   e. Teach client to avoid restrictive clothing, including girdles, garters, and socks

2. Goal: relief of pain

   a. Assess pain on a 1 to 10 scale and provide analgesics as ordered

   b. Teach relaxation techniques because stress increases vasoconstriction

   c. Keep feet warm and in a dependent position; do not elevate feet if pain is present

3. Goal: intact, healthy skin on extremities

   a. Teach client skills in skin care and daily inspection of feet

   b. Teach client to always wear shoes/slippers and avoid trauma to the feet; bath water should be checked with the hands, not the feet, to prevent burns to tissue at high risk for injury that may also have decreased sensation

   c. Teach client to have toenail care performed by a professional only

   d. If an ulcer develops, healing will be slow unless arterial blood flow to the affected limb is improved through a surgical revascularization procedure

4. If surgery is indicated, provide appropriate postoperative care

   a. Angioplasty

      1) Monitor **neurovascular status** (color, motion, sensitivity, temperature, and presence of distal peripheral pulses) to the affected extremity every 15 min × 4, every 30 min × 4, then q 1–4 hr(s) after sheath removal

      2) Notify physician if client experiences weak or thready pulses, coolness, numbness, or tingling in the extremity

      3) Monitor the sheath site for signs of external and subcutaneous bleeding

      4) Instruct the client to notify the nurse and apply manual pressure to the site should a sensation of warmth or wetness be felt at the site

      5) Maintain immobilization of affected extremity for at least 6 hours by reminding client to keep extremity still or lightly immobilize ankle with sheet tucked under both sides of mattress

      6) Maintain a pressure dressing and sand bag at site

  b. Bypass grafting

   1) Provide standard postoperative care

   2) Assess for occlusion of graft by assessing for severe ischemic pain, loss of pulses, decreasing ankle-brachial index, numbness/tingling in extremity, coolness of the extremity

  c. **Endarterectomy** (opening the artery and removing obstructing plaque) or amputation in severe cases; use same principles of care

F. Medication therapy

 1. Aspirin inhibits platelet aggregation

 2. Pentoxifylline (Trental) decreases blood viscosity to increase blood flow to the microcirculation and tissues of the extremities

 3. Cilostazol (Pletal) inhibits platelet aggregation and enhances vasodilation

G. Client education

 1. Promote vasodilation: provide warmth (never by direct heat to the limb) and prevent long periods of exposure to cold; avoid use of restrictive clothing

 2. Proper positioning: keep feet dependent to increase blood flow to legs; may elevate feet at rest but not above level of the heart; never cross legs or ankles; following bypass surgery, may keep legs level with rest of body

 3. Stop smoking

 4. Meticulous foot care as would be performed by clients with diabetes mellitus

 5. Trental should be taken with food and any effects may take 6 to 8 weeks to notice

 6. Exercise program with weight reduction is helpful (see Box 4-1 for client education points for managing peripheral arterial disease)

NCLEX!

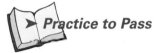

Practice to Pass

You are assigned a client scheduled for angiography. What will you tell your client about this procedure? What are the nursing implications?

Box 4-1

Client and Family Education for Peripheral Arterial Disease

- Stop smoking.
- Lose weight and eat a low-fat diet.
- Do not cross legs while sitting.
- Elevate feet at rest, but not above heart level.
- Do not stand or sit for long periods of time.
- Do not wear restrictive clothing.
- Keep affected extremity warm but never apply direct heat.
- Inspect feet daily and keep them clean and dry.
- Avoid walking barefoot; wear proper-fitting shoes.
- Avoid mechanical or thermal injury to the legs at feet.
- Begin and maintain an exercise and walking program.
- Notify healthcare provider of any changes in color, sensation, temperature, or pulses in extremities.

H. Expected outcomes/evaluation

1. Improved peripheral tissue perfusion manifested by palpable or audible pedal pulses and the absence of claudication

2. Absence of arterial ulcers

3. Improved activity tolerance

VI. Arterial Embolism

A. Description: arterial emboli usually arise from thrombi that developed in the heart as a result of atrial fibrillation, myocardial infarction, prosthetic valves, or congestive heart failure

B. Etiology and pathophysiology

1. Thrombi become detached and are carried from the left side of the heart into the arterial system where they may lodge and cause obstruction

2. The symptoms may be abrupt and will depend on the size and location of the embolus

3. Ischemia will progress to necrosis and gangrene within hours

C. Assessment: the "six Ps"

1. Pain

2. Pallor (pale color)

3. Pulselessness (diminished or absent pulses)

4. Parasthesias (altered local sensation)

5. Paralysis (weakness or inability to move extremity)

6. **Poikilothermia** (body temperature that varies with environment)

D. Priority nursing diagnoses: Ineffective peripheral tissue perfusion, Impaired protection

E. Planning and implementation

1. Assess peripheral pulses and neurovascular status every 2 to 4 hours

2. Place affected extremity in a neutral position with no restrictive bedding/clothing

3. Assess level of pain using a 1 to 10 scale

4. Change position every 2 hours to increase or improve collateral circulation

5. Assess for and report unusual bleeding from anticoagulant therapy

6. Monitor lab values, including APTT, PT, and INR levels

7. If necrosis is present, surgical treatment is required; an emergency cmbolectomy needs to be performed within 4 to 5 hours of embolism to prevent necrosis and permanent damage to the extremity

F. Medication therapy (if no necrosis present): thrombolytic therapy with streptokinase, t-PA or heparin; coumadin therapy at home

G. Client education

1. Pre- and post-operative teaching if embolectomy is performed

2. Measures to promote peripheral circulation and maintain tissue integrity (refer back to Box 4-1)

H. Expected outcomes/evaluation

1. Peripheral pulses strong bilaterally

2. No tissue damage or necrosis

3. Therapeutic lab values for anticoagulant therapy

    a. Warfarin: monitor INR value

        1) normal 0.75 to 1.25

        2) therapeutic 2.0 to 3.0

    b. Heparin: monitor PTT value; therapeutic value is 1.5 to 2.5 times the control

VII. Buerger's Disease (Thromboangiitis Obliterans)

A. Description: an inflammatory disease of the small- and medium-sized veins and arteries accompanied by thrombi and sometimes vasospasm of arterial segments; may occur in upper or lower extremities but is most common in the leg or foot

B. Etiology and pathophysiology

1. The cause of Buerger's disease is unknown, but since it occurs mostly in young men who smoke, it is currently thought to be a reaction to something in cigarettes and/or to have a genetic or autoimmune component

2. Inflammation occurs; microthrombiform; these can lead to vasospasm, and this process ultimately obstructs bloodflow

C. Assessment

1. The first signs and symptoms are usually a bluish cast to a toe or finger and a feeling of coldness in the affected limb

2. Since the nerves are also inflamed, there may be severe pain and constriction of the small blood vessels controlled by them; rest pain is common

3. Overactive sympathetic nerves also may cause the feet to sweat excessively, even though they feel cold

4. As the blood vessels become blocked, intermittent claudication and other symptoms similar to those of chronic obstructive arterial disease often appear

5. Ischemic ulcers and gangrene are common complications of progressive Buerger's disease

D. Priority nursing diagnoses: Ineffective tissue perfusion; Pain

E. Planning and implementation

1. Arrest progress of disease by smoking cessation

2. Take measures to promote vasodilation (similar to other arterial disorders)

3. Provide for pain relief

4. Provide emotional support

F. Medication therapy: analgesic pain medications, calcium channel blockers to ease vasospasm, pentoxifylline (Trental) to reduce blood viscosity

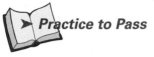

▶ Practice to Pass

Acute arterial occlusion may be caused by a thrombus or an embolus. What is the difference between the two causes? Are there any differences in treatment?

NCLEX!

NCLEX!

NCLEX!

G. Client education

1. Stop smoking

2. Take measures to promote peripheral circulation and maintain tissue integrity (refer back to Box 4-1)

H. Expected outcomes/evaluation

1. Absence of ulcers/impaired skin integrity

2. Relief of pain

3. Cessation of smoking

VIII. Raynaud's Disease

A. Description: localized, intermittent episodes of vasoconstriction of small arteries of the hands and less commonly the feet, causing color and temperature changes

B. Etiology and pathophysiology

1. A vasospastic disorder of unknown origin that primarily affects young women

2. Vasospastic attacks tend to be bilateral and manifestations usually begin at the tips of the digits causing pallor, numbness, and the sensation of cold

NCLEX!

3. Attacks are triggered by exposure to cold, emotional stress, caffeine ingestion, and tobacco use

C. Assessment

1. Symptoms usually appear in the hands after exposure to cold and/or stress; are bilateral and symmetrical

NCLEX!

2. Classic triphasic color changes (pallor, cyanosis, and rubor) in the hands with accompanying reduction in skin temperature

3. The intensity of pain increases as disease progresses

4. The skin of the fingertips may thicken and nails may become brittle

D. Priority nursing diagnoses: Ineffective tissue perfusion, Chronic pain

E. Planning and implementation

1. Keep hands warm and free from injury

2. Avoid stressful situations

3. In severe cases, a **sympathectomy** (surgical dissection of the nerve fibers that allows vasoconstriction to occur) may be performed to relieve symptoms associated with vasospasm

F. Medication therapy

1. Analgesics for pain

2. Vasodilators may provide some relief of symptoms, as well as vascular smooth muscle relaxants and calcium channel blockers

NCLEX!

G. Client education

1. Keep hands warm: wear gloves when out of doors, in air-conditioned environments, or when handling cold food

2. Avoid injury to hands

3. Lifestyle changes: stop smoking; employ stress relief, such as biofeedback

H. Expected outcomes/evaluation

1. Decrease in or absence of attacks

2. No injury to hands and/or wounds heal quickly

IX. Aortic Aneurysm

A. Description: a localized dilation or outpouching of a weakened area in the aorta that is classified by region as thoracic or abdominal, or as dissecting

B. Etiology and pathophysiology

1. The aorta is particularly susceptible to aneurysm formation because of constant stress on the vessel wall

2. Aneurysms occur in men more often than women and their incidence increases with age

3. Most aneurysms are found in the abdominal aorta below the level of the renal arteries

4. The growth rate of an aneurysm is unpredictable

5. Half of all aneurysms greater than 6 cm in size will rupture within 1 year

6. The major risk factor is atherosclerosis

C. Assessment

1. Thoracic aneurysms are often asymptomatic with the first sign being rupture

   a. Symptoms may include pain in the back, neck, and substernal area that may only occur when lying supine

   b. The client may experience dysphagia and dyspnea, stridor, or cough when pressing on the esophagus or laryngeal nerve

2. Abdominal aneurysms may also be asymptomatic until rupture

   a. The client may report a "heartbeat" in the abdomen when lying down

   b. A pulsating abdominal mass may be present

   c. Moderate to severe abdominal or lumbar back pain may be present (severe pain may be a sign of impending rupture)

   d. The client may experience claudication

   e. Cool or cyanotic extremities may be noted

   f. Systolic bruit may be heard

3. Dissecting aneurysms present with sudden, severe, and persistent pain described as "tearing" or "ripping" in the anterior chest or the back

   a. Pain may extend to the shoulder, epigastric area, or abdomen

   b. Pallor, sweating, and tachycardia will be evidenced

   c. Initially the client may have an elevated BP that may be different in one arm from the other

   d. Possible syncope and paralysis of lower extremities may be present

NCLEX!

NCLEX!

D. Priority nursing diagnoses: Ineffective tissue perfusion; Pain; Anxiety

E. Planning and implementation

1. Diagnostic tests that may be ordered

    a. Chest x-ray

    b. Transesophageal echocardiography

    c. Aortography

    d. Ultrasound

    e. CT scan or MRI

2. The overall goals for a client with an aneurysm

    a. Normal tissue perfusion

    b. Intact motor and neurologic function

    c. Reduction in anxiety

    d. No complications of surgical repair

3. Surgical care

    a. Surgical management may be performed on an emergency or elective basis (surgery not usually performed on aneurysms less than 4 to 5 cm in size)

    b. Emergency surgery is the only intervention for clients with a ruptured aneurysm

    c. Hematomas into the scrotum, perineum, flank, or penis indicate retroperitoneal rupture

    d. Once the aorta ruptures anteriorly into the peritoneal cavity, death is almost certain

    e. Surgical technique involves excision of the aneurysm with replacement of the excised segment with a synthetic graft

    NCLEX!

    f. Preoperatively the nurse marks and assesses all peripheral pulses for comparison postoperatively

    NCLEX!

    g. Postoperatively the nurse assesses for complications, which may include:

        1) Graft occlusion

        2) Hypovolemia/renal failure

        3) Respiratory distress

        4) Cardiac dysrhythmias

        5) Paralytic ileus

        6) Paraplegia/paralysis

F. Medication therapy

    NCLEX!

1. The goal of nonsurgical management is to maintain blood pressure at a normal level to decrease the pressure on the arterial system and reduce the risk of rupture

2. Antihypertensive therapy and diuretics may be prescribed

3. Pulsatile flow may be reduced by medications that reduce cardiac contractility

4. Postoperatively clients will be placed on anticoagulant therapy: heparin while the client is in the hospital and warfarin (Coumadin) when discharged to home

G. Client education

1. Clients who do not undergo operative repair must be urged to receive routine physical examinations to monitor the status of the aneurysm

2. Teach the client signs and symptoms of impending rupture (see assessment of dissecting aneurysms above)

3. Teach the client to monitor blood pressure and report any increases immediately

4. Provide teaching about anticoagulant therapy (see Box 4-2)

5. For postoperative clients, teach routine postoperative care

   a. Do limited lifting for 4 to 6 weeks after surgery (no heavy lifting at all)

   b. Monitor the incision site for bleeding/infection

   c. Assess neurovascular status of the extremities and presence of pulses

   d. Clients who receive a synthetic graft may require prophylactic antibiotics before invasive procedures

H. Expected outcomes/evaluation

1. Client has normal tissue perfusion

2. The aneurysm does not rupture

3. For surgical clients, absence of postoperative complications and maintenance of normal tissue perfusion post-surgical grafting

X. Thrombophlebitis

A. Description: the formation of a thrombus (clot) in association with inflammation of the vein; classified as superficial or deep

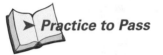

NCLEX!

NCLEX!

▶ Practice to Pass

Your plan of care for a client having repair of an aortic aneurysm includes monitoring of the graft site and prevention of hypovolemic or hemorrhagic shock. What specifically will be included in your plan of care?

Box 4-2
Client and Family Education for Anticoagulant Therapy

- Wear a medical identification bracelet.
- Take medication at approximately the same time each day.
- Stress the importance of routine lab work.
- Do not use aspirin-containing products or nonsteroidal antiinflammatory drugs (NSAIDs).
- Avoid trauma.
- Shave with an electric razor.
- Use a soft toothbrush.
- Report possible adverse side effects immediately to healthcare provider:
  - Any bleeding that does not stop within several minutes.
  - Unusual bleeding from gums, skin, vagina, rectum, or nose.
  - Weakness or dizziness.

B. Etiology and pathophysiology

    1. Etiology: Virchow's triad (at least 2 of 3 present for thrombosis to occur)

        a. Stasis of venous flow

        b. Damage to the inner lining of the vein (endothelial layer)

        c. Hypercoagulability of the blood

    2. Pathophysiology

        a. RBCs, WBCs, and platelets adhere to form a thrombus (usually in valve cusps of veins)

        b. As thrombus enlarges it eventually occludes the lumen of the vein

        c. If only partial occlusion of the vein occurs, blood flow continues and the thrombotic process stops; if detachment does not occur, it will become firmly organized and attached within 24 to 48 hours

        d. If detachment occurs, emboli form which generally flow through the venous system, back to the heart, and into the pulmonary circulation

C. Assessment

    1. Subjective: history of thrombophlebitis, pelvic/abdominal surgery, obesity, neoplasm (hepatic and pancreatic), congestive heart failure (CHF), atrial fibrillation, prolonged immobility, myocardial infarction (MI), pregnancy and/or postpartum period, IV therapy, hypercoagulable states (polycythemia, dehydration/malnutrition)

    2. Objective: signs vary according to thrombus size, location, and adequacy of collateral circulation

        a. Superficial

            1) Palpable, firm, subcutaneous, cord-like vein

            2) Surrounding area warm, red, tender to the touch

            3) Edema may or may not be present

            4) Most common cause in the arms is IV therapy; in the legs it is often related to varicose veins

        b. Deep

            1) Unilateral edema

            2) Pain

            3) Warm skin and elevated temperature

            4) If the inferior vena cava is involved, both legs will be edematous

            5) If the superior vena cava is involved, both upper extremities, neck, back, and face may become edematous or cyanotic

            6) If the calf is involved, **Homan's sign** may be present (pain on dorsiflexion of the foot, especially when the leg is raised)

    3. Diagnostic studies

        a. Venous duplex scanning

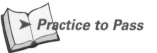

► *Practice to Pass*

You are caring for a 57-year-old client admitted for thrombophlebitis. The client's wife rushes into the hall stating, "My husband can't breathe. It happened all of a sudden." On assessment you note the client to be experiencing severe dyspnea, tachycardia, and chest pain. What do you suspect is occurring? What nursing actions will you implement?

    b. Doppler ultrasonic flowmeter

    c. D-dimer, a product of fibrin degradation, indicates fibrinolysis (that occurs as a reaction to thrombosis)

    d. Venography and plethysmography, former 'gold standards' for diagnosis, are rarely used today

    e. MRI

    f. Lung scan

D. Priority nursing diagnoses: Pain; Ineffective tissue perfusion; Risk for Impaired skin integrity

E. Planning and implementation

    1. Educate client about diagnostic tests that may be performed

    2. Provide for relief of pain

        a. Assess pain on a scale of 1 to 10

        b. Elevate affected leg higher than the heart to promote venous drainage

        c. Provide analgesics as ordered

    3. Decrease edema

        a. Apply warm, moist compresses, intermittent or continuous, to affected extremity

        b. Measure and monitor leg/arm circumference when edema is present

        c. Monitor status of peripheral pulses

    4. Prevent skin ulceration

        a. Keep bed covers from touching affected limb by using an overbed cradle

        b. Do not allow use of restrictive clothing

    5. Prevent pulmonary emboli

        a. Maintain strict bedrest

        b. Never massage affected extremity

        c. Instruct client to report any pink-tinged sputum and monitor for tachypnea, tachycardia, shortness of breath, chest pain, and apprehension, which may indicate a pulmonary embolism

F. Medication therapy

    1. Anticoagulant therapy

        a. Inhibits clotting factors that would extend thrombus formation

        b. Will not induce thrombolysis but prevents clot extension

        c. Heparin: intravenously or subcutaneous while in the hospital

        d. Warfarin: home therapy for 2 to 4 months

    2. Thrombolytics

        a. Dissolve blood clots by imitating natural enzymatic processes

      b. Approved drugs include streptokinase (Streptase), and alteplase (Activase)

      c. Is usually effective in less than 72 hours

      d. Higher risk for hemorrhage exists than when using heparin therapy

  3. Analgesics: NSAIDs are usually prescribed to reduce pain and relieve inflammation

G. Client education

  1. Prevention

      a. Early ambulation postoperatively

      b. Use of compression stockings

      c. Low dose anticoagulant therapy

      d. Avoid prolonged standing or sitting; avoid sitting with crossed legs

      e. Avoid restrictive clothing

      f. Stop smoking

  2. Provide education about anticoagulant therapy (see Box 4-2)

H. Expected outcome/evaluation

  1. No pain, edema, or tenderness

  2. No impaired skin integrity

  3. No embolus

XI. Venous Insufficiency

A. Description: inadequate venous return over a long period of time that causes pathologic changes as a result of ischemia in the vasculature, skin, and supporting tissues

B. Etiology and pathophysiology

  1. Venous insufficiency occurs after prolonged venous hypertension, which stretches the veins and damages the valves, preventing blood return

  2. Venous insufficiency also occurs after thrombus formation or when valves are not functioning correctly, which may result from:

      a. Prolonged standing/sitting (teachers, waitresses, nurses, office workers)

      b. Pregnancy and obesity

  3. With time, stasis results in edema of the lower limbs, discoloration to the skin of the legs and feet, and venous stasis ulceration

C. Assessment

  1. Subjective

      a. Past history of thrombophlebitis, hypertension, varicosities

      b. Past history of long periods of sitting and/or standing

  2. Objective

      a. Edema of the lower legs, may extend to the knee

    b. Thick, coarse, brownish skin around the ankles ("gaiter" area) and feet

    c. Stasis ulcers, usually in the malleolar area

  3. See Table 4-2 for a general comparison of manifestations of arterial and venous disorders

D. Priority nursing diagnoses: Impaired skin integrity, Risk for infection related to skin ulcerations, Disturbed body image, Ineffective tissue perfusion

E. Planning and implementation

  1. Increase venous blood return, decrease venous pressure

    a. Bedrest

    b. Keep legs elevated above heart level

    c. Avoid long periods of standing

    d. Wear elastic support or compression stockings

      1) Apply stockings *before* getting out of bed and placing the leg in a dependent position

      2) Wear stockings during the day and evening, remove at night

      3) Never push stockings down around the leg—they will further impair circulation

      4) Handwash stockings daily and air dry; machine washing or drying will damage elastic fibers

  2. Treat venous stasis ulcer(s)

    a. Open lesions are treated with a hydrocolloid dressing and compression wraps; a topical ointment, such as low-dose hydrocortisone, zinc oxide, or an antifungal may also be indicated

    b. Ulcers may be treated with an Unna Boot or other compression wrap that is changed every 1 to 2 weeks and is usually applied over a base dressing

    c. Severe ulcers may need surgical debridement

Table 4-2

Comparison of Arterial and Venous Vascular Disease

Assessment	Arterial Disease	Venous Disease
Color	Pale	Ruddy; cyanotic if dependent
Edema	None or minimal	Usually present
Nails	Thick and brittle	Normal
Pain	Worse with elevation and exercise; may be sudden or severe; rest pain; claudication	Better with elevation; positive Homan's sign, dullness or heaviness
Pulses	Decreased, weak, or absent	Normal
Temperature of extremity	Cool	Warm
Ulcers	Dry and necrotic	Moist; malleolar

F. Medication therapy

1. Topical agents to skin ulcers, such as hydrocortisone, antifungals or zinc oxide, may be prescribed

2. Oral or IV antibiotics may be prescribed when ulcers become infected or cellulitis occurs

3. Sclerosing agents (called sclerotherapy) may be used to occlude bloodflow in a vein, causing disappearance of the varicosity; this may be followed up with use of compression bandage for a short period of time

NCLEX!

G. Client education

1. Elevate legs for at least 20 minutes four times a day

2. Keep legs above the level of the heart when in bed

3. Avoid prolonged sitting or standing

4. Do not cross legs when sitting

5. Do not wear tight, restrictive pants, socks, or boots; avoid girdles and garters that restrict circulation in the upper leg

6. Wear support stockings as instructed above

H. Expected outcomes/evaluation

1. Reduction in edema

2. Healing/prevention of stasis ulcers

XII. Varicose Veins

A. Description: a vein or veins in which blood has pooled, producing distended, tortuous, and palpable vessels

B. Etiology and pathophysiology

1. One in five people worldwide will develop varicosities

2. They are more common in women over thirty-five, obesity, those with a positive family history of varicosities, and in those who stand for long periods of time

3. Varicose veins may develop after trauma or damage to a vein or valve or from gradual venous distension, which diminishes the action of the muscle pump, and increases the pull of gravity on blood within the legs

4. As the vein swells, increased hydrostatic pressure will push plasma through the stretched vessel walls and edema of surrounding tissue may occur

C. Assessment

NCLEX!

1. Subjective: the client may complain of aching, heaviness, itching, swelling and unsightly appearance to the leg(s)

NCLEX!

2. Objective

a. Dilated, tortuous superficial veins will be seen along the upper and lower leg

b. Superficial inflammation may develop along the path of the varicose vein

c. Positive Trendelenburg test (done to evaluate valve competence)

         1) Client is placed in a supine position with elevated legs

         2) As the client sits up, the veins would normally fill from the distal end

         3) If there are varicosities, the veins fill from the proximal end

D. Priority nursing diagnoses: Pain, Ineffective tissue perfusion, Risk for impaired skin integrity, Risk for peripheral neurovascular dysfunction

E. Planning and implementation

    1. Assess and provide pain relief

      a. Assess pain on a scale of 1 to 10

      b. Provide analgesics as needed

    2. Improve venous circulation

      a. Assess pulses and neurovascular status of lower extremities

      b. Teach/apply support stockings

      c. Avoid prolonged sitting and standing; never cross legs; walking is encouraged

      d. Elevate feet above heart level when lying down

      e. Avoid restrictive clothing/shoes

    3. Prevent skin breakdown; teach proper skin care and importance of avoiding trauma to legs

    4. Teach preoperative and postoperative care if surgery is chosen

      a. Sclerotherapy involves injecting a sclerosing agent into the varicosed vein, usually in the physician's office

         1) Procedure is palliative but not curative

         2) Elastic bandages may need to be worn for up to 6 weeks

      b. Vein ligation surgery involves ligation (tying off) of the entire vein (usually the saphenous) and dissection and removal of the incompetent tributaries

         1) Perform hourly circulation checks postoperatively

         2) Elevate extremity to a 15-degree angle to prevent stasis and edema

         3) Apply compression gradient stockings from foot to groin

F. Medication therapy: no specific medications are used

G. Client education

    1. Prevention

      a. Avoid sitting or standing for long periods

      b. Change position often

      c. Avoid constrictive clothing

      d. Elevate legs when sitting to promote venous return

      e. Maintain ideal body weight

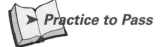

Practice to Pass

A 53-year-old teacher is seen in the ambulatory care center with complaints of leg pain from her varicose veins. She asks you why the varicosities cause pain. How do you respond?

H. Expected outcomes/evaluation

1. Relief of discomfort

2. Improved circulation

3. Avoidance of complications such as thrombophlebitis and ulcerations

---

Case Study

Mr. B. comes into your community health clinic with a large, weeping ulcer on the malleolus of the right foot that he claims is not painful. He has 2+ edema in both feet. Vital signs are within normal limits. Lab results are remarkable for a WBC of 12.3/mm^3. He states that his occupation is a collector in a toll booth, that he stands most of the time, and reports often working 10- and 12-hour shifts. He denies taking any medication other than an occasional acetaminophen (Tylenol) for headache.

❶ What is the likely cause of the ulcer on Mr. B.'s foot?

❷ What are the usual signs and symptoms for this disorder?

❸ State three nursing diagnoses appropriate for this client.

❹ What are the primary nursing interventions?

❺ On Mr. B.'s followup appointment in 2 months, what would you look for to evaluate your nursing care?

For suggested responses, see page 736.

Posttest

1   The nurse is performing an assessment on a 50-year-old male who is a cashier at a local store, and who often stands 6 to 8 hours at a time. The nurse should inspect the client for:

(1) Capillary dysfunction.
(2) Buerger's disease.
(3) Varicosities.
(4) Aneurysms.

2   The nurse is conducting a screening clinic for hypertension in the community. For which of the following clients should the nurse pay particular attention to blood pressure?

(1) Caucasian adult female
(2) Latino/Hispanic adult male
(3) Asian adult male
(4) African-American adult male

3   When assessing a client, the nurse determines the capillary refill time to be 7 seconds. The nurse determines the client may be experiencing:

(1) Normal signs of aging.
(2) Impending stroke.
(3) Decreased cardiac output.
(4) Hypokalemia.

4   After the first dose of an antihypertensive agent, your client suddenly becomes hypotensive. You should position the client:

(1) In a semi-Fowler's position.
(2) In a side-lying position.
(3) In Trendelenburg position.
(4) With legs elevated 30 degrees.

5	The nurse is planning to instruct a client on the side effects of nifedipine (Procardia) for hypertension. Which side effect should the nurse include?	(1) Hypokalemia (2) Dizziness (3) Bleeding (4) Tachycardia
6	A client taking spironolactone (Aldactone) complains of irregular heart rate, diarrhea, and stomach cramping. The client's potassium level is 7.1 mEq/L. The nurse concludes that the client is experiencing:	(1) Hyponatremia. (2) Hypercalcemia. (3) Hyperkalemia. (4) Hypernatremia.
7	The nurse explains to a client that the goal of anti-coagulant therapy in a client with a deep vein thrombosis is to:	(1) Prevent embolization. (2) Dissolve the clot. (3) Allow immediate ambulation. (4) Prevent infection.
8	The nurse needs to explore with a client her understanding of treatment options for varicose veins that were just described by the physician. Which treatment would the nurse plan to include in this discussion?	(1) Endarterectomy (2) Venography (3) Sclerotherapy (4) Plethysmography
9	Which of the following medications is likely to be administered on a daily basis to a client newly admitted to the clinical nursing unit who has a history of peripheral arterial disease?	(1) Acetaminophen (Tylenol) (2) Ibuprofen (Motrin) (3) Aspirin (4) Heparin
10	Which of the following statements would indicate a positive outcome for a client with chronic arterial occlusive disease?	(1) "I will keep my feet elevated above the level of my heart when I sleep." (2) "I will wear my compression stockings when awake." (3) "I will keep walking even when I feel pain in my legs to increase circulation." (4) "I will check the temperature of my bathwater with my hands before getting into the water."

See pages 164–165 for Answers and Rationales.

Answers and Rationales

Pretest

1 **Answer: 4** *Rationale:* Blood pressure should be consistently below 140/90. Lifestyle modification must be used in all hypertensive clients with or without medication therapy.
Cognitive Level: Application
Nursing Process: Planning; *Test Plan:* PHYS

2 **Answer: 1** *Rationale:* Pain of arterial occlusive disease is related to interrupted blood flow, which causes tissue hypoxia. An increase in blood supply, then,

should reduce the client's ischemic pain. The other options list additional manifestations of peripheral arterial disease.
Cognitive Level: Analysis
Nursing Process: Evaluation; *Test Plan:* PHYS

3 **Answer: 3** *Rationale:* Beta adrenergic blocking agents, such as propranolol, cause a decrease in heart rate and decreased contractility, which can result in bradycardia or heart failure. Constipation is a side effect of therapy with some of the calcium channel

blockers, while hypokalemia increases risk of digitalis toxicity.
Cognitive Level: Application
Nursing Process: Planning; *Test Plan:* PHYS

4 **Answer: 4** *Rationale:* The classic manifestations of a deep vein thrombosis are calf or groin pain, which may or may not be associated with leg swelling. The other options describe symptoms of arterial disease.
Cognitive Level: Application
Nursing Process: Assessment; *Test Plan:* PHYS

5 **Answer: 4** *Rationale:* Orange juice is an excellent source of potassium. Coffee will adversely elevate blood pressure. Milk is high in sodium. Cranberry juice is not as high in potassium as orange juice.
Cognitive Level: Analysis
Nursing Process: Evaluation; *Test Plan:* HPM

6 **Answer: 1** *Rationale:* The primary symptom of a dissecting aneurysm is sudden, severe pain. Abdominal dissections commonly cause back pain. The other responses don't address this emergency.
Cognitive Level: Application
Nursing Process: Implementation; *Test Plan:* PHYS

7 **Answer: 2** *Rationale:* Heparin dose concentration and number of units per milliliter per hour are ordered to maintain a therapeutic PTT. The other responses are incorrect.
Cognitive Level: Application
Nursing Process: Analysis; *Test Plan:* PHYS

8 **Answer: 3** *Rationale:* Intermittent claudication caused by muscle ischemia is a primary symptom of peripheral arterial disease. Pain occurs with activity but is relieved with rest. The other options are not associated with this disorder.
Cognitive Level: Analysis
Nursing Process: Analysis; *Test Plan:* PHYS

9 **Answer: 1** *Rationale:* Clients with orthostatic hypotension are at risk for dizziness and syncope if they arise quickly. Option 3 is a correct action but does not relate directly to orthostatic hypotension. Blood pressure should also be taken while the client is sitting and standing (option 2). Option 4 is unrelated to the question.
Cognitive Level: Application
Nursing Process: Planning; *Test Plan:* PHYS

10 **Answer: 4** *Rationale:* A common complication of hypertensive disease is target organ disease, including retinal damage to the eye. The appearance of the

retina can provide important information about the severity of the hypertensive process.
Cognitive Level: Analysis
Nursing Process: Implementation; *Test Plan:* HPM

Posttest

1 **Answer: 3** *Rationale:* 50 percent of people over the age of 50 develop varicose veins and a major risk factor is standing for long periods of time at work. The other responses do not address this concern.
Cognitive Level: Application
Nursing Process: Assessment; Test plan: HPM

2 **Answer: 4** *Rationale:* Primary hypertension is more common in African-Americans than in people of other ethnic backgrounds. For this reason, this client should be carefully evaluated.
Cognitive Level: Application
Nursing Process: Assessment; *Test Plan:* HPM

3 **Answer: 3** *Rationale:* Blanching of the nailbed for more than 3 seconds after release of pressure may indicate reduced arterial capillary perfusion, which may be an indication of decreased cardiac output. The other options are incorrect for the time frame indicated or do not apply.
Cognitive Level: Analysis
Nursing Process: Analysis; *Test Plan:* PHYS

4 **Answer: 4** *Rationale:* Elevating the legs increases venous return to the heart and will assist in raising the blood pressure. A semi-Fowler's position could lower the blood pressure even further. A side-lying position will have no beneficial effect, and the Trendelenburg position could impair respirations by causing upward pressure on the diaphragm by gravity.
Cognitive Level: Application
Nursing Process: Implementation; *Test Plan:* PHYS

5 **Answer: 2** *Rationale:* Calcium channel blockers relax arterial smooth muscle, which lowers peripheral resistance through vasodilation. Dizziness is a common side effect because of orthostatic hypotension. Clients need to be taught to change position slowly to prevent falls.
Cognitive Level: Application
Nursing Process: Planning; *Test Plan:* PHYS

6 **Answer: 3** *Rationale:* Spironolactone is a potassium-sparing diuretic. Hyperkalemia (potassium greater than 5.5 mEq/L) is a possible side effect. The other responses are incorrect.
Cognitive Level: Analysis
Nursing Process: Analysis; *Test Plan:* PHYS

7 **Answer: 1** *Rationale:* Anticoagulant therapy is used for deep vein thrombosis to prevent propagation of the clot, development of a new thrombus, and embolization. It does not dissolve the clot. It has no effect on infection and does not allow for immediate ambulation.
Cognitive Level: Analysis
Nursing Process: Implementation; *Test Plan:* PHYS

8 **Answer: 3** *Rationale:* Sclerotherapy, the injection of a sclerosing agent into a varicose vein followed by compression with a compression bandage for a period of time, is a common procedure for varicose veins.
Cognitive Level: Application
Nursing Process: Planning; *Test Plan:* PHYS

9 **Answer: 3** *Rationale:* Because of the risk for inflammation or a blood clot, low doses of aspirin are recommended for all clients with peripheral vascular disease. Aspirin has antiplatelet activity; without platelet aggregation, a clot cannot form.
Cognitive Level: Analysis
Nursing Process: Analysis; *Test Plan:* PHYS

10 **Answer: 4** *Rationale:* Sensation in the feet may be diminished in clients with arterial occlusive disease. Teach the client to check the bathwater with the hands to prevent the risk of a burn injury. The client should stop and rest when pain is experienced (option 3). Options 1 and 2 are useful treatments for venous disease.
Cognitive Level: Analysis
Nursing Process: Evaluation; *Test Plan:* HPM

References

Daugherty, J. (2000). Nursing management: Vascular disorders. In S. Lewis, M. Heitkemper, & S. Dirksen (Eds.), *Medical-surgical nursing: Assessment and management of clinical problems* (5th ed.). St. Louis, MO: Mosby, Inc., pp. 978–1009.

Deglin, J. H. & Vallerand, A. H. (2003). *Davis' drug guide for nurses* (8th ed.). Philadelphia: F.A. Davis.

DeMartinis, J. E. (2001). Clients with hypertensive disorders: Promoting positive outcomes. In J. Black, J. Hawks, & A. Keene. *Medical-surgical nursing: Management for positive clinical outcomes* (6th ed.). Philadelphia: W. B. Saunders, pp. 1379–1398.

LeMone, P. & Burke, K. (2004). *Medical-surgical nursing: Critical thinking in client care* (3rd ed.). Upper Saddle River, NJ: Prentice-Hall, pp. 1176–1263.

Levine, B. (2000). Nursing management: Hypertension. In S. Lewis, M. Heitkemper, & S. Dirksen (Eds.), *Medical-surgical nursing: Assessment and management of clinical problems* (5th ed.). St. Louis, MO: Mosby, Inc., pp. 817–840.

Lueckenotte, A. (2000). *Gerontologic nursing* (2nd ed.). St Louis, MO: Mosby, Inc., pp. 439–478, 501–511, 543–559.

Nunnelee, J. D. (2001). Management of clients with vascular disorders. In J. Black, J. Hawks, & A. Keene (Eds.), *Medical-surgical nursing: Management for positive clinical outcomes* (6th ed.). Philadelphia: W. B. Saunders, pp. 1399–1432.

Sellers, J. B., & Brubaker, M. L. (1999). Cardiovascular disorders. In E. Youngkin, K. Sawin, J. Kissinger, & D. Israel (Eds.), *Pharmacotherapeutics: A primary care clinical guide*. Stamford, CT: Appleton & Lange, pp. 309–367.

Sieggreen, M. (2001). Assessment of the vascular system. In J. Black, J. Hawks, & A. Keene (Eds.), *Medical-surgical nursing: Management for positive clinical outcomes* (6th ed.). Philadelphia: W. B. Saunders, pp. 1368–1378.

CHAPTER 5

Neurological Disorders

Eileen Reilly-Mitchell, MSN, RN, BC-APN

CHAPTER OUTLINE

Overview of Anatomy and Physiology of the Nervous System
Diagnostic Tests and Assessments of the Nervous System

Acute Disorders of the Nervous System
Chronic Disorders of the Nervous System

OBJECTIVES

- Identify basic structures and functions of the neurological system.

- Describe the pathophysiology and etiology of common neurological disorders.

- Discuss expected assessment data and diagnostic test findings for selected neurological disorders.

- Identify priority nursing diagnoses for selected neurological disorders.

- Discuss therapeutic management of selected neurological disorders.

- Discuss nursing management of a client experiencing a neurological disorder.

- Identify expected outcomes for a client experiencing a neurological disorder.

[*Media Link*]

Use the CD-ROM enclosed with this text, or log onto the address given to access the free, interactive Companion Website created for this series. The CD-ROM and Companion Website accompanying this book offer additional practice opportunities and information—NCLEX Review, Case Studies, Glossary, In Depth with NCLEX, and more.

www.prenhall.com/hogan

REVIEW AT A GLANCE

agnosia *the inability to recognize familiar subjects; agnosia may be visual, auditory or tactile*

aphasia *a language disorder*

apraxia *the inability to carry out motor pattern (i.e., drawing a figure, getting dressed) even with strength and coordination*

autonomic dysreflexia *an exaggerated sympathetic response that occurs in clients with T-6 injuries or above; the response is seen after spinal shock occurs when a stimuli cannot ascend the cord, a*

stimulus such as the urge to void or abdominal discomfort triggers massive vasoconstriction below the injury, vasodilation above the injury, and bradycardia

bradykinesia *slow movements caused by muscle rigidity*

Broca's area *motor control of speech in the temporal lobe of the dominant hemisphere*

dysarthria *defective articulation of speech*

dysphagia *difficulty swallowing*

hemianopsia *the loss of half of the visual field in one or both eyes*

intrathecal *through the theacal of the spinal cord into the subarachnoid space*

paraplegia *paralysis of the lower extremities*

tetraplegia *formally called quadriplegia, is paralysis of the arms, trunk, legs, and pelvis*

Wernicke's area *the section of the temporal lobe responsible for the primary auditory reception area and auditory association areas of speech*

Pretest

1 Which of the following nursing actions would be contraindicated when performing mouth care with an unconscious client?

(1) Give oral care using toothettes
(2) Brush the teeth with a small (child-size) toothbrush
(3) Position the client to one side or the other
(4) Use an alcohol-based product for better cleansing

2 A nurse monitoring a client who has sustained a head injury would determine that the intracranial pressure (ICP) is rising if which of the following vital sign trends is noted during the course of the work shift?

(1) ↑ temperature, ↓ pulse, ↑ respirations, ↓ BP
(2) ↓ temperature, ↑ pulse, ↓ respirations, ↑ BP
(3) ↓ temperature, ↑ pulse, ↑ respirations, ↓ BP
(4) ↑ temperature, ↓ pulse, ↓ respirations, ↑ BP

3 The client has been intubated and placed on a mechanical ventilator to reduce intracranial pressure (ICP) by decreasing the carbon dioxide level. Which of the following carbon dioxide values would indicate that the optimal amount of hyperventilation has been achieved?

(1) $PaCO_2$ 18 mm Hg
(2) $PaCO_2$ 29 mm Hg
(3) $PaCO_2$ 38 mm Hg
(4) $PaCO_2$ 46 mm Hg

4 A client who experienced a thrombotic stroke and has residual hemiparesis of the right side is undergoing rehabilitation. The nurse caring for this client reinforces occupational therapy recommendations by placing items for personal hygiene:

(1) On the overbed table on the right side.
(2) On the overbed table on the left side.
(3) One foot away from the bed on the right side.
(4) One foot away from the bed on the left side.

5 A client with spinal cord injury is at risk for experiencing autonomic dysreflexia. The nurse would carefully monitor for which of the following manifestations?

(1) Tachycardia
(2) Hypotension
(3) Severe, throbbing headache
(4) Cyanosis of the head and neck

6 A nurse is caring for a client who just experienced a seizure. While doing follow-up documentation, the nurse would include which of the following items in the nursing progress note?

(1) The amount of lighting in the room when the seizure began
(2) Utterance of sounds
(3) Amount of sleep the client had during the night prior to the seizure
(4) Food and fluid intake just before onset of the seizure

7 The nurse has implemented a teaching plan for the client with Parkinson's disease. The nurse evaluates the teaching as effective if the client states to do which of the following to help combat manifestations of the disease?

(1) Plan the most strenuous activities for the evening hours when bedtime is near
(2) Use a rocking motion to get up out of chairs
(3) Sit in a soft reclining chair to support joints while watching television
(4) Choose clothing with several snaps and buttons to increase the benefits of physical therapy

8 A client who is in Stage II of Alzheimer's disease has memory impairment. The nurse should plan to do which of the following at the beginning of the upcoming work shift?

(1) Check to ensure that the client is wearing an ID badge
(2) Place the client in a quiet, calm environment
(3) Write a note on the cover of the chart asking for a p.r.n. order for restraints
(4) Instruct ancillary caregivers to assess the client's level of consciousness hourly

9 A client newly diagnosed with trigeminal neuralgia asks the nurse to explain why it hurts so much when an episode occurs. The nurse would explain that the pain of trigeminal neuralgia is the result of which of the following?

(1) Stimulation of the nerve by temperature or pressure
(2) Irritation due to cellular effects of hypoglycemia
(3) Release of epinephrine during the fight-or-flight response
(4) An immune system reaction to cold and influenza viruses

10 A client is scheduled for an electroencephalogram (EEG) early in the morning. The nurse working the night shift prior to the procedure would write a note to do which of the following per protocol order in the early morning on the day of the test?

(1) Instruct the client to refrain from washing the hair
(2) Hold the daily dose of anticonvulsant
(3) Place the client on NPO status
(4) Reinforce client teaching that the test is only mildly uncomfortable

See pages 208–209 for Answers and Rationales.

I. Overview of Anatomy and Physiology of the Nervous System

A. Basic structure and function of cells in the nervous system

1. Neurons are the basic anatomical and functional units in the nervous system; each neuron has three parts:

   a. The cell body, which is the major part of the neuron

   b. The axon, which carries the stimulus away from the cell body

      1) Axons extend a long way from the cell body and do not branch until the very end

      2) Axons in the peripheral nervous system (PNS) are covered with a insulating lipid layer called myelin sheath for rapid conduction of nerve impulses

      3) Each axon terminates at a synapse where neurotransmitters and other chemical substances are released

   c. The dendrites direct impulses toward the cell body; they usually extend a short distance from the cell body and branch copiously

    d. Nerve cells are separated by a synaptic cleft; neurotransmitters are secreted into the cleft by one neuron to stimulate the dendrites of another neuron

    e. Conduction of a nerve impulse is initiated when a stimulus is sufficient to create an action potential (a summation of impulses from the dendrites); it is then sent down the axon by depolarization; in myelinated nerves the action potential hops from one node of Ranvier to the next for rapid conduction

  2. Glial cells: supportive structures of the nervous system that nourish, support and protect the brain neurons; because these cells divide by mitosis, they are a source of primary tumors of the nervous system; there are four main types of glial cells in the brain and one in the PNS:

    a. Astrocytes: star-like cells that provide nutrition to neurons, regulate synaptic connectivity, remove cellular debris, and control movement of molecules in the blood–brain barrier

    b. Oligodendrocytes: produce the myelin sheath within the central nervous system (CNS) that insulates the neuron allowing for fast transmission of impulses

    c. Ependymal cells: line the ventricular system and the choroid plexuses; they produce cerebral spinal fluid (CSF) and act as a barrier between the fluid-filled ventricles and cerebral tissue

    d. Microglia: small phagocytic cells scattered in the CNS that disintegrate and remove cellular debris and waste products

    e. Schwann cells: these cells in the PNS produce insulating myelin sheaths, just as the oligodendrocytes do in the CNS, which facilitates rapid conduction of impulses

B. The central nervous system

  1. Consists of the brain and spinal cord

  2. The brain is composed of divisions

    a. The cerebrum, the largest division, composes the top of the brain and enables individuals to reason, function intellectually, express personality and mood, and interact with the environment

      1) Includes two hemispheres, each of which is divided into a frontal lobe, a temporal lobe, a parietal lobe, and an occipital lobe; each lobe has specific functions

      2) The right hemisphere generally controls the left side of the body and the left controls the right side of the body; usually one hemisphere is considered dominant

      3) The frontal lobe performs high level cognitive function, has memory storage, influences somatic motor control, controls voluntary eye movements and controls motor aspect of speech in **Broca's area,** which is located in the dominant hemisphere (usually the left)

      4) The temporal lobe is located behind the frontal and under the parietal lobe and has the primary auditory receptive areas and the auditory association area (**Wernicke's area**), which is usually found on the dominant side and is responsible for interpreting speech; another important area

in the temporal lobe is the interpretive area that integrates somatic, auditory and visual data (this impacts perception, learning, memory, emotions, and intellectual abilities)

    5) The parietal lobe holds the primary sensory cortex and sensory association areas; in these areas, sensations such as size, shape, weight, texture and consistency are defined and localized; it also processes visual–spatial information and controls spatial orientation

    6) The occipital lobe is the visual center for the eyes; it controls both eye reflexes and interpretation of sight

  b. The diencephalons and hypophysis are located at the bottom of the cerebrum near the midbrain; this includes the thalamus and related structures and the pituitary gland; this area has many functions including temperature control, water metabolism, pituitary secretion, visceral and somatic activities, visible physical expressions in response to emotions, sleep-wake cycle and food-getting reflex

  c. The cerebellum is a double-lobed area posterior to the pons that is responsible for muscle synergy and coordination, and maintains balance through feedback loops

  d. The brainstem is an integration system that also controls basic functions; there are three major divisions of the brainstem, the midbrain, pons and medulla; the reticular activating system (RAS) is responsible for alertness; the substantia nigra is affected in Parkinson's disease; most of the cranial nerves originate in the brainstem

3. The spinal cord is an elongated mass of nerve tissue that runs most of the length of the vertebral column

  a. The spinal cord is divided into four areas: the cervical area (C1 to C7) transverses the neck; the thoracic area (T1 to T12) goes through the chest; the lumbar area (L1 to L5) goes through the lower back; the sacral area (S1 to S4) is in the sacrum

  b. Sensory tracts (dorsal roots) carry afferent impulses from the periphery to the dorsal root ganglia where the cell bodies of the sensory components are located; from this point they are then sent to the brain; there are two types of sensory fibers

    1) General somatic afferent fibers carry pain, temperature, touch and proprioception from the body wall, tendon and joints

    2) General visceral fibers carry sensory input from the organs of the body

  c. Motor tracts (ventral roots) convey efferent impulses from the spinal cord to the body; there are two types of fibers:

    1) General somatic fibers that innervate voluntary striated muscles

    2) General visceral efferent fiber that innervate smooth and cardiac muscle and regulate glandular secretions

C. The peripheral nervous system

1. Has 31 pairs of spinal nerves, 12 pairs of cranial nerves, and the autonomic system that is divided into the sympathetic and parasympathetic nervous system

2. Each pair of spinal nerves has dorsal and ganglion roots that exit the spinal cord by way of an intervertebral foramina that corresponds with the spinal level; these nerves carry input between specific areas called dermatomes and the spine

3. Cranial nerves (CN): the 12 pairs of cranial nerves arise from the brain; there are 3 pure sensory nerves, 5 pure motor nerves and 4 mixed (sensory and motor) nerves; the olfactory nerve (CN I) and optic nerve (CN II) arise from the cerebrum; CN III and IV arise in the midbrain; CN V through VIII arise in the pons, while CN IX to XII arise in the medulla (see Table 5-1 for overview of cranial nerves)

4. Autonomic nervous system: is a collection of motor nerves that regulate activities of the viscera, smooth muscles, and glands to maintain a stable internal environment; the two parts of the system (sympathetic and parasympathetic) work antagonistically

   a. The sympathetic nervous system (SNS) is active during times of stress, such as the fright, flight or fight response; it increases heart rate and blood pressure and vasoconstricts the peripheral blood vessels

   b. The parasympathetic system is a conservation, restoration, and maintenance system; it decreases heart rate and increases gastrointestinal (GI) activity

D. Blood supply

1. The brain is unique in that it can only use glucose for its energy supply; a lack of glucose for 5 minutes results in irreversible brain damage; the brain receives 750 mL/min of blood or 15 to 20 % of the resting cardiac output; blood flow rates for specific sites correspond directly with the rate of metabolism

2. The cerebral arteries are thinner, have more internal elasticity and less smooth muscle than the arteries in the rest of the body; the brain is supplied with blood by two sets of arteries that divide it into anterior and posterior circulation

   a. The anterior circulation, fed by the internal and external carotids, delivers blood to a central area at the base of the cerebrum called the circle of Willis; from there it feeds the anterior cerebrum via anterior cerebral, the

Table 5-1	**Cranial Nerve Name**	**Type of Nerve**	**Physiological Functions**
Overview of Cranial Nerves	Olfactory (I)	Sensory	Ability to smell
	Optic (II)	Sensory	Visual fields, visual acuity
	Oculomotor (III)	Motor	Extraocular movements (EOM)
	Trochlear (IV)	Motor	Extraocular movements (EOM)
	Trigeminal (V)	Mixed	Movement of eyelids, ability to clench jaw
	Abducens (VI)	Motor	EOM
	Facial (VII)	Mixed	Movement of eyelids, facial symmetry
	Acoustic (VIII)	Sensory	Hearing ability
	Glossopharyngeal (IX)	Mixed	Gag, swallow, and cough reflexes, voice quality
	Vagus (X)	Mixed	Gag, swallow, and cough reflexes, voice quality
	Spinal Accessory (XI)	Motor	Neck strength and shoulder shrug
	Hypoglossal (XII)	Motor	Tongue movement

middle of the cerebrum via the middle cerebral artery, and the posterior cerebrum via posterior cerebral artery; the tissues that are at the terminal areas fed by the two circulations are called watershed zones because they are subject to marginally adequate blood supply; during times of hypoperfusion, these may be the first affected

    b. The posterior circulation, fed by the vertebral arteries, delivers blood to the posterior fossa; at the bottom of the posterior fossa, blood flows together into one basilar artery and delivers it to the cerebellum, midbrain, pons, and medulla

    c. The meninges are supplied with blood from branches of the external carotid arteries that ascend into the brain at the base of the skull

  3. The venous system of the brain is unique

    a. Vessel walls are thinner than other veins of the body

    b. In addition, they do not follow the path of arteries but follow their own course

    c. There are no valves in the brain's venous system and therefore drainage depends on venous pressure and gravity

    d. Dural sinuses collect blood from the brain and empty it into the jugular veins

E. The blood-brain barrier

  1. Is a descriptive term that refers to a network of endothelial cells in the wall of the capillaries and astrocyte projections in close proximity that do not have pores between them

  2. This tight junction does not allow the normal nonspecific filtering process that occurs in the rest of the body; therefore, molecules must enter the brain by active transport, endocytosis and exocytosis, which creates a highly selective barrier that guards the entrance to the neurons

  3. The movement of substances across this barrier depends on particle size, lipid solubility, chemical dissociation and protein-binding potential

  4. The barrier is very permeable to water, oxygen, carbon dioxide, other gases, glucose and lipid soluble compounds

F. Protective structures

  1. Meninges: cover the brain and spinal cord to protect and support; it is divided into three layers from outer to inner (dura mater, arachnoid, and pia mater)

    a. The dura is a tough membranous tissue that surrounds and extends into the brain tissue that provides important landmarks, such as the falx cerebri and the tentorium cerebelli, which is an important structure to note because nursing care differs based whether an injury is supratentorial (above the tentorium) or infratentorial (below the tentorium)

    b. The arachnoid membrane lies below the dura and is a network of delicate, elastic tissue that contains blood vessels of varying sizes

    c. The pia mater is a vascular membrane that covers the entire brain with tiny vessels that extend into the gray matter of the brain

    d. Within the meninges, there are important potential spaces (epidural, subdural, subarachnoid) where bleeding can occur

  2. Skull: the bony structure of the head that includes 8 fused cranial bones and 14 facial bones; the cranium encloses the brain in a protective vault; many of the internal cranial surfaces are irregularly shaped; the foramen magnum is the large hole at the base of the skull through which the spinal cord runs

  3. Spine: a flexible column that encloses the spinal cord, formed from the stacking of 33 bones called vertebrae; each vertebra has a body anteriorly and an arch that has 2 laminae and 2 pedicles that form 7 processes; this interlocking support structure provides protection and flexibility; the spine is divided into 7 cervical, 12 thoracic, 5 lumbar, and 4 sacral vertebrae

  4. Cerebrospinal fluid (CSF) and the ventricular system

    a. CSF is a clear colorless, odorless solution that fills the ventricular system and subarachnoid space of the brain and spinal cord; it acts as a shock absorber to cushion the brain from injuries caused by movement; it also has electrolytes, glucose, protein, oxygen, and carbon dioxide dissolved in solution

    b. The ventricular system is composed of two lateral ventricles (one in each hemisphere of the cerebrum), a third ventricular that lies midline in the thalamic area, and a fourth ventricle that lies below the third, anterior to the cerebellum and the subarachnoid space

    c. The flow of CSF starts in the choroid plexus in each lateral ventricle and travels to the third ventricle via the Foramina of Monro; this landmark is used as the zero point in ventricular drainage systems; from the third ventricle the CSF flows into the fourth ventricle via the aqueduct of Sylvius, through two lateral foramen of Luschka, midline through the foramen of Mafendie into the subarachnoid space, down to the spinal cord and up again to the subarachnoid space on the top of the brain, where it is absorbed by arachnoid villi

II. Diagnostic Tests and Assessments of the Nervous System

  A. Assessment of the nervous system

    1. Assess circumstances of injury and admission, pertinent family and social history

    2. Assess chief complaint

      a. A—any associated symptoms with chief complaint

      b. P—what provokes (makes worse) or palliates (makes better) symptoms

      c. Q—quality of pain

      d. R—region and radiation

      e. S—severity of pain on a scale of 1–10

      f. T—timing—when did it stop and start, intermittent or constant, duration

    3. Health information: including past medical history, current medications, recent surgeries or other treatments

NCLEX!

4. Physical assessment of neurological functioning

a. Mental status

NCLEX!

1) A screening mental status examination includes orientation to person, place and time, appearance and behavior, mood, speech pattern, and thought and perception including insight, thought, content and judgment

2) In order to conduct this examination, the client must be awake, alert and able to understand and respond to questions

3) A client with an altered level of consciousness (LOC) may have a range of behaviors; terms used to describe this range vary from confused to comatose (see Table 5-2)

4) Acute confusion or delirium should be recognized and treated by eliminating the cause; try to avoid confusing delirium with dementia (a chronic problem)

NCLEX!

b. Cranial nerves: assessment of cranial nerves can be performed as described in Table 5-3; some methods of assessment test more than one cranial nerve at a time

c. Motor function

1) Inspect all body muscles for size, tone, movement, and strength

NCLEX!

2) Compare left and right side for symmetry and equality

3) Assess for tremors (rhythmic movements) and fasciculations (twitching)

Table 5-2	Term	Description
Terms Used to Describe Level of Consciousness	Full consciousness	Alert, oriented to person, place, and time, and comprehends written and spoken words
	Confusion	Disoriented to person, place, and/or time; misinterprets environment; has poor judgment; unable to think clearly
	Lethargic	Oriented but slow and sluggish in speech, mental processes, and motor activity
	Obtundation	Readily arousable to stimuli; responds with one or two words; can follow simple commands when asked, but quickly drifts back to sleep
	Stupor	Lies quietly with minimal movement; responds with a groan or eye opening only to vigorous and repeated verbal with tactile stimuli; usually localizes painful stimuli
	Coma	Unarousable to stimuli; nonverbal; may exhibit nonpurposeful response to stimuli
	Light coma	Unarousable; withdraws nonpurposefully to pain; may decerebrate or decorticate; brainstem reflexes intact
	Deep coma	Unarousable; unresponsive to painful stimuli; brainstem reflexes usually absent; decerebrate posturing usually noted
	Delirium	Has rapid onset; brief impairment of cognition including a clouding of consciousness and difficulty sustaining and shifting attention
	Dementia	A generalized, long-term decline in cognitive abilities such as memory, language, and clear consciousness

Source: Adapted from LeMone, P. and Burke, M. (2000), *Medical surgical nursing: Critical thinking in client care* (2nd ed.). Upper Saddle River, NJ: Prentice Hall.

	Cranial Nerve	Assessment
Table 5-3		
Cranial Nerve Assessment Tests	Cranial nerve I (Olfactory)	Assess ability to identify common odors
	Cranial nerve II (Optic)	Use Snellen chart to assess vision
	Cranial nerves III, IV, and VI (Oculomotor, Trochlear and Abducens)	EOM: extraocular movements; have client follow finger through all visual fields Ptosis (III): a droopy eyelid PEARLA: assess pupils equal and reactive to light and accommodation Nystagmus: the pupil movement choppy Doll's Eyes: in the comatose client it is present when eyes stay center while moving head left and right; absent when eyes move with the head
	Cranial nerve V (Trigeminal)	Jaw clench: palpate the masseter and temporal muscles when the client's jaw is clenched; note differences on left or right Compare light, dull, and sharp sensations on both side of the face Corneal reflex: on an unconscious client a wisp of cotton is touched to the cornea. The normal response is to blink Lids (V, VII): stroke each lid to elicit a blink response
	Cranial nerve VII (Facial)	Facial symmetry: note droopiness of nasal labia fold, lower eyelid or corner of mouth when asking client to grin, raise eyebrows and sniff; assess accuracy of tasting sweet, sour, and salty items on anterior two-thirds of the tongue
	Cranial nerve VIII (Acoustic)	Assess hearing of each ear with a ticking watch or whispering; cold caloric testing: irrigating ear in ice cold water causes a slow movement of the eyes toward the irrigated side with a rapid return to midline; this is called the oculovestibular reflex and indicates an intact brainstem
	Cranial nerves IX and X (Glossopharyngeal and Vagus)	Swallow reflex: can the client swallow water or is there dysphagia (difficulty swallowing)? Gag reflex: assess gag by touching the back of both side of the throat; a unilateral loss may be noted Hoarseness: is the client's voice hoarse? Cough reflex: is the client's cough strong, weak or absent? Assess sweet, salty, and sour taste on the posterior third of the tongue
	Cranial nerve XI (Spinal Accessory)	Neck strength: have client turn head against resistance Shoulder shrug: have client shrug shoulders against resistance
	Cranial nerve XII (Hypoglossal)	Tongue deviation: have client stick out tongue and move it side to side against resistance; if there is a weakness, the tongue will go to the stronger side

4) Criteria for grading muscle strength (see Box 5-1)

5) Common terms that are used when describing motor function are found in Table 5-4

d. Cerebellar examination: balance and coordination are under the control of the cerebellum

NCLEX!

1) To assess gait, have the client walk normally and then on on heels and toes and assess coordination; perform a Romberg's test by having the client stand with feet together and eyes closed while you stand close by to prevent falling; there should be minimal swaying for 20 seconds

2) To assess coordination, observe the client's ability to touch own nose and then touch one of your fingers, then his or her nose again; next observe the client's ability to touch each finger to the thumb of the same

Box 5-1

**Criteria for Grading
Muscle Strength**

0 = No contraction

1 = Trace of contraction

2 = Active movement with gravity

3 = Active movement against gravity

4 = Active movement against gravity and resistance

5 = Normal power

Note: Findings are recorded as a fraction with 5 (highest possible score) as the denominator; ex. normal finding is 5/5.

hand; finally, observe the client's ability to run the heel down the shin on each side while lying in the supine position

e. Sensory function

1) Have the client close the eyes while you touch the client on all dermatomes with objects that are sharp, dull, light to touch, and that vibrate (over bony prominence); the client should be able to discriminate the location and type of touch

2) To assess a client's sense of position (kinesthesia) have the client close the eyes and move the client's finger or toe up or down and ask the client to describe the movement

3) To assess for stereognosis, have the client identify an object in his or her hand with the eyes closed

4) To assess for graphesthesia have the client identify a number or letter traced on the palm of the hand

5) Test two-point discrimination by touching a client with two simultaneous pinpricks and asking how many pinpricks there were; use dull points on a caliper and begin on finger pads

f. Reflexes

1) The deep tendon reflexes (patellar, biceps, brachioradialis, triceps and Achilles) are assessed with a reflex hammer and scored; see Box 5-2 for the criteria for scoring

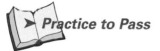

Practice to Pass

A client newly admitted to a long-term care facility exhibits confusion. What client assessments would be necessary to determine whether the client is experiencing delirium (acute confusion) versus dementia (chronic confusion)?

Table 5-4

**Common Terms
Associated with Motor
Function**

Term	Common Meaning
Strong	Normal strength
Weak	Not as strong as expected; moves against resistance but weak
Unable to lift	Can't bring limb off the bed; can't move against gravity
Withdraws	Pulls back from pain source
Reflex	Involuntary contraction of muscle or groups of muscles in response to pain
Decorticate	To painful stimuli, flexes arms, wrists, and fingers with adduction of the upper extremities and extension, internal rotation and plantar flexion of lower extremities
Decerebrate	To painful stimuli, extends, adducts, and hyperpronates arms and stiffly extends legs and planter flexes feet
Flaccid	No response to pain; no muscle tone
Ataxia	Incoordination of voluntary muscle groups

Box 5-2

**Standard Criteria for
Grading Reflexes**

0 = absent or no response

1 = hypoactive; weaker than normal (+)

2 = normal (++)

3 = stronger than normal (+++)

4 = hyperactive (++++)

2) The superficial abdominal reflex is assessed by lightly stroking the abdomen from the side to the midline; normally the side stroked will contract

3) The cremasteric reflex is assessed by lightly stroking the inside of the thigh on a male client to raise the testicle on that side

4) The Babinski reflex is assessed by stroking the lateral aspect of the sole of the foot from heel to ball, curving medially in the ball; its presence is noted with dorsiflexion of the big toe and fanning of the other toes, and is considered normal in infants but abnormal in adults; in adults, the normal response is curling of the toes (called a negative Babinski)

g. Speech: is usually described from the interview

1) Clear: normal fluent speech

2) **Dysarthria:** ineffective articulation of speech; may be a motor deficit of the tongue and speech muscles

3) Aphasia: a language disorder that is classified by type:

a) Expressive, motor, or nonfluent aphasia: is sometimes called Broca's aphasia; it is an inability to express one's self using motor aspects of speech

b) Receptive, fluent or sensory aphasia: is sometimes called Wernicke's aphasia; it is an inability to comprehend spoken words

c) Global aphasia: a client can neither express nor comprehend language (mixed receptive and expressive)

B. Diagnostic studies of the nervous system

1. Cerebrospinal fluid analysis: CSF is collected for analysis via lumbar puncture; the CSF is then studied for color, clarity, glucose, protein, blood, white cells, and bacteria; normal CSF is colorless, clear, and without blood or bacteria (white cells 0 to 5 cells/mm^3), glucose 40 to 80 mg/dL, and protein 16 to 45 mg/dL; assess site for leakage of CSF and for signs of infection after the procedure; following lumbar puncture, position head elevated with water-based contrast and flat with oil-based contrast

2. Radiological studies

a. Cerebral angiography: used to view the vascular structure of the brain; can be used to find arterio-venous malformations and/or aneurysms; use standard measures associated with use of contrast media (assess for allergy to iodine or shellfish; force fluids following to aid in excretion)

        b. Computed tomography (CT): the brain is scanned in layers for density and digitally converted to images of the layers; CT's are painless and readily available; it is very helpful in detecting bleeding, hydrocephalus, and ischemic strokes older than 48 hours; may be done with or without contrast; see precautions noted above

        c. Magnetic resonance imaging (MRI): the brain is scanned in layers by using a magnet to line up hydrogen atoms and then converts the findings of the scan into images; it can view the images on several planes; it is used to detect soft tissue changes including necrotic tissue, tumors, edema, congenital disorders, and degenerative diseases; assess client for implanted sources of metal that would contradict use of this procedure as a diagnostic method

   3. Electrographic studies

        a. Electroencephalography (EEG): a diagnostic procedure that measures brain waves with multiple scalp electrodes that is then interpreted by a neurologist; patterns of brain waves may suggest epilepsy, herpes simplex, encephalitis and dementia disorders; it is also an important criterion in determining brain death

           1) Teach client that the test will not deliver electric shock

           2) Shampoo the hair before the procedure for cleanliness and following the procedure to remove residual electrode gel or paste

           3) Withhold anticonvulsants and other medications as ordered for 12 to 24 hours prior

           4) Have the client eat regular meals to avoid hypoglycemia that could affect results

        b. Electromyography (EMG) and nerve conduction studies: these tests are used to differentiate between peripheral nerve and muscle disorders; conduction velocity of muscles is measured between 2 points and recording/measurements are taken at rest, with movement, and with electrical stimulation

   4. Ultrasound

        a. Carotid doppler scan: a noninvasive ultrasound of the carotids that detects occlusions and stenosis; ultrasound procedures cause no discomfort

        b. Transcranial doppler ultrasonography (TCD): a portable non-invasive technique used to assess intracranial circulation by measuring blood flow velocity; it is used to assess vasospasm, transient ischemic attack (TIA), headache, subarachnoid hemorrhage (SAH), head injury, and arteriovenous malformations (AVM)

III. Acute Disorders of the Nervous System

  A. Altered level of consciousness (LOC)

   1. Description: an altered LOC is a change in arousal or alertness and/or a change in cognition or solving complex problems (thought processes, memory, perception, problem solving and emotion); it is often the first sign of a change in neurologic status

2. Etiology and pathophysiology

   a. Causes for unconsciousness vary from primary CNS disorders (such as damage to the reticular activating system or the cerebrum) to dysfunction of other organ systems

   b. In addition, metabolic disorders may alter the cellular environment enough to inhibit neuronal activity

   c. The term coma is reserved for those who have long periods of unconsciousness, lasting from hours to months; neurological origin of coma results from damage to both hemispheres of the brain, damage to the brainstem, or both

3. Assessment

   a. Clinical manifestations

   1) Except for cases where there is damage to the brainstem, brain function deterioration and changes in LOC follow a predictable pattern from higher functions to primitive functions

   2) Confusion, forgetfulness, disorientation to time, then person, then place, agitation, poor problem solving abilities, or any change in behavior may be an early change in cerebrum function

   3) Changes of lethargy, obtundation, and stupor result from greater cerebral deterioration

   4) A change from purposeful movements to decorticate posturing (see Figure 5-1a), small reactive pupils, and positive doll's eyes manifest midbrain deterioration

   5) Decerebrate posturing (see Figure 5-1b), fixed pupils, and positive cold caloric tests show deterioration at the pons

   6) Finally, fixed pupils, flaccidity, and negative cold caloric tests indicate involvement at the medulla level

   7) Glasgow Coma Scale assessment includes components of eye opening (scored from 1 to 4), best verbal response (scored from 1 to 5), and best motor response (scored from 1 to 6); total score ranges from 3 to 15; a score of 8 or lower usually indicates coma

   b. Diagnostic and laboratory test findings

   1) CT and MRI may detect hemorrhage, tumor, cysts, edema, or brain atrophy

Figure 5-1

A. Decorticate rigidity.
B. Decerebrate rigidity.

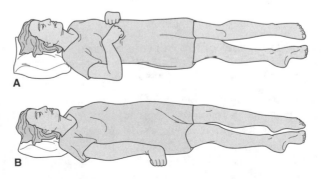

    2) EEGs evaluate unrecognized seizures as a cause for an altered LOC

    3) Cerebral angiography evaluates cerebral circulation for aneurysm and arterial-venous malformations

    4) Transcranial doppler study is a less invasive method to study blood flow

    5) A lumbar puncture with CSF analysis is done for infection

    6) Laboratory tests such as glucose, serum electrolytes, osmolarity, and creatinine, liver function, complete blood count (CBC), arterial blood gases (ABGs) and toxicology screens may be ordered to rule out metabolic, toxic, or drug-induced disorders

4. Therapeutic management: depends on the cause of the altered mental status; in addition to treating the cause of the problem, ongoing care focuses on airway maintenance, skin integrity, preventing contractures, and maintaining nutrition

5. Priority nursing diagnoses: Ineffective airway clearance; Risk for aspiration; Risk for impaired skin integrity; Impaired physical mobility; Risk for Imbalanced nutrition: less than body requirements

6. Planning and implementation

a. Assess for ability to clear secretions; assess breath sounds; maintain patent airway in the unconscious client; maintain client with ineffective airway in side-lying position; provide tracheostomy care every 4 hours if client has one

b. Assess swallowing and gag reflex; provide intervention to prevent aspiration; monitor for and report possible aspiration

c. Assess skin integrity every shift; reposition client every 2 hours; provide interventions to prevent skin breakdown; keep linens clean, dry, and wrinkle-free

d. Provide proper support devices to maintain extremities in functional condition perform passive range of motion (ROM) regularly

e. Monitor nutritional status and assess daily weight; assess need for alternative methods of nutritional support

7. Medication therapy: depends on the cause of the altered mental status

8. Client education: family anxiety is common when clients have altered mental status, especially if the prognosis is uncertain

a. Reinforce information provided by the physician

b. Encourage the family to talk to the client

c. Evaluate and provide information about client's care when the family is ready

d. Offer support services as needed

9. Evaluation: clients should maintain a clear and patent airway, remain aspiration free, maintain skin integrity, maintain functional status, and maintain nutritional status

B. Increased intracranial pressure (ICP)

1. Description

a. Increased intracranial pressure (ICP) is defined as a prolonged pressure greater than 15mm Hg or 180 mm H$_2$O measured in the lateral ventricles

NCLEX!

NCLEX!

b. Coughing, sneezing, straining, and bending forward cause a transient increase in ICP that does not cause significant tissue ischemia

c. Cushing's triad/response: involves three classic signs or responses to increased ICP: increased systolic blood pressure while diastolic remains the same, widening pulse pressure, and reflex bradycardia from stimulation of the carotid bodies

d. A prolonged increase in ICP causes tissue ischemia because cerebral blood flow and perfusion are compromised

e. Autoregulation, a compensatory mechanism to maintain cerebral blood flow, is disrupted and can lead to cellular hypoxia and ischemia

f. Untreated increased ICP leads to herniation and ultimately death

2. Etiology and pathophysiology: because the brain is encased in a closed cavity, expansion any of the contents of the cavity can cause increased ICP

a. Cerebral edema is an increase in volume of brain tissue due to alterations in capillary permeability (vasogenic edema), changes in functional or the structural integrity of the cell membrane (cytotoxic edema) or an increase in interstitial fluids (interstitial cerebral edema); edema is usually proportional to the size of the injury and may be localized or generalized

b. Hydrocephalus is an increase in the volume of CSF within the ventricular system; it may be noncommunicating hydrocephalus where drainage from the ventricular system is impaired (as when a mass blocks the flow of CSF) or communicating hydrocephalus, such as when blood blocks the arachnoid villi from absorbing CSF in a subarachnoid hemorrhage

3. Assessment

a. Clinical manifestations: the earliest signs of increased ICP may be blurred vision, decreased visual acuity, and diplopia because of pressure on the visual pathways; headache, papilledema or swelling of the optic disk and vomiting are the next signs; the most significant sign of increased ICP is a change in LOC; as pressure increases from front to back of the brain, the LOC deteriorates)

b. Diagnostic and laboratory test findings are directed to identifying and treating the underlying cause of the increased ICP

1) CT or MRI scanning is generally the initial test

2) In general a lumbar puncture is not performed because of the possibility of brain herniation caused by the sudden release of pressure

3) Laboratory tests are performed to augment and monitor treatment approaches; serum osmolarity monitors hydration status and ABGs measure pH, oxygen, and carbon dioxide (hydrogen ions and carbon dioxide are vasodilators that can increase ICP)

4. Therapeutic management

a. Increased ICP is a medical emergency with little time for lengthy diagnostic studies; it centers on restoring normal pressure and can be accomplished through medications, surgery, and drainage of CSF from the ventricular system

b. A drainage catheter, inserted via ventriculostomy into the lateral ventricle, can be done to monitor ICP and to drain CSF to maintain normal pressure;

if used, the system is calibrated with the trasducer is leveled 1 inch above the ear (height of foramen of Munro); sterile technique is of utmost importance

5. Priority nursing diagnoses: Altered cerebral tissue perfusion, Risk for infection, Impaired physical mobility, Risk for ineffective airway clearance

6. Planning and implementation

    a. Assess neurological status every 1 to 2 hours and report any deterioration; assessment areas include LOC, behavior, motor/sensory function, pupil size and response, vital signs with temperature

    b. Maintain airway; elevate head of bed 30° or keep flat as prescribed; maintain head and neck in neutral position to promote venous drainage

    c. Assess for bladder distention and bowel constipation; assist client when necessary to prevent Valsalva maneuver

    d. Plan nursing care so it is not clustered because prolonged activity may increase ICP; provide for a quiet environment (lights kept low also) and limit noxious stimuli; limit stimulants such as radio, TV, and newspaper; avoid ingesting stimulants such as coffee, tea, cola drinks, and cigarette smoke

    e. Maintain fluid restriction as prescribed

    f. Keep dressings over catheter dry and change dressings as prescribed; monitor insertion site for CSF leakage or infection; monitor clients for signs and symptoms of infection; use aseptic technique when in contact with ICP monitor

7. Medication therapy

    a. Osmotic diuretics such as mannitol (Osmitrol) and loop diuretics such as furosemide (Lasix) are mainstays used to decrease ICP; they work by drawing water from edematous tissues and into the vascular system; they can also disturb glucose and electrolytes so it is necessary to monitor their effect

    b. Corticosteroids have been shown to be effective in decreasing ICP, especially with tumors, although its mechanism of action is unclear

8. Client education

    a. Teach the client at risk for increased ICP to avoid coughing, blowing the nose, straining for bowel movements, pushing against the bed side rails, or performing isometric exercises

    b. Advise the client to maintain neutral head and neck alignment

    c. Encourage the family to maintain a quiet environment and minimize stimuli

    d. Educate the family that upsetting the client may increase ICP

9. Evaluation: normal intracranial pressure is maintained; ischemia is minimized; airway patency and functional status are maintained

C. Head trauma: skull fractures

1. Description: skull fracture is a break in the skull that occurs with or without intracranial trauma; the force of the impact significantly increases the risk of hematoma formation; the disruption of the skull can lead to infection and cranial nerve injury

2. Etiology and pathophysiology: skull fractures occur from trauma; they may be labeled as open or closed, depending on whether or not the skin is broken; there are four classifications of fractures:

   a. *Linear* fractures are the most common; risk of infection and CSF leakage is minimal because the dura remains intact; hematoma formation is possible

   b. *Comminuted* and *depressed* skull fractures have a higher risk of brain tissue damage and infection especially if the overlying skin and dura is torn or damaged; the risk of secondary brain injury is reduced because, impact energy caused bone fracture instead of being transferred to brain tissue

   c. *Basilar* skull fractures involve the base of the skull and are usually secondary injuries; most are uncomplicated, but those that disrupt the sinuses and middle ear bones can lead to infection and CSF leakage

3. Assessment

   a. Clinical manifestations associated with skull fractures may give clues to area of fracture; basilar skull fracture may produce the following manifestations

      1) Battle's sign, ecchymosis over the mastoid process

      2) Hemotympanum, blood visible behind the tympanic membrane

      3) Raccoon eyes, bilateral periorbital ecchymosis

      4) Rhinorrhea, CSF leakage through the nose

      5) Otorrhea, CSF leakage through the ear

   b. Diagnostic and laboratory test findings: diagnosis of skull fractures may be done with plain x-ray films, and CT or MRI scans; basilar skull fractures may be difficult to identify on plain x-ray

4. Therapeutic management: treatment depends on the type and location of the injury

   a. Linear skull fractures generally require bed rest and observation for underlying brain injury; no specific treatment is necessary

   b. Commuted and depressed skull fractures require surgical intervention within 24 hours

   c. Basilar skull fractures do not require surgery unless there is persistent CSF leakage; regular neurological assessments and observations for meningitis are required

5. Priority nursing diagnoses: Risk for infection, Risk for injury

6. Planning and implementation

   a. Observe client for otorrhea or rhinorrhea

   b. Test clear ear drainage and sinus drainage for glucose; only CSF has glucose; mucous secretions do not

   c. Observe blood tinged drainage for halo sign; glucose-containing CSF dries in concentric rings on gauze or tissues

   d. Keep nasopharynx and external ear clean; use sterile technique and supplies when cleaning drainage from nose and/or ears

e. Instruct client not to blow nose, cough, or inhibit sneeze and to sneeze through an open mouth

    f. Use aseptic technique when changing head dressings

  7. Medication therapy

    a. Dexamethasone may be administered to decrease cerebral edema

    b. Antibiotics may be given when there is a risk of infection

  8. Client education: instruct client and family to go to the emergency department if the client experiences drowsiness or confusion, difficulty waking, vomiting, blurred vision, slurred speech, prolonged headache, blood or clear fluid leaking from ears or nose, weakness in an arm or leg, stiff neck, or convulsions

  9. Evaluation: client recovers without complications or complications are recognized quickly

D. Head trauma: intracranial hemorrhage

  1. Description: intracranial hemorrhage is an escape of blood into the cranium, most commonly associated with blunt trauma; hemorrhage may cause a very slow to very rapid neurological deterioration

  2. Etiology and pathophysiology: intracranial hemorrhage results directly from trauma or from the shearing forces on cerebral arteries and veins from acceleration-deceleration injuries; they are classified by location

    a. Epidural hematoma

      1) Develops between the dura and the skull

      2) As the hematoma forms, it strips the dura away from the skull

      3) Epidural hematomas usually develop from a tear in the meningeal artery

      4) Because this is an arterial bleed, it rapidly expands, leading to a rapid deterioration in neurological status

    b. Subdural hematoma

      1) Forms between the dura mater and the arachnoid-pia mater layers of the meninges

      2) Usually involves veins but may involve small arteries as well

      3) As blood collects, pressure is applied to the underlying brain tissue

      4) Subdural hematomas may be acute (developing within 48 hours after an acute injury), subacute (developing 2 days to 3 weeks after lesser injury) or chronic (developing 3 weeks to months after a minor injury), or they may develop spontaneously

    c. Intracerebral hemorrhage

      1) Is bleeding into the brain tissue

      2) It can occur anywhere in the brain but is most common in the frontal or temporal lobes

3) It may be the result of closed head trauma, where shearing forces are applied deep in the brain; an example of this is in a motor vehicle accident where an individual hits the head on the windshield, resulting in coup and contrecoup injury

3. Assessment

    a. Clinical manifestations

        1) Epidural hematoma: the client may initially lose consciousness then have a short period of lucidness, followed rapidly by deterioration from drowsiness to coma; other manifestations include headache, fixed dilated pupil on affected side, hemiparesis, hemiplegia, and possible seizures; this condition is a surgical emergency

        2) Subdural hematoma: manifestations may develop slowly and may be mistaken for dementia in the elder client; slow thinking, confusion, drowsiness, or lethargy are common; headaches, ipsilateral pupil dilation and sluggishness, and possible seizures are other signs

        3) Intracerebral hematomas vary in initial presentation depending on the location; headache is common; as the hematoma progresses, a decreased LOC, hemiplegia, and ipsilateral pupil dilation occurs; an expanding clot may lead to herniation

    b. Diagnostic and laboratory test findings: diagnosis may be made with CT and MRI scanning; laboratory values are of little use in establishing diagnosis, but may be used as baseline data for client's overall state of health

4. Therapeutic management: small hematomas will reabsorb spontaneously and may be treated conservatively; surgical intervention is needed for epidural hematomas and larger subdural hematomas; surgery is less successful in intracerebral hematomas because of widespread tissue damage; supportive care and preventing complications are goals of therapy

5. Priority nursing diagnoses: Ineffective airway clearance, Ineffective breathing pattern, Risk for injury, Risk for disuse syndrome (if unable to purposely move in environment), Altered cerebral tissue perfusion

6. Planning and implementation

    a. Assess neurological signs on a regular schedule; clear the client's nose and mouth of secretions; suction airway as needed

    b. Monitor respiratory pattern for rate, depth and rhythm if client is not ventilated; prepare for oxygen administration and endotracheal intubation for respiratory distress

    c. Prepare for cranial surgery for deteriorating neurological condition

    d. Provide appropriate preoperative and postoperative care as needed

    e. Provide previously discussed measures to manage increased intracranial pressure

7. Medication therapy: no medication is indicated specific to hematomas; medication such as anticonvulsants and steroids could be used as indicated to treat seizures and increased ICP if they occur as complications

8. Client education: the family needs to be informed of the possibility of surgery to evacuate the hematoma

9. Evaluation: client maintains adequate respiratory rate and rhythm, adequate cerebral perfusion, and remains free of neurological complications

E. Inflammatory conditions: meningitis

1. Description: an inflammation of the meninges of the brain and spinal cord; besides infectious disease exposure, risk factors include basilar skull fracture, otitis media, sinusitis, mastoiditis, neurosurgery or other invasive procedures, systemic sepsis, and impaired immune function

2. Etiology and pathophysiology: most frequently is caused by infection of the meninges and CSF (rarely chemicals are the cause); infection (bacterial, viral, fungal or parasitic) causes an inflammatory response in the meninges; bacterial meningitis may be complicated by hydrocephalus, cerebral edema, arthritis, and cranial nerve damage; viral meningitis is usually less severe; the course of the disease is usually shorter and more benign

3. Assessment

   a. Clinical manifestations

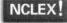

   1) Restlessness, agitation, and irritability

   2) Abdominal and back pain

   3) Nausea and vomiting

   4) Severe headaches

   5) Signs of meningeal irritation, nuchal rigidity (stiff neck), positive Brudzinski's sign (pain, resistance and hip and knee flexion occur when the neck is flexed to the chest while lying supine) and positive Kernig's sign (pain and/or resistance occurs with flexion of the knee and hip and straightening of the knee in the supine position) and photophobia

   6) Chills and high fever

   7) Confusion, altered LOC

   8) Seizures

   9) Signs and symptoms of increasing ICP

   b. Diagnostic and laboratory test findings: lumbar puncture with CSF analysis including gram stain and cultures is the definitive diagnostic measure for meningitis; cultures of blood, urine, throat, and nose are collected to identify possible source of infection

4. Therapeutic management: bacterial meningitis is a medical emergency that, if not treated, can be fatal within days; successful treatment depends on accurate diagnosis and aggressive treatment; treatment focuses on eradicating infection with antibiotics, supportive treatment and managing symptoms; surgical treatment may include placement of an Ommaya reservoir to allow **intrathecal** (into the subarachnoid space) administration of antibiotics

5. Priority nursing diagnoses: Altered protection, Risk for deficient fluid volume

6. Planning and implementation

   a. Assess neurological status and vital signs (with temperature) regularly

   b. Assess and report changes in neurological status or presence of cranial nerve dysfunction

c. Assess, prepare for, and report any seizure activity

d. Assess for signs of increased ICP

e. Administer prescribed medications and maintain fluid restrictions

f. Assess for fluid volume deficits, monitor intake and output and daily weights, skin turgor, laboratory values, and urine concentration

7. Medication therapy: high-dose broad-spectrum antibiotics initially (bacterial meningitis) to cross the blood-brain barrier; when cultures are reported a more specific antibiotic may be used; anticonvulsants (usually phenytoin [Dilantin]) are prescribed to prevent or control seizures; antipyretic, antiemetic and analgesic medications are used for symptom relief; IV fluid replacement is continued until client can resume oral intake

8. Client education

a. Teach the client the name and purpose of prescribed antibiotics and to take them until they are gone; teach client about other ordered medications as well

b. Teach the client and family to recognize and report signs and symptoms of ear, throat, and upper respiratory infections so they can be assessed for meningitis

9. Evaluation: neurological status improves; symptoms of infection disappear; close contacts with symptoms receive proper and prompt medical care

F. Guillain Barré syndrome

1. Description: an acute, rapidly-progressive inflammation of peripheral motor and sensory nerves characterized by motor weakness and paralysis that ascends from lower extremities in a majority of cases; outcome is generally excellent if care is appropriate

2. Etiology and pathophysiology: occurs most frequently between ages of 30 and 50 years; etiology is unknown, but autoimmune reaction is suspected, because it often develops after viral infection, immunizations, fever, injury, and sometimes surgery; antibody (IgM) formation targets peripheral nerve myelin, which damages myelin sheath and disrupts nerve conduction; the nerve re-myelinizes in the opposite direction of the demyelination

3. Assessment

a. Clinical manifestations

1) Weakness/paresis or partial paralysis progressing upward from lower extremities (paralysis in Guillain Barré is "**g**round to the **b**rain") and then to total paralysis requiring ventilatory support

2) Paresthesias (numbness and tingling) and pain

3) Muscle aches, cramping and nighttime pain

4) Respiratory compromise and/or failure (dyspnea, diminished vital capacity and breath sounds), decreasing O_2 saturation, abnormal ABGs

5) Difficulty with extraocular eye movements, dysphagia, diplopia, difficulty speaking

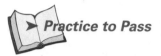

Practice to Pass

A college student visits health service complaining of a headache that does not ever go away. What other assessments would the nurse make to determine whether the client could be developing meningitis, which has been on the rise in this college community?

NCLEX!

6) Autonomic dysfunction (orthostatic hypotension), hypertension, change in heart rate, bowel and bladder dysfunction, flushing, and diaphoresis

b. Diagnostic and laboratory findings: nerve conduction test results are diminished, CSF examination shows elevated protein

4. Therapeutic management

a. Supportive care to maintain function of all body systems, including respiratory, cardiac, GI, renal, and skin; medications as discussed below

b. Plasmapheresis: plasma is removed and separated from whole blood; blood cells are then returned without the plasma to removed antibodies that cause disorder; monitor for complications of this therapy, which include bleeding from loss of clotting factors and fluid and electrolyte imbalance

5. Priority nursing diagnoses: Risk for disuse syndrome; Altered protection; Ineffective breathing pattern; Risk for impaired gas exchange; Imbalanced nutrition: less than body requirements

6. Planning and implementation

NCLEX!

a. Monitor respiratory status: rate, depth, breath sounds, vital capacity, note secretions, and check gag, cough, and swallowing

b. Monitor cardiac status: heart rate, BP, dysrhythmias

c. Administer chest physiotherapy and pulmonary hygiene measures

NCLEX!

d. Maintain adequate nutrition as appropriate: administer enteral or parenteral nutrition as needed; if client can swallow, assist with small frequent feedings of soft foods; weigh client weekly; check electrolyte status; provide mouth care every 2 hours

e. Monitor bowel and bladder function: assess bowel sounds and frequency, amount, color of bowel movements; offer bedpan; check for distention and residuals in client who cannot void spontaneously; perform intermittent catheterization as needed; encourage fluid intake to 3500 mL/day

NCLEX!

f. Prevent complications of immobility: encourage use of weak extremities as able; provide assistance with ROM and exercises prescribed by PT; protect immobile extremities with use of air mattress or special bed, and elbow and heel protectors; turn and reposition every 2 hours; elevate extremities to prevent dependent edema; use antiembolism compression devices/stockings

g. Provide eye care for the client with inability to close eyelids completely; instill artificial tears, cleanse eyes as needed, use eye shields and tape eyes closed if needed

h. Provide comfort and analgesics as needed

i. Promote communication with client and family, using alternative means of communication if client is on ventilator or is unable to speak because of weak speech muscles

j. Initiate discharge planning at time of admission

7. Medication therapy: IV immunoglobulins (may result in low-grade fever, muscle aches, headache, or (rarely) acute renal failure or retinal necrosis; adrenocorticotropic hormone (ACTH) and corticosteroids or anti-inflammatory drugs; supportive medications that include stool softeners, antacids or H_2 receptor antagonists, and analgesics

8. Client education: explain all care with rationales and provide information about the progression of the disease; encourage client and family to express feelings and participate in care as much as possible

9. Evaluation: client maintains satisfactory respiratory, cardiac, GI, and renal status; client resumes ability to move extremities and recovers from illness with no permanent loss of function

G. Cerebrovascular accident (CVA, brain attack, stroke)

1. Description: a CVA is a condition where neurological deficits occur as a result of decreased blood flow to a localized area of the brain; hypertension, diabetes mellitus, sickle cell disease, substance abuse, and atherosclerosis are risk factors for stroke; onset of stroke may be rapid or gradual

2. Etiology and pathophysiology: ischemia followed by cell death is the result of severe and prolonged cerebral blood flow obstruction; resulting deficits predict the location of the stroke; there are four types of brain attacks:

   a. Transient ischemic attack (TIA) is a brief period of neurological deficits that resolve within 24 hours; they are frequently precursors to a permanent CVA; the causes of TIAs may be inflammatory arterial disorders, sickle cell anemia, atherosclerotic changes in cerebral vessels, thrombosis, and emboli

   b. Thrombotic CVA is caused by a thrombus (blood clot) occluding a cerebral vessel thrombi tend to form on atherosclerotic plaque in the larger arteries while the blood pressure is lower (such as during sleep or rest); thrombosis occurs quickly but deficits progress slowly

   c. Embolic CVA is caused by a traveling blood clot; the source of the clot is elsewhere in the body; the CVA has a sudden onset with immediate symptoms; if the embolus is not absorbed, deficits will be persistent

   d. Hemorrhagic CVA or intracranial hemorrhage occurs when a blood vessel ruptures; this most often occurs in the presence of long-term, poorly controlled hypertension; other factors that may cause a hemorrhagic CVA include a ruptured intracranial aneurysm, embolic CVA, tumors, arteriovenous malformations, anticoagulant therapy, liver disease, and blood disorders; this form of CVA is most often fatal because of rapidly increasing ICP; onset of symptoms is rapid; loss of consciousness occurs in about half the cases

3. Assessment

   a. Clinical manifestations: vary according to cerebral vessel involved

      1) Internal carotid: contralateral motor and sensory deficits of the arm, leg and face; in dominant hemispheric CVA, **aphasia** (loss of ability to use language); in nondominant hemispheric CVA, **apraxia** (inability to perform known tasks), **agnosia** (inability to recognize) and unilateral neglect and homonymous **hemianopsia** (loss of one half of the visual field in each eye)

2) Middle cerebral artery: drowsiness, stupor, coma, contralateral hemiplegia and sensory deficits of arm and face, aphasia, and homonymous **hemianopsia**

3) Anterior cerebral artery: contralateral weakness or paralysis and sensory loss of the foot and leg, loss of decision making and voluntary action abilities, and urinary incontinence

4) Vertebral artery: pain in face, nose or eye, numbness or weakness of face on ipsilateral side, problems with gait, **dysphagia** (difficulty swallowing), and **dysarthria** (difficulty speaking)

b. Diagnostic and laboratory test findings: a CT and MRI demonstrate hemorrhage, tumors, ischemia, edema, and tissue necrosis; cerebral angiography detects abnormal vessel structure, vasospasm, stenosis of the carotid artery and loss of vessel wall integrity; ultrasound evaluates blood flow

4. Therapeutic management

a. Drug therapy is the most common treatment for CVAs; if it is a thrombotic stroke, medications could include thrombolytics and/or heparin

b. It is imperative not to disrupt a clot that has formed following hemorrhagic CVA

c. Surgery is not usually indicated as a treatment modality

d. Rehabilitation is crucial to improve deficits

5. Priority nursing diagnoses: Impaired physical mobility, Self-care deficit, Impaired verbal communication

6. Planning and implementation

a. Encourage active range of motion on unaffected side and passive range of motion on affected side

b. Turn client every 2 hours

c. Monitor lower extremities for thrombophlebitis

d. Encourage use of unaffected arm for ADLs

e. Teach client to put clothing on affected side first

f. Resume diet orally only after successfully completing a swallowing evaluation; clients may need thickened liquids, foods with the consistency of oatmeal, and to chew on unaffected side of mouth; this is sometimes referred to as a dysphagia diet

g. Collaborate with occupational and physical therapy for rehabilitation

h. Try alternate methods of communication with aphasia clients

i. Accept client's frustration and anger as normal to loss of function

j. Teach client with homonymous hemianopsia to overcome the deficit by turning the head side to side to be able to fully scan the visual field

7. Medication therapy

a. Antiplatelet agents are used to treat TIAs and previous CVA clients (except hemorrhagic CVAs)

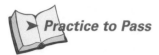

Practice to Pass

What are the key differences in nursing management of a client who had a hemorrhagic stroke versus an ischemic stroke?

b. During the acute phase of thrombotic and embolic stroke, thrombolytic therapy using tissue plasminogen activator may be administered within 3 hours to dissolve the clot

c. Anticoagulant therapy with heparin initially and then continued with an oral anticoagulant after the acute phase

d. In clients with cerebral edema, hyperosmolar solutions (mannitol) or diuretics (furosemide or Lasix) may be given

e. In clients with seizures, anticonvulsants, such as phenytoin (Dilantin), barbiturates, diazepam (Valium) and lorazepam (Ativan) may be given

8. Client education

a. Educate client and family about CVA and CVA prevention

b. Educate client and family about community resources

c. Educate client and family about physical care and need for psychosocial support

d. Educate client and family about medications

9. Evaluation

a. Client understands CVA and CVA prevention

b. Client maximizes self-care

c. Motor function is maximized

G. Spinal cord trauma

1. Description

a. Spinal cord injuries are usually due to trauma; young adults and adolescents are most commonly affected

b. The injury affects motor and sensory function at the level of injury and below

c. Spinal cord injuries are classified by complete or incomplete cord injury, cause of injury, and level of injury; in clinical practice, these overlap

d. Perception, sexual function, and elimination are also affected

e. Risk factors include age, gender, and alcohol and drug abuse

2. Etiology and pathophysiology: spinal injuries are usually the result of excessive force applied to the spinal cord and vertebral column; four types of injuries occur:

a. Hyperflexion compresses vertebral bodies and disrupt ligaments and discs

b. Hyperextension disrupts ligaments and causes vertebral fractures

c. Axial loading is the application of excessive vertical force and may cause compression fractures

d. Excessive rotation tears ligaments and fractures articualar surfaces and causes compression fractures (see Figure 5-2)

Figure 5-2 Spinal cord injury mechanisms. A. Hyperflexion; B. Hyperextension; C. Axial loading, a form of compression.

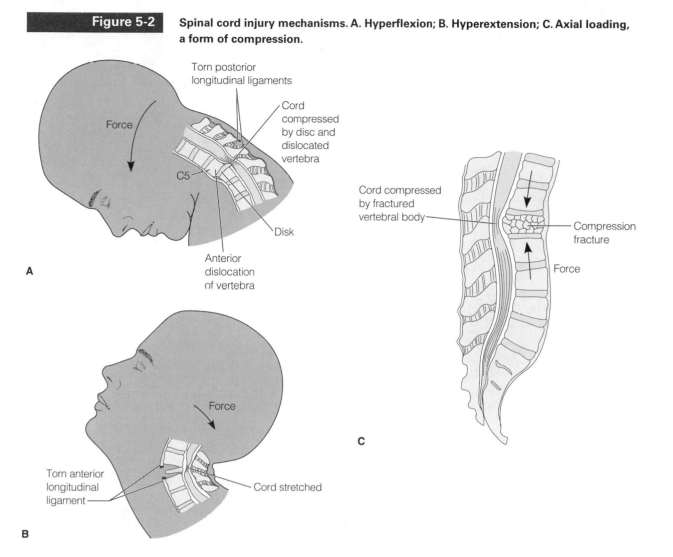

3. Assessment

   a. Clinical manifestations

NCLEX!

1) Spinal shock, the temporary loss of reflex function, may occur following a spinal cord injury: symptoms include bradycardia, hypotension, flaccid paralysis of skeletal muscles, loss of pain, touch, temperature, pressure, visceral and somatic sensations, bowel and bladder dysfunction and loss of ability to perspire; spinal shock has resolved once spinal reflexes return

2) **Paraplegia** is paralysis of the lower portion of the body; it occurs when the injury level is in the thoracic spine or lower

3) **Tetraplegia,** formally quadriplegia, is paralysis of the arms, trunk, legs and pelvic portion; it occurs when the level of injury is in the cervical spine

NCLEX!

4) **Autonomic dysreflexia** is an exaggerated sympathetic response that occurs in clients with T6 injuries or higher; the response is seen after spinal shock occurs when a stimuli cannot ascend the cord; a stimulus such as the urge to void or abdominal discomfort triggers massive vasoconstriction below the injury, vasodilation above the injury, and bradycardia

b. Diagnostic and laboratory test findings: x-ray films are done to visualize fractures; CT and MRI scans show changes in the vertebrae, spinal cord and tissues surrounding the cord; an EMG is done after the acute injury to locate the level of injury

NCLEX!

4. Therapeutic management: acute management of spinal cord injuries involves immobilizing injury and treating complications of respiratory distress, atonic bladder, paralytic ileus, and cardiovascular alterations; high-dose steroid protocol is initiated to prevent secondary cord injury from edema and ischemia; stabilization with devices such as halo traction and Gardner-Wells tongs or surgery is done when indicated

5. Priority nursing diagnoses: Impaired gas exchange, Dysreflexia, Disturbed self-esteem

6. Planning and implementation

a. Monitor vital capacity and respiratory effectiveness; high cervical cord injuries may inhibit respiratory function

b. Monitor for signs of ascending edema; may cause respiratory compromise

c. Assist client with quad coughing by pushing in and up at the xiphoid process when client is coughing

d. Treat autonomic dysreflexia immediately

NCLEX!

NCLEX!

1) Elevate head of bed and remove TEDS

2) Assess blood pressure every 2 to 3 minutes while assessing for stimuli that initiated response; remove the stimulus immediately when found

3) With severe hypertension unresolved by removing the offending stimulus notify the physician and administer antihypertensives as ordered per protocol

e. Encourage client to verbalize feelings about loss of function and care

f. Institute bowel and bladder training programs to restore a regular schedule for elimination

g. Encourage self-care and independent decision making

h. Include family and important others in discussions

i. Clients with spinal cord injury because of fracture or dislocation of cervical vertebrae may benefit from a Halo brace; it is an external fixation device that allows earlier mobility because skeletal cervical traction by Gardner-Wells tongs or other apparatus is not needed

7. Medication therapy: corticosteroids (such as methylprednisolone, Solu-Medrol) are used to decrease or control edema of the cord; vasopressors are used to treat hypotension or hypertension due to spinal shock or autonomic

Practice to Pass

A client with recent spinal cord injury is beginning the rehabilitative phase of care. What ancillary services are needed to support the client's efforts to return to independent living?

dysreflexia; antispasmodics (baclofen or Lioresal and diazepam or Valium are used to treat spasticity in clients); analgesics and tricyclic antidepressants are used to treat pain

8. Client education

   a. Teach client and family to promote independence in self-care, such as self-catheterization technique, bowel evacuation, activities of daily living, etc.

   b. Educate client and family about the variety of community resources that will be needed

   c. If client has a Halo vest, teach that it raises the center of gravity; avoid bending over to reduce risk of falls; neck is immobilized in midline so client needs to learn to turn entire body to scan environment; driving is prohibited; food is cut into small pieces and a straw is used for liquids

9. Evaluation

   a. Client maintains adequate respiratory status

   b. Autonomic dysreflexia resolves

   c. Feelings about loss of function are verbalized

   d. Client makes satisfactory adjustments in lifestyle

IV. Chronic Disorders of the Nervous System

A. Seizures

1. Description

   a. A seizure is an episode of excessive and abnormal electrical activity of all or part of the brain

   b. This abnormal electrical activity is manifested by disturbances in skeletal motor activity, sensation, autonomic dysfunction of the viscera, behavior or consciousness

   c. Seizures may be isolated from acute febrile state, head injury, infection metabolic or endocrine disorders or exposure to toxins

   d. If the seizure activity is chronic, (i.e., they reoccur within minutes, days or even years), the diagnosis of epilepsy is given

2. Etiology and pathophysiology

   a. The exact initiating factor for seizures is unknown

   b. All people have a seizure threshold; when that threshold is exceeded a seizure ensues

   c. Metabolic needs, oxygen requirements, metabolic by-products, and cerebral blood flow increase dramatically

   d. As long as cerebral blood flow can meet the demands of the seizure, the brain is protected from cellular exhaustion and destruction

   e. Epilepsy may be idiopathic (without identifiable cause) or may occur secondary to a known cause such as birth trauma, infection, vascular abnormalities, trauma, or tumors

  f. Seizures are classified as partial or generalized; partial seizures begin in one area of the cortex and generalized involve both hemispheres and deeper brain structures

 3. Assessment

  a. Clinical manifestations

   1) *Simple partial seizures* are limited to one hemisphere; manifestations include alterations in motor function, sensory signs or autonomic or psychic symptoms

   2) *Complex partial seizures* originate in the temporal lobe and may be preceded by an aura: an impaired level of consciousness and repetitive nonpurposeful movements such as lip-smacking, picking, or aimless walking are noted; amnesia is common

   3) *Generalized partial seizure* is a partial seizure that has spread to both hemispheres and deeper structures of the brain

   4) *Absence seizure* is a generalized seizure that lasts 5 to 30 seconds; there is a sudden brief cessation of motor activity and a blank stare; they may occur occasionally or up to a 100 per day; they may be accompanied by eyelid fluttering or automatisms such as lip-smacking; more common in children than adults

   5) Tonic-clonic seizures (grand mal) are the most common type of seizure

    a) They may be preceded by an aura but are often without warning

    b) Typically the seizure starts with a loss of consciousness and sharp muscle contractions

    c) The client falls to the floor, and may have urinary and/or bowel incontinence

    d) Breathing ceases and cyanosis develops during the tonic phase (about 15 sec to 1 min)

    e) The clonic phase (60 to 90 sec) follows with alternating muscle contraction and relaxation in all extremities, hyperventilation, and eyes rolled back in the head (see Figure 5-3)

    f) In the next phase (postictal period) the client is relaxed with quiet breathing, unconscious and unresponsive; the client gradually regains consciousness and may have transient confusion and disorientation; clients often complain of head and muscle aches, fatigue and may sleep several hours

    g) Clients will have amnesia of the seizure and events just prior to the seizure

   6) *Status epilepticus* is a life-threatening emergency that can occur during seizure activity; it is characterized by continuous cycles of tonic-clonic activity with short periods of calm between them; this cumulative effect can interfere with respiration; the client is in great danger of developing hypoxia, hyperthermia, hypoglycemia, and exhaustion if seizure activity is not stopped

  b. Diagnostic and laboratory test findings: diagnostic testing is done to confirm diagnosis and to determine treatable causes and precipitating factors;

NCLEX!

NCLEX!

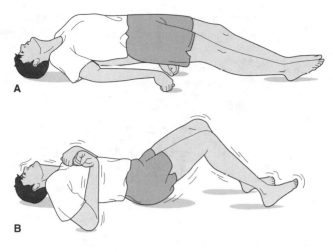

Figure 5-3

Tonic-clonic contractions in grand mal seizures. A. Tonic phase; B. Clonic phase.

these include a complete neurological examination, EEG, skull X-ray scries, CT scan, lumbar puncture with CSF analysis, blood studies and electrocardiogram

4. Therapeutic management: pharmacological interventions are the mainstay of controlling seizure activity; when all attempts fail, then surgery for excision of tissue involved in the seizure activity may be the safest alternative

5. Priority nursing diagnoses: Risk for ineffective airway clearance, Risk for injury, Anxiety

6. Planning and implementation

   a. Provide interventions during seizure to maintain airway patency; turn client to side if needed to maintain airway and promote drainage of secretions without aspiration; have oxygen and suction equipment at the bedside for use following a seizure if needed; do not try to force an object, such as a bite stick, into the mouth of a client who is seizing, as this may break teeth or cause other injury

   b. Provide interventions during a seizure to reduce the risk of injury; do not restrain client but provide an environment that will not create further injury; teach family members how to protect the client during seizures

   c. Document seizure activity promptly and report it as appropriate

   d. Provide support to client that concerns are normal; help the client identify leisure activities that are safe; provide information about resources and support groups; provide accurate information about hiring practices and legalities of driving or operating heavy/dangerous equipment

7. Medication therapy

   a. Anticonvulsants that raise seizure threshold or limit the spread of abnormal electrical activity are the mainstay of epilepsy treatment

   b. Some commonly used anticonvulsants are phenytoin (Dilantin), divalproex sodium (Depakote), valproic acid (Depakene), carbamazepine (Tegretol), gabapentin (Neurontin), and lamotrigine (Lamictal)

    c. Diazepam (Valium), lorazepam (Ativan) and phenobarbital are also used intermittently to stop seizure activity during acute episodes

  8. Client education

    a. Correct misconceptions, fears, and myths about epilepsy

    b. Encourage client and family to express feelings

    c. Provide information about community and national resources for epilepsy

    d. Stress the importance of follow-up care

    e. Review any laws (such as driving a motor vehicle) that apply to people with epilepsy

    f. Refer for employment or vocational counseling as needed

    g. Stress the importance of wearing a medical alert band

    h. Emphasize aura alert

    i. Stress the importance of continuing anticonvulsant therapy

    j. Stress the importance of avoiding physical and emotional stress

    k. Help client focus on positive aspects of life

    l. Teach to avoid alcohol and limit caffeine; and to take showers instead of baths to avoid drowning

    m. Discuss factors that may trigger seizure activity, such as increased stress, lack of sleep, emotional upset, and alcohol use

  9. Evaluation

    a. Client has reduced or absent seizure activity

    b. Client is protected from harm during seizure

    c. Client verbalizes importance of continuing anticonvulsant drug therapy

    d. Client obtains a medical alert band

B. Parkinson's disease (PD)

  1. Description: Parkinson's disease is a progressive, degenerative neurological disease characterized by bradykinesia, muscle rigidity, and nonintentional tremor; it commonly affects older adult and is usually diagnosed between the ages of 50 to 60; as the disease progresses the burden of care increases

  2. Etiology and pathophysiology: in PD, atrophy occurs in the substantia nigra that produces the neurotransmitter dopamine; as dopamine decreases, acetylcholine is no longer inhibited; this imbalance in neurotransmitter is the clinical basis for symptoms

  3. Assessment

    a. Clinical manifestations: begin subtly; fatigue and a slight resting tremor may be the only initial symptoms; in a small population of clients dementia may be the presenting symptom

      1) **Bradykinesia** is slow movements caused by muscle rigidity; they affect also the eyes, mouth, and voice; there is also a staring gaze

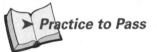

Practice to Pass

A client with seizure disorder is started on anticonvulsant therapy with phenytoin (Dilantin). What are the key elements that should be included in a teaching plan about this medication?

NCLEX!

NCLEX!

2) Uncoordinated movements

3) Short stepped, shuffling and propulsive gait, which leads to increased risk of falls

4) Postural disturbance, trunk tilted forward

5) Seborrhea

6) Excessive sweating of face and neck with absence of sweating on trunk and extremities

7) Heat intolerance

8) Constipation

9) Anxiety

10) Depression

11) Sleep disturbances

12) Dysphagia

   b. Diagnostic and laboratory test findings

1) CBC may show anemia

2) Chemistry profile may show low albumin and protein

3) Drug screens may be done to rule out toxic causes

4) An EEG may show a slow pattern and disorganization

5) An upper GI series may show delayed emptying, distention, and mega-colon

6) A video fluoroscopy may show a slowed response of the cricopharyngeal muscles when swallowing

4. Therapeutic management: management includes medications, surgery, and rehabilitation aimed at optimizing functional level; a team approach is essential to quality care of PD clients

5. Priority nursing diagnoses: Impaired physical mobility; Impaired verbal communication; Imbalanced nutrition: less than body requirements

6. Planning and implementation

   a. Perform active ROM twice a day

   b. Ambulate at least four times a day

   c. Use assistive devices when recommended

   d. Assess communication skills, speech, hearing, and writing

   e. Consult with a speech pathologist if necessary

   f. Assess nutritional status and self-feeding abilities

   g. Monitor diet for foods high in bulk and fluids

7. Medication therapy: drugs used to treat PD include monoamine oxidase (MAO) inhibitors, dopaminergics, dopamine agonists, and anticholinergics to treat PD; eventually all these drugs lose effectiveness; the fluctuating response to drugs is called the on-off response; antidepressants, especially amitriptyline, are used to treat depression; propranolol may be used to treat tremors

8. Client education

    a. Teach preventive measures for malnutrition, falls, and other environmental hazards, constipation, skin breakdown from incontinence and joint contractures

    b. Teach gait training and exercises for improving ambulation, swallowing, speech, and self-care

9. Evaluation: client maintains adequate nutritional status, client remains free from falls; constipation is controlled

C. Multiple sclerosis

1. Description: a chronic disorder of the CNS where the myelin and nerve axons in the brain and spinal cord are destroyed; there are four forms based on the rate of progression: benign, relapsing-remitting, primary progressive, and secondary progressive

2. Etiology and pathophysiology

    a. Unknown etiology, possibly an autoimmune or genetic basis or may be caused by childhood viral infections

    b. The destruction of myelin and nerve axons causes a temporary, repetitive, or sustained interruption in the conduction of nerve impulses which causes the symptoms of MS

    c. Plaque formation occurs throughout the white matter of the CNS, which also affects the nerve impulses of optic nerves, cervical spinal cord, thoracic and lumbar spine

    d. Inflammation occurs around the plaques as well as normal tissue

    e. Astrocytes appear in the lesions and scar tissue forms, replacing the axons and leading to permanent disability

3. Assessment

    a. Clinical manifestations: visual disturbances or blindness (retrobulbar neuritis), sudden, progressive weakness of one or more limbs, spasticity of muscles, nystagmus, tremors, gait instability, fatigue, bladder dysfunction (UTIs, incontinence), depression

    b. Diagnostic and laboratory findings: lumbar puncture for CSF (clonal IgG bands present); MRI, CT scans, muscle testing show characteristic changes

4. Therapeutic management: no cure is available; supportive care is indicated

5. Priority nursing diagnoses: Risk for disuse syndrome, Altered protection, Disturbed body image, Risk for infection

6. Planning and implementation

    a. Overall goal of care is to maintain as much independent function as possible

b. Include rest periods to prevent fatigue in the client, which is an exacerbating factor

c. Assist the client to have choices in care and set priorities on a day-to-day basis whenever possible to maintain sense of control and independence

d. Assist client with ADLs on an as-needed basis; provide adaptive utensils or other assistive devices as needed

e. Maintain a fluid intake of at least 2000 mL/day to maintain bowel and bladder function and prevent impaction and/or urinary tract infection

f. Communicate with client about issues of concern, such as coping skills, sexuality, changing body image, or other issues perceived by the client

g. Avoid sources of infection; illness can act as a stressor and trigger an exacerbation

7. Medication therapy: immunosuppressant therapy, antiviral drugs, corticosteroids, antibiotics for urinary tract infections, interferon-alpha, glatiramer (Copaxone), anticholinergic drugs, and antispasmodics

8. Client education: medications, symptoms, bladder training, intermittent self-catheterization, sexual functioning, avoiding complications, and possible triggers (fatigue, temperature extremes, illness)

9. Evaluation: client maintains independence to degree allowed by symptoms; is free of infection; verbalizes importance of preventing fatigue that would exacerbate disease process

D. Myasthenia gravis

1. Description: a chronic progressive disorder of the peripheral nervous system affecting transmission of nerve impulses to voluntary muscles; causes muscle weakness and fatigue that increases with exertion and improves with rest; eventually leads to fatigue without relief from rest

2. Etiology and pathophysiology

a. Causes include unknown etiology, family history of autoimmune disorders, thyroid tumors

b. An autoimmune process triggers the formation of autoantibodies that decrease the number of acetylcholine receptors and widen the gap between the axon ending and the muscle fiber in the neuromuscular (myoneural) junction

c. Muscle contraction is hindered because the IgG autoantibodies prevent acetylcholine from binding with the receptors; destruction of the receptors at the neuromuscular junction occurs

d. Is associated with continued production of autoantibodies by the thymus gland in 75 percent of cases

e. Onset is usually slow but can be precipitated by emotional stress, hormonal disturbance (pregnancy, menses, thyroid disorders), infections/vaccinations, trauma and surgery, temperature extremes, excessive exercise, and drugs that block or decrease neuromuscular transmission (opioids, sedatives, barbiturates, alcohol, quinidine, anesthetics), and thymus tumor

3. Assessment

   a. Clinical manifestations

      1) Mild diplopia (double vision) and unilateral ptosis (eyelid drooping) caused by weakness in the extraocular muscles; weakness may also involve the face, jaw, neck, and hip

      2) Complications arise when severe weakness affects the muscles of swallowing, chewing and respiration; respiratory distress is manifested by tachypnea, decreased depth, abnormal ABGs, O_2 sat < 92 percent, and decreased breath sounds

      3) Bowel and bladder incontinence, paresthesias and pain in weak muscles

      4) Myasthenic crisis: sudden motor weakness; risk of respiratory failure and aspiration; most often caused by insufficient dose of medication or an infection

      5) Cholinergic crisis: severe muscle weakness caused by over medication; also cramps, diarrhea, bradycardia, and bronchial spasm with increased pulmonary secretions and risk of respiratory compromise

   b. Diagnostic and laboratory findings

      1) ABGs and pulmonary function tests may show respiratory insufficiency

      2) Electromyography (EMG) shows decreased amplitude when motor neurons are stimulated

      3) Confirmation of the clinical diagnosis can be made by IV administration of edrophonium chloride (Tensilon), which allows voluntary muscle contraction; Tensilon allows acetylcholine to bind with its receptors, which temporarily improves symptoms; weakness returns after the effects of Tensilon are discontinued; a positive Tensilon test confirms diagnosis of myasthenia gravis

4. Therapeutic management: focuses on medication management with anticholinesterases: neostigmine (Prostigmin), pyridostigmine (Mestinon); immunosuppressants: corticosteroids, azathiopirine (Imuran), and cyclosporine (Cytoxan); antiinflammatory drugs; thymectomy (removal of the thymus gland); plasmapheresis—removes IgG antibodies, atropine sulfate (Atropine) for cholinergic crisis

5. Priority nursing diagnoses: Ineffective airway clearance, Impaired swallowing, Activity intolerance, Risk for injury, Disturbed body image

6. Planning and implementation

   a. Maintain effective breathing pattern and airway clearance; thoroughly assess for respiratory distress

   b. Monitor meals and teach client to bend head slightly forward while eating/drinking to improve swallowing

   c. Teach client to avoid exposure to infections, especially respiratory

    d. Teach client effective coughing, use chest physiotherapy and incentive spirometry; have oral suction available, teach client how to use it; be prepared to intubate if needed

NCLEX!

    e. Provide adequate nutrition: schedule meds 30 to 45 minutes before eating for peak muscle strength while eating; offer food frequently in small amounts that are easy to chew and swallow—soft or semisolid as needed; administer IV fluids and nasogastric tube feedings if client is unable to swallow

    f. Promote improved physical mobility with referrals to physical therapy/occupational therapy

    g. Provide eye care: instill artificial tears; use a patch over one eye for double vision; wear sunglasses to protect eyes from bright lights

    h. Promote positive body image and coping skills: encourage participation in treatment plan; plan time for active listening and encourage client to express feelings; reinforce progress and explain all care

7. Medication therapy: anticholinesterases such as neostigmine (Prostigmin), pyridostigmine (Mestinon); immunosuppressants such as corticosteroids, azathioprine (Imuran), and cyclosporine (Cytoxan); anti-inflammatory drugs

8. Client education

    a. Instruct client to plan rest periods and to conserve energy; plan major activities early in day; schedule activities during peak medication effect

NCLEX!

    b. Instruct client to avoid extremes of hot and cold, exposure to infections, emotional stress and meds that may worsen or precipitate an exacerbation (alcohol, sedatives, local anesthetics)

    c. Instruct client in signs of crisis

    d. Encourage client to wear a Med-Alert bracelet

    e. Instruct in alternative methods of communication if needed: eye blink, finger wiggle for yes/no; flash cards or communication board; teach to support lower jaw with hands to assist with speech

9. Evaluation

    a. Maintains patent airway and breathing without aspiration

    b. Maintains activities of daily living with assistance

    c. Demonstrates adequate coping skills for managing chronic and debilitating illness

E. Alzheimer's disease

1. Description: Alzheimer's disease (AD) is a progressive dementia with irreversible deterioration of general intellectual function; it affects adults in middle to late life; AD incidence increases with age

2. Etiology and pathophysiology: The cause of AD is unknown; chemical changes in the brain are found in the hippocampus, and frontal and temporal lobes of the cerebral cortex; the clients lose nerve cells; perfusion to affected areas is decreased; the brain atrophies; amyloid, a starch-like protein accumulates in brain tissue; as AD progresses more areas of the brain are affected

3. Assessment

    a. Clinical manifestations: AD is classified into three stages based on manifestations and abilities

        1) Early stage: lasts 2 to 4 years; the client appears healthy and alert but may be restless or uncoordinated; cognitive impairment is not apparent; memory impairment, subtle changes in personality, and problems doing simple calculations may be the first manifestations of AD

        2) Middle stage: lasts 2 to 12 years; memory impairment is more evident (recent memory is lost before remote memory); the client is less able to behave spontaneously; the client may wander or get lost; increasing confusion and disorientation is apparent even though there are periods of lucidity; language deficits including paraphasia (using the wrong word) and echolalia (repetition of words or phrases) are common; judgment is impaired; self-care is compromised because sequencing of tasks is lost; sensorimotor deficits of apraxia, astereognosis, and agraphia are common

        3) Late stage: lasts 2 to 4 years; this is characterized by increasing dependence, aphasia, incontinence, loss of motor skills and gross loss of cognitive abilities

    b. Diagnostic and laboratory test findings: AD is a diagnosis of exclusion, meaning that other causes of symptoms are ruled out; CBC may reflect anemia; EEG may show slowing in the later stages of AD; CT and MRI may show atrophy; psychometric evaluations reflect memory and cognitive impairment

4. Therapeutic management: AD clients and their families require extensive follow-up and support; because there is no cure for AD, the main objective of care is to match function with environment; safety and least restrictive environment are high priorities

5. Priority nursing diagnoses: Altered thought processes, Anxiety, Hopelessness

6. Planning and implementation

    a. Label room, drawers, or other items as needed

    b. Orient client to person, place, and time as needed

    c. Keep daily routine consistent as possible

    d. Remove client from activities that increase anxiety

    e. Avoid criticizing or judging expressed feelings

    f. Provide realistic information about disease process

    g. Use therapeutic communication and listening skills to reduce agitation; listening to client's recollection of past events is helpful for client's psychosocial status

7. Medication therapy: reversible acetylcholinesterase inhibitors, such as tacrine (Cognex), donazepil (Aricept), and rivastigmine (Exelon) improve memory in AD client; antihistamine and tricyclic antidepressants are avoided because of high anticholinergic activity; occasionally tranquilizers are necessary to treat agitation

8. Client education

    a. Avoid stopping reversible acetylcholinesterase inhibitors suddenly because it can trigger behavior problems

    b. Teach caregivers about community resources

    c. Educate client and caregivers about expectations for client's disease process

9. Evaluation: safety is maintained, the least restrictive environment is provided, frequent follow-up care is provided

F. Cranial nerve disorders

1. Description: cranial nerve (CN) disorders involve dysfunction of the cranial nerves, the most commonly affected are the trigeminal nerves (CN V) and the facial nerve (CN VII); trigeminal neuralgia and Bell's palsy are the respective disorders; trigeminal neuralgia is a chronic disease of the trigeminal nerve that causes severe facial pain; Bell's palsy is a unilateral paralysis of the facial muscles

2. Etiology and pathophysiology

    a. Trigeminal neuralgia has an unknown cause; it affects one or more of the three divisions of the trigeminal nerve; the ophthalmic, the maxillary and the mandibular; the maxillary and the mandibular divisions are affected most often

    b. Bell's palsy also has an unknown cause; inflammation of the nerve and a viral cause has been suggested; 80 percent of clients recover completely within a few weeks to months; of those remaining 15 percent will recover some function but have permanent facial paralysis

3. Assessment

    a. Clinical manifestations

        1) Trigeminal neuralgia: brief, intense, skin surface pain is the characteristic symptom; episodes may occur as frequently as 100 times a day or as little as a few times each year; pain typically starts peripherally and advances centrally; motor or sensory deficits do not occur; some clients may have trigger zones that initiate the onset of pain; in others, pain may be triggered by light touch, eating, swallowing, talking, shaving, sneezing, brushing teeth, or washing the face

        2) Bell's palsy: manifestations include one-sided paralysis of the facial muscles, paralysis of the upper eyelid with loss of the corneal reflex on the affected side, loss or impairment of taste over the anterior portion of the tongue on affected side, and increased tearing from lacrimal gland on the affected side

    b. Diagnostic and laboratory test findings: there are no specific laboratory tests specific to cranial nerve disorders

4. Therapeutic management

    a. Trigeminal neuralgia treatment is centered on controlling pain with anticonvulsant medications such as carbamazepine (Tegretol); surgical procedures include microvascular decompression (removal of blood vessel from posterior trigeminal root) or rhizotomy, (surgical severing of the nerve root)

NCLEX!

b. Bell's palsy: the only medical treatment that influences outcome is administration of corticosteroids, but their use has been questioned; antiviral medication is also currently very popular

5. Priority nursing diagnoses: Risk for imbalanced nutrition: less than body requirements; Pain; Risk for injury

NCLEX!

6. Planning and implementation

a. Encourage client to chew on unaffected side

b. Monitor dietary intake

c. Assist with physiotherapy, including moist heat, gentle massage, and facial nerve stimulation with faradic current

d. Protect cornea with artificial tears, sunglasses, eye patch at night, and gentle intermittent closure of eye

7. Medication therapy

a. Trigeminal neuralgia: the most useful drug for controlling pain is carbamazepine (Tegretol); when this is not effective, phenytoin (Dilantin) is tried

b. Bell's palsy: a corticosteroid such as prednisone (Deltasone) influences outcome by decreasing edema of nerve tissue; antivirals are also used

8. Client education

a. Wear an eye patch at night

b. Wear protective glasses when outside

c. Inspect the inside of mouth on affected side for food that may collect between mouth and teeth

9. Evaluation: the eye is protected; pain is controlled

Case Study

A 24-year-old male is admitted to the neuroscience nursing unit following a motor vehicle accident in which he suffered a head injury after hitting the windshield while unrestrained in the front passenger seat. He is being evaluated for a possible intracranial hemorrhage secondary to the injury. You are the admitting nurse for this client.

❶ What will you include in a focal neurological assessment of this client?

❷ What diagnostic tests will confirm the presence of intracranial hemorrhage?

❸ What signs would indicate that the client is developing increased intracranial pressure?

❹ How will you plan care to minimize elevations in intracranial pressure?

❺ What medications do you anticipate being ordered for this client?

For suggested responses, see page 736.

Posttest

1 An unconscious client who is not receiving mechanical ventilation and who does have enteral feeding infusing has sudden onset of adventitious breath sounds. The nurse would first gather additional data to determine the presence of which of the following nursing diagnoses?

(1) Risk for aspiration
(2) Risk for fluid volume deficit
(3) Risk for imbalanced nutrition: less than body requirements
(4) Altered thought processes

2 A client has undergone insertion of an intracranial pressure (ICP) monitoring device. The nurse would become most concerned if the ICP readings measured which of the following for a prolonged period of time?

(1) 3 mm Hg
(2) 7 mm Hg
(3) 10 mm Hg
(4) 22 mm Hg

3 The nurse is admitting a client from the emergency department following a fall that resulted in increased intracranial pressure (ICP). The nurse interprets that the client's Glasgow Coma Scale score has improved the most after making which of the following latest assessments?

(1) Best eye opening response 5, best motor response 4, best verbal response 8
(2) Best eye opening response 4, best motor response 6, best verbal response 5
(3) Best eye opening response 6, best motor response 5, best verbal response 4
(4) Best eye opening response 3, best motor response 8, best verbal response 6

4 The nurse planning care for a client who suffered a cerebrovascular accident (CVA) with residual dysphagia would write on the care plan to avoid doing which of the following during meals?

(1) Feed the client slowly
(2) Give the client thin liquids
(3) Give foods with the consistency of oatmeal
(4) Place food on the unaffected side of the mouth

5 A client who experienced a spinal cord injury at the level of T5 rings the call bell for assistance. Upon entering the room, the nurse finds the client to have a flushed head and neck, complaining of severe headache, and being diaphoretic. The pulse is 47 and BP is 220/114 mm Hg. The nurse concludes that immediate treatment is needed for:

(1) Malignant hypertension.
(2) Pulmonary embolism.
(3) Autonomic dysreflexia.
(4) Spinal shock.

6 A nurse is preparing to admit a client from the emergency department who experienced seizure activity. The nurse would omit placing which of the following pieces of equipment in this client's room?

(1) Padded tongue blade
(2) IV equipment
(3) Oxygen and suction equipment
(4) Padded bedrails

7 The home care nurse is doing an admission assessment on a client discharged from the hospital with a diagnosis of Parkinson's disease. When assessing the client's neurological status, the nurse would find the client's gait to be:

(1) Staggering and unsteady.
(2) Shuffling and propulsive.
(3) Waddling but broad-based.
(4) Accelerating with walking on tips of toes.

8 A client with Alzheimer's disease begins to speak to the nurse about life in the 1930s. Which of the following actions by the nurse is most appropriate?

(1) Orient the client to time, place, and person.
(2) Distract the client by inviting him to watch television.
(3) Encourage the client to talk about recent events in the news.
(4) Listen to the client's anecdotes.

9 The nurse reads in an admission note that the physical examination of a client revealed an impairment of cranial nerve II. The nurse instructs ancillary caregivers to do which of the following when caring for this client?

(1) Whisper to the client
(2) Serve food at room temperature
(3) Clear the client's path of obstacles
(4) Test the temperature of any running water

10 The nurse is instructing the client with Bell's palsy information regarding medications that might reduce nerve tissue edema. The nurse would explain the actions and side effects of which of the following medications?

See pages 209–210 for Answers and Rationales.

(1) Acetaminophen (Tylenol)
(2) Ibuprofen (Advil)
(3) Dexamethasone (Decadron)
(4) Prednisone (Deltasone)

Answers and Rationales

Pretest

1 Answer: 4 *Rationale:* Alcohol is a drying agent and should not be used when performing mouth care (lemon-glycerin products should also be avoided). Use a small toothbrush to make cleaning easier. Place the client on the right or left side and avoid the supine position to reduce the risk of aspiration. Toothettes can be used on the gums, tongue, and mucous membranes to reduce drying and subsequent breakdown.
Cognitive Level: Application
Nursing Process: Implementation; *Test Plan:* PHYS

2 Answer: 4 *Rationale:* Vital signs changes are late indicators of rising intracranial pressure. Trends include an increase in temperature and blood pressure, and a decrease in pulse and respirations. The level of consciousness would also deteriorate before these manifestations arise.
Cognitive Level: Application
Nursing Process: Assessment; *Test Plan:* PHYS

3 Answer: 2 *Rationale:* Hyperventilation to achieve a $PaCO_2$ of 25 to 30 mm Hg causes cerebral vasoconstriction that will lead to reduced intracranial blood volume and reduced ICP. Option 1 is excessive; option 3 is normal, and option 4 indicates hypercarbia (excess carbon dioxide).
Cognitive Level: Analysis
Nursing Process: Evaluation; *Test Plan:* SECE

4 Answer: 2 *Rationale:* Hemiparesis is a one-sided weakness that often occurs following stroke. The client will have maximum return of function and the least amount of frustration with relearning new tasks when objects are placed within easy reach on the un-

affected side. This will also decrease the risk of client injury because the client will not have to reach for objects needed for self-care. Unilateral neglect is not a problem when the client has right-sided deficits, so objects do not need to be placed on the affected side.
Cognitive Level: Application
Nursing Process: Implementation; *Test Plan:* SECE

5 Answer: 3 *Rationale:* Clients who have a spinal cord injury above the level of T7 are at risk for autonomic dysreflexia, an exaggerated autonomic response to a noxious stimulus. This complication can be assessed by noting the presence of severe, throbbing headache, flushed face and neck, bradycardia, and severe hypertension that is sudden in onset. Other signs to assess for are nausea, sweating, nasal stuffiness, and blurred vision.
Cognitive Level: Application
Nursing Process: Assessment; *Test Plan:* PHYS

6 Answer: 2 *Rationale:* Documentation about seizure activity includes the time the seizure began, changes in pupil size, eye deviation or nystagmus, body part(s) affected, utterance or sounds (epileptic cry), the type of movements and progression, client condition during the seizure, and post-ictal status. The other items listed are unnecessary.
Cognitive Level: Application
Nursing Process: Implementation; *Test Plan:* PHYS

7 Answer: 2 *Rationale:* Clients with Parkinson's disease have bradykinesia (slow movements that are hard to initiate), which can be offset to some degree by rocking back and forth to initiate movement. Activities should be interspersed with rest periods throughout the day to minimize fatigue. Chairs

should be high and firm rather than soft and deep. Velcro fasteners and slide buckles will be of most use to a client who is trying to maintain independence with dressing and grooming.
Cognitive Level: Analysis
Nursing Process: Evaluation; *Test Plan:* HPM

8 **Answer: 1** *Rationale:* Nurses caring for clients who have Alzheimer's disease should ensure that these clients are wearing an identification bracelet so they do not become lost if they wander. It is unnecessary to assess LOC hourly, and restraints are also not indicated. It is not essential that the client be placed in a quiet, calm environment; rather, they often prefer to be allowed to move about at will.
Cognitive Level: Application
Nursing Process: Planning; *Test Plan:* SECE

9 **Answer: 1** *Rationale:* The pain of trigeminal neuralgia is triggered by stimulation of the sensory fibers of the trigeminal nerve. Examples of pressure-related triggering events include shaving, toothbrushing, washing the face, and eating or drinking. Examples of temperature-related triggers include environmental changes and hot or cold food and drink. The other options listed do not initiate the pain of this disorder.
Cognitive Level: Application
Nursing Process: Implementation; *Test Plan:* PHYS

10 **Answer: 2** *Rationale:* Antidepressants, tranquilizers, and anticonvulsants are generally withheld for 24 to 48 hours before an EEG. The client does not have to be NPO, but should avoid stimulants such as coffee, tea, cola, alcohol, and cigarettes. Preprocedure care for EEG involves teaching that there is no discomfort, and shampooing the hair.
Cognitive Level: Application
Nursing Process: Implementation; *Test Plan:* SECE

Posttest

1 **Answer: 1** *Rationale:* Oral or gastrointestinal secretions can enter the client's airway and cause aspiration. The onset of adventitious breath sounds indicates this risk clearly. The other options are incorrect because they do not relate to the client's airway.
Cognitive Level: Analysis
Nursing Process: Analysis; *Test Plan:* PHYS

2 **Answer: 4** *Rationale:* Normal ICP readings extend up to 10 mm Hg pressure (options 1, 2, and 3). Sustained elevations above 15 mm Hg are of concern, as they are abnormally high. The client's neurological status is probably deteriorating as well.
Cognitive Level: Analysis
Nursing Process: Analysis; *Test Plan:* PHYS

3 **Answer: 2** *Rationale:* As outlined in the options, the Glasgow Coma Scale is divided into three subsets. Each subset has a range of scores within it, and for the total scale the highest possible score is 15 while the lowest is 3. The higher the score, the more optimal should be the recovery. Scores in the "best eye opening response" category range from spontaneously (4), to speech (3), to pain (2), no response (1). Scores in the "best motor response" category range from obeys verbal commands (6), localizes pain (5), flexion-withdrawal (4), flexion-abnormal (3), extension-abnormal (2), no response (1). Scores in the "best verbal response" category range from oriented $\times$ 3 (5), conversation-confused (4), speech-inappropriate (3), sounds-incomprehensible (2), and no response (1).
Cognitive Level: Analysis
Nursing Process: Assessment; *Test Plan:* PHYS

4 **Answer: 2** *Rationale:* A client who experienced a CVA may have involvement of the cranial nerve responsible for swallowing (XII), and generally undergoes a swallowing evaluation to determine whether a diet can be taken. The client with some residual dysphagia may be started on a diet once the gag and swallow reflexes have returned. In this instance, liquids should be thickened to avoid aspiration. The other options represent helpful actions for the client with dysphagia.
Cognitive Level: Application
Nursing Process: Implementation; *Test Plan:* PHYS

5 **Answer: 3** *Rationale:* Above the level of T6, clients with spinal cord injury are at risk for autonomic dysreflexia. It is a life-threatening syndrome triggered by a noxious stimulus below the level of the injury. This complication is characterized by severe, throbbing headache, flushing of the face and neck, bradycardia, and sudden severe hypertension. A client may also exhibit nasal stuffiness, blurred vision, nausea and sweating.
Cognitive Level: Analysis
Nursing Process: Analysis; *Test Plan:* PHYS

6 **Answer: 1** *Rationale:* It is highly controversial whether or not to use a bite stick when a client is experiencing seizure activity. The greatest risk is that teeth could be damaged if it is inserted during a seizure. The other pieces of equipment listed are useful in the care of the client and should be made ready at the bedside.
Cognitive Level: Application
Nursing Process: Implementation; *Test Plan:* SECE

7 Answer: 2 *Rationale:* The Parkinsonian gait is characterized by short, shuffling, accelerating steps. The head leans forward, the hips and knees flexed, and the client has difficulty starting (bradykinesia) and stopping. Options 1, 3, and 4 describe ataxic, dystrophic, and festinating gait, respectively.
Cognitive Level: Application
Nursing Process: Assessment; *Test Plan:* PHYS

8 Answer: 4 *Rationale:* Since long-term memory is retained for a longer period of time than short-term memory, clients with Alzheimer's disease will be able to recollect events from long ago. It is helpful to allow clients to reminisce. The other options represent nontherapeutic techniques for this client as described.
Cognitive Level: Analysis
Nursing Process: Implementation; *Test Plan:* PSYC

9 Answer: 3 *Rationale:* The optic nerve, which governs vision, is cranial nerve II. For this client it would be most helpful to clear the area of objects that may not be perceived by the client but that could lead to falls. The actions described in the other options are unnecessary.
Cognitive Level: Analysis
Nursing Process: Planning; *Test Plan:* SECE

10 Answer: 4 *Rationale:* Prednisone is often used to treat Bell's palsy. The drug is a steroid, which will reduce inflammation and edema and thereby allow the return of normal circulation in the area of the nerve. It can help preserve a significant amount of function, and is effective against pain, when given early in the course of treatment.
Cognitive Level: Analysis
Nursing Process: Evaluation; *Test Plan:* PHYS

References

Barker, L., Burton, J., & Zieve, P. (1999). *Principles of ambulatory medicine* (5th ed.). Media, PA: Williams and Wilkins, pp. 1230–1250, 1274–1295.

Brillhart, B. (2000). Nursing management: Patient with a stroke. In S. Lewis, M. Heitkemper, & S. Dirksen (Eds.), *Medical surgical nursing: Assessment and management of clinical problems* (5th ed.). (pp. 1645–1671). St. Louis, Mosby.

Bruegge, M. (2001). Assessment of the neurologic system. In J. Black, J. Hawks, & A. Keene (Eds.), *Medical-surgical nursing: Clinical management for positive outcome* (6th ed.). Philadelphia: Saunders, pp. 1874–1904.

Hickey, J. (2001) *The clinical practice of neurological and neurosurgical nursing* (5th ed.). Philadelphia: Lippincott, pp. 35–168, 275–327, 543–566, 613–634, 666–667.

Kerr, M. (2000). Nursing management: Intracranial problems. In S. Lewis, M. Heitkemper, and S. Dirksen (Eds.), *Medical-surgical nursing: Assessment and management of clinical problems* (5th ed.). St. Louis: Mosby, pp. 1608–1643.

LeMone, P. & Burke, K. (2000). *Medical-surgical nursing: Critical thinking in client care* (2nd ed.). Upper Saddle River, NJ: Prentice Hall, Inc., pp. 1672–1868.

McCance, K. & Huether, S. (2002). *Pathophysiology: The biological basis for disease in adults and children* (4th ed.). St. Louis, MO: Mosby-Year Book Inc., pp. 460–473, 489–492.

Minton, M. (2001). Management of clients with cerebral disorders. In J. Black, J. Hawks, & A. Keene (Eds.), *Medical-surgical nursing: Clinical management for positive outcomes* (6th ed.). Philadelphia: Saunders, pp. 1923–1949.

Seidel, H., Ball, J., Dains, J., & Benedict G. (1999). *Mosby's guide to physical examination* (4th ed.). St. Louis, MO: Mosby Inc., pp. 775–804.

Shpritz, D. W. (2002). Interventions for clients with problems of the central nervous system. The brain. In. D. Ignatavicius & M. Workman *Medical-surgical nursing: Critical thinking for collaborative care* (4th ed.). Philadelphia: Saunders, pp. 897–924.

Shpritz, D. W. (2002). Interventions for clients with problems of the central nervous system: The spinal cord. In D. Ignatavicius & M. Workman (Eds.), *Medical-surgical nursing: Critical thinking for collaborative care* (4th ed.). Philadelphia: W. B. Saunders, pp. 925–952.

Smeltzer, S. & Bare, B. (2000). *Brunner & Suddarth's textbook of medical-surgical nursing* (9th ed.). Philadelphia: Lippincott, pp. 1607–1631, 1633–1670, 1674–1698, 1700–1760.

Renal and Urinary Disorders

Sammie L. Justesen, RN

CHAPTER OUTLINE

OBJECTIVES

▌ Identify basic structures and functions of the renal and urinary systems.

▌ Describe the pathophysiology and etiology of common renal and urinary disorders.

▌ Discuss expected assessment data and diagnostic test findings for selected renal and urinary disorders.

▌ Identify priority nursing diagnoses for selected renal and urinary disorders.

▌ Discuss therapeutic management of selected renal and urinary disorders.

▌ Discuss nursing management of a client experiencing a renal or urinary disorder.

▌ Identify expected outcomes for the client experiencing a renal or urinary disorder.

[Media Link]

Use the CD-ROM enclosed with this text, or log onto the address given to access the free, interactive Companion Website created for this series. The CD-ROM and Companion Website accompanying this book offer additional practice opportunities and information—NCLEX Review, Case Studies, Glossary, In Depth with NCLEX, and more.

www.prenhall.com/hogan

REVIEW AT A GLANCE

acute renal failure *sudden interruption of renal function caused by obstruction, poor circulation, or kidney disease*

chronic renal failure *slow, progressive loss of kidney function and glomerular filtration*

cystectomy *partial or total removal of the urinary bladder and surrounding structures*

cystitis *inflammation of the bladder*

glomerulonephritis *inflammation of the renal glomerulus characterized by decreased urine production, blood and protein in the urine, and edema*

hematuria *presence of blood in the urine*

hemodialysis *procedure to remove wastes from the blood by filtering the client's blood through a machine*

intravenous pyelography (IVP) *a radiology technique that involves injecting a contrast medium into a vein and taking x-ray films of the kidneys as the medium is cleared from the blood into the urinary system*

lithotripsy *procedure that breaks up stones within the urinary system*

nephrotic syndrome *renal disease characterized by massive edema and excess protein excretion*

oliguria *diminished urine production in relation to intake, usually less than 400 mL in 24 hours*

peritoneal dialysis *procedure during which blood is filtered through the peritoneal membrane to remove waste products*

polycystic kidney disease *a disorder characterized by multiple cysts of the kidney*

polyuria *excess production of urine*

proteinuria *presence of protein in the urine*

pyelonephritis *a pus-forming infection of the kidney that usually moves upward from the lower urinary tract*

pyuria *pus in the urine*

urinary diversion *procedure that provides an alternative route for urine excretion when normal channels are damaged or defective*

vesicoureteral reflux *backflow of urine from the bladder into the ureter*

Pretest

1 The nurse has admitted a client with uremia. The nurse plans care for which of the following underlying disorders?

(1) Polycystic kidney disease
(2) End-stage renal failure
(3) Pyelonephritis
(4) Cystitis

2 A client receiving peritoneal dialysis (PD) has outflow that is less than the inflow for two consecutive exchanges. Which of the following actions would be best for the nurse to take first?

(1) Check the client's blood pressure.
(2) Change the client's position.
(3) Irrigate the dialysis catheter.
(4) Continue to monitor the third exchange.

3 The nurse is planning to teach the client with acute glomerulonephritis about dietary restrictions. The nurse should include in the plan to make which of the following dietary changes?

(1) Limit fluid intake to 500 mL per day.
(2) Restrict protein intake by limiting meats and other high-protein foods.
(3) Increase intake of high-fiber foods, such as bran cereal.
(4) Increase intake of potassium-rich foods such as bananas or cantaloupe.

4 A client develops a renal disorder after taking an antibiotic that has nephrotoxicity as an adverse effect. The nurse adds to the client's medical record a standardized care plan for which of the following disorders?

(1) Polycystic kidney disease
(2) Glomerulonephritis
(3) Acute renal failure
(4) Chronic renal failure

5 A client with a chronic urinary tract infection is scheduled for a number of laboratory tests. The nurse would review results of which of the following tests to best evaluate whether the kidneys are being adversely affected?

(1) Serum potassium
(2) Urinalysis
(3) Serum creatinine
(4) Urine culture

6 A female client with recurrent cystitis has been told to follow an acid-ash diet. The client demonstrates understanding of diet instruction if she states to avoid which of the following foods?

(1) Fish
(2) Corn
(3) Eggs
(4) Milk

7 The nurse is teaching the client to perform peritoneal dialysis (PD). The nurse reviews in detail which of the following essential actions that will help to prevent the major complication of peritoneal dialysis?

(1) Monitor the client's post-void residuals.
(2) Maintain strict aseptic technique during connection and disconnection.
(3) Add heparin to the dialysate at least once per day.
(4) Change catheter site dressing twice daily.

8 The nurse would assess a client with kidney stones for which of the following to best determine whether the client is developing renal colic?

(1) Flank pain
(2) Difficult urination
(3) Absence of urine
(4) Headache

9 A client seen in the emergency department complains of painful urination, frequency, and urgency. Which of the following conditions would the nurse suspect?

(1) Renal calculi
(2) Cystitis
(3) Glomerulonephritis
(4) Polycystic kidney disease

10 Which of the following is the priority nursing diagnosis for a client with urinary tract infection (UTI)?

(1) Anxiety
(2) Disturbed sleep pattern
(3) Disturbed body image
(4) Pain

See pages 254–255 for Answers and Rationales.

I. Overview of Anatomy and Physiology of the Renal and Urinary Systems

A. Renal structures (see Figure 6-1)

1. Kidneys: bean-shaped organs located on either side of spinal column behind the peritoneal cavity; regulate fluid and acid-base balance in the body

2. Adrenal glands: located atop each kidney; influence blood pressure and sodium and water retention

3. Renal cortex: outer region of kidneys; contains blood-filtering mechanisms

4. Renal medulla: middle region of kidneys; contains renal pyramids

5. Renal pyramids: triangular wedges containing tubular structures

   a. Apex: tapered section of each pyramid; empties into the calyx (calyces)

   b. Calyx (calyces): channel urine from renal pyramids to renal pelvis

6. Renal pelvis: expansion of the upper end of the ureters, formed as calyces join together

7. Nephrons: basic functional units of kidneys; selectively secrete and reabsorb ions; perform mechanical filtration of fluid, wastes, electrolytes, acids, and bases

   a. Glomerular capsule (Bowman's capsule): surrounds glomeruli

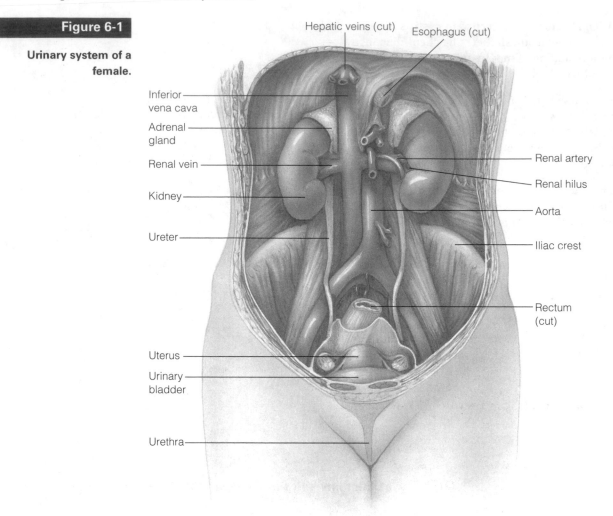

Figure 6-1

Urinary system of a female.

Hepatic veins (cut)

Esophagus (cut)

Inferior vena cava

Adrenal gland

Renal vein

Kidney

Ureter

Uterus

Urinary bladder

Urethra

Renal artery

Renal hilus

Aorta

Iliac crest

Rectum (cut)

b. Glomerulus (glomeruli): tuft of capillaries within each nephron; filter large plasma proteins and blood cells

c. Glomerular filtrate: fluid filtered by the glomeruli; similar to plasma; made up of water, electrolytes, glucose, amino acids, and metabolic wastes

8. Proximal convoluted tubule: unit of the nephron, located in renal cortex; receives filtrate from glomerular capsules; reabsorbs water and electrolytes

9. Loop of Henle: forms renal pyramid in the medulla; U-shaped portion of renal tubule

a. Descending loop of Henle: removes water from filtrate

b. Ascending loop of Henle: removes sodium and chloride from filtrate; helps maintain osmolality

10. Distal convoluted tubule: convoluted portion of tubule beyond loop of Henle; located in renal cortex; removes more sodium and water

B. Blood vessels of the kidneys

1. Renal artery: large branch of abdominal aorta that delivers blood to each kidney

2. Interlobar arteries: branches of the renal artery within each kidney

3. Peritubular capillaries: surround the renal tubules

4. Renal vein: returns filtered blood to the circulation; empties into inferior vena cava

C. Function of the kidneys

1. Kidneys filter waste products as well as needed materials, such as electrolytes, from the blood; necessary items are returned to the blood through reabsorption; this mechanism allows fine-tuning of blood homeostasis

2. Filtration: first step in blood processing; water and solutes move from plasma in the glomerulus into Bowman's capsule; depends on pressure gradient between blood in glomeruli and filtrate in Bowman's capsule

3. Reabsorption: second step in urine formation; molecules move from the tubules into blood through tubule cells; active and passive transport mechanisms are used in all parts of renal tubules

   a. Proximal tubules: reabsorb sodium and other major ions through active and passive transport

   b. Loop of Henle: reabsorbs through counter-current mechanism (passive); contents flow in opposite directions

   c. Distal tubules: reabsorb sodium by active and passive transport in smaller amounts than proximal tubules

   d. Collecting ducts: prevent water from leaving the filtrate; use active and passive reabsorption

4. Tubular secretion: movement of substances out of the blood into the tubular fluid; tubule cells secrete certain substances in addition to performing reabsorption

5. Regulation of urine volume: hormones play a central part in urine regulation

6. Osmolality: osmotic pressure of a solution expressed as the number of osmols of pressure per kg of water; active transport and reabsorption mechanisms are based on osmolality of solutions

D. Renal hormones and enzymes

1. *Antidiuretic hormone (ADH):* regulates urine volume by acting in distal tubule and collecting ducts to increase water reabsorption and urine concentration

2. *Atrial natriuretic hormone (ANH):* secreted by muscle fibers in atrium of heart; promotes loss of sodium via the urine

3. *Aldosterone:* secreted by adrenal cortex; increases sodium absorption in distal and collecting tubules and controls potassium secretion, leading to osmotic imbalance that causes reabsorption of water; works in conjunction with ADH

   a. Increased serum potassium levels lead to increased aldosterone secretion

      b. Increased aldosterone secretion increases sodium and water retention and depresses formation of renin

    4. Renin: enzyme secreted by kidneys; helps regulate sodium retention and, therefore, blood pressure and fluid volume

      a. Renin-angiotensin system: converts angiotensinogen to angiotensin I in the liver

      b. Angiotensin II: formed in the lungs from angiotensin I; vasoconstrictor that stimulates adrenal cortex to produce aldosterone

    5. Erythropoietin: hormone produced by kidneys in response to low oxygen levels in arterial blood; travels to bone marrow and stimulates increased red blood cell (RBC) production

E. Urinary excretion

    1. Ureters: extend from renal pelvis of kidney to urinary bladder; conduct urine to the bladder

    2. Bladder: elastic sac located behind symphysis pubis; stores and excretes urine

      a. Ruggae: ridges formed by mucous membrane on bladder wall

      b. Detrussor muscle: muscular layer of bladder

    3. Urethra: tube that carries urine from bladder to exterior of body

      a. Female urethra: embedded in anterior wall of vagina

      b. Male urethra: passes through prostate gland, urogenital diaphragm (a ligament), and the penis; passes both urine and semen

    4. Urinary meatus: exterior opening of urethra

    5. Urination: an involuntary or voluntary reflex allowing urine to leave the body

      a. Micturition reflex: parasympathetic response that stimulates relaxation and contraction of external sphincter, allowing urine to pass

      b. Internal sphincter muscle: helps control urine passage into urethra; relaxes in response to parasympathetic nerve fibers in bladder wall

      c. External sphincter muscle: voluntary muscle that allows urine to pass into urethra; controlled by micturition reflex

    6. Characteristics of normal urine

      a. Color: clear, pale amber

      b. Consistency: 95 percent water with many dissolved substances

      c. Output: 1,000 to 2,000 mL per 24-hour period

      d. Specific gravity: commonly 1.015 to 1.025

      e. Odor: faint ammonia

II. Diagnostic Tests and Assessments of the Urinary System

A. Urine studies

    1. Urinalysis: examines urine for specific gravity, color (light to dark yellow or amber, depending on concentration), pH (5 to 9, with an average of 6), protein (negative), glucose (negative), and ketone bodies (negative); examines urine sediment for blood cells, casts, and crystals

2. Urine culture: checks urine for bacteria; urine is normally sterile

3. 24-hour urine specimen: urine is collected over 24 hours for the following tests:

   a. Creatinine: nitrogenous waste product excreted by muscle tissue; normally found in urine (normal = 15 to 25 mg/kg in 24 hours)

   b. Creatinine clearance: test to assess how well the kidneys remove creatinine from the blood (male = 95 to 135 mL/min; female = 85 to 125 mL/min)

   c. Protein: less than 150 mg/24 hours

   d. Urea nitrogen: end product of protein metabolism (normal 6 to 17 g/24 hours)

4. Urine osmolality: osmotic pressure (concentration) of urine; average is 500 to 800 mOsm/kg water, with an extreme range of 50 to 1,400 mOsm/kg water

B. **Renal scan:** intravenous radioactive substance (radionuclide) is injected, then observed passing through kidneys; evaluates renal blood flow, nephron and collecting system function, and renal structures

C. **Radiographic studies**

   1. Kidney-ureter-bladder radiography (KUB): x-ray series that shows kidney size, position, and structure; provides limited diagnostic information

   2. Renal angiography: x-ray images of renal blood vessels and tissues, obtained by injecting contrast medium into the femoral artery; detects abnormalities such as cysts, renal artery stenosis, and renal infarction

   3. Renal venography: x-ray images of renal veins, obtained by injecting contrast medium in a large vein; detects renal vein thrombosis

   4. Retrograde cystography: contrast medium instilled into bladder, followed by x-ray examination; helps diagnose ruptured or neurogenic bladder and other conditions

D. **Computerized tomography (CT) scan:** generates a three-dimensional, computerized image of kidneys; identifies masses and other lesions; contrast medium may be injected

E. **Magnetic resonance imaging (MRI):** passes magnetic energy through body to produce three-dimensional images of renal tissue; also called nuclear magnetic resonance (NMR)

F. **Ultrasonography:** high-frequency sound waves are directed through the body and reflect back to the source; a computer evaluates the reflection (echo) and records/displays it; useful for clients with renal failure and those allergic to contrast medium; evaluates kidney size, shape, and position

G. **Blood studies**

   1. *Blood urea nitrogen (BUN):* measures nitrogenous urea in the blood; urea is produced by protein metabolism; insufficient excretion causes levels to rise and may indicate renal disorders; also rises with dehydration and intake of high-protein diet or other conditions where excess protein is metabolized

      a. Normal: 8 to 25 mg/dL

      b. BUN levels best evaluated in conjunction with serum creatinine levels

2. Serum creatinine: creatinine is a nitrogenous waste resulting from muscle metabolism of creatine; creatinine levels reflect glomerular filtration rate

a. Measures renal damage more reliably than BUN, because severe renal damage is the only cause of significant elevation

b. Normal: 0.6 to 1.5 mg/dL for adult males; 0.6 to 1.1 mg/dL for adult females

H. Hemodynamic studies

1. **Intravenous pyelography (IVP):** x-ray of kidneys and urinary tract after IV injection of contrast medium; also called excretory urography

2. Cystoscopy or cystourethroscopy: insertion of a cystoscope with a fiberoptic light source and telescopic lens into the urethra; procedures include biopsy of bladder and prostate, lesion resection, calculi collection, or passage of catheter to renal pelvis

3. Percutaneous renal biopsy: client is positioned on abdomen while needle is inserted into kidney to remove tissue; x-ray may be used to guide the needle

   a. Tissue studies (histology) can reveal renal disease, malignant tumors, and other conditions

   b. Risks include bleeding, hematoma, arteriovenous fistula, and infection

III. Common Nursing Techniques and Procedures

A. Urinary catheterization: introduction of a catheter into the urinary bladder

1. Indwelling urinary catheter: a retention (Foley) catheter with balloon is inserted and remains in place

   a. Explain procedure to client and ensure privacy

   b. *Female:* assist client to supine position, with knees flexed and thighs externally rotated; drape the client

   c. Wearing disposable gloves, cleanse perineal area; remove gloves

   d. Prepare equipment and set up sterile field; don sterile gloves

   e. Drape client with sterile drape

   f. Lubricate sterile cotton balls with antiseptic solution (agency policy may differ concerning use of antiseptic)

   g. Lubricate insertion tip of catheter

   h. Clean meatus with antiseptic (check agency policy)

   i. Use non-dominant hand to separate labia minor and expose urinary meatus; assess meatus for swelling, discharge, or redness

   j. Grasp catheter near the insertion end with sterile, gloved hand

   k. Gently insert catheter into meatus and advance the catheter until urine flows; do not use forceful pressure; ask client to take deep breaths to relax external sphincter

   l. Advance the catheter farther into bladder (1 to 2 inches) and inflate balloon by injecting contents of prefilled syringe

m. Apply slight tension by pulling back on catheter until resistance is felt to confirm that balloon is in the bladder

n. Anchor catheter to client's thigh with non-allergic tape

o. Secure drainage bag to bed frame in a dependent position

p. *Male:* use same positioning except knees do not need to be flexed

q. Wearing disposable gloves, wash penis, and dry it well

r. Follow steps d, e, f, g, and h described above

s. Grasp insertion end of catheter with sterile, gloved hand

t. Lift penis to 90-degree angle with body and exert slight traction

u. Insert catheter steadily about 20 cm (8 inches) until urine begins to flow; ask client to take deep breaths to relax external sphincter; rotate catheter during insertion if slight resistance is met because of curvature of the urethra

v. Advance catheter farther into bladder (1 to 2 inches) and inflate balloon by injecting contents of prefilled syringe

w. Follow steps l, m, n, and o described above

2. Intermittent catheterization: used for clients with neurogenic bladder dysfunction; may be done by the nurse or by the client at home after proper instruction; teach the client the following procedure

a. Catheterize as often as needed; may be every 2 to 3 hours at first, then every 4 to 6 hours

b. Encourage to void before procedure if appropriate; use catheter to obtain residual urine if amount voided is less than 100 mL

c. Assemble all supplies and use good lighting

d. Wash hands

e. Clean urinary meatus with towelette or soapy washcloth, then rinse and dry; female clients should clean perineum from front to back

f. Assume comfortable position, such as standing with one foot elevated, semi-reclining in bed, or sitting on chair or toilet

g. Apply lubricant to catheter tip

h. *Female:* locate meatus using a mirror or touch; separate labia with dominant hand; direct catheter through meatus, then forward and upward

i. *Male:* hold penis with slight upward tension to 90-degree angle and insert catheter

j. Hold catheter in place until all urine is drained, then withdraw slowly

k. Wash catheter with soap and water; store in clean container

l. Notify care provider of cloudy urine, sediment, bleeding, fever, or difficulty passing catheter

m. Drink at least 2,000 to 2,500 mL of fluid daily; cranberry and prune juices help to acidify the urine to possibly reduce bacterial growth in the bladder

B. Urine collection

1. 24-hour urine collection

   a. Obtain specimen container with preservative from laboratory

   b. Provide clean receptacle to collect urine (bedpan, urinal, commode, or collection device on toilet) unless client already has an indwelling urinary catheter

   c. Post signs in client's room, on chart, and in bathroom alerting personnel to save urine

   d. Have client void and discard this urine at beginning of collection period, if indwelling catheter used, empty the collection bag at the start time

   e. During collection period, save all urine in container; place container on ice or refrigerate as indicated; don't contaminate urine with bathroom tissue or feces

   f. Instruct client to empty bladder at end of collection period and save this urine

   g. Send collected urine to laboratory with completed requisition

   h. Document collection of specimen, time started and completed, and any observations

2. Clean catch (midstream)

   a. Many clients can obtain specimen themselves after instruction

   b. Male clients void directly into container, while females hold container between their legs during voiding

   c. Ask client to wash genital and perineal area with soap and water

   d. Instruct how to clean meatus with antiseptic towelettes

   e. Female clients: use three towelettes, clean perineal area from front to back; use each towelette only once

   f. Male clients: clean meatus with circular motion and distal portion of penis; use each towelette only once

   g. For client who needs assistance: nurse may don gloves, clean perineal area, assist client to a comfortable position, and open clean-catch kit

   h. Instruct client to begin voiding, then place specimen container in stream of urine; collect 30 to 60 mL of urine

   i. Cap the container, touching only the outside

   j. Label container, place in biohazard bag along with requisition, and immediately send to laboratory

   k. Document pertinent data, such as difficulty voiding, strong odor to urine, or sediment

C. Peritoneal dialysis: removes toxins from blood of client with acute or chronic renal failure; uses peritoneal membrane as semipermeable dialyzing membrane

1. Hypertonic dialyzing solution (dialysate) is instilled through a catheter in peritoneal cavity

2. Excess concentrations of electrolytes and uremic toxins move by diffusion across peritoneal membrane into dialysis solution; excess water moves into solution by osmosis

3. Dialysate is drained after appropriate dwelling time

4. Procedure is performed manually, or by use of a cycler machine; client may also perform continuous ambulatory peritoneal dialysis (CAPD)

5. Possible complications

   a. Peritonitis from bacteria entering peritoneal cavity (use aseptic technique when handling catheter or tubing); this is critical to prevent because it could result in client having to change therapy to hemodialysis

   b. Catheter obstruction from clots or kinking (keep all lines unobstructed; add heparin to dialysate perprotocol)

   c. Insufficient outflow (reposition client as needed to bring fluid into contact with catheter; allow to ambulate if advisable due to condition)

   d. Hypotension and hypovolemia from excess fluid removal (carefully monitor I & O records; report accordingly)

   e. Hyperglycemia (from glucose in dialysate; monitor diabetic clients closely; do not allow fluid to dwell longer than ordered)

6. Peritoneal dialysis procedure

   a. Explain procedure and check vital signs and weight

   b. Have client urinate if able to avoid bladder puncture or discomfort; perform catheterization if client unable to void

   c. Warm dialysate to body temperature in a warmer

   d. Use 1.5-, 2.5- or 4.25-percent dextrose solution, usually with heparin added to prevent catheter clotting; dialysate should be clear and colorless; add prescribed medication as ordered

   e. Put on surgical mask and prepare dialysis administration set, maintaining strict sterile technique at all times

   f. Place drainage bag below client and connect outflow tubing

   g. Connect dialysis infusion line to dialysate bags and hang on IV pole

   h. Place client in supine position, prime the tubing with solution, close the clamps, and connect infusion line to abdominal catheter

   i. Test catheter by instilling 500 mL of dialysate into peritoneal cavity; clamp tubing; unclamp outflow line and drain fluid into collection bag; if outflow is brisk, the catheter is patent

   j. Unclamp infusion lines and infuse prescribed amount of dialysate; close clamps when bag is empty

   k. Allow solution to dwell for prescribed time (usually up to 4 hours)

   l. Open outflow clamps and allow solution to drain

   m. Repeat cycle according to prescribed number of times; when completed, clamp peritoneal catheter and disconnect inflow line while wearing sterile gloves

n. Apply sterile dressing to catheter site

o. During procedure, monitor vital signs every 10 minutes until stable, then every 2 to 4 hours

p. Observe for signs of peritonitis: fever, persistent abdominal pain and cramping; slow or cloudy dialysate drainage; swelling, redness, or tenderness around catheter; increased WBC count

q. Wear protective eyewear when draining or handling outflow solution

r. Check outflow tubing periodically for clots or kinks; having client change position may increase flow

s. Clients lose protein during peritoneal dialysis and require fewer or no dietary restrictions of protein

t. Calculate fluid balance at end of each exchange (with manual dialysis) or at end of each session or every 8 hours, depending on protocol; include oral and IV intake, urine output, and wound drainage in calculations

D. Urinary diversion stoma care

1. Collection device should fit snugly around stoma; allow no more than 1/8-inch margin of skin between stoma and faceplate

2. Stoma should appear light or bright red; suspect a problem if it is deep red or bluish in color

3. Check peristomal skin for breakdown; main cause of irritation is urine leakage; change device and cleanse skin if leakage occurs

a. Cleanse area with warm water and pat dry; apply light coating of karaya powder and thin layer of protective dressing

b. Notify physician if severe skin excoriation occurs

4. Assess intake and output; note changes in urine color, odor, or clarity

5. Home care by client

a. Expect stoma shrinkage within 8 weeks after surgery; may require different pouch size

b. Encourage client to change appliance as needed early in the morning when urine production is less following sleep

c. Appliance is often a one-piece unit (faceplate and collection bag), and needs to be emptied regularly and changed according to product directions

d. Instruct client to report fever, chills, flank pain, abdominal pain, and pus in the urine (**pyuria**) or blood in urine (**hematuria**)

e. Refer client to support group, such as United Ostomy Association

E. Care of an arteriovenous fistula

1. An arteriovenous fistula provides vascular access to a vein and an artery for hemodialysis; the most common sites are the radial or brachial artery and the cephalic vein

2. Assess circulation at access site by auscultating for bruits and palpating for thrills; lack of bruit may indicate blood clot and requires immediate surgical intervention

NCLEX!

3. Avoid using accessed arm for other procedures, such as IV insertion, blood pressure monitoring, or venipuncture

4. Monitor site for bleeding after completion of hemodialysis

5. Home care instructions for client

    a. Keep fistula area clean and dry

    b. Notify health provider of pain, swelling, redness, or drainage in accessed arm

    c. Exercise is beneficial and helps stimulate vein enlargement

NCLEX!

    d. Don't allow any treatments or procedures on accessed arm

NCLEX!

    e. Avoid excessive pressure to arm; don't sleep on it, wear constrictive clothing or jewelry, or lift heavy objects

    f. Avoid showering, bathing, or swimming for several hours after dialysis

F. Hemodialysis: a procedure to remove wastes from the body by filtering the client's blood using a machine

1. Nurses who have undergone specialized instruction and training perform hemodialysis

2. Before the procedure, weigh client and take vital signs; check blood pressure in lying and standing positions (orthostatic blood pressures)

NCLEX!

3. Wear protective eyewear, gown, and gloves for protection during hemodialysis procedure

4. Dialysis is continued usually for 3 to 4 hours, depending on client's condition; monitor partial thromboplastin time or other standard laboratory studies as ordered according to protocol (heparin is used as an anticoagulant during the procedure)

5. At end of treatment, obtain blood samples as ordered, return blood remaining in dialyzer to client, and remove needles from vascular access device

6. Monitor access device for bleeding and maintain pressure on site as needed

NCLEX!

7. Early in the course of hemodialysis, assess for and report disequilibrium syndrome, a condition in which cerebral edema forms from less rapid excretion of wastes behind the blood-brain barrier, and subsequent uptake of fluid by brain cells

    a. Assess client for headache, mental confusion, decreasing level of consciousness, nausea, vomiting, twitching, and possible seizure activity

    b. Call physician to obtain necessary orders for anticonvulsant medication

    c. It is prevented by dialyzing for shorter times or at reduced blood flow rates early in the course of therapy

IV. Nursing Management of the Client Having Renal or Bladder Surgery

A. Lithotripsy: also called extracorporeal shock-wave lithotripsy (ESWL); uses high-energy shock waves to break up calculi, allowing normal passage of urine to resume

1. Perform preoperative teaching about procedure and postoperative course and care

    a. Treatment takes 30 minutes to 1 hour

      b. Client will receive a general or epidural anesthetic

  2. Postprocedure care

      a. Perform baseline assessment and check vital signs following agency policy

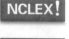

      b. Maintain patency of indwelling urinary catheter and monitor intake and output

      c. Strain urine for calculi fragments and send these to laboratory for analysis

      d. Slight hematuria is common, but report persistent bleeding

      e. Encourage ambulation to aid passage of calculi fragments

      f. Increase fluid intake as ordered to aid passage of calculi fragments

      g. Give analgesics as needed; severe pain may indicate presence of new calculi—report such findings immediately

  3. Home care instructions for client

      a. Drink 3 to 4 L of fluid daily up to 1 month after treatment

      b. Strain urine during first week and save any calculi fragments; bring these to first followup visit with physician

      c. Expect blood-tinged urine, mild GI upset, and pain in the treated side as calculi fragments pass

      d. Report severe pain, persistent blood in urine, inability to void, fever and chills, or nausea and vomiting

      e. Review prescribed medications or dietary regimen

B. Ureterolithotomy, pyelolithotomy, nephrolithotomy: involve making an incision into the ureter, renal pelvis, or renal calyx to remove urinary calculi

  1. Preoperative period

      a. Explain procedure to client

      b. Explain postoperative care, including presence of a urinary catheter

      c. Administer pre-anesthetic medications as ordered

  2. Postoperative period

      a. Perform baseline assessments as for all postoperative clients (vitals signs, level of consciousness, status of dressing)

      b. Monitor urine output for amount, color, and clarity; urine may be bright red initially, but amount of bleeding should diminish; cloudy urine may indicate infection

      c. Maintain placement and patency of urinary catheters; irrigate gently as ordered

      d. Assess for pain and administer analgesics as needed

      e. Increase client's fluid intake, as ordered, to aid passage of calculi fragments

      f. Strain urine for calculi fragments and send these to laboratory for analysis

  3. Home care for client

      a. Follow agency policy for home incision care

b. Drink 3 to 4 liters of fluid daily up to a month after treatment

c. Report bloody, cloudy, or foul-smelling urine

d. Report inability to void, fever, chills, and redness, swelling, or purulent drainage from incision

e. Strain urine during first week and save any calculi fragments; bring these to first followup visit with physician

f. Avoid strenuous exercise, sexual activity, heavy lifting, or straining until advised otherwise by physician

g. Mild activity aids passage of any retained calculi fragments

h. Review prescribed medications or dietary regimen

i. Outline catheter care if client is discharged with indwelling catheter

C. Cystectomy with urinary diversion

    1. Complete radical **cystectomy** involves surgical removal of the bladder, plus adjacent muscles and tissues

        a. In men, the prostate and seminal vesicles are removed, which results in impotence

        b. In women, the uterus, uterine tubes, and ovaries are removed, resulting in sterility

        c. A urinary diversion is created to provide for urine collection and drainage

    2. **Urinary diversion:** a procedure that provides an alternative route for urine excretion when normal channels are damaged or defective

        a. Ileal conduit: also called ileal loop; reroutes urine from kidneys to pouch in abdominal wall created from a segment of the ileum; urine drains continuously from the ileal pouch

        b. Nephrostomy: drains urine through a catheter placed directly into the kidney; used when a ureter is blocked or damaged; may be temporary

    3. Preoperative period

        a. Reduce anxiety through preoperative teaching about procedure and postoperative course and care

        b. Client may awaken with nasogastric tube, IV, indwelling urinary catheter, Penrose drain, or other drains

        c. Assess client's support systems and ability to care for self after surgery

        d. Address concerns about changes in body image and loss of sexual or reproductive function

        e. Administer preanesthetic medications as prescribed

        f. Administer antibiotics (usually erythromycin and neomycin) for 24 hours before surgery, as prescribed

        g. Begin bowel preparations about 4 days prior to surgery

        h. Administer enema on night before surgery to clear fecal matter from the bowel as prescribed or per protocol

4. Postoperative period

a. Perform baseline assessments as for all postoperative clients (vital signs, level of consciousness, status of dressing, and patency of urinary catheter)

b. Monitor amount and character of urine drainage every hour; report output less than 30 mL/hour; irrigate catheter as ordered

c. Observe for signs of hypovolemic shock, such as pallor, hypotension, and tachycardia

d. Inspect stoma and incision for bleeding and observe urine for frank bleeding and clots; expect slight hematuria for several days

e. Observe incision for signs of infection (redness and purulent drainage); change dressing according to agency policy or surgeon's order

f. Encourage frequent position changes, coughing and deep breathing, and early ambulation, if appropriate

g. Assess respiratory status frequently

h. Administer prescribed analgesic and antispasmodic medications as needed

5. Home care instructions for clients

a. Report signs of infection, including fever, chills, cloudy urine, purulent drainage or redness of incision

b. Report persistent blood in urine, inability to void, or painful urination

c. Instruct in care of stoma and provide supplies as needed; refer client to support organization, such as the United Ostomy Association

d. Weakness, incisional pain, and fatigue may persist for several weeks

D. **Ureteral stent:** catheter used to maintain patency and promote healing of the ureters; may be temporary after surgery or used for long periods in clients with a damaged ureter

1. Stent is positioned during surgery or cystoscopy

2. Nursing care

a. If stent has been brought to surface, secure it and maintain its position

b. Monitor urine output, including color, consistency, and odor

c. Observe for signs of infection, obstruction, or bleeding, including fever, tachycardia, cloudy urine, pain, hematuria

d. Maintain fluid intake

e. If stent is semi-permanent, instruct client and family in its care

E. **Nephrectomy:** removal of the kidney

1. Preoperative period

a. Reduce anxiety through preoperative teaching about procedure and postoperative course and care

b. Client may awaken with nasogastric tube, IV, indwelling urinary catheter, Penrose drain, or other drains

     c. Assess client's support systems and ability to care for self after surgery

     d. Administer preanesthetic medications as ordered

     e. Assess baseline urinary status

  2. Postoperative period

     a. Perform baseline assessments as for all postoperative clients (vital signs, level of consciousness, status of dressing, and patency of urinary catheter)

     b. Assess client's fluid and electrolyte status, because significant amount of blood is lost during nephrectomy; monitor hemoglobin and hematocrit results and urine specific gravity

     c. Monitor amount and character of urine drainage every hour; report output less than 30 mL/hour; irrigate catheter as ordered.

     d. Observe for signs of urinary infection: fever, redness at surgical site, cloudy urine, or discharge

     e. Assess patency of urinary or wound drainage tubes; reinforce or change dressing as needed

     f. Encourage frequent position changes, coughing and deep breathing, and early ambulation, if appropriate

     g. Assess respiratory status frequently

     h. Administer analgesic medications as needed

F. Renal transplantation

  1. Preoperative period

     a. Reduce anxiety through preoperative teaching about procedure and postoperative course and care; encourage client to express feelings and ask questions

     b. Assess client's support systems and ability to care for self after surgery and follow medical regime

     c. Instruct client that rejection of the donated organ by the recipient's body is the major obstacle in transplantation; reassure client that rejection usually isn't life-threatening and the client can resume dialysis if needed (see Table 6-1)

     d. Begin administering immunosuppressant drugs; discuss their purpose and possible adverse effects with client; monitor for signs of anaphylaxis

     e. Plan for the client to undergo dialysis the day before surgery, a cleansing enema, and many laboratory tests

  2. Postoperative period

     a. Perform baseline assessments as for all postoperative clients (vital signs, level of consciousness, status of dressing)

     b. Encourage frequent position changes, coughing and deep-breathing, and early ambulation, if appropriate

     c. Use special infection control measures: strict aseptic technique when changing dressings or performing catheter care; limit client's contact with

Table 6-1	**Description**	**Manifestations**	**Management**
Renal Transplant Rejection	**Hyperacute** Occurs within hours of surgery; results from antibody reaction to donor antigens; occurs rarely now due to better histocompatibility assessments	Urine output stops; examination of kidney shows a blue, flaccid appearance	Transplanted kidney must be removed; client must resume hemodialysis until (possibly) another kidney is available
	Acute Occurs within days to months after surgery; body mounts an immune system defense against tissue in donor organ	Urine output drops sharply and BUN and creatinine rise; possible fever, graft tenderness, swelling	Increased dosage of immunosuppressant drugs, including steroids and monoclonal antibodies
	Chronic Occurs from months to years after surgery; etiology is unclear, but may involve immune response to donor tissue	More gradual decline in kidney function, including urine output, BUN, and creatinine; proteinuria may occur	No specific treatment; client must resume hemodialysis caused by loss of graft until or unless another donor kidney is transplanted

staff and visitors; wear a surgical mask when in the client's room; monitor white blood cell (WBC) count and notify physician of significant drop

    d. Observe for signs of tissue rejection: fever; redness, tenderness, and swelling at surgical site; elevated WBC count; decreased urine output with increased **proteinuria** (protein in urine); sudden weight gain; hypertension; elevated BUN and creatinine levels

    e. Provide analgesic medications as needed; pain should decrease after 24 hours

    f. Monitor urine output closely; report output less than 100 mL/hour; decreased urine may indicate thrombus formation at renal artery anastomosis site

    g. Expect blood-tinged urine for several days; irrigate catheter as ordered, using strict aseptic technique

    h. With a living donor transplant, urine flow should begin immediately after revascularization and connection of ureter to client's bladder; with a cadaver transplant, expect anuria for 2 days to 2 weeks (client will need dialysis during this period)

    i. Monitor daily renal function tests: creatinine clearance, and BUN; urine creatinine, electrolytes, urine pH, and specific gravity

    j. Observe for signs of hyperkalemia (weakness and irregular pulse, tall peaked T-waves on cardiac rhythm strip)

    k. Weigh client daily; rapid weight gain may indicate fluid retention

  3. Home care for client

    a. Carefully measure and record intake and output; notify physician if urine output falls below 600 mL for any 24-hour period

b. Instruct client how to collect 24-hour urine samples

c. Advise client to weigh self at least twice weekly

d. Drink at least 1 liter of fluid daily, unless advised otherwise

e. Report signs of rejection: redness, warmth, tenderness, or swelling over the kidney; fever; decreased urine output; elevated blood pressure

f. Avoid crowds and persons with known infections for 3 months after surgery

g. Practice regular, moderate exercise, but avoid heavy lifting or contact sports for at least 3 months; beware of lap-style seat belts

h. Wait at least 6 weeks before engaging in sexual activity

IV. Disorders of the Urinary System

A. Urinary calculi

1. Description

    a. Presence of stones in the urinary tract

    b. One of the most common urologic problems

2. Etiology and pathophysiology

    a. Stones form when chemicals and other elements of urine become concentrated and form crystals; usually related to metabolic or dietary causes

    b. Types of stones

      1) Calcium phosphate and/or oxalate—most common type

      2) Struvite

      3) Uric acid

      4) Cystine—least common type

    c. Most stones form in the kidneys, but bladder stones are common in clients with indwelling urinary catheters or those with inability to empty the bladder completely (see Figure 6-2)

    d. Stones may be single or multiple and vary in size; large calculi cause pressure necrosis and can also lead to obstruction

    e. Risk factors

      1) Dehydration: concentrates calculus-forming substances

      2) Infection: damaged tissue and changing pH provide an environment for calculi to develop; bacteria may form the nucleus of calculi

      3) Obstruction: urine stasis allows solid materials to collect; also promotes infection, which worsens the obstruction

      4) Metabolic factors: hypoparathyroidism, renal tubular acidosis, elevated uric acid levels, defective oxalate metabolism, and excessive vitamin D or dietary calcium intake

Figure 6-2

Development and location of calculi within the urinary tract.

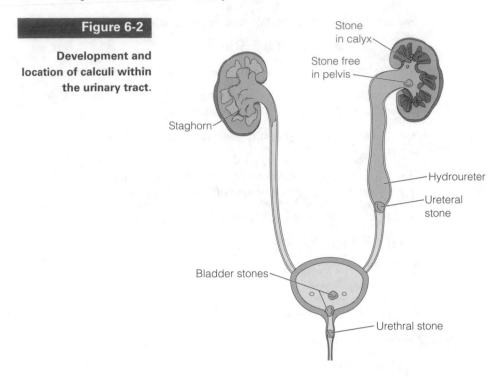

Stone in calyx

Stone free in pelvis

Staghorn

Hydroureter

Ureteral stone

Bladder stones

Urethral stone

3. Assessment

    a. Clinical manifestations

        1) Pain is the most common symptom

        2) Renal calculi cause flank pain on side of affected kidney; may radiate to groin, called renal colic

        3) Fluctuates in intensity and may be severe; nausea and vomiting sometimes accompany severe pain

        4) Other symptoms: abdominal distention, fever, and chills

    b. Diagnostic and laboratory test findings

        1) Urinalysis (may reveal hematuria, pyuria, and crystal fragments)

        2) 24-hour urine levels for calcium, uric acid, and oxalate

        3) Serum levels for calcium, phosphorus, and uric acid

        4) Chemical analysis of stones passed for content and type

        5) KUB, IVP, retrograde pyelography, renal ultrasound, CT scan, cystoscopy, and MRI

4. Therapeutic management

    a. Stones that are too large to be passed spontaneously (usually more than 5 mm in diameter), multiple stones, and those that obstruct the urinary tract usually require surgical intervention

        1) Extracorporeal shock-wave lithotripsy (ESWL) uses externally generated waves to pulverize or shatter urinary stones/calculi, which are then excreted in the urine

NCLEX!

NCLEX!

2) Ureterolithotomy, pyelolithotomy, or nephrolithotomy: utilizes a surgical incision used to remove calculi from affected areas; requires a large flank incision and an extended recovery time

3) Percutaneous nephrostomy: small incision in flank allows insertion of an endoscope to visualize renal pelvis; stones are removed with forceps or a basket device, or lithotripsy is used to crush stones

4) Transurethral uroscopy: a ureteral catheter is passed via a cystoscope to drain urine proximal to a stone and dilate the ureter, allowing the stone to pass; a basket catheter passed through the cystoscope can also remove the calculus

   b. Treatment for calcium phosphate and/or oxalate stones

1) Acid-ash diet with limitations of foods high in calcium and oxalates; foods high in oxalates include dark green leafy vegetables, rhubarb, beets, nuts, chocolate, and others, while dairy products are high in calcium

2) Increase hydration and exercise

   c. Treatment for struvite stones: acid-ash diet

   d. Treatment for uric acid stones

1) Alkaline-ash and low-purine diet

2) Increase hydration

   e. Treatment for cystine stones

1) Alkaline-ash diet

2) Increase hydration

5. Priority nursing diagnoses: Pain; Impaired urinary elimination; Deficient knowledge; Risk for infection; Urinary retention

6. Planning and implementation

   a. Treatment is geared toward relief of symptoms, removal or destruction of calculi, and prevention of future stone formation

   b. 90 percent of calculi pass out of the urinary system without invasive treatment

   c. Treatments are carried out as described in section 4 above on therapeutic management

   d. Provide pain relief measures and treat other symptoms as they occur

   e. Assess urinary function and monitor intake and output

   f. Strain all urine and save solid material for analysis

   g. Encourage ambulation and vigorous fluid intake to help client pass calculi

   h. Record daily weights to assess fluid status and renal function

7. Medication therapy: antimicrobial therapy for infection; analgesics for pain; and diuretics to prevent urine stasis

8. Client education

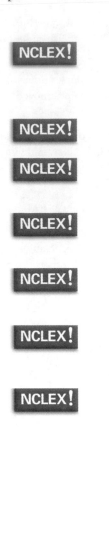

   a. Proper diet is essential to prevent recurrence of stones; teach dietary needs related to type of calculus

   1) Acid-ash foods include cranberries, plums, grapes, and prunes; tomatoes; eggs and cheese; whole grains; meat and poultry

   2) Alkaline-ash foods include legumes, milk and milk products, green vegetables, rhubarb, fruits except those acid-ash fruits noted above

   3) High-calcium foods include milk and other dairy products, beans and lentils, dried fruits, canned or smoked fish (except tuna), flour, chocolate, and cocoa

   4) Foods high in oxalate include asparagus, beets, celery, cabbage, fruits, tomatoes, green beans, chocolate and cocoa, beer, cola beverages, nuts, and tea

   5) High-purine foods include organ meats, sardines and herring, venison, and goose; other meats also contain purines and should be limited in quantity

   b. Increase fluid intake to 2,500 to 3,500 mL/day

   c. Maintain activity at level that will prevent urinary stasis and resorption of calcium from bone

   d. If discharged prior to stone passage, collect and strain all urine and bring stones to followup visit; observe amount and character of urine and report to healthcare provider at followup visit also

   e. Report increased pain, persistent blood in urine, inability to void, significant decrease in urine output

   f. Report signs of infection: burning with urination, cloudy urine, or fever

   g. Review specific drug information and procedures for self-administration

9. Evaluation: client verbalizes understanding of medications and correctly demonstrates their use; has recovered stone; identifies dietary and lifestyle measures to prevent calculi; has relief of pain; and exhibits no sign of complications

B. Urinary retention

1. Description: inability to empty the bladder that leads to bladder distention, poor contractility of the detrussor muscle, and further inability to urinate

2. Etiology and pathophysiology

   a. Mechanical obstruction of bladder outlet is most often caused by benign prostatic hypertrophy or acute inflammation

   b. Functional problems

   1) Surgery may disrupt function of the detrussor muscle, leading to retention of urine

   2) Many medications can interfere with detrussor muscle function, including anticholinergics, antidepressant and antipsychotic agents, anti-Parkinson drugs, antihistamines, and some antihypertensives

3. Assessment

    a. Clinical manifestations

        1) Firm, distended bladder that may be displaced to one side of midline

        2) Overflow voiding or incontinence may occur, with 25 to 50 mL of urine eliminated at frequent intervals

    b. Diagnostic and laboratory test findings

        1) Residual urine (post-voiding catheterization) in amounts over 50 mL obtained from bladder catheterization

        2) Positive urine culture indicates presence of urinary tract infection (UTI)

        3) Elevated serum creatinine and BUN levels indicate disturbances in renal function

        4) Elevated blood glucose may indicate diabetes

        5) Cystometrography evaluates muscle function

4. Therapeutic management: surgical correction of any condition causing mechanical obstruction of urine flow, including benign prostatic hyperplasia (BPH) and calculi

5. Priority nursing diagnoses: Urinary retention; Risk for infection; Deficient knowledge

6. Planning and implementation

    a. Palpate bladder for distention at regular intervals

    b. Monitor intake and output and observe urine

    c. Attempt to stimulate relaxation of urethral sphincter by running water, providing warm water in which client could place fingers, pour warm water over perineum, or provide warm sitz bath

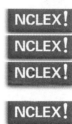

    d. Perform intermittent straight catheterization as ordered

    e. Evaluate client's medication regime for drugs that cause urinary retention

    f. Clients with mechanical obstruction need surgery to remove or repair obstruction; men with BPH may require resection of prostate gland

7. Medication therapy: cholinergic medications to promote detrussor muscle contraction and bladder emptying; anticholinesterase drugs to increase detrussor muscle tone

8. Client education

    a. Teach client to perform straight catheterization at home, if needed

    b. Recognize and report signs of urinary tract infection: burning with urination, cloudy urine, pelvic pain, fever, and strong urine odor

    c. Recommend moderate to high fluid intake and a diet that acidifies the urine; cranberry juice is one item that helps maintain acidity

    d. Review specific drug information and procedures for self-administration

9. Evaluation: client maintains a normal voiding pattern or is able to self-catheterize at home; has normal urine output; and verbalizes signs and symptoms of infection

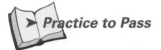

Practice to Pass

A female client who voids 50 mL of urine at a time tells you, "This is normal for me." How should you respond?

C. Urinary incontinence

1. Description: involuntary urination

   a. The North American Nursing Diagnosis Association (NANDA) identifies five types of incontinence (2001)

      1) Stress incontinence: loss of urine with increased abdominal pressure

      2) Reflex incontinence: involuntary loss of urine at somewhat predictable intervals when a specific bladder volume is reached

      3) Urge incontinence: involuntary passage of urine soon after a strong urge to void

      4) Functional incontinence: involuntary, unpredictable passage of urine

      5) Total incontinence: continuous and unpredictable loss of urine

   b. Incontinence is a symptom of other problems, not a disease in itself, although it has a significant impact on client's life

2. Etiology and pathophysiology

   a. May be acute or chronic, and the cause may be congenital or acquired

   b. Occurs when pressure within urinary bladder exceeds urethral resistance, allowing urine to escape; any condition causing higher than normal bladder pressure or reduced urethral resistance may lead to incontinence

   c. Common causes: relaxation of pelvic musculature, disruption of cerebral and nervous system control, and disturbances of bladder musculature

   d. Risk factors for incontinence in older clients: decreased bladder capacity, laxity of pelvic muscles in females, immobility, chronic degenerative diseases, low fluid intake, diabetes, and stroke

3. Assessment

   a. Clinical manifestations: involuntary passage of urine

   b. Diagnostic and laboratory test findings

      1) Weak abdominal and pelvic muscle tone in women

      2) Enlarged prostate in men

      3) Post-voiding residual urine greater than 50 mL

      4) Cystometrography: reduced muscle function and tone

      5) Ultrasonography and cystoscopy identify possible causes of the incontinence

4. Therapeutic management

   a. Surgical suspension of the bladder neck to treat stress incontinence associated with urethrocele

   b. Prostatectomy to treat overflow incontinence due to enlarged prostate

   c. Implantation of an artificial sphincter to treat clients with neurogenic bladder

5. Priority nursing diagnoses: Impaired urinary elimination; Reflex incontinence; Stress incontinence; Urge incontinence; Functional incontinence; Total incon-

tinence; Risk for infection; Disturbed body image; Risk for impaired skin integrity; and Self-care deficit

6. Planning and implementation

   a. Goal is to identify and correct cause of incontinence; if unable to correct underlying problem, client may learn techniques to manage urine output

   b. Monitor diagnostic tests to evaluate cause of incontinence

   c. Employ behavioral techniques, such as bladder training, for clients who are cognitively and functionally intact

   d. Insert urinary catheter as ordered and monitor client's urinary output

7. Medication therapy: anticholinergics for stress incontinence to increase bladder capacity and inhibit detrussor muscle contractions; antihistamines to enhance contraction of smooth muscles of bladder neck; estrogen therapy for incontinence associated with postmenopausal atrophic vaginitis

8. Client education

   a. Teach client to care for indwelling urinary catheter at home

   b. Teach client to recognize and report signs of urinary tract infection: burning with urination, cloudy urine, pelvic pain, fever; and strong urine odor

   c. Recommend moderate to high fluid intake and a diet that acidifies the urine; cranberry juice helps maintain acidity

   d. Review specific drug information and procedures for self-administration

   e. Some clients may be instructed to keep a voiding diary to help diagnose the cause(s) of incontinence

   f. Teach Kegel exercises to strengthen pelvic floor muscles (see Box 6-1)

   g. Instruct in dietary and fluid intake modifications to reduce stress and urge incontinence; consume most fluids during times of day client is most able to remain continent

   h. Teach client to wear clothing that is easily removed for ease in toileting

   i. Teach client to use assistive devices, such as raised toilet seats, bedside commode, and urinal or bedpan, as needed

9. Evaluation: client verbalizes understanding of medications and demonstrates their use; utilizes safety measures; reports reduction of incontinent episodes; monitors urinary output; verbalizes a state of dryness that is personally satis-

---

Box 6-1

Teaching Kegel Exercises

- First, sit or stand with the legs apart.
- Tense your muscles to pull your rectum, urethra, and vagina up inside, and hold for a count of 3 to 5 seconds. The pull should be felt at the cleft of your buttocks.
- Try to stop and start your stream of urine.
- Develop a schedule that will help remind you to do these exercises.
- To control episodes of stress incontinence, brace the muscles and use the Kegel maneuver when doing any activity that increases intra-abdominal pressure, such as coughing, laughing, sneezing, or lifting.

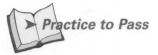

Practice to Pass

A female client reports dribbling of urine when she laughs, sneezes, or coughs. What advice should you give this client based on the type of incontinence she describes?

factory; verbalizes diet and fluid modifications to reduce stress and urge incontinence, and demonstrates care of indwelling urinary catheter

D. Urinary tract infections

1. Description: presence of microorganisms in the urinary tract leading to inflammation

2. Etiology and pathophysiology

   a. Infections are classified according to the region and primary site affected

   b. Urinary tract is sterile above the urethra; pathogens enter by ascending from the perineal area or from the bloodstream; the ascending route is most common

   c. *Escherichia coli* is the most frequent infective organism, causing about 80 percent of all cases; 5 to 15 percent are caused by *staphylococcus*

   d. Free urine flow, large urine output, and pH are antibacterial defenses

   e. Microscopic examination provides identification of the organism (especially important for chronic infections)

   f. Females are prone to urinary tract infections because the urethra is shorter than the male urethra

3. Assessment

   a. Clinical manifestations: burning, frequency, fever, cloudy urine, strong odor to urine, and pain in pelvic area

   b. Diagnostic and laboratory findings

      1) Urine cultures and Gram stain determine presence and number of bacteria

      2) WBCs are elevated with an increase in neutrophils

      3) Blood or urine tests are also performed to rule out STDs, which produce similar symptoms

4. Therapeutic management

   a. Surgical intervention may be necessary if recurrent UTI is caused by structural abnormalities

   b. These procedures may include:

      1) Ureteroplasty (surgical repair of the ureter) for stricture

      2) Ureteral stent (catheter in the ureter to provide free flow of urine)

5. Priority nursing diagnoses: Infection; Impaired patterns of urinary elimination; Deficient knowledge; Pain

6. Planning and implementation

   a. Increase fluid intake to 3,000 mL per day

   b. Administer urinary antimicrobials as ordered

   c. Administer analgesic and antispasmodic medications as needed

   d. Encourage client to void every 2 to 3 hours and to completely empty bladder to reduce urinary stasis

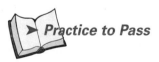

Practice to Pass

How would you respond to a female client who asks you why she seems to have more urinary tract infections as compared to her husband?

      e. Monitor intake and output and observe urine characteristics

  7. Medication therapy

      a. Antimicrobials to eradicate bacteria

      b. Antispasmodics and analgesics to relieve pain, frequency, and burning

  8. Client education

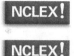

      a. Avoid beverages that irritate bladder: carbonated or caffeinated drinks and alcohol

      b. Teach women about hygiene measures to prevent reoccurrence: wipe from front to back, keep perineum clean and dry, do not douche, avoid tight-fitting pants; void after sexual intercourse

      c. Finish the complete course of antibiotics, even if symptoms subside

      d. Teach correct use, purpose, and effects of medication

      e. Phenazopyridine (Pyridium), a urinary analgesic, turns the urine reddish orange; teach the client to protect clothing and not to mistake this discoloration for bleeding (hematuria)

      f. Instruct in signs of infection: frequency, burning, cloudy urine, fever, and malodorous urine

      g. Maintain acidic urine by drinking cranberry juice daily (helps prevent bacteria from clinging to bladder wall)

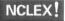

      h. Maintain fluid intake of at least 8 to 10 glasses per day

  9. Evaluation: client verbalizes understanding of medications and demonstrates their use; identifies measures to prevent infection; identifies signs of infection; normal voiding pattern is restored

E. Cystitis

  1. Description: inflammation (infection) of the bladder

  2. Etiology and pathophysiology

      a. Infection or obstruction of urethra is the most common cause

      b. Noninfectious cystitis results from exposure to radiation, chemical agents, or a metabolic disorder

      c. Gram-negative bacteria from the lower GI tract usually cause infectious cystitis

      d. Females are more prone to cystitis because:

          1) The urethra is short and straight

          2) The urinary meatus is close to the vagina and anus

          3) Tissue trauma and potential contamination occurs during sexual intercourse

          4) In some cases, poor personal hygiene and voluntary urinary retention contribute to the risk

      e. Males are more likely to develop urinary infection with aging because of prostatic hypertrophy, which impedes urine flow leading to incomplete bladder emptying and urinary stasis

3. Assessment

   a. Clinical manifestations

      1) Older clients may have nonspecific symptoms, such as nocturia, incontinence, confusion, lethargy, or anorexia

      2) See previous section on urinary tract infection

   b. Diagnostic and laboratory test findings: see previous section on urinary tract infection

4. Therapeutic management: see previous section on urinary tract infection

5. Priority nursing diagnoses: Impaired patterns of urinary elimination; Deficient knowledge; Pain

6. Planning and implementation

   a. Assist in identifying and removing cause of condition (infection, obstruction, etc.)

   b. Administer antimicrobial medications as ordered

   c. Collect uncontaminated urine specimens as needed

   d. Maintain acid urine (pH 5.5)

   e. Encourage bedrest or decreased activity during acute stage

   f. Increase fluid intake to 3,000 mL/day

7. Medication therapy

   a. Antimicrobials to eradicate bacteria if that is the cause

   b. Antispasmodics and analgesics to relieve pain, frequency, and burning

8. Client education

   a. See section on urinary tract infections

   b. Practice frequent voiding (every 2 to 4 hours) to flush bacteria from the urethra

   c. Avoid harsh soaps, bubble bath, powder, or sprays in the perineal area

   d. Take showers rather than baths if recurrent infection is a problem

9. Evaluation: client verbalizes medication instruction and demonstrates its use; identifies measure to prevent infection; identifies signs of infection; normal voiding pattern is restored; verbalizes three methods to prevent recurrence of infection

F. Pyelonephritis

1. Description: infection of one or both kidneys that usually begins in the renal pelvis; may be acute or chronic

2. Etiology and pathophysiology

   a. Affects the renal pelvis and parenchyma, the functional portion of the kidney

   b. Infection develops in scattered areas and spreads from renal pelvis to cortex; kidney becomes edematous and abscesses may develop; tissue destruction primarily affects the tubules; with healing, scar tissue replaces normal tissue and affected tubules atrophy

c. *E. coli* causes 85 percent of cases; *Proteus* and *Klebsiella* bacteria are examples of less common causes

d. Acute form is a bacterial infection, usually caused by bacteria that ascend from lower urinary tract

e. Risk factors: pregnancy, urinary tract obstruction, congenital malformation, urinary tract trauma, calculi, and diabetes

f. Asymptomatic bacteriuria or cystitis may lead to acute pyelonephritis

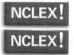

g. Chronic form is associated with nonbacterial infections and noninfectious processes caused by metabolic, chemical, or immunologic disorders

1) Often results from an autoimmune process leading to inflammation

2) Acute episodes may contribute to the inflammation and scarring associated with the chronic form

3) Fibrosis and scarring lead to dilation of renal pelvis and gradual destruction of tubules

4) May lead to chronic renal failure and end-stage renal disease

h. **Vesicoureteral reflux** (urine moves from bladder back toward the kidneys) is a common risk factor in children who develop pyelonephritis; it is also seen in adults when bladder outflow is obstructed

3. Assessment

a. Clinical manifestations: urinary frequency, dysuria, flank pain, costovertebral tenderness, tachypnea, GI symptoms, muscle tenderness, fever, chills, malaise

b. Diagnostic and laboratory findings: hematuria, pyuria, bacteriuria, leukocyte casts in urine, and leukocytosis

4. Therapeutic management: same as for urinary tract infection

5. Priority nursing diagnoses: Impaired patterns of urinary elimination; Deficient knowledge deficit; Pain

6. Planning and implementation

a. Administer and monitor drug therapy

b. Maintain bedrest until symptoms subside

c. Force fluids to maintain urine output of 1,500 mL/day

d. Continue monitoring for presence of bacteria

e. Monitor urinalysis: concentration and electrolytes

f. If oliguria present, maintain diet low in protein and high in calories and vitamins

g. Observe for edema and signs of renal failure

7. Medication therapy: antimicrobial therapy; urinary antiseptics; and analgesics for pain

8. Client education

   a. Instruct client to monitor urine output and notify care provider if less than 1,500 mL/day

   b. Instruct in methods to prevent chronic renal insufficiency

   c. Advise client to take high-calorie, low-protein diet if oliguria present

   d. Teach hygiene to prevent further infections

   e. Encourage bedrest during acute stage

   f. Finish complete course of antibiotics, even if symptoms resolve

   g. Teach correct use, purpose, and effects of medication

9. Evaluation: client verbalizes understanding of medications and demonstrates proper use; identifies measure to prevent further infection; identifies signs of infection; normal voiding pattern is restored; and verbalizes methods to prevent recurrence of infection

G. Neoplastic disease

1. Description

   a. Neoplastic disease is a pathologic tissue overgrowth that may be benign or malignant

   b. Other classifications: solid, cystic, superficial, invasive, primary, or metastatic

2. Etiology and pathophysiology

   a. Most urinary tract tumors arise from the epithelial tissue that lines the entire urinary tract

   b. Even nonmalignant tumors may lead to obstruction, renal failure, hemorrhage, and invasion and inflammation of surrounding tissues

   c. Tissue destruction may cause fistulas, which can allow urine to leak into the pelvis, vagina, or bowel

   d. Bladder cancer is fifth most common malignancy; occurs most often after age 50, and is more common in men than women

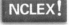

   e. Major factors in bladder cancer

      1) Presence of carcinogens in the urine

      2) Chronic inflammation or infection of bladder mucosa

   f. Other risk factors: cigarette smoke, exposure to chemicals and dyes used in certain industries, chronic use of phenacetin-containing analgesic agents; carcinogenic agents from these materials are excreted in urine and stored in the bladder between voidings, leading to abnormal cell development

3. Assessment

   a. Clinical manifestations

      1) Observe for painless hematuria, which is the presenting symptom in 75 percent of cases; hematuria may be gross or microscopic, and is often intermittent

NCLEX!

      2) Inflammation surrounding tumor may cause signs of urinary tract infection, such as frequency, urgency, and dysuria

      3) With ureteral tumors, observe for colicky pain from obstruction

      4) Neoplasms cause few outward symptoms and may not be discovered until urinary obstruction occurs or a fistula develops

   b. Diagnostic and laboratory test findings

      1) Urinalysis shows gross or microscopic hematuria

      2) Urine cytology shows abnormal tumor or pre-tumor cells; see Table 6-2 for information about renal cell cancer staging

      3) Visualization of tumors via intravenous pyelography, ultrasound, CT scan, cystoscopy, or ureteroscopy

  4. Therapeutic management

   a. Radiation therapy

   b. Surgical intervention for bladder tumors

      1) Tumor resection

      2) Partial cystectomy: resection of tumor

      3) Radical cystectomy: removal of the bladder and adjacent structures

   c. Urinary diversion may also be created

      1) Cutaneous ureterostomy: one or both ureters excised from the bladder and brought to a stoma

      2) Ileal conduit: portion of ileum is isolated from the small intestine that is formed into a pouch; ureters are attached to the pouch; pouch has open stoma

      3) Colon conduit: same as ileal conduit but a portion of the sigmoid colon is used

      4) Kock pouch: same as ileal conduit but nipple valves are formed preventing leakage and reflux (see Figure 6-3)

      5) Indiana continent urinary reservoir: reservoir is formed from colon and cecum and portion of the ileum is brought to the surface

      6) Ileocystoplasty: section of the ileum is used; this procedure is ideal for men because it allows the client to void

  5. Priority nursing diagnoses: Impaired patterns of urinary elimination; Deficient knowledge; Anxiety; Disturbed body image; and Risk for infection

Table 6-2	Stage of Tumor	Extent of Tissue Involvement
Renal Cell Cancer Staging	I	Kidney capsule only
	II	Kidney capsule with invasion through capsule into local fascia only
	III	Kidney, regional lymph node, ipsilateral renal vein, and possibly inferior vena cava
	IV	Kidney, as well as local invasion or distant metastases

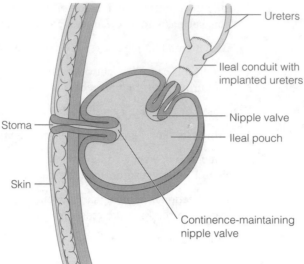

Figure 6-3

A continent urinary diversion. A segment of ileum is separated from the small intestine and formed into a pouch. Nipple valves are formed at each end of the pouch by intussuscepting tissue backward into the reservoir to prevent leakage.

6. Planning and implementation

  a. Monitor urinary status, including intake and output, signs of infection, hematuria, and BUN and creatinine levels

  b. Monitor urinary output from all catheters, stents, and tubes for amount, color, and clarity

  c. Prepare client for invasive tests to confirm location and size of neoplasm

  d. Follow guidelines for care before and after surgery, chemotherapy, and radiation treatments

  e. Encourage increased fluid intake, unless contraindicated

  f. Provide analgesics as needed for pain

  g. Encourage client to express feelings about potentially life-threatening illness and ask questions

7. Medication therapy: chemotherapeutic agents may be given IV or administered by intravesical instillation (into the bladder)

8. Client education

  a. Explain all nursing and medical interventions, including benefits and possible adverse effects

  b. Provide information about diagnosis and the client's specific neoplasm

  c. Stress importance of compliance with long-term treatment plan and followup care

  d. Instruct client in methods to prevent infection

  e. For clients with a stoma or indwelling catheter, teach home care procedures and when to consult care provider

NCLEX!

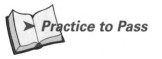

Practice to Pass

During a routine assessment, a client tells you, "I've been noticing blood in my urine." What would be your appropriate nursing action?

    f. For clients with a continent ileostomy, teach how to catheterize pouch (approximately every four hours) and wear a small dressing to protect the stoma and clothing

    g. Teach relaxation techniques and other coping mechanisms

  9. Evaluation: client verbalizes understanding of the disorder and proposed treatment plan; client's fluid intake and output is balanced; client communicates fears and concerns about diagnosis; and client demonstrates appropriate care of stoma or catheter

H. Glomerulonephritis

  1. Definition: a group of kidney diseases caused by inflammation of the capillary loops in the glomeruli of the kidney

  2. Etiology and pathophysiology

    a. Caused by an immunologic reaction to an antigen

    b. Endogenous antigens are already present in glomerulus or other body tissues

    c. Exogenous antigens come from infections occurring in the body

    d. Antigen-antibody complexes trapped within the glomeruli produce an inflammatory response that damages the glomeruli

    e. Most often follows infections with group A beta-hemolytic streptococcus

    f. Upper respiratory infection, skin infection, and autoimmune processes (systemic lupus erythematosus) predispose to glomerulonephritis

    g. Symptoms appear 2 to 3 weeks after original infection

    h. Has higher incidence in men than women; may occur at any age

  3. Assessment

    a. Clinical manifestations

      1) Early symptoms may be mild: pharyngitis, fever, and malaise

      2) Recent upper respiratory or skin infections, pericarditis, or lower UTI

      3) Weakness and fatigue

      4) Anorexia, nausea, and vomiting

      5) Cocoa-colored urine

      6) Peripheral edema

      7) Hypertension

    b. Diagnostic and laboratory test findings

      1) Hematuria, proteinuria (most important indicator of glomerular injury), hypoalbuminemia

      2) Pulmonary infiltrates

      3) Positive antibody response tests for streptococcal exoenzymes

      4) Elevated erythrocyte sedimentation rate (ESR)

5) Elevated BUN and creatinine

6) Decreased serum sodium, elevated potassium, and decreased phosphate

7) Decreased creatinine clearance

8) Delayed uptake and excretion of radioactive dye in renal scan

9) Positive renal biopsy findings

4. Therapeutic management

   a. Plasmapheresis: removal of harmful components in the plasma

   b. Sodium restriction

   c. Dialysis if the disease progresses to renal failure

5. Priority nursing diagnoses: Impaired urinary elimination; Activity intolerance; Excess fluid volume

6. Planning and implementation

   a. Administer penicillin as prescribed for residual infection

   b. Provide appropriate diet: protein restriction if oliguria is severe; high carbohydrate to provide energy; potassium usually restricted; sodium restriction for hypertension and edema

   c. Maintain fluid restriction as needed

   d. Encourage complete bedrest during acute stage

   e. Monitor vital signs frequently; observe for hypertension

   f. Monitor intake and output and daily weight

   g. Evaluate for signs of renal failure: oliguria, azotemia, and acidosis

7. Medication therapy: antimicrobials for infection; analgesics for pain relief; and vitamin and electrolyte replacement as needed

8. Client education

   a. Instruct in the need to maintain strict bedrest during acute phase

   b. Instruct in dietary changes and importance of maintaining diet

   c. Advise of the importance of fluid restriction if oliguria present

   d. Explain the purpose of laboratory tests and other procedures

9. Evaluation: client is able to resume usual activities of daily living; signs and symptoms of fluid overload are absent; client demonstrates knowledge of therapeutic diet and fluid restriction; client maintains desired weight; and nausea and vomiting are absent

I. Nephrotic syndrome

1. Description: renal disease characterized by massive edema and albuminuria

2. Etiology and pathophysiology

   a. Seen with any renal condition that damages glomerular capillary membrane: glomerulonephritis, lipoid nephrosis, syphilitic nephritis, amyloidosis, or systemic lupus erythematosus

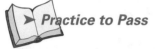

Practice to Pass

The nurse is preparing a client with glomerulonephritis for discharge. What dietary instructions should be included in the teaching plan?

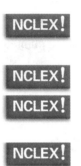

b. Allows plasma proteins to escape into the urine, resulting in hypoalbuminemia, with decreased oncotic pressure in plasma and fluid shifts from intravascular to interstitial spaces; this leads to edema

c. Salt and water retention also contribute to edema, which may be severe

d. Kimmelstiel-Wilson syndrome, a specific form of intercapillary glomerulosclerosis, is associated with diabetes mellitus

e. Thromboemboli (mobilized blood clots) are a common complication and may occlude peripheral veins and arteries, pulmonary arteries, and renal veins

f. Prognosis is poor for adults with this syndrome; less then 50 percent experience complete remission; at least 30 percent develop end-stage renal failure

3. Assessment

  a. Clinical manifestations

    1) Severe generalized edema

    2) Symptoms of renal failure

    3) Loss of appetite and fatigue

    4) Amenorrhea

  b. Diagnostic and laboratory test findings

    1) Pronounced proteinuria, hypoalbuminemia, and hyperlipidemia

    2) Positive renal biopsy finding

4. Therapeutic management

  a. No specific treatment

  b. Since 30 percent of adults with nephrotic syndrome progress to end-stage renal failure, see section on therapeutic management of renal failure

5. Priority nursing diagnoses: Excess fluid volume; Fatigue; Ineffective protection; Ineffective role performance

6. Planning and implementation

  a. Provide nursing care to control edema

    1) Sodium-restricted diet

    2) Avoidance of sodium-containing drugs (such as several OTC products)

    3) Diuretics that block aldosterone formation (Lasix and Edecrin)

    4) Administer salt-poor albumin to reduce fluid retention

  b. Provide high-protein diet to restore body proteins, high-calorie diet, and a restricted sodium diet if edema is present

  c. Administer drug therapy as prescribed

  d. Maintain bedrest until edema begins to subside

  e. Monitor laboratory and diagnostic test results, including BUN, creatinine, serum electrolytes, urinalysis, hemoglobin, and hematocrit

    f. Observe for signs of pulmonary edema: tachypnea, dyspnea, crackles in the lungs

    g. Total intake and output records every 4 to 8 hours and weigh client daily

    h. Maintain fluid restriction; offer ice chips and provide frequent mouth care

    i. Provide for adequate rest and energy conservation

    j. Be aware that immune system depression increases risk of infection

        1) Assess for signs of infection, such as purulent wound drainage and signs of UTI

        2) Monitor CBC, with close attention to WBC and differential

NCLEX!

        3) Use good handwashing and infection control techniques

        4) Avoid or minimize invasive procedures

7. Medication therapy: immunosuppressive therapy for clients with autoimmune disorders; angiotensin converting enzyme (ACE) inhibitors to reduce protein loss; NSAIDs to reduce proteinuria; penicillin or other broad-spectrum antibiotics to eradicate bacteria; and antihypertensives to maintain normal blood pressure if needed

8. Client education

NCLEX!

    a. Take measures to maintain general health, as disorder may persist for months or years

    b. Avoid sources of infection such as people with upper respiratory infections

    c. Nutritious diet (low-sodium, high-protein)

    d. Activity as tolerated

    e. Use and potential effects of medications

    f. Signs, symptoms, and implications of improving or declining renal function

9. Evaluation: client maintains blood pressure within normal limits; returns to usual weight with no evidence of edema; consumes adequate calories while following dietary limitations; and demonstrates understanding of disease and prescribed management regimen

J. Polycystic kidney disease

    1. Description

        a. Hereditary disease characterized by cyst formation and massive kidney enlargement, affecting both children and adults

        b. Autosomal dominant form affects adults

        c. Autosomal recessive form usually diagnosed in childhood

    2. Etiology and pathophysiology

        a. Renal cysts are fluid-filled sacs affecting the nephron; they develop in the tubular epithelium of the nephron and fill with glomerular filtrate or secreted solutes and fluid

        b. Cysts range in size from microscopic to several centimeters

c. As cysts enlarge and multiply, the kidneys also enlarge; renal blood vessels and nephrons are compressed and obstructed, and functional tissue is destroyed

d. The disorder is slow and progressive; adult symptoms usually manifest themselves by age 30 to 40

e. Clients with this disorder often develop cysts elsewhere in the body, including liver, spleen, pancreas, brain, and other organs

3. Assessment

   a. Clinical manifestations

     1) Flank pain

     2) Polyuria

     3) Nocturia

     4) Signs of UTI

     5) Signs of renal calculi

     6) Hypertension

     7) Palpable, enlarged, and knobby kidney

     8) Signs of chronic renal failure as the client approaches 50 to 60 years of age

   b. Diagnostic and laboratory test findings

     1) Gross hematuria, proteinuria

     2) Positive findings in renal ultrasonography, IVP, and CT scan

4. Therapeutic management

   a. Largely supportive

   b. Eventually will require dialysis or transplantation

5. Priority nursing diagnoses: Excess fluid volume; Anticipatory grieving; Deficient knowledge; Ineffective individual coping

6. Planning and implementation

   a. Provide supportive care to help client cope with symptoms; no effective treatment is available

   b. Encourage fluid intake of 2,000 to 2,500 mL/day to help prevent UTI and calculi

   c. Administer antihypertensive agents as prescribed

   d. Discuss that hemodialysis and possibly renal transplant will be indicated as disease progresses

   e. Provide nursing care directed toward edema control

     1) Sodium restriction in diet

     2) Diuretics that block aldosterone formation

7. Medication therapy: ACE inhibitors to control hypertension; diuretics to control edema; and antibiotics if infection develops

8. Client education

   a. Instruct in maintenance of general health status, as disorder is chronic and progressive

   b. Teach client how to avoid UTI and to recognize early signs of infection

   c. Instruct to avoid medications that are potentially toxic to kidneys and check with care provider before taking any new drug

   d. Discuss genetic counseling and screening of family members for evidence of disease

   e. Teach client to maintain fluid intake of at least 2,500 mL/day

9. Evaluation: client demonstrates knowledge of measures to prevent urinary tract infection; recognizes early signs of infection; verbalizes need to avoid medications that are toxic to kidneys; maintains fluid intake of 2,500 mL/day; and verbalizes knowledge of disease and its consequences

K. Acute renal failure

1. Description: a sudden loss of kidney function caused by failure of renal circulation or damage to the tubules or glomeruli

2. Etiology and pathophysiology

   a. Usually reversible, with spontaneous recovery in a few days to weeks

   b. Ischemia is primary cause; when allowed to continue for more than 2 hours, it produces irreversible damage to tubules

   c. Etiologic categories

      1) Prerenal: accounts for 55 percent of renal failure; caused by decreased blood flow to kidneys; readily reversible when recognized and treated early; may be caused by severe dehydration, diuretic therapy, circulatory collapse; hypovolemia, or shock

      2) Intrarenal: caused by a disease process, ischemia, or toxic conditions such as acute glomerulonephritis, vascular disorders, toxic agents, or severe infection

      3) Postrenal: caused by any condition that obstructs urine flow such as in benign prostatic hyperplasia, renal or urinary tract calculi, or tumors

3. Assessment

      a. Clinical manifestations follow three phases: initiation, maintenance, and recovery; the initiation stage has very few manifestations; the maintenance phase is characterized by **oliguria** (urine output < 400 mL/24 hours); signs of improving renal function characterize the recovery stage

      1) Muscle weakness, nausea, vomiting, and diarrhea may occur

      2) Neurologic symptoms such as confusion, agitation, disorientation, seizures, and coma may also be present

   b. Diagnostic and laboratory test findings

      1) Hyperkalemia, hyperphosphatemia, and hypocalcemia

2) Metabolic acidosis

3) Azotemia

4) Anemia

5) Elevated creatinine and BUN levels

6) Proteinuria

7) Urinalysis show specific gravity equal to the specific gravity of plasma; presence of casts, RBC, WBC, and renal tubular epithelial cells

8) Positive renal biopsy findings

4. Therapeutic management

   a. Fluid and electrolyte management

   b. Supportive therapy with dialysis

5. Priority nursing diagnoses: Excess fluid volume; Imbalanced nutrition: less than body requirements; Deficient knowledge; Risk for infection

6. Planning and implementation

   a. Monitor intake and urinary output

   b. Observe for oliguria followed by **polyuria** (excess urine output from diuresis)

   c. Weigh daily and observe for edema

   d. Monitor for complications of electrolyte imbalances, such as acidosis and hyperkalemia

   e. Allow client to verbalize concerns regarding disorder

   f. Encourage prescribed diet: moderate protein restriction, high in carbohydrates, restricted potassium

   g. Once diuresis phase begins, evaluate slow return of BUN, creatinine, phosphorus, and potassium to normal

7. Medication therapy

   a. Avoid nephrotoxic drugs

   b. Use volume expanders as prescribed to restore renal perfusion in hypotensive clients and Dopamine IV to increase renal blood flow

   c. Use loop diuretic to reduce toxic concentration in nephrons and establish urine flow

   d. Use ACE inhibitors to control hypertension

   e. Use antacids or histamine H_2-receptor antagonists to prevent gastric ulcers

   f. Use Kayexalate to reduce serum potassium levels and sodium bicarbonate to treat acidosis

8. Client education

   a. Dietary and fluid restrictions, including those that may be continued after discharge

b. Signs of complications, such as fluid volume excess, CHF, and hyper-kalemia

c. Monitor weight, blood pressure, pulse, and urine output

d. Avoid nephrotoxic drugs and substances: NSAIDs, some antibiotics, radio-logic contrast media, and heavy metals; consult care provider prior to taking any OTC drugs

e. Recovery of renal function requires up to 1 year; during this period, nephrons are vulnerable to damage from nephrotoxins

9. Evaluation: client verbalizes understanding of dietary and fluid restrictions; verbalizes need to avoid nephrotoxic substances; verbalizes signs of infection and when to notify health care provider; demonstrates ability to monitor blood pressure, pulse, and urine output; maintains weight, and vital signs are within normal range

L. End-stage renal disease (ESRD)

1. Definition

a. Loss of renal function characterized by a glomerular filtration rate (GFR) less than 20 percent of normal

b. The final stage of **chronic renal failure** (slow, progressive loss of kidney function and glomerular filtration); ends fatally with uremia

2. Etiology and pathophysiology

a. Most common causes of chronic renal failure are diabetic neuropathy, hypertension, glomerulonephritis, systemic lupus erythematosus, and cystic kidney disease

b. Progressive loss of renal function occurs in four stages; fourth stage ends with ESRD (uremia)

c. As 90 percent or more of nephrons are destroyed, BUN and creatinine clearance rise, and urine specific gravity is fixed at 1.010 (normal up to 1.025)

d. Uremia: "urine in blood"; term used for symptoms associated with ESRD

e. Loss of erythropoietin leads to chronic anemia and subsequent fatigue

f. There is inadequate clearance of fluid and electrolytes, leading to fluid and sodium retention, as well as hyperkalemia, hypermagnesemia, hyperphosphatemia, and hypocalcemia; metabolic acidosis occurs because of impaired hydrogen ion excretion

3. Assessment

a. Clinical manifestations

1) Early: nausea, apathy, weakness, and fatigue

2) Late: client may experience frequent vomiting, increasing weakness, lethargy, and confusion

3) Client may complain of "restless leg syndrome," paresthesia, and sensory loss

4) Personality changes, such as anxiety, irritability, and hallucinations; seizures and coma may occur in late stages

5) Respirations may change to Kussmaul pattern, with deep coma following

6) Skin becomes pale and dry, with yellowish hue; metabolic wastes cause itching and uremic frost (crystallized deposits of urea on the skin)

b. Diagnostic and laboratory test findings

1) Urinalysis shows fixed specific gravity approximately 1.010, equivalent to plasma; abnormal proteins, blood cells, and casts are present.

2) Elevated creatinine and BUN

3) Decreased creatinine clearance

4) Abnormal electrolyte values as noted above

5) Moderate anemia

6) Decreased platelets

7) Decreased renal size by ultrasonography

8) Positive renal biopsy if damage caused by cancer

5. Priority nursing diagnoses: Impaired tissue perfusion: renal; Imbalanced nutrition: less than body requirements; Risk for infection; Disturbed body image; Excess fluid volume; Activity intolerance

6. Planning and implementation

a. Provide diet low in protein with supplemented amino acids; restrict fluids as ordered

b. Provide electrolyte replacement or restriction

1) Sodium restriction

2) Potassium restriction

3) Replacement of bicarbonate stores to treat acidosis

c. Monitor and plan nursing care for hypertension and heart failure

d. Prepare client for dialysis or kidney transplant

e. Administer medications with caution because of inability to excrete properly

f. Monitor intake and output and vital signs

g. Monitor laboratory results for BUN and serum creatinine, pH, electrolytes, and CBC

h. Provide symptomatic relief for nausea and vomiting

i. Observe for signs of infection

j. Provide rest periods to combat fatigue, which is chronic in nature

k. Help client learn about and adjust to diagnosis; support coping strategies and work with client to develop realistic goals

7. Medication therapy: limited by kidneys' inability to excrete; diuretics to reduce volume of extracellular fluid; ACE inhibitors to maintain normal blood pressure; electrolyte replacement; phosphate binding agents; Kayexalate to reduce serum potassium levels; folic acid and iron supplements to combat anemia; and multivitamins

8. Client education

   NCLEX!

   a. Monitor weight, vital signs, and urine output at home

   b. Fluid and dietary restrictions (low-sodium, low-potassium, low-protein) need to be followed carefully

   c. Monitor symptoms of uremia

   d. Avoid nephrotoxic drugs and substances: NSAIDs, some antibiotics, radiologic contrast media, and heavy metals

   NCLEX!

   e. Teach strategies to avoid thirst, yet continue fluid restrictions, such as frequent mouth care, sugarless hard candy, using ice chips instead of liquids, or using a spray bottle instead of a cup to limit fluids ingested

   f. Discuss hemodialysis or renal transplant therapies as indicated

   g. Recommend methods to combat nausea: antiemetics; mouth care; small, frequent meals

   h. Provide referral to mental health counseling or support group

9. Evaluation: client verbalizes understanding of dietary and fluid restrictions; verbalizes need to avoid nephrotoxic substances; verbalizes signs of infection; takes medications as ordered

Case Study

C. S., a 60 year old truck driver, has been an insulin-dependent diabetic for the past 20 years. Diabetic neuropathy has led to several complications, including end-stage renal disease, which he developed two years ago. He now receives hemodialysis three times a week and has an AV fistula in his left forearm. Yesterday, C. S. presented in the Emergency Department with a respiratory infection and was hospitalized with pneumonia, hypertension, and fluid overload. He will receive dialysis while on your nursing unit.

❶ It is appropriate to administer an aminoglycoside antibiotic for his respiratory infection? Why or why not?

❷ What changes would you expect to see in this client's blood glucose levels during and after hemodialysis?

❸ C. S. missed his dialysis treatment on the day of admission. How might this be evidenced in his respiratory status?

❹ His wife comments on the fruity odor of his breath. What complication would cause this sign?

❺ C. S. complains of dry, itching skin. How would you explain this symptom to him? What nursing measures for skin care would you provide?

For suggested responses, see page 736.

Posttest

1 When caring for a client diagnosed with end-stage renal failure, which of the following diets should the nurse recommend?

(1) Increased protein, decreased carbohydrates
(2) Restricted protein, increased carbohydrates
(3) Increased potassium and sodium
(4) Restricted phosphorus and magnesium

2 The client diagnosed with cystitis will be given a prescription for an antibiotic. The nurse explains to the client that which of the following medications that is combined with the antibiotic will reduce the symptom of dysuria?

(1) Phenazopyridine (Pyridium)
(2) Bethanechol chloride (Urecholine)
(3) Oxybutinin chloride (Ditropan)
(4) Propantheline bromide (Pro-Banthine)

3 The client has developed urolithiasis, and it is determined that the client has uric acid stones. The nurse instructs the client to limit which of the following foods in the diet that was previously eaten regularly?

(1) Oranges
(2) Cheese
(3) Liver
(4) Eggs

4 In gathering data on an elderly male client the nurse suspects that the most likely cause of his urinary retention is:

(1) Benign prostatic hyperplasia (BPH).
(2) Urinary tract infection.
(3) Voluntary urinary retention.
(4) Anticholinergic medications.

5 A client complains of inability to inhibit urine flow long enough to reach the toilet. The nurse documents the presence of which type of urinary incontinence?

(1) Stress
(2) Reflex
(3) Urge
(4) Functional

6 Which of the following nursing actions is most appropriate when caring for a client with a nursing diagnosis of Excess fluid volume?

(1) Teaching clients about sodium content of foods
(2) Administration of vitamin D supplements
(3) Assessing and documenting client's energy level
(4) Observing for signs of hypocalcemia

7 Which of the following types of liquid should the nurse recommend for a client who has frequent urinary tract infections?

(1) Soda drinks
(2) Caffeine drinks
(3) Citrus juices
(4) Cranberry juice

8 A client has undergone creation of an ileal conduit. Which of the following instructions to the client about ostomy care would be appropriate to include in the teaching plan?

(1) Cut the faceplate of the appliance so that the opening is slightly smaller than the stoma.
(2) Plan to do appliance changes just before bedtime.
(3) Limit fluids to minimize odor from urine breakdown to ammonia.
(4) Cleanse the skin around the stoma using gentle soap and water; rinse and dry well.

9 The nurse is caring for a client with a history of renal disease. The nurse most closely monitors the client for signs of nephrotoxicity if the client is ordered to receive which of the following medications?

(1) Aminoglycoside antibiotics
(2) Aspirin-containing drugs
(3) Loop diuretics
(4) Potassium supplements

10 A client underwent cystectomy for cancer of the bladder and had a Kock pouch created for urinary diversion. The home care nurse would follow up with the client about which of the following instructions for self-care?

(1) Application and care of external pouch
(2) Technique for catheterizing the Kock pouch
(3) Proper administration of prophylactic antibiotics
(4) Foods that must be restricted in the diet

See pages 255–256 for Answers and Rationales.

Answers and Rationales

Pretest

1 Answer: 2 *Rationale:* Uremia is a syndrome, or group of symptoms, associated with end-stage renal disease. The normal function of the kidney is altered, resulting in various metabolic and systemic effects including fluid and electrolyte disturbances. Pyelonephritis (inflammation of the kidney and renal pelvis) and cystitis (inflammation of the urinary bladder) do not lead to uremia. Polycystic kidney disease is a hereditary disease characterized by kidney enlargement and cyst formation.
Cognitive Level: Analysis
Nursing Process: Planning; *Test Plan:* PHYS

2 Answer: 2 *Rationale:* If outflow drainage is less than inflow, the nurse should change the client's position to shift abdominal fluid, and hopefully move the catheter into contact with the fluid in the abdomen. Although vital signs are monitored, the blood pressure is not a concern at this time (option 1). The catheter does not need to be irrigated (option 3). A direct nursing intervention is needed, while continuing to monitor is an assessment and does not correct the current problem (option 4).
Cognitive Level: Application
Nursing Process: Implementation; *Test Plan:* PHYS

3 Answer: 2 *Rationale:* A client with glomerulonephritis should eat a diet that is high in calories but low in protein to inhibit protein catabolism, and allow the kidneys to rest by diet (since they have fewer nitrogenous wastes to clear). It is important to protect the kidneys while they are recovering their function. The other responses are incorrect.
Cognitive Level: Application
Nursing Process: Implementation; *Test Plan:* PHYS

4 Answer: 3 *Rationale:* Acute renal failure is a condition that may be caused by nephrotoxic drugs such as aminoglycoside antibiotics. Acute renal failure has a rapid onset and is potentially reversible. The condition usually responds to treatment if diagnosed early. Chronic renal failure develops insidiously and requires dialysis or transplantation.
Cognitive Level: Application
Nursing Process: Analysis; *Test Plan:* PHYS

5 Answer: 3 *Rationale:* Serum creatinine measures the amount of creatinine in the blood. Creatinine is the end product of creatine phosphate, used in skeletal muscle contraction. Blood urea nitrogen (BUN), another common laboratory test, measures the nitrogen portion of urea and helps detect dehydration. These tests are often ordered together when assessing renal function.
Cognitive Level: Application
Nursing Process: Assessment; *Test Plan:* PHYS

6 Answer: 4 *Rationale:* An acid-ash diet lowers urine pH, which may reduce bacterial growth. An acid-ash diet includes the following foods: meat, fish, shellfish, poultry, cheese, eggs, cranberries, prunes, plums, corn, lentils, grains, and foods high in chlorine, phosphorus, and sulfur. Foods to be avoided include milk and milk products; all vegetables except corn and lentils; all fruits except cranberries, plums, and prunes; and foods containing high amounts of sodium, potassium, calcium, and magnesium.
Cognitive Level: Application
Nursing Process: Implementation; *Test Plan:* PHYS

7 Answer: 2 *Rationale:* Peritonitis is the major complication of PD. The nurse should use strict aseptic technique and should teach the client to use it whenever accessing the catheter. The client does not need post-void residuals (option 1). Heparin is added to dialysate as ordered, but it would be added to each bag, not to one bag per day randomly; the catheter site dressing is changed daily (options 3 and 4).
Cognitive Level: Analysis
Nursing Process: Implementation; *Test Plan:* PHYS

8 **Answer: 1** *Rationale:* Renal colic is an acute, severe pain in the flank and upper abdominal quadrant on the affected side, generally associated with renal calculi that obstruct a ureter. Clients experiencing renal colic describe it as sudden in onset and may be accompanied by nausea, diaphoresis, and vomiting.
Cognitive Level: Application
Nursing Process: Assessment; *Test Plan:* PHYS

9 **Answer: 2** *Rationale:* Painful urination, frequency, and urgency are common signs of cystitis, or bladder infection. In addition, the urine may have a foul odor and appear cloudy. Bacteria, virus, parasites, or fungi may cause the condition, with GI tract bacteria being the most common cause.
Cognitive Level: Analysis
Nursing Process: Assessment; *Test Plan:* PHYS

10 **Answer: 4** *Rationale:* Pain is the most common sign of UTI and is usually the most distressing symptom for the client. The pain may be caused by inability to void or by bladder spasms. The client may have manifestations of the other nursing diagnoses as well, but pain is the highest priority.
Cognitive Level: Analysis
Nursing Process: Planning; *Test Plan:* PHYS

Posttest

1 **Answer: 2** *Rationale:* With end-stage renal disease the kidneys have difficulty excreting protein and the build-up of toxins in the system causes systemic problems. Clients must usually restrict dietary protein while increasing carbohydrate intake to meet energy needs and prevent tissue breakdown. Potassium and sodium are restricted in clients with end-stage renal failure. Protein-rich foods are also high in phosphorus, which is restricted to avoid osteodystrophy. Magnesium is not specifically restricted.
Cognitive Level: Application
Nursing Process: Implementation; *Test Plan:* PHYS

2 **Answer: 1** *Rationale:* The pain experienced with cystitis usually resolves as antibiotic therapy becomes effective. However, clients may be treated for urinary tract pain with phenazopyridine, which is a urinary analgesic. Bethanechol chloride is a cholinergic agent used with neurogenic bladder or urinary retention. Oxybutinin and propantheline bromide are antispasmodics used to treat bladder spasm.
Cognitive Level: Application
Nursing Process: Implementation; *Test Plan:* PHYS

3 **Answer: 3** *Rationale:* Clients who have urinary stones of the uric-acid type should avoid foods containing high amounts of purines, including the following: organ meats (liver, brain, heart, kidney, and sweetbreads), herring, sardines, anchovies, meat extracts, consommés, and gravies. Foods that are low in purines include all fruits, many vegetables, milk, cheese, eggs, refined cereals, sugars and sweets, coffee, tea, chocolate, and carbonated beverages.

4 **Answer: 1** *Rationale:* Benign prostatic hyperplasia (BPH) is a common cause of urinary retention when the enlarged prostate gland obstructs urinary flow. The other answers may also cause retention, but are less common than BPH.
Cognitive Level: Application
Nursing Process: Assessment; *Test Plan:* PHYS

5 **Answer: 3** *Rationale:* This type of incontinence is called urge incontinence, caused by a hypertonic or overactive detrussor muscle that leads to increased pressure within the bladder. Stress incontinence is loss of urine with abdominal pressure. Reflex incontinence refers to loss of urine at somewhat predictable intervals when a specific bladder volume is reached. Functional incontinence is an involuntary, unpredictable passage of urine.
Cognitive Level: Analysis
Nursing Process: Assessment; *Test Plan:* PHYS

6 **Answer: 1** *Rationale:* Clients with Excess fluid volume need to have restrictions in sodium intake because of the relationship of water and sodium. Elevated serum sodium will cause water to be retained. The client should be instructed to avoid foods that are high in sodium such as cured meats, preserved foods, and canned goods. In addition, developing a schedule for oral intake and offering limited ice chips and frequent mouth care helps in the water restriction necessary for these clients. The other options are not appropriate interventions for the nurse to implement specific for the nursing diagnosis Excess fluid volume.
Cognitive Level: Application
Nursing Process: Implementation; *Test Plan:* PHYS

7 **Answer: 3** *Rationale:* Cranberry juice reduces bacteria by acidifying urine and making it more difficult for bacteria to remain attached to the bladder wall. Citrus fruits should not be used because they make the urine alkaline. Drinks containing caffeine, including sodas, may irritate the bladder and worsen the urinary frequency.
Cognitive Level: Application
Nursing Process: Implementation; *Test Plan:* PHYS

8 **Answer: 4** *Rationale:* Peristomal skin should be cleansed with each appliance change using a gentle soap and water, and then should be rinsed and dried thoroughly. The client should change the appliance early in the morning, when urine production is slowest from lack of fluid intake during sleep. The opening of the appliance should be cut no larger than 3 mm greater than the opening of the stoma; an opening smaller than the stoma would prevent proper application. Fluids are encouraged to dilute the urine and decrease the odor.
Cognitive Level: Application
Nursing Process: Planning; *Test Plan:* HPM

9 **Answer: 1** *Rationale:* Nephrotoxicity can be caused by aminoglycoside antibiotics. This type of drug accumulates in tubular cells, eventually killing

them. Options 2 and 3 are ototoxic, while option 4 is avoided in renal disease.
Cognitive Level: Analysis
Nursing Process: Analysis; *Test Plan:* PHYS

10 **Answer: 2** *Rationale:* A Kock pouch is a continent internal ileal reservoir, eliminating the need for an external pouch. The nurse needs to instruct the client about the technique for catheterizing the pouch to empty the urine. Antibiotics are not required unless an infection is present and dietary restrictions are unnecessary.
Cognitive Level: Application
Nursing Process: Implementation; *Test Plan:* PHYS

References

Berger, K. J. & Williams, M. (1999). *Fundamentals of nursing: Collaborating for optimal health* (2nd ed.). Stamford, CT: Appleton & Lange.

Christensen, B. L. & Kockrow, E. O. (1999). *Adult health nursing.* St. Louis, MO: Mosby, pp. 337–378.

Corbett, J. (2000). *Laboratory tests and diagnostic procedures with nursing diagnoses* (5th ed.). Upper Saddle River, NJ: Prentice Hall, Inc., pp. 62–109.

Dudek, S. (2001). *Nutrition essentials for nursing practice* (4th ed). Philadelphia: Lippincott Williams & Wilkins, pp. 634–660.

Kozier, B., Erb, G., Berman, A., & Burke, K. (2003). *Fundamentals of nursing: Concepts, process, and practice* (7th ed.). Upper Saddle River, NJ: Prentice Hall, Inc., pp. 1203–1247.

LeMone, P. & Burke, K. (2000). *Medical-surgical nursing: Critical thinking in client care* (2nd ed.). Upper Saddle River, NJ: Prentice-Hall, Inc., pp. 882–1012.

Lewis, S., Heitkemper, M., & Dirksen, S. (2004). *Medical-surgical nursing: Assessment and management of clinical problems* (6th ed.). St. Louis: Mosby, pp. 1152–1244.

North American Nursing Diagnosis Association (2001). *Nursing Diagnosis: Definitions and Classification,* 2001–2002. Philadelphia: NANDA.

Pierson, C. A. & Mishler, M. A. (1999). Interventions for clients with urinary problems. In D. Ignatavicius, M. Workman, & M. Mishler (Eds.), *Medical-surgical nursing across the health care continuum* (3rd ed.). Philadelphia: W. B. Saunders, pp. 1819–1852.

Visovsky, C. (1999). Interventions for clients with chronic and acute renal failure. In D. Ignatavicius, M. Workman, & M. Mishler (Eds.), *Medical-surgical nursing across the health care continuum* (3rd ed.). Philadelphia: W. B. Saunders, pp. 1879–1926.

CHAPTER 7

Hepatobiliary and Pancreatic Disorders

Debera Jane Thomas, DNS, FNP/ANP, RN-CS
Lynn L. Fletcher, MSN, FNP, RN-CS

CHAPTER OUTLINE

OBJECTIVES

▌ Identify basic structures and functions of the hepatobiliary and pancreatic systems.

▌ Describe the pathophysiology and etiology of common hepatobiliary and pancreatic disorders.

▌ Discuss expected assessment data and diagnostic test findings for selected hepatobiliary and pancreatic disorders.

▌ Identify priority nursing diagnoses for selected hepatobiliary and pancreatic disorders.

▌ Discuss therapeutic management of selected hepatobiliary and pancreatic disorders.

▌ Discuss nursing management of a client experiencing a hepatobiliary or pancreatic disorder.

▌ Identify expected outcomes for the client experiencing a hepatobiliary or pancreatic disorder.

[Media Link]

Use the CD-ROM enclosed with this text, or log onto the address given to access the free, interactive Companion Website created for this series. The CD-ROM and Companion Website accompanying this book offer additional practice opportunities and information—NCLEX Review, Case Studies, Glossary, In Depth with NCLEX, and more.

www.prenhall.com/hogan

REVIEW AT A GLANCE

ascites *accumulation of fluid that is rich in proteins in the peritoneal cavity*

asterixis *flapping tremor of the hands from an increased serum ammonia level*

cholecystectomy *surgical removal of the gallbladder either through a laparoscope or an abdominal incision*

cholecystitis *acute or chronic inflammation of the gallbladder*

cholelithiasis *gallstones in the biliary tree most commonly formed from cholesterol*

cirrhosis *fibrosis of the liver from chronic inflammation*

esophageal tamponade *direct pressure applied to bleeding esophageal varices using a special nasogastric tube with esophageal and gastric balloons that are inflated to apply pressure*

esophageal varices *distended tortuous veins in the esophagus that are prone to rupture*

hepatic encephalopathy *accumulation of ammonia in the blood from chronic liver disease that results in neurological symptoms of confusion, irritability, coma, and asterixis*

hepatitis *inflammation of the liver caused by numerous viruses, bacteria, toxic chemicals, and drugs*

hepatorenal syndrome *renal failure caused by alterations in circulation resulting from chronic liver disease without primary renal disease*

hyperbilirubinemia *elevated serum bilirubin, both indirect and direct bilirubin*

hypoalbuminemia *low serum albumin resulting from chronic liver disease*

icteric *second phase of acute viral hepatitis marked by jaundice and lasting from 2 to 6 weeks*

jaundice *yellow-orange discoloration of the skin and mucous membranes caused by a serum bilirubin greater than 2.5 mg/dL*

lithotripsy *a procedure in which sound waves are passed through the calculi to disintegrate the stones*

pancreatitis *acute or chronic inflammation of the pancreas*

paracentesis *a procedure used to remove excess fluid from the abdominal cavity*

portal hypertension *abnormally high blood pressure in the portal venous circulation contributing to ascites formation and esophageal varices*

sclerotherapy *treatment for esophageal varices in which a sclerosing agent is injected in the bleeding vessel causing the vein to thrombose*

Pretest

1 A client asks the nurse how she can live without her gallbladder. In order to respond to this client, the nurse must have which understanding of the hepatobiliary system?

(1) The liver produces about 1,000 mL of bile per day.
(2) The gallbladder makes about 90 mL of bile per day.
(3) The liver concentrates bile more than 10 times.
(4) The gallbladder dilutes and releases bile.

2 The nurse reviews a client's laboratory tests and notices that the total serum bilirubin is 2.5 mg/dL. The nurse should assess the client for which of these clinical manifestations?

(1) Ascites
(2) Diarrhea
(3) Scleral icterus
(4) Hypertension

3 The client is diagnosed with obstructive jaundice. The nurse should ask the client about which of these manifestations?

(1) Clear, pale urine
(2) Clay-colored stools
(3) Lactose intolerance
(4) Ankle edema

4 A client has jaundice. Which of the following comfort measures would be appropriate for the nurse to implement?

(1) Offer hot beverages frequently
(2) Encourage taking a hot bath or shower
(3) Keep the air temperature at approximately 68° to 70°F
(4) Suggest the use of alcohol-based skin lotion

5 The client is exposed to hepatitis A. When teaching this client about infection control, the nurse explains that the client is most infectious to others at which of these times?

(1) 7 days after exposure
(2) 10 days before the onset of symptoms
(3) 2 months after exposure
(4) 14 days after symptoms begin

6 The client with cirrhosis of the liver asks the nurse why she has edema. The nurse would use which of the following statements to explain how edema results from pathophysiologic changes in cirrhosis?

(1) "The edema occurs because your liver produces fewer proteins that help draw fluid into the bloodstream."
(2) "The high osmotic pressure of proteins in your blood pushes fluid into body tissues."
(3) "Because of the liver disease, the kidneys are able to filter less fluid, so the body cannot excrete it as urine very easily."
(4) "Your body is metabolizing sex hormones more quickly, leading to fluid retention."

7 The client has just had a liver biopsy. Which of the following nursing actions would be the priority after the biopsy?

(1) Monitor pulse and blood pressure every 30 minutes until stable and then hourly for up to 24 hours.
(2) Ambulate every 4 hours for the first day as long as client can tolerate this.
(3) Measure urine specific gravity every 8 hours for the next 48 hours.
(4) Maintain NPO status for 24 hours post-biopsy.

8 Lactulose (Cephulac) is ordered for the client with cirrhosis. Which of the following serum laboratory tests should the nurse monitor to determine if the drug is having the desired effect?

(1) Albumin
(2) Ammonia
(3) Sodium
(4) Lactate

9 The client is admitted to the hospital for possible cholelithiasis. While taking the history, the nurse notes that the client has which of the following risk factors for development of gallstones?

(1) Black race
(2) History of hypertension
(3) Age of 37 years
(4) Use of oral contraceptives

10 The client is diagnosed with chronic pancreatitis, and pancrelipase (Lipancreatin) is prescribed. Which of the following instructions should the nurse give to this client about the administration of this medication?

(1) "Take the drug with meals."
(2) "Take the drug with a large glass of milk."
(3) "Take the drug between meals."
(4) "Take the drug after it is crushed and mixed with ice cream."

See pages 296–297 for Answers and Rationales.

I. Overview of Anatomy and Physiology

A. Basic structures of the hepatobiliary system (see Figure 7-1)

1. Liver: located in the right upper quadrant (RUQ) of the abdomen, beneath the diaphragm and weighing 1,200 to 1,600 grams

   a. Composed of two lobes; right is larger than the left

   b. The right and left lobes are separated by the falciform ligament, which anchors the liver to the abdominal wall; the right lobe is divided into the caudate and quadrate lobes

   c. Covered with a fibroclastic capsule called the Glisson capsule that contains blood vessels, lymphatics, and nerves

2. Biliary tract: composed of gallbladder and associated ducts; cystic, hepatic, and common bile ducts

   a. Bile is synthesized in the liver and transported to the bile ducts via the bile canaliculi that surround each hepatic cell

Figure 7-1

Anatomy of hepatobiliary-pancreatic system.

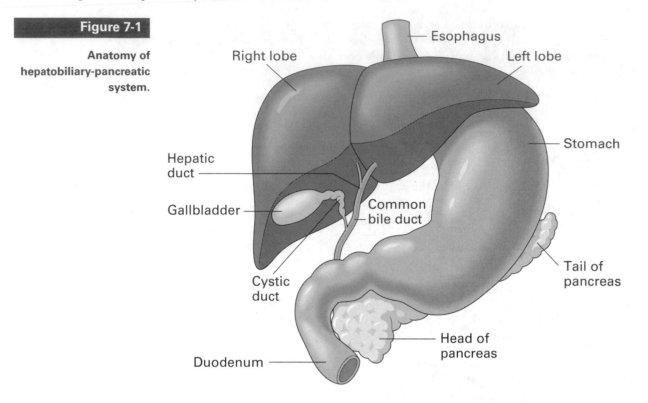

b. Bile canaliculi drain into the right or left hepatic bile ducts which come together to form the common hepatic duct

c. The sphincter of Oddi is at the distal end of the common hepatic duct and controls the flow of bile into the duodenum

d. The cystic duct connects the gallbladder to the hepatic duct and they merge to form the common bile duct

e. The common bile duct opens into the duodenum allowing secretion of bile necessary for digestion

3. Gallbladder: sac-like organ located on the inferior surface of the liver

   a. Mucosa of the gallbladder wall absorbs water and electrolytes resulting in a high concentration of bile salts, bile pigments, and cholesterol

   b. Primary purpose of the gallbladder is to store and concentrate bile; about 90 mL

4. Pancreas: primary enzyme-producing gland of the digestive system with both exocrine and endocrine functions that is located along the upper quadrants of the abdomen; the head is located within the curve of the duodenum; the tail touches the spleen; the body lies behind the stomach

B. Basic functions of the hepatobiliary system

1. Liver: produces 700 to 1200 mL of bile per day, which is a bitter-tasting alkaline, yellow-green fluid containing bile salts (conjugated bile acids),

cholesterol, bilirubin, electrolytes, and water; formed by the hepatocytes and secreted into the biliary caniculi; it also is responsible for the following functions:

a. Stores fat-soluble vitamins (A, D, E, and K)

b. Metabolizes bilirubin, by-product of the destruction of old red blood cells

c. Stores and releases blood during hemorrhage

d. Synthesizes plasma proteins to maintain plasma oncotic pressure

e. Synthesizes prothrombin, fibrinogen, and clotting factors I, II, VII, IX, X

f. Synthesizes phospholipids and cholesterol necessary for the production of bile salts, steroid hormones, and plasma membranes

g. Converts amino acids to carbohydrates through deamination

h. Stores and releases glucose

i. Stores and releases copper

j. Stores iron as ferritin

k. Detoxifies alcohol and certain drugs

l. Phagocytosis

m. Produces bile; contains salts necessary for digestion of fat

2. Biliary tract: functions to transport bile formed in the liver to the bile ducts and eventually to the duodenum

3. Gallbladder: stores and concentrates bile; stores about 90 mL of bile

   a. Contracts and releases bile into the cystic duct that joins the hepatic duct and together form the common bile duct

   b. Common bile duct terminates in the duodenum

   c. The sphincter of Oddi controls the release of bile into the duodenum; gallbladder contraction is regulated by hormones secreted by the duodenal mucosa in the presence of fat, which act to relax the sphincter of Oddi and allow flow of bile into the duodenum

4. Pancreas: produces enzymes (exocrine) and hormones (endocrine) that assist in the digestive process

   a. Pancreatic secretions flow through the ducts of the pancreas and empty into the duodenum through the common bile duct or one of the accessory ducts

   b. The endocrine pancreas secretes insulin and glucagon hormones from islets of Langerhans

      1) Insulin: protein hormone that promotes the storage and utilization of food, primarily glucose and fats

      2) Glucagon: stimulates glycogenolysis in the liver

   c. Exocrine pancreas secretes enzymes; composed of secretory units called acini and a series of ducts that secrete enzymes and alkaline fluids into the pancreatic duct (Wirsung duct), which empties into the common bile duct at the ampulla of Vater; the pancreas produces about 1 to 1.5L of pancreatic juice/day, which is alkaline and neutralizes the acidic chyme as it empties into the duodenum

1) Lipase promotes fat breakdown

2) Pancreatic α-amylase promotes carbohydrate breakdown

3) Trypsin, chymotrypsin, and carboxypeptidase break down proteins

4) Hormonal and vagal stimuli control the secretion pancreatic juices; secretin, a hormone secreted from the small intestine, stimulates the acinar and duct cells to secrete the alkaline-rich fluid that neutralizes chyme and prepares it for further enzymatic digestion

II. Disorders of the Hepatobiliary System: Liver

A. Jaundice: also referred to as icterus

1. Description

   a. Yellow-orange discoloration of the skin and mucous membranes; caused by a disturbance of bilirubin metabolism causing **hyperbilirubinemia** (serum bilirubin greater than 2.5 mg/dL)

   b. Associated with diffuse hepatocellular disorders or present in newborns because of impaired bilirubin uptake and conjugation

2. Etiology and pathophysiology

   a. Hyperbilirubinemia and jaundice can result from hemolysis or from disorders of the bile ducts (obstruction) or liver cells

   b. Jaundice is caused by the accumulation of bilirubin pigments in the skin and can be classified as obstructive or hemolytic

   c. Obstructive jaundice is classified as extrahepatic or intrahepatic

      1) Intrahepatic jaundice: disturbance of hepatocyte function and obstruction of the bile canaliculi, which decreases the flow of conjugated bilirubin into the common bile duct and thus into the intestine; if caused by the failure of the liver cells (hepatocytes) there will be a primary increase in the unconjugated form of bilirubin; common causes are drug reactions (phenothiazines) or hepatitis

      2) Extrahepatic jaundice: the common bile duct is occluded by gallstones or a tumor, preventing transport of bile into the duodenum; the accumulation of bile within the liver overflows into the blood causing hyperbilirubinemia; because the liver conjugates this bilirubin (direct), it is water-soluble and can be found in the urine

   d. Hemolytic jaundice is caused by excessive breakdown of red blood cells

      1) The amount of bilirubin produced exceeds the ability of the liver to conjugate it, so there is a subsequent increase in unconjugated or indirect bilirubin within the serum

      2) Unconjugated bilirubin is insoluble in water and will not be found in the urine; causes include blood transfusion reactions, membrane defects of erythrocytes, severe infection, or toxic substances

3. Assessment

   a. General assessments

      1) Vital signs and full physical exam; focused on the examination of the skin, mucous membranes, and eyes looking for signs of yellowish discoloration

      2) Abdominal swelling, pain in the right upper quadrant, and presence of hepatomegaly

      3) Questions regarding appetite and color of urine and stool

   b. Clinical manifestations

      1) Yellowish discoloration of the skin and mucous membranes caused by the deposition of bilirubin

      2) Scleral icterus (the yellowish discoloration of the sclera)

      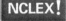

      3) Pruritus (severe itching) secondary to the accumulation of bilirubin in the skin

      4) Elevation of conjugated bilirubin that causes urine to be dark (tea- or cola-colored); may be present before jaundice appears

      5) Complete obstruction of the flow of bile into the duodenum causes light or clay-colored stools

      6) Jaundice caused by an infectious process may be accompanied by fever and chills

      7) Any client with liver dysfunction or injury may complain of nausea, anorexia, and/or fatigue

   c. Diagnostic and laboratory test findings

      1) Laboratory findings depend on whether hyperbilirubinemia is caused by elevations of direct (conjugated) or indirect (unconjugated) bilirubin; serum bilirubin is reported as total bilirubin and is further divided into direct and indirect portions

         a) Total bilirubin (serum)—0.1 to 1.0 mg/dL; indirect (unconjugated) bilirubin—0.2 to 0.8 mg/dL; direct (conjugated) bilirubin—0.1 to 0.3 mg/dL

         b) Urine bilirubin—0 to 0.2 mg/dL

         c) Jaundice caused by hepatocellular failure will increase the level of indirect bilirubin

         d) Jaundice resulting from obstructive causes will increase the level of direct bilirubin

         e) Hemolytic jaundice increases the level of indirect bilirubin

         f) An elevated level of bilirubin in the urine is always caused by an increased level of direct bilirubin (it is water-soluble, and indirect bilirubin is not)

      2) Other liver function tests help diagnose the cause of jaundice

         a) Alanine aminotransferase (ALT)—5 to 35 IU/L; used to identify hepatocellular diseases of the liver; elevation of ALT indicates damage to liver cells and helps eliminate hemolysis as the cause of jaundice

  b) Aspartate aminotransferase (AST)—5 to 40 IU/L (adults); levels vary depending on the type of jaundice; with hepatitis, the levels can be elevated 20 times above normal, gallstones can cause levels 10 times above normal

  c) ALT and AST ratios; used to help diagnose causes of liver dysfunction

  d) Alkaline phosphatase (ALP)—30 to 85 ImU/mL (adult); found in the liver and bone; ALP is increased with both extrahepatic and intrahepatic biliary obstructive processes

  e) Radiologic procedures can help confirm infiltrative or cholestatic processes; abdominal ultrasound and CT scans can detect tumors, stones, and other focal liver lesions that may be causing the jaundice

4. Therapeutic management

   a. Aimed at symptom management and includes keeping the client comfortable

   b. Often clients will be kept NPO pending diagnostic testing and because the introduction of food will increase pain secondary to stimulation of the digestive tract

   c. IV hydration and pain management are important aspects of care

   d. Management is aimed at treating the cause of the jaundice

5. Priority nursing diagnosis: Altered comfort: itching

6. Planning and implementation

   a. Cool or tepid baths containing colloidal substances (oatmeal, cornstarch, soybean powder) can reduce or ease pruritus (itching)

   b. Cool room (68 to 70°F) with 30 to 40 percent humidity

   c. Use an emollient lotion rather than one containing alcohol, which is too drying

7. Medication therapy: there is no specific medication therapy for jaundice

   a. Topical corticosteroids may provide some relief

   b. Bile-sequestering agents remove excess bile from the fat deposits under the skin decreasing pruritus

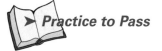

A client with jaundice is complaining of severe itching. What instructions can the nurse give to help relieve the itching?

8. Client education

   a. Educate the client about diagnostic tests required to diagnose the cause of jaundice

   b. Once the cause of jaundice is determined, educate the client regarding the disease process and future management

   c. Help the client understand that the causes of jaundice are usually correctable

   d. Advise the client with liver problems to avoid alcohol and acetaminophen, since both can cause further liver damage

9. Evaluation

   a. The client verbalizes the disease process and identifies appropriate dietary adjustments as indicated

   b. The client identifies ways to reduce itching

B. **Hepatitis A (HAV)**

   1. Description

      a. Viral infection of the liver causing diffuse inflammation of hepatic tissue; self-limiting

      b. Most common type of viral hepatitis, causing approximately 40 percent of reported cases worldwide

   2. Etiology and pathophysiology

      a. Transmitted by the fecal-oral route, particularly in overcrowded and unsanitary conditions; sources include contaminated food, water, and shellfish

      b. Also be transmitted by intimate contact with a person infected with the virus or through blood transfusion

      c. Virus can be isolated from feces, bile, and serum of infected individuals

      d. Many adults have HAV antibodies in their blood without knowledge of having the disease

      e. Incubation period is 4 to 6 weeks

      f. The client is most contagious 10 to 14 days prior to the onset of symptoms when fecal shedding of the virus is greatest

      g. Antibodies (anti-HAV) form 4 weeks postinfection; during the acute phase (2 to 3 months postinfection) IgM anti-HAV is elevated followed by elevation of IgG anti-HAV that persists for several years postinfection and creates immunity to the disease

      h. Can cause hepatic cell necrosis and swelling; inflammation, degradation, and regeneration of the liver cells occur simultaneously

      i. In the acute phase, swelling of the hepatic cells causes obstruction of the flow of bile within the bile canaliculi causing jaundice

   3. Assessment

      a. General assessment includes physical exam for dehydration (secondary to nausea, vomiting, anorexia), jaundice, and abdominal pain; review of laboratory studies for evaluation of progression or regression of disease

      b. Clinical manifestations

         1) A range of symptoms occurs, including anorexia, nausea, vomiting, malaise, fever, jaundice, and abdominal pain secondary to liver swelling

         2) Course of acute viral hepatitis is divided into three phases

            a) Prodromal (preicteric) phase (most contagious) occurs before jaundice appears, about 2 weeks after exposure to the virus, and includes flu-like symptoms (general malaise, gastrointestinal [GI] complaints, nausea, vomiting, diarrhea, and anorexia), headache, fatigue, myalgia, joint pain, and low-grade fever; food odors, smoking, or alcohol may cause nausea

b) **Icteric** phase is marked by the onset of jaundice; occurs about 2 weeks after the prodromal phase and lasts 2 to 6 weeks; includes dark-colored urine and clay-colored stools prior to the appearance of jaundice and pruritis; liver remains enlarged and may be tender to touch

c) Recovery (posticteric) phase begins with the resolution of jaundice and lasts several weeks, during which symptoms improve, energy levels increase, and serum enzymes normalize

c. Diagnostic and laboratory test findings

1) Anti-HAV is the antibody to HAV and is present from the onset of symptoms and persists for a lifetime

2) IgM anti-HAV is the serum immunoglobulin M HAV antibody; it is found in clients with recent infection and persists for up to 6 months postinfection

3) IgG anti-HAV is the serum immunoglobulin G HAV antibody; is present during the recovery phase and remains elevated for years postinfection; contributes to immunity to the disease

4) Alkaline phosphatase (ALP); nonspecific test to evaluate liver or bone dysfunction; can be elevated with hepatitis

5) Gamma-glutamyl transferase (GGT); acutely elevated with alcohol consumption and hepatotoxic drugs

6) Transaminases: ALT and AST; elevated to varying degrees with hepatitis caused by hepatocyte injury

7) Bilirubin; both direct and indirect levels can be elevated secondary to liver cell injury

8) Prothrombin time (PT); prolonged if the liver is injured to the point that it can no longer produce the proteins necessary for blood coagulation

4. Therapeutic management: includes both pre- and post-exposure prophylaxis as well as symptom management

a. Transmission is prevented through proper handwashing and the use of gloves for disposal of contaminated items (bedpans, fecal matter, bed linens)

b. Contact precautions should be instituted if there is fecal incontinence

c. Clinical illness is avoided in 90 percent of the cases with the HAV vaccine; the vaccine can be given prior to exposure or during the early incubation period

d. Most clients with HAV infection are managed as outpatients and rarely are admitted to the hospital

5. Priority nursing diagnoses

a. Risk for transmission of infection

b. Imbalanced nutrition: less than body requirements related to nausea, vomiting, anorexia, diarrhea

    c. Activity intolerance

    d. Altered comfort related to pain, arthralgia, abdominal pain, pruritis, headache

6. Planning and implementation

    a. Use of universal precautions and meticulous handwashing by client, family, and staff are imperative

    b. Clients should have a private bathroom

    c. Proper bagging, cleansing, and disposal of contaminated items is needed

    d. Provide anti-emetic medications as ordered and encourage a diet high in carbohydrates and low in fat

    e. Abstinence from alcohol is essential

    f. If liver function is compromised, protein and salt should be restricted

    g. Encourage a good breakfast; clients tend to become more nauseous later in the day

    h. Initiate intravenous (IV) fluids as ordered

    i. Assess for signs of dehydration and monitor electrolyte status

    j. Encourage gradual increase of activity as tolerated

    k. Plan nursing activities to allow for adequate rest

    l. Inform clients they may never donate blood

    m. Observe for blood in stool or urine, multiple ecchymosis, or petechiae, or oozing of blood from gums or minor cuts, which may indicate a complication

7. Medication therapy

    a. Is aimed at symptom relief; consist of anti-emetics and analgesics; because most analgesics are metabolized in the liver, their use must be limited

    b. IV fluids may be necessary if the client is unable to tolerate oral fluids

    c. Prophylaxis may be considered if known HAV exposure has occurred and it is early within the incubation period

    d. Vitamin K is indicated if prothrombin time is prolonged

    e. Antihistamines can be given for pruritis

8. Client education

    a. Since most clients with acute viral hepatitis are not hospitalized, they require detailed education about the disease and prevention of transmission; meticulous handwashing must be used and they must avoid sharing eating utensils, bath towels, and other personal care items that are in contact with body fluids

    b. Instruct client to avoid alcohol and any drugs that may be hepatotoxic (such as acetaminophen)

    c. Educate client about safe sex practices as a general health measure

9. Evaluation

   a. Client demonstrates understanding of disease process and the necessary steps to avoid transmitting the infection both in the hospital and after discharge

   b. Resumes normal bowel elimination pattern

   c. Activity progressively increases to a level normal for the client

   d. Client is able to meet daily caloric intake and maintain a stable weight

C. Hepatitis B (HBV)

   1. Description: DNA hepadenovirus

      a. Another form of viral hepatitis

      b. HBV is a vaccine-preventable disease

      c. Infects about 5 percent of the world's population; about 59 percent of the cases in the United States occur in heterosexuals with multiple sex partners, homosexual males, and IV drug users; healthcare workers comprise about 3 percent of all reported cases

      d. Can progress to a chronic form of the disease

   2. Etiology and pathophysiology

      a. Transmitted parenterally and through sexual contact with infected individuals

      b. Transmitted through contaminated blood or blood products or sharing of needles with persons infected with the virus; clients who require hemodialysis are also at risk

      c. The incubation period is 30 to 160 days

      d. Onset is insidious and is associated with a wide spectrum of liver involvement ranging from subclinical carrier state to fulminant hepatitis

      e. Can be severe and chronic

      f. The pathophysiological changes are the same with all types of viral hepatitis (previously discussed)

   3. Assessment

      a. Clinical manifestations for all forms of viral hepatitis are similar (see previous discussion) and may vary only in degrees

      b. Specific assessments

         1) Vital signs, including weight and reported weight loss

         2) Assessment of the skin and integument looking for jaundice, signs of pruritis, signs of bleeding, petechiae or ecchymotic areas, dehydration, and scleral icterus

         3) Lymphadenopathy

         4) Abdominal assessment for pain (location, type), hepatomegaly, swelling of the abdomen (may indicate **ascites**)

         5) Edema

6) Current nutritional state (adequate intake, nausea, anorexia, and vomiting) and elimination pattern (diarrhea)

7) Activity level, fatigue, ability to perform ADLs

8) Risk factors: IV drug use, homo/bisexual lifestyle, unprotected sexual contact, blood transfusion, tattoos

  c. Diagnostic and laboratory tests

1) HBsAg; hepatitis surface antigen, present during active disease; first test to become abnormal; rises prior to the onset of symptoms; peaks during the first week of symptoms and normalizes prior to the resolution of jaundice; if it remains elevated for a prolonged period of time, the client is considered to be a carrier

2) HBsAb; appears about 4 weeks after the disappearance of HbsAg and signifies the end of the acute phase of the infection as well as immunity to subsequent infection; in its concentrated form it is given as HBV vaccine

3) HBcAg; hepatitis core antigen

4) HBcAb; hepatitis core antibody; appears about 1 month after infection; remains in the serum of clients with chronic hepatitis; remains elevated during the time when HBsAg disappears and HBsAb appears; this is called the "core window," and HBcAb is the only detectable marker of recent infection

5) HBeAg; hepatitis B e-antigen; not usually used as a diagnostic test; marker used to determine client's index of infectivity; its presence in a client with acute HBV infection indicates early and active disease with high infectivity; used to predict the development of chronic HBV infection

6) HBeAb; this antibody indicates that the acute HBV infection is over or nearly over; infectivity is low

7) Anti-HBs-antibody to HBsAg is the IgG immunoglobulin that creates immunity and is present for a lifetime

8) Anti-HBe-antibody to HBeAg

9) Anti-HBc-antibody to hepatitis B core antigen, present for a lifetime

10) Alkaline phosphatase (ALP); nonspecific test to evaluate liver or bone dysfunction; can be elevated with hepatitis

11) Gamma-glutamyl transferase (GGT); acutely elevated with alcohol consumption and hepatotoxic drugs

12) Transaminases: ALT and AST; elevated to varying degrees with hepatitis caused by hepatocyte injury

13) Bilirubin; both direct and indirect levels can be elevated secondary to liver cell injury

14) Prothrombin time (PT); prolonged if the liver is injured to the point that it can no longer produce the proteins necessary for blood coagulation

4. Therapeutic management: the goal of management is to prevent transmission and support the liver's ability to heal itself

5. Priority nursing diagnoses: as previously discussed in section on hepatitis A

6. Planning and implementation

   a. Use universal precautions, which include wearing goggles, gown, and gloves when splattering of blood or body fluids is likely

   b. Proper labeling and disposal of contaminated items is essential

7. Medication therapy

   a. Vaccination is available; given as a series of three intramuscular injections to adults, children and infants; the second and third injections are given at 1 and 6 months after the initial injection; efficacy of the vaccination approaches 95 percent

   b. Routine vaccination is recommended for all infants in the United States

   c. Pre-exposure vaccination is recommended for individuals in high-risk occupations, including healthcare workers, individuals living in group homes, hemodialysis clients, individuals who are sexually active (especially those with multiple partners), IV drug users, individuals who require frequent transfusions of blood or blood products, inmates, and international travelers who reside in endemic areas

   d. Postexposure vaccination is recommended for individuals who come in contact with infected blood or body fluids, who have sexual contact with infected individuals, and infants exposed to a caregiver with known HBV infection or born to a mother with known HBsAg

   e. HBIG is given to newborns exposed prenatally and to unvaccinated individuals who have been exposed (percutaneously or mucosally) to infected blood or body fluids

   f. If a person with prior vaccination has had percutaneous or mucosal exposure to infected blood or body fluids, the blood should be tested for anti-HBs and the client should be given HBIG as well as a booster dose of HBV vaccine

8. Client education

   a. Instruct client about the possibility of developing chronic active hepatitis and the importance of follow-up

   b. Reinforce the use of safe sex practices and vaccination

9. Evaluation: identifies ways to prevent transmission and practices safe sex

D. Hepatitis C (HCV)

1. Description: HCV is an RNA flavirus

   a. Previously known as non-A non-B

   b. Is the cause of most posttransfusion hepatitis

   c. Is responsible for about 20 percent of all cases of viral hepatitis

   d. Up to 80 percent of individuals develop chronic hepatitis, which is a risk factor for liver failure and hepatocellular carcinoma

2. Etiology and pathophysiology

   a. Incubation period is between 2 and 20 weeks postexposure

   b. Transmission occurs parenterally and possibly sexually since the virus has been isolated from feces and semen

   c. Most cases of HCV have no known risk factors

   d. The pathophysiology is the same for all forms of hepatitis, previously discussed

3. Assessment

   a. Clinical manifestations

      1) Acute infection is generally asymptomatic

      2) 25 to 35% develop malaise, weakness, and anorexia

      3) Symptoms in chronic hepatitis generally only occur when liver disease is advanced; fatigue and malaise most commonly occur

   b. Diagnostic and laboratory tests

      1) Anti-HCV; antibody to hepatitis C virus; most accurate in detecting chronic hepatitis C

      2) There is an HCV viral titer; HCV IgG indicates prior infection

      3) Liver biopsy to determine extent of liver damage and response to treatment

      4) General laboratory tests for hepatitis as previously discussed

4. Therapeutic management

   a. The hallmark of treatment now is medication therapy to prevent chronic hepatitis development

   b. A goal of treatment is to prevent transmission of the virus

5. Priority nursing diagnoses: as previously discussed for other forms of hepatitis

6. Planning and implementation: as previously discussed for other forms of hepatitis

7. Medication therapy

   a. Combination therapy is used for 12 to 18 weeks or as long as 48 weeks

   b. The combination of interferon alfa-2b and ribavirin therapy produces a more sustained response than when interferon is used alone

   c. Cost of therapy is high in terms of both dollars and adverse effects (fever, chills, fatigue, myalgia, headache, arthralgia, leukopenia, neutropenia, thrombocytopenia, anemia, anorexia, nausea, dizziness, confusion, paresthesia, numbness, depression, hypotension, chest pain, and heart failure)

8. Client education

   a. Is aimed at transmission prevention (previously discussed)

   b. Reinforce the possibility of chronic disease and the importance of maintaining the medication therapy

9. Evaluation

    a. Client indicates understanding of modes of transmission and prevention

    b. Client follows through with medication therapy

E. Hepatitis D (HDV); defective RNA virus

1. Description: also known as "delta hepatitis" and occurs only in individuals with HBV because it depends upon the HBV virus to replicate

2. Etiology and pathophysiology

    a. Incubation period is 4 to 24 weeks

    b. Transmitted parenterally; there is a question of whether it can be transmitted via the fecal-oral route and sexually

    c. Must have HBV from a past or simultaneously occurring infection

    d. In the United States, it is most often transmitted through infected blood

3. Assessment

    a. Clinical manifestations: similar to all viral hepatitis infections

    b. Diagnostic and laboratory studies

        1) HDV antigen can be detected by immunoassay within a few days of infection

        2) IgM HDV; present during early infection

        3) Persistent elevation of antibodies indicates a chronic/carrier state

4. Therapeutic management: because HDV requires the presence of HBV, vaccination of individuals not infected with HBV is recommended

5. Priority nursing diagnoses: as previously discussed for hepatitis A

6. Planning and implementation: as previously discussed for hepatitis A

7. Medication therapy: there are no medications specific to the treatment of HDV

8. Client education: same followup appointment schedule as for those for hepatitis A

9. Evaluation: outcomes same as for Hepatitis A

F. Cirrhosis

1. Description

    a. Irreversible and chronic liver disease characterized by diffuse inflammation and fibrosis of liver tissue

    b. These structural changes lead to loss of liver function because of scarring and obstruction of hepatic blood flow

2. Etiology and pathophysiology (see Figure 7-2)

    a. Three classifications: Laënnec's, biliary, and post-necrotic

        1) Laënnec's cirrhosis, also called as alcoholic cirrhosis, is the most prevalent type in the United States, and is highest among middle-aged men

► *Practice to Pass*

What information should the nurse give to a client with viral hepatitis about its transmission?

NCLEX!

Figure 7-2 Multisystem effects of cirrhosis.

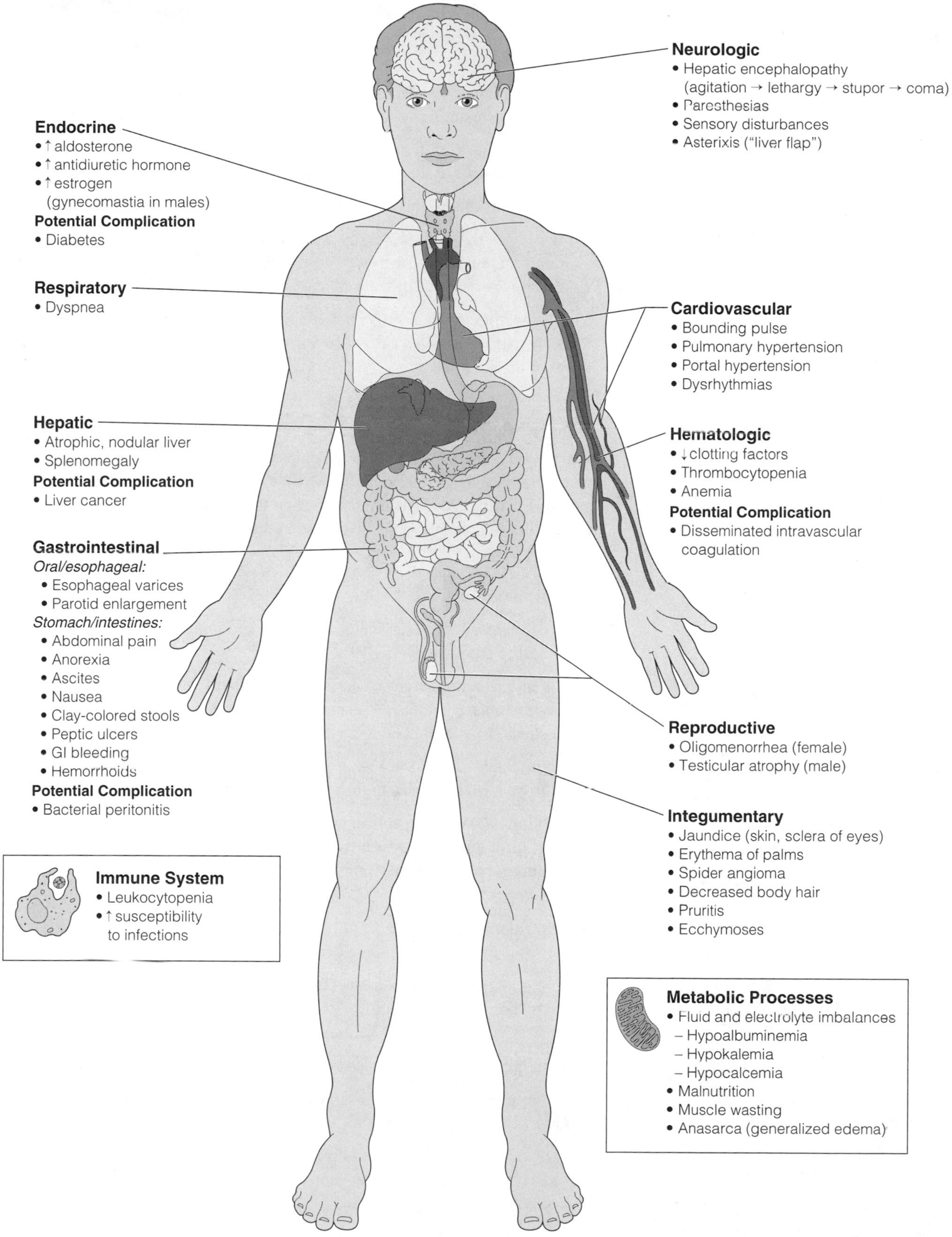

Neurologic
- Hepatic encephalopathy (agitation → lethargy → stupor → coma)
- Paresthesias
- Sensory disturbances
- Asterixis ("liver flap")

Endocrine
- ↑ aldosterone
- ↑ antidiuretic hormone
- ↑ estrogen (gynecomastia in males)

Potential Complication
- Diabetes

Respiratory
- Dyspnea

Cardiovascular
- Bounding pulse
- Pulmonary hypertension
- Portal hypertension
- Dysrhythmias

Hepatic
- Atrophic, nodular liver
- Splenomegaly

Potential Complication
- Liver cancer

Hematologic
- ↓ clotting factors
- Thrombocytopenia
- Anemia

Potential Complication
- Disseminated intravascular coagulation

Gastrointestinal
Oral/esophageal:
- Esophageal varices
- Parotid enlargement
Stomach/intestines:
- Abdominal pain
- Anorexia
- Ascites
- Nausea
- Clay-colored stools
- Peptic ulcers
- GI bleeding
- Hemorrhoids

Potential Complication
- Bacterial peritonitis

Reproductive
- Oligomenorrhea (female)
- Testicular atrophy (male)

Integumentary
- Jaundice (skin, sclera of eyes)
- Erythema of palms
- Spider angioma
- Decreased body hair
- Pruritis
- Ecchymoses

Immune System
- Leukocytopenia
- ↑ susceptibility to infections

Metabolic Processes
- Fluid and electrolyte imbalances
  - Hypoalbuminemia
  - Hypokalemia
  - Hypocalcemia
- Malnutrition
- Muscle wasting
- Anasarca (generalized edema)

273

a) It is caused by prolonged, excessive alcohol intake with or without malnutrition; is directly related to the toxic effects of alcohol on the liver

b) Alcohol is metabolized to acetaldehyde, which is toxic to hepatocytes, resulting in inflammation, necrosis, and collagen formation

c) It begins with fatty infiltration of the liver causing a large firm liver (reversible at this stage if alcohol intake is stopped)

d) In late stages, the liver becomes small and nodular (irreversible)

2) Biliary cirrhosis is caused by obstruction of the bile canaliculi and ducts and results in necrosis and fibrosis; the cause can be autoimmune in nature or caused by tumors, gallstones, or chronic pancreatitis

3) Postnecrotic cirrhosis results from a chronic, severe liver disease such as hepatitis; it is also caused by inherited metabolic liver disorders such as Wilson's disease

b. Regardless of the cause, cirrhosis develops slowly; the severity and rate of progression depend on the cause and repeated injury to the hepatocytes

c. Disruption of portal blood flow secondary to structural changes in the liver results in edema, ascites, splenomegaly (caused by splanchnic venous congestion), portal hypertension (see section that follows), hemorrhoids, varicose veins, and esophageal varices (see section that follows)

3. Assessment

a. Specific assessments

1) Vital signs: orthostatic measurement of blood pressure and pulse, temperature and weight

2) Integument/skin: signs of jaundice and scleral icterus, bruises, hematomas, petechiae, evidence of pruritus, spider angiomata, telangiectasia, hair loss, palmar erythema, caput medusa, and edema

3) Pulmonary: decreased breath sounds in the bases (may indicate pleural effusion) or crackles (might indicate development of heart failure)

4) Abdomen: swelling, shifting dullness, fluid wave, or increasing abdominal girth that are indicative of ascites; change in bowel sounds, pain or tenderness in the right-upper quadrant (RUQ), hepatomegaly, splenomegaly

5) Nutritional status: muscle atrophy and wasting; check color and character of urine (dark) and stool possibly (clay-colored)

6) Neurological: decreased level of consciousness, disorientation, tremor, **asterixis** (flapping tremor of hand from increased ammonia levels), and decreased deep tendon reflexes (DTRs)

b. Clinical manifestations (see Box 7-1)

1) GI symptoms include nausea, vomiting, anorexia, constipation, weight loss

2) Decreased ability to metabolize carbohydrates (CHOs) leads to hypoglycemia, decreased energy, and alterations in glycogenolysis, gluconeogenesis, and glycogenesis

Box 7-1	
Signs and Symptoms of Cirrhosis	

- General malaise
- Skin
  Pruritis
  Spider angiomata
  Ecchymosis
  Propensity for bleeding
  Edema
- Gastrointestinal
  Nausea
  Vomiting
  Anorexia
  Pyrosis
  Weight loss/malnutrition
  Constipation
  Flatulence
- Abdomen
  Ascites (increasing abdominal girth)
  Abdominal pain (RUQ)

  Positive fluid wave
  Shifting dullness
  Caput medusa
- Neurological
  Fatigue
  Encephalopathy
  Asterixis
- Gynecomastia
- Loss of body hair
- Testicular atrophy
- Erectile dysfunction
- Menstrual irregularities
- Palmar erythema
- Anemia
- Hemorrhoids
- Clay-colored stools
- Dark urine

3) Alteration in fat metabolism causes increased synthesis of fatty acids and triglycerides leading to fatty liver and hepatomegaly

4) Alteration in protein metabolism leads to low albumin levels and with the decrease in osmotic pressure, development of edema and ascites; decreased protein also decreases the production of clotting factors that increases the risk of bleeding

5) Decreased metabolism of sex steroids (estrogen, progesterone, and testosterone) leads to gynecomastia, loss of body hair, development of palmar erythema and spider angiomata, erectile dysfunction, and menstrual disorders

6) Decreased metabolism of aldosterone results in sodium and water retention and adds to development of edema and ascites

7) Decreased metabolism of ammonia leads to increased serum ammonia levels and hepatic encephalopathy (manifests as lack of coordination, decreased memory, lack of orientation, and coma)

8) Decreased stores of vitamins and minerals leads to malnutrition, fatigue, and anemia

9) Obstruction of the flow of bile leads to hyperbilirubinemia and jaundice, clay-colored stools, dark-colored urine

10) Splenomegaly leads to pancytopenia

11) Fibrosis and scarring continue, resulting in increased portal pressure that causes ascites, hemorrhoids, esophageal varices, caput medusa (superficial abdominal veins)

12) Involuntary tremor or flapping of the hands is called liver flap or asterixis

13) Malnutrition: leads to muscle atrophy and bitemporal wasting

c. Diagnostic and laboratory findings

NCLEX!

1) Biopsy is the only definitive way to diagnose the type of cirrhosis; may not be necessary if clients have clinical manifestations with supportive risk factors; may not be advisable because prolonged PT would place the client at increased risk for bleeding; Figure 7-3 illustrates the biopsy procedure, and Box 7-2 describes nursing care after liver biopsy

2) No laboratory tests will diagnose cirrhosis; lab tests are similar to those discussed for clients with hepatitis

3) Findings include varying degrees of increased transaminases, decreased albumin, prolonged PT, hyperbilirubinemia, hyponatremia from excess-free water, hypokalemia from diuretic therapy, and hypomagnesemia.

4) Complete blood count (CBC) reflects pancytopenia (anemia, thrombocytopenia, leukopenia)

5) Elevated serum ammonia level

6) Liver ultrasound may reveal an enlarged fibrofatty liver or a small fibrotic and nodular liver; highly dense areas may reflect possible hepatocellular carcinoma

Figure 7-3

Liver biopsy procedure. A. The client exhales completely and holds the breath to elevate the liver and diaphragm to highest position; B. Physician inserts needle into liver; C. Approximately 1 mL of saline is injected to clear needle of blood and tissue; D. Needle is guided further into liver and sample is aspirated. After withdrawing the needle, pressure is applied to site. Specimen is placed in formalin (preservative) and sent for laboratory analysis.

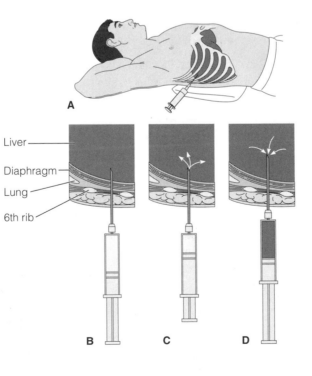

Box 7-2	
Nursing Care after Liver Biopsy	• Vital signs q 15 min × 4; q 30 min × 2; q 1 hr × 2; q 4 hr × 4; then q 6 hr • Observe dressing for oozing on same schedule as vital signs • Monitor for signs and symptoms of bleeding • Apply direct pressure to biopsy site immediately after procedure • Position on right side for compression over biopsy site • Maintain NPO for 2 hr postprocedure • Bedrest for 24 hr • Avoid activities that increase intra-abdominal pressure (coughing, lifting, straining) for 1 to 2 weeks

4. Therapeutic management

   a. Abdominal **paracentesis** is performed on clients with severe ascites; it is an invasive procedure that is accomplished by draining fluid from the abdomen via a needle; fluid is often sent for culture

   b. Surgical intervention to prevent the reaccumulation of ascitic fluid includes insertion of a LeVeen shunt or transjugular intrahepatic portosystemic shunt (TIPS); these shunts help to relieve portal hypertension

5. Priority nursing diagnoses

   a. Excess fluid volume related to **hypoalbuminemia** (low serum albumin levels) and hyperaldosteronism

   b. Imbalanced nutrition: less than body requirements related to anorexia, liver failure, and dietary restrictions

   c. Risk for injury related to bleeding, fatigue, and activity intolerance

   d. Risk for ineffective breathing pattern related to ascites

   e. Risk for impaired skin integrity related to jaundice, malnutrition, edema, and prolonged bleeding time, pruritis

   f. Ineffective individual coping related to health crisis (and for those with cirrhosis related to alcohol, inability to cope with life pressures)

6. Planning and implementation

   a. Clients with ascites are fluid-restricted to prevent further accumulation of ascitic fluid

   b. Diet restrictions include low sodium intake to prevent further ascitic fluid accumulation and decreased protein intake

   c. Provide small frequent meals

   d. Administer antiemetics and diuretics as ordered

   e. Weigh daily, and monitor intake and output (I & O)

   f. Measure abdominal girth to assess progression of ascites

g. For respiratory support, use high Fowler's position and use supplemental O_2 as ordered; encourage deep-breathing; allow activity as tolerated; measure oxygen saturation, and arterial blood gases as ordered

h. Maintain skin integrity; remove moist linens promptly; keep client's skin clean and moistened with emollient; administer antihistamines as ordered; encourage activity as tolerated or reposition every 2 hours

NCLEX!

i. Institute bleeding precautions: prevent constipation, avoid injections, observe for signs and symptoms of bleeding, encourage use of soft toothbrush, monitor labs (CBC, PT)

j. Assess understanding of illness; identify support system; assess coping skills; offer clergy support; encourage Alcoholics Anonymous for those with cirrhosis secondary to alcohol dependence; provide substance abuse consultation as indicated

7. Medication therapy

a. Diuretics; these are given cautiously to promote excretion of excess fluid to decrease ascites; most commonly used drugs are spironolactone (Aldactone), a potassium-sparing diuretic, and furosemide (Lasix), a loop diuretic

b. Lactulose (Cephulac); a disaccharide laxative that is not absorbed by the GI tract; it pulls water into the bowel and helps to decrease the absorption of ammonia

c. Other medications include vitamin K to treat prolonged PT, antihistamines, and antiemetics

8. Client education

NCLEX!

a. Lifestyle changes include dietary restrictions, abstinence from alcohol, fluid restrictions; suggest nutrition consultation

b. Teach client to reduce intake of foods that are high in sodium; canned and frozen foods, highly processed cheeses, potato chips, etc. must be avoided

c. Instruct clients to limit intake of foods high in protein: eggs, cheese, milk, and meats

NCLEX!

d. Instruct clients to avoid taking any over-the-counter medications without checking with healthcare provider first since many medications are hepatotoxic (such as acetaminophen)

e. Review signs and symptoms that require medical attention after discharge: weight gain, increased abdominal girth, respiratory distress, bleeding gums, blood in the stool or urine, fever, abdominal pain

f. Teach the client how to adjust dose of lactulose according to number of loose stools per day (usually three)

g. Involve family and other support persons in the client's care

9. Evaluation

a. Client demonstrates understanding of illness and the importance of making lifestyle changes after discharge from the hospital

b. Client participates in care while hospitalized such as charting I & O, daily weights

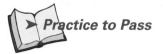

Practice to Pass

The client with cirrhosis has just had a liver biopsy. What does the usual post-biopsy care include?

NCLEX!

c. Client demonstrates understanding of dietary restrictions by verbalizing foods high in protein and sodium

d. Client contacts Alcoholics Anonymous if appropriate

e. Client verbalizes understanding of bleeding precautions

f. Client demonstrates good skin care

G. **Complications of cirrhosis** (see Box 7-3)

1. **Portal hypertension;** an abnormally high blood pressure (BP) within the portal venous system; most commonly caused by cirrhosis but can be caused by anything that impedes blood flow through the portal venous system or through the vena cava, such as fibrosis or inflammation of liver tissue secondary to cirrhosis, hepatitis or infection, hepatic vein thrombus, tumor, or right heart failure

   a. Clinical manifestations

      1) Includes all the findings described with cirrhosis

      2) Other potentially fatal conditions that can develop as a result of portal hypertension are varices, ascites, hepatic encephalopathy leading to coma, and hepatorenal syndrome; each of these is discussed in more detail below

      3) Most common clinical manifestation is vomiting of blood secondary to rupture of esophageal varices; clients with oozing varices may present with anemia and melanotic stools

      4) Splenomegaly can result from increased pressure within the splenic vein, which branches off the portal vein

      5) Clients may complain of irritation from hemorrhoids or may present with bright red rectal bleeding secondary to hemorrhoids

   b. Therapeutic management: parallels that for the treatment of cirrhosis and is based on symptomatic treatment of varices, ascites, encephalopathy, and hepatorenal syndrome, which are discussed in more detail below

   c. Planning and implementation: similar to care given for esophageal varices, ascites, encephalopathy, and hepatorenal syndrome, discussed in the following sections

   d. Medication therapy: is aimed at decreasing portal venous pressure without precipitating hypotensive crisis; diuretics and fluid restriction are treat-

NCLEX!

Box 7-3	

Complications of Cirrhosis	• Portal hypertension
	   Right-sided heart failure
	   Esophageal varices
	   Varicose veins
	• Ascites
	• Encephalopathy/coma
	• Hepatorenal syndrome

ments of choice; propranolol (Inderal), a beta-blocker, has also been used to decrease portal venous pressures

2. **Esophageal varices:** develop as a result of increased portal pressure; are distended and tortuous vessels that can rupture secondary to coughing, sneezing, vomiting, or ingestion of foods high in roughage; bleeding can be abrupt and painless with mortality reaching 50 percent; ruptured esophageal varices are considered a medical emergency

NCLEX!

a. Clinical manifestations: if the bleeding is slow, melena and decreasing hemoglobin and hematocrit are present, but if bleeding is abrupt, severe hematemesis and signs of hypovolemic shock (tachycardia, hypotension) can occur

b. Therapeutic management: includes stopping the bleeding either by **sclerotherapy** or esophageal tamponade (direct pressure by use of a special nasogastric tube with esophageal and gastric balloons)

c. Planning and implementation

1) Maintain airway, breathing, and circulation and measure VS

2) Start two large-bore IVs with infusion of normal saline (NS) as ordered

3) Draw serum laboratory tests (CBC, type and cross-match, chemistries)

4) Begin gastric lavage if ordered

NCLEX!

5) Esophageal tamponade/balloon tamponade is done via placement of Sengstaken-Blakemore or Minnesota tubes, which are multi-lumen gastric tubes, placed nasally and extend into the stomach; there are two balloons, one in the esophageal area which, when inflated, tamponades the bleeding varices in the esophagus and the gastric balloon, which serves as an anchor (see Chapter 8)

6) Sclerotherapy and banding are accomplished via endoscopy; physician locates the bleeding vessel via endoscope and injects a sclerosing agent (causes thrombosis and hemostasis); may be done emergently or as an elective procedure

7) Keep clients NPO for either of the above procedures (if elective); provide an explanation regarding the procedure, and give a mild sedative as ordered before the procedure

8) Prepare the client for transfer to a setting with cardiac monitoring capability

d. Medication therapy

1) Vasopressin: IV infusion, usually given when a cardiac monitor is in place; can be given intermittently or via continuous infusion; lowers portal pressure by causing splanchic vasoconstriction and thus helps control bleeding from esophageal varices; used with caution in clients with cardiac disease because of vasoconstriction

2) Propranolol (Inderal); beta-blocker that reduces portal pressure, not effective in all clients; given in low doses such as 10 mg QID

3) Sandostatin (Octreotide) decreases splanchnic blood flow and thus reduces bleeding from esophageal varices

3. Ascites: an accumulation of plasma-rich fluid within the peritoneal cavity secondary to portal hypertension, increased aldosterone, and decreased oncotic pressure (hypoalbuminemia); cirrhosis is the most common cause; kidneys retain sodium and thus water, further increasing third-spaced fluid and anasarca

   a. Clinical manifestations: abdominal distention, weight gain, increased abdominal girth, dilation of venous system over the abdomen (caput medusa), generalized edema, and respiratory distress if accumulation of ascitic fluid is large

   b. Therapeutic management

      1) Paracentesis to remove fluid; diuretics; shunting devices (to treat portal hypertension)

      2) Diagnostic testing to identify liver disease: abdominal ultrasound, paracentesis with fluid examination, liver biopsy

      3) Comfort measures

   c. Planning and implementation

      1) Monitor fluid and electrolyte status

      2) Give fluids as ordered

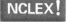

      3) Monitor daily weights and measure abdominal girth every 8 to 24 hrs

      4) Restrict intake of dietary protein and sodium

      5) Provide education about disease process and diagnostic tests

      6) Assess for respiratory distress, monitor vital signs for hypotension and/or tachycardia

      7) Keep scissors at bedside of client with Sengstaken-Blakemoore tube for use in cutting tube if respiratory distress occurs because of balloon displacement

   d. Medication therapy: there are no specific medications for treatment of ascites; management is aimed at treating the cause; beta blockers may help to decrease portal hypertension

4. **Hepatic encephalopathy:** a neurological complication caused by the accumulation of toxic substances (primarily ammonia) in the blood

   a. Clinical manifestations: loss of memory, irritability, confusion, lethargy, sleep disturbances, stupor, coma, and asterixis

   b. Therapeutic management: aimed at reducing the production of nitrogenous wastes (urea) and ammonia, correcting fluid and electrolyte imbalances, and eliminating use of sedating drugs and drugs metabolized by the liver

   c. Planning and implementation

      1) Perform frequent neurologic assessment to note progression of lethargy

      2) Administer medications to reduce ammonia levels and intestinal bacteria as ordered

3) Restrict dietary protein

4) Avoid sedating medications

5) Monitor for fluid and electrolyte imbalances and implement corrective measures as ordered

6) Treat the cause of liver disease by implementing ordered therapies

d. Medication therapy

1) Lactulose (Cephulac) is a hyperosmolar laxative that passes unabsorbed into the large intestine where it is hydrolyzed to an acid, which renders ammonia unabsorbable and produces diarrhea; diarrhea limits the amount of time feces are available for intestinal bacteria to act on and form more ammonia

2) Neomycin is sometimes used to sterilize the bowel thus limiting further ammonia production; use with caution because of nephrotoxicity

5. Hepatorenal syndrome: renal failure associated with advanced liver failure and caused by alterations in circulation without primary renal disease; most commonly found in Laënnec's cirrhosis and fulminant hepatitis; results in sudden renal failure possibly from diuretics characterized by intrarenal vasoconstriction, oliguria, azotemia, anorexia, and fatigue; is associated with a poor prognosis

a. Clinical manifestations include decreased urine output, hyponatremia, decreased urine osmolality and hypotension; usually associated with advanced liver disease thus jaundice, ascites, GI bleeding occur; increased BUN, creatinine levels are present

b. Therapeutic management

1) Fluid and electrolyte imbalances and encephalopathy are treated with the aim of restoring renal and liver function

2) Drugs that are nephrotoxic or hepatotoxic drugs are eliminated (such as neomycin sulfate)

3) Liver transplantation is the definitive treatment

4) Hemodialysis is used to treat hyperkalemia and fluid overload

c. Planning and implementation involves carefully assessing I & O daily weights, monitoring electrolyte status, educating client about hemodialysis and/or preparing client for liver transplant

d. Medication therapy includes stopping use of all nephrotoxic and hepatotoxic medications

H. Cancer of the liver

1. Description

a. Most common types are metastases from lung, breast, kidney, and other forms of GI cancers

b. Primary liver cancer (hepatoma) is uncommon in the United States, but is more prominent in areas with increased chronic liver disease (Africa, Asia)

c. Prognosis is poor; there is < 20 percent survival rate for those with primary liver cancer

---

▶ Practice to Pass

The client with hepatic encephalopathy is ordered to receive lactulose. What is the purpose of this medication?

2. Etiology and pathophysiology

   a. Tumors arise in the liver cell (hepatocellular) or the bile duct (cholangiocellular)

   b. Primary liver cancer is more common in the presence chronic liver disease

   c. Tumors can be diffuse, nodular, or single nodule

   d. The tumor compresses surrounding cells and can invade the blood supply causing necrosis or hemorrhage

   e. Most primary hepatic cancers in the United States result from Laënnec's cirrhosis or HBV; other etiologic agents are nitrosamines, prolonged androgen therapy, pesticides, and contraceptive steroids

3. Assessment

   NCLEX!

   a. Clinical manifestations: RUQ pain or mass, fullness in the epigastric region, fatigue, general malaise, anorexia and weight loss; later signs can include ascites, fever, jaundice, variceal bleeding, liver failure, and splcnomegaly

   b. Diagnostic and laboratory test findings: the degree of laboratory abnormalities varies depending on the degree of liver damage

      1) CBC: anemia

      2) Hyperbilirubinemia

      3) Prolonged PT

      4) Elevated erythrocyte sedimentation rate (ESR) due to inflammation of the liver

      5) Hypoalbuminemia-malnutrition, liver failure

      6) Elevated alkaline phosphatase, AST, ALT when there is liver failure/damage

      7) Alteration of blood glucose due to liver damage

      8) AFP (alpha-fetoprotein): high elevations in 70 percent of those with hepatocellular cancer

      9) Ultrasound, CT scan, or MRI may reveal focal liver lesions

      10) Definitive diagnosis is made through biopsy or aspiration of lesion

4. Therapeutic management

   a. Partial hepatectomy for individuals with solitary lesions and without extrahepatic manifestations; serial AFPs are done following the procedure to assess effects of intervention

   b. Liver transplantation may be done for those meeting established criteria for the procedure

   c. Radiation therapy may be a palliative measure employed to shrink the tumor or reduce pain or pressure on surrounding structures

   d. Chemotherapy as a primary therapy has limited response; sometimes chemotherapy is infused via hepatic arterial pump

   e. Pain control is important

   f. Follow principles of therapeutic management of other liver disorders when other manifestations of liver failure are present

5. Priority nursing diagnoses

   a. Grieving related to loss, poor prognosis

   b. Risk for infection related to altered immune response and malnutrition

   c. Risk for injury related to weakness, prolonged bleeding, and malnutrition (see other sections related to liver failure)

6. Planning and implementation

   a. Provide care as outlined for other complications of liver failure/disorders

   b. Provide education regarding liver cancer and chemotherapy

   c. Refer to other sections for measures related to liver failure/complications

7. Medication therapy

   a. Chemotherapy can include 5-fluorouracil, methotrexate, and doxorubicin

   b. Other medications may be used, as discussed in prior sections related to liver failure/complications

8. Client education

   a. Teach about the disease process, expected outcomes, and chemotherapy

   b. Educate client regarding etiologic agents that cause or contribute to the development of hepatic cancer

   c. Refer to prior sections on liver disorders/complications for other teaching points related to liver disease

9. Evaluation

   a. Demonstrates effective coping skills

   b. Has stable or decreasing serial AFP levels

   c. Demonstrates appropriate knowledge regarding complications of liver failure

III. Disorders of the Hepatobiliary System: Gallbladder

A. Cholelithiasis

NCLEX!

1. Description: gallstones can occur anywhere within the biliary tree, although stones within the gallbladder are most common; 80 percent are composed of cholesterol, while 20 percent are pigmented; 20 to 25 million adults have gallstones and most are asymptomatic; they affect 10 percent of males and 15 percent of females over age 55

2. Etiology and pathophysiology

   a. Cholesterol gallstone formation is enhanced by production of mucin glycoprotein, which traps cholesterol leading to stasis of bile, and contributes to stone formation; cholesterol stones (usually several) develop slowly, are hard, white, or yellow-brown, radiolucent, and can be up to 4 centimeters in size

b. Pigmented stones form because of an increase in unconjugated bilirubin and calcium with a concurrent decrease in bile salts; usually develop within the intra- and extrahepatic ducts and are preceded by bacterial invasion

c. Increased bile concentration, bile stasis, and hypercholesterolemia contribute to stone formation

d. Most stones are formed within the gallbladder and migrate out through the ducts of the biliary tree; symptoms are consistent with location of stone; many clients are asymptomatic

e. Risk factors associated with the formation of gallstones are listed in Box 7-4

3. Assessment

a. Clinical manifestations

1) Depend on the location of the stones

NCLEX!

2) Classic manifestations include severe and steady right upper quadrant (RUQ) pain that radiates to the right scapula or shoulder; sudden onset, lasting 1 to 3 hours

3) May occur after a high-fat meal

4) Other symptoms include nausea, vomiting, heartburn, and flatulence

5) Fever and chills occur with development of acute cholecystitis

NCLEX!

6) Biliary colic or cramping-type pain occurs when the stone is lodged in the cystic or common bile duct; if the stone blocks the duct, edema and inflammation of gallbladder (cholecystitis) occur and may be associated with jaundice

NCLEX!

7) Physical exam findings include positive Murphy's sign—palpation of the RUQ causes severe pain with inspiratory arrest; bowel sounds may be absent

---

Box 7-4

Risk Factors for Gallstones

- Female gender
- Family history (may be related to familial high dietary fat intake and sedentary lifestyle)
- Obesity
- Very-low-calorie diet with rapid weight loss
- Pregnancy
- Use of estrogen-containing medications (oral contraceptives, hormone replacement therapy)
- Crohn's disease
- Jejunal bypass surgery
- Type 1 diabetes mellitus
- Aging
- Congenital malformation of biliary duct
- Hyperlipidemia
- Cirrhosis
- Caucasian race

8) Jaundice is not usually seen unless there is blockage of the common bile duct

b. Diagnostic and laboratory test findings

1) CBC to evaluate presence of infection

2) Serum bilirubin: levels increase when there is a stone in biliary ductal system causing obstruction

3) Electrolytes: assess for dehydration or electrolyte depletion secondary to vomiting, anorexia

4) Liver function tests (LFTs) to assess for hepatic involvement/damage caused by obstruction of the bile ducts

5) Alkaline phosphatase: increases with biliary obstruction

6) Serum amylase and lipase to assess for pancreatitis

7) Abdominal x-rays (flat plate) may reveal stones; however, most stones are not radiopaque

8) Ultrasonography is used to identify stones, gallbladder and ductal dilatation in non-obese clients

9) Oral cholecystogram is not used as frequently as ultrasound for diagnosis of stones; involves ingestion of oral dye to assess the ability of the gallbladder to concentrate and excrete bile; outlines stones for visualization

10) Gallbladder scans (HIDA): cholescintigraphy-nuclear medicine scan to evaluate for acute cholecystitis

4. Therapeutic management

a. Oral dissolution therapy using ursodeoxycholic acid for clients who are poor surgical risks or refuse surgery; given orally to dissolve cholesterol stones; effective for small stones < 2 cm in diameter, full treatment can take up to 3 years and 50 percent of clients experience reoccurrence of stones within 5 years

b. Extracorporeal shock wave **lithotripsy** uses shock waves to disintegrate stones; oral dissolution therapy is used postprocedure to dissolve stone fragments; clients may experience biliary colic postprocedure when the gallbladder is contracting to pass the stone fragments

c. Endoscopic retrograde cholangiopancreatography (ERCP) is used for both diagnostic and treatment purposes; involves use of fiberoptic endoscope to visualize the biliary tree, remove stones, drain bile sludge, and collect biopsies

d. Laparoscopic cholecystectomy is less invasive and involves shorter hospital stay; abdomen is insufflated with CO_2; laparoscope is introduced through a small incision, and the gallbladder is deflated and removed through the small abdominal incision

e. **Cholecystectomy:** surgical removal of the gallbladder; T-tube placement may accompany surgery, in which a T-tube is placed in the common bile duct to assist passage of bile until edema has decreased; bile collects in a bag by gravity drainage

5. Priority nursing diagnoses

   a. Acute pain

   b. Risk for impaired gas exchange related to pain and ineffective inspiratory effort

   c. Risk for infection related to bile duct obstruction and/or postoperative complications

   d. Imbalanced nutrition: less than body requirements related to nausea, vomiting, and anorexia

   e. Anxiety related to lack of knowledge about disease process and treatment measures

6. Planning and implementation

   a. Implement comfort measures including administration of analgesics and antiemetics as ordered

   b. Provide education regarding diagnostic tests and disease process

   c. Maintain NPO status preprocedure as ordered; institute IV fluids as ordered

   d. Provide diet instruction regarding low-fat diet, frequent small meals

   e. Encourage obese individuals to lose weight

   f. Monitor fluid and electrolyte balance

   g. Also see section below for surgical intervention for disorders of the gallbladder

7. Medication therapy

   a. Symptomatic treatment of pain and nausea with analgesics and antiemetics as ordered

   b. Meperidine (Demerol) is the preferred opioid analgesic because morphine can cause spasms of the sphincter of Oddi

   c. Cholestyramine (Questran) is used for severe cases of pruritus; binds bile salts to hasten excretion through the feces

   d. Oral dissolution medications

      1) Chenodeoxycholic acid (CDCA): a bile acid, taken orally for dissolving cholesterol stones

      2) Urodeoxycholic acid (UDCA): similar to CDCA—less hepatotoxic and does not cause fatty diarrhea as does CDCA

8. Client teaching

   a. Provide instruction about disease process and gallstone formation

   b. Give information about diagnostic procedures and expected outcomes

   c. Provide diet instruction, particularly a review of foods high in fat

9. Evaluation

   a. Client is pain-free

   b. Clients understands the disease process including dietary restrictions

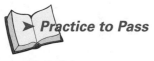

Practice to Pass

What dietary instructions should the nurse give to the client with cholelithiasis?

B. Cholecystitis

1. Description: an acute or chronic disorder, most often caused by gallstones obstructing the cystic duct resulting in distention and inflammation of the gallbladder; pain is similar to that of gallstones

2. Etiology and pathophysiology

   a. Most commonly caused by gallstone obstructing the cystic or common bile duct

   b. Approximately 5 percent of clients develop acalculous cholecystitis precipitated by trauma, prolonged hyperalimentation, fasting, or surgery

3. Assessment

   NCLEX!

   a. Clinical manifestations: include all of those previously identified for cholelithiasis; also fever, leukocytosis, elevation of serum bilirubin (possible jaundice) and alkaline phosphatase, elevation of amylase if pancreatic ducts are involved; abdominal guarding, rigidity, and rebound tenderness suggest peritoneal involvement

   b. Diagnostic and laboratory testing as outlined for cholelithiasis

4. Therapeutic management

   NCLEX!

   a. Clients are usually kept NPO and are given IV fluids for hydration until the pain subsides

   b. Opioid analgesics are used for pain control

   c. IV antibiotics are administered

   d. Surgical intervention is postponed until the acute infectious process has subsided

5. Priority nursing diagnoses are the same as those outlined for cholilithiasis

6. Planning and implementation: see section for cholelithiasis

7. Medication therapy includes opioid analgesics for pain control and IV antibiotics

8. Client teaching

   a. Clients will require preoperative teaching as discussed in section 3 below

   b. Some clients will be discharged to home and return after a period of convalescence for elective cholecystectomy

9. Evaluation

   a. Client experiences no pain

   b. Client is afebrile and has no signs of infection

   c. Client verbalizes understanding of disease process and surgical intervention

C. Surgical intervention for disorders of the gallbladder

1. Types of surgical intervention

   a. Laproscopic cholecystectomy: removal of the gallbladder through a small abdominal incision guided by a fiberoptic endoscope

      b. Cholecystectomy: surgical removal of the gallbladder through an abdominal incision in the RUQ

      c. Cholecystectomy with T-tube placement: gallbladder is removed and a T-tube is placed within the common bile duct to facilitate bile flow through edematous ducts postprocedure

    2. Postoperative nursing care

      a. Prevent infection: administer IV antibiotics as ordered, keep incision clean and dry; perform abdominal assessment for peritonitis q 4 hr; monitor vital signs, report any temperature > 100°F

      b. Prevent pain: administer pain medication as ordered; instruct client to request pain medication before pain becomes too intense; medicate for pain prior to postop exercise/ambulation; keep client comfortable to promote deep-breathing, turning, and coughing

NCLEX!

      c. Prevent pulmonary infection: keep client comfortable to promote q 2 hr turning, coughing, deep-breathing; reinforce the importance of incentive spirometry q 1 hr postoperatively

NCLEX!

      d. Maintain clients who have had T-tube placement in a Fowler's position to promote gravity drainage of bile

        1) Keep the collection container below the level of the incision

        2) Assess bile drainage and record amount

        3) Assess the skin for inflammation secondary to bile leakage

        4) Instruct client about proper handling of the tube for turning and ambulating

        5) Report bile drainage in excess of 500 mL after 3 days to surgeon

        6) Instruct client that T-tube is removed when bile drainage has subsided and stools have returned to a normal brown color

Practice to Pass

The client has just returned from surgery following a cholecystectomy. What should be included in the postoperative care?

      e. Maintain NPO status as ordered; advance diet as tolerated

      f. Monitor bowel sounds and encourage ambulation to promote peristalsis

      g. Prevent deep vein thrombosis with leg exercises and frequent ambulation; assess Homan's sign with vital signs

      h. Provide general postoperative instruction prior to discharge regarding wound care, analgesia, diet, and signs of infection

IV. Disorders of the Hepatobiliary System: Pancreas

  A. Acute pancreatitis

NCLEX!

    1. Description

      a. Occurs when there is obstruction to flow of pancreatic enzymes resulting in inflammation of the pancreas

      b. Can be mild, severe, or fulminant

      c. The inflammatory process can be associated with alcoholism, obstructive biliary disease, peptic ulcer disease (PUO), medications (thiazide diuretics, NSAIDs, estrogens, steroids, salicylates) or hyperlipidemia

      d. Alcohol abuse and gallbladder disease constitute 80 percent of acute pancreatitis cases in the United States

  2. Etiology and pathophysiology

      a. Exact pathophysiologic mechanism is unknown; most likely it is the result of a combination of factors

      b. Injury to the pancreas or obstruction of the pancreatic duct results in leakage of the pancreatic enzymes into the pancreatic tissue, leading to autodigestion of pancreatic tissue and acute pancreatitis

      c. Pain is caused by edema and stretching of pancreatic capsule and chemical irritation; pain may be referred to the back because of the retroperitoneal location of gland

      d. Obstructing cholelithiasis causing reflux of bile into the pancreas can also precipitate acute pancreatitis

      e. Enzymes break down pancreatic tissue causing inflammation, edema, damage to vasculature, hemorrhage, and necrosis of pancreatic tissue

      f. Leakage of these enzymes into the bloodstream can cause further systemic complications, which can result in death

      g. Excess hydrochloric acid secretion from chronic alcohol ingestion causes spasms of the sphincter of Oddi and ampulla of Vater, which can also obstruct flow of pancreatic enzymes

      h. Fatty necrosis is normally present with fulminant disease and involves the pancreas as well as the thoracic and abdominal cavities

      i. Necrotic tissue can form walled off abscesses and systemic complications

      j. Acute interstitial pancreatitis: diffuse inflammation and edema of the pancreas is present but the pancreas maintains anatomical features; there is no necrosis or hemorrhage within the gland; it is less severe than hemorrhagic

      k. Acute hemorrhagic pancreatitis: a more severe form of interstitial pancreatitis with inflammation, hemorrhage, and necrosis of pancreatic tissue

      l. Biliary pancreatitis: more common in females 55 to 65 years of age caused by transient obstruction of the ampulla of Vatter by a gallstone or biliary sludge

      m. Alcoholic pancreatitis; more common in younger males, cause is not understood but is most likely toxic in nature

  3. Assessment

      a. Clinical manifestations vary with severity of attack

        1) Acute epigastric pain, steady and severe, can occur in the umbilical area and radiate into the back; it may be temporally associated with ingestion of alcohol or a fatty meal

        2) Pain is greater when lying supine and improves with sitting up and leaning forward, flexion of the knee, or fetal positioning

        3) Nausea and vomiting is common and is worse with any oral intake and does not relieve abdominal pain

NCLEX!

4) Vital signs: fever (rarely above 102ºC), hypotension, and tachycardia

5) Leukocytosis, hyperglycemia, and elevated amylase and lipase

6) Abdominal tenderness, rigidity, progressive distention, and decreased bowel sounds

7) Fulminant disease can progress to hypovolemic shock, ascites, jaundice, and renal failure

8) Grey Turner's sign is a bluish discoloration over the flank area and represents accumulation of blood in that area

9) Cullen's sign is a bluish discoloration around the umbilicus

b. Diagnostic and laboratory test findings

1) Amylase levels increase early and may return to normal levels within 48 hours

2) Lipase levels increase with pancreatitis and psuedocyst, and persist for 5 to 7 days

3) Urine amylase increases in acute pancreatitis

4) Leukocytosis

5) Hyperglycemia, as high as 500 to 900 mg/dL

6) Hypocalcemia if calcium is sequestered by fat necrosis in the abdomen, sign of severe pancreatitis

7) Elevated C reactive protein indicates severity of disease

8) Alcohol abusers may have hypomagnesemia and hypoalbuminemia

9) Pancreatitis with liver involvement; elevated bilirubin and LFTs

10) Abdominal x-ray: identifies ascites, gallstones

11) Abdominal ultrasound to identify gallstones, pancreatic mass, or pseudocyst

12) CT scan: gold standard to visualize size of pancreas, and to identify fluid collections, abscesses, masses, and areas of hemorrhage or necrosis

13) Chest x-ray identifies pleural effusion resulting from enzymatic irritation from leaking pancreatic fluid

NCLEX!

4. Therapeutic management: treatment is aimed at supportive care, preventing further autodigestion of pancreatic tissue, and preventing systemic complications

a. Nothing by mouth (NPO) status with nasogastric tube if ileus or protracted vomiting

b. IV hydration to prevent hypotension and shock

c. Total parenteral nutrition (TPN) if needed for prolonged episodes; reverses catabolic state

d. Possible peritoneal lavage to remove toxic exudates from the abdominal cavity

e. ERCP to remove retained/obstructing gallstones or perform a sphincterotomy

f. Surgical removal of gallbladder for gallstones after acute pancreatitis is resolved

g. Surgical removal/drainage of pseudocyst or abscess may be necessary for recovery

5. Priority nursing diagnoses: Acute pain related to pancreatic edema, stretching, and chemical irritation; Imbalanced nutrition: less than body requirements related to poor oral intake and malabsorption; Risk for fluid imbalance; Risk for infection related to adverse effects of malnutrition

6. Planning and implementation

a. Administer pain medications as ordered and on regular schedule

b. Keep NPO with nasogastric suction to decrease gastric secretions that stimulate pancreatic secretions

c. Monitor lab results for increase leukocytosis, signs of increased catabolism, malnutrition

NCLEX!

d. Monitor vital signs, daily weights, hourly urine outputs, bowel sounds, and stool chart (frequency, color, odor, and consistency)

e. Assess respiratory function; provide pulmonary hygiene measures to prevent pneumonia

f. Educate client regarding disease process and therapeutic procedures

g. Provide diet instruction when oral feeding is resumed (usually when amylase level returns to normal and abdominal pain subsides)

h. Maintain bedrest during acute phase and increase as tolerated

7. Medication therapy

NCLEX!

a. Meperidine (Demerol) for pain; causes less spasm of sphincter of Oddi than morphine

b. Antiemetics

c. Gastric protection with IV H_2 blocker: cimetidine (Tagamet) or ranitidine (Zantac)

d. Antispasmodics such as dicyclomine (Bentyl)

e. Electrolyte replenishment as indicated by laboratory tests

f. Insulin as required to regulate serum glucose levels

g. Antibiotics as ordered for infection

NCLEX!

h. Some clients with chronic pancreatic involvement may require long-term treatment with the pancreatic enzyme replacement pancrelipase (Lipancreatin)

8. Client education

a. Instruction regarding the disease process and expected outcomes

b. Nutrition; explain necessity for NPO status during the acute phase and once oral feeding resumes, provide several small meals with no alcohol allowed

    c. Importance of taking enzyme replacement to prevent malnutrition and weight loss

  9. Evaluation

    a. Client verbalizes understanding of disease process and necessary steps to prevent future attacks

    b. Follows dietary restrictions in accordance with etiologic factors, no alcohol and low cholesterol

B. Cancer of the pancreas

  1. Description: most involve cancer of the ductal epithelium and are adenocarcinomas; comprises 3 to 4 percent of all cancers and can occur at any age but most often after age 50

  2. Etiology and pathophysiology

    a. Is associated with cigarette smoking and in women with long history of diabetes

    b. Other risk factors include exposure to industrial chemicals, environmental toxins, high-fat diet, and pancreatitis

    c. Incidence is 30 percent higher in men than in women, 65 percent greater in African Americans than Caucasians

    d. Is usually located in the head of the pancreas, deep within the tissue, often causing obstruction of the common duct

    e. Metastasis almost always occurs prior to symptoms with invasion of the tumor into the posterior wall of the stomach, the duodenal wall, colon, and common bile duct

  3. Assessment

    a. Clinical manifestations

      1) Slow onset with anorexia, nausea, weight loss, flatulence, and dull epigastric pain

      2) Later pain is severe, is worse when lying down, and is unrelated to meals

      3) Jaundice, pruritis, clay-colored stools, and dark urine when there is involvement of bile ducts

      4) Some clients may have a palpable abdominal mass or ascites

      5) Diarrhea and steatorrhea late in disease

      6) Diabetes

    b. Diagnostic and laboratory test findings

      1) See those listed for pancreatitis, jaundice, and cholelithiasis

      2) CT scan will reveal a mass and a histological diagnosis can be made via CT-guided needle biopsy

4. Therapeutic management

   a. Most clients do not present for treatment until the cancer is too advanced, and thus treatment is in most cases aimed at supportive or palliative care

   b. Pancreatic cancer is usually fatal within 6 months regardless of treatment

   c. ERCP may be performed to place stents within the ductal system to facilitate bile drainage

   d. Surgical management

      1) Gastrojejunostomy: bypasses the duodenum

      2) Choledochojejunostomy: relieves biliary obstruction

      3) Pancreatoduodenectomy (Whipple's procedure): surgical removal of the head of the pancreas, the entire duodenum, the distal third of the stomach, a portion of the jejunum, and the lower half of the common bile duct

   e. Chemotherapy and radiation therapy are usually adjuncts to surgical intervention

5. Priority nursing diagnoses: Deficient knowledge related to disease process and treatment options; Imbalanced nutrition: less than body requirements related to decreased intake and disease process; Acute pain related to disease process; Anxiety and/or fear related to diagnosis; Hopelessness related to diagnosis

6. Planning and implementation

   a. Provide supportive care and education regarding treatment options and assistance with educated decision making

   b. Pain management is integral to quality of life; administer analgesics as ordered and assess effectiveness for appropriate discharge regimen

   c. Provide preoperative teaching should the client opt for surgical intervention

   d. Provide information about support groups in the geographical area

7. Medication therapy

   a. No specific medications for treatment of pancreatic cancers

   b. All medications are aimed at controlling symptoms: pain, nausea, vomiting

   c. Chemotherapy is rarely effective and is used most often for palliative treatment

8. Client education

   a. Instruct about the disease process and poor prognosis

   b. Reinforce the importance of pain control and symptom relief

   c. Reinforce the importance of abstinence from smoking and alcohol

9. Evaluation

   a. Client verbalizes understanding of the potential for developing tolerance and physical dependence to opioid analgesics

NCLEX!

   b. Client has support system in place prior to discharge

   c. Client verbalizes importance of ample rest and proper nutrition

   d. Client is comfortable with decisions regarding treatment choices

   e. Client has adequate control of pain allowing for optimal amount of activity

---

Case Study

S. D., a 60-year-old male, is admitted to the hospital with cirrhosis. He has a history of alcoholism and hepatitis B.

❶ What should the nurse expect to find on his initial laboratory results?

❷ S. D. is scheduled for a liver biopsy. What are the priorities of care for this procedure?

❸ What are the complications of cirrhosis and hepatitis B, and what assessments should the nurse make to determine the presence of complications?

❹ What instructions about diet modifications should the nurse give to S. D.?

❺ If S. D. asks the nurse about the long-term outcome of cirrhosis, what should be included in the response?

For suggested responses, see pages 736–737.

Posttest

1   A client with cirrhosis is admitted to the hospital. Which of the following assessments made by the nurse would indicate the development of portal hypertension?

(1) Hematemesis
(2) Asterixis
(3) Elevated blood pressure
(4) Confusion

2   The nurse should teach the client with liver disease to avoid which of these over-the-counter medications after discharge?

(1) Ranitidine (Zantac)
(2) Psyllium (Metamucil)
(3) Ascorbic acid (Vitamin C)
(4) Acetaminophen (Tylenol)

3   The nurse is doing discharge teaching for a client who has cirrhosis and ascites. Which of the following foods used by the client as snacks should the nurse instruct the client to avoid?

(1) Whole wheat bread
(2) Cookies
(3) Potato chips
(4) Hard candy

4   The client who has liver disease asks the nurse why he bruises so easily. Which of the following information should the nurse include in the response?

(1) "Your liver is unable to make the proteins that are needed to make clotting factors."
(2) "Your liver can no longer metabolize drugs and render them inactive."
(3) "Your liver is breaking down blood cells too rapidly."
(4) "Your liver can't store vitamin C any longer."

5 A client is seen in the clinic for a routine physical examination and the laboratory test results indicate an elevated HBsAg. In order to plan teaching for this client, the nurse interprets this lab result to mean:

(1) The client has immunity to hepatitis B.
(2) The client has active hepatitis B.
(3) The client has resolving hepatitis B.
(4) The client has had the hepatitis B vaccine.

6 The client who has esophageal varices is receiving a vasopressin infusion. Which of these findings would indicate a complication of this therapy?

(1) Chest pain
(2) Tinnitus
(3) Flushed skin
(4) Polyuria

7 The client who has cholelithiasis is scheduled for extracorporeal shock wave lithotripsy. The nurse should tell the client about which of these symptoms that may occur after this procedure?

(1) Colic-type pain
(2) Headache
(3) Diarrhea
(4) Hiccups

8 The client who has acute cholecystitis tells the nurse, "I just want my gallbladder taken out now." Which of the following is the best response by the nurse?

(1) "I don't blame you, but they want your pain under control first."
(2) "Would you like me to ask if your physician will schedule surgery today?"
(3) "The symptoms are distressing, but the surgeon must wait until your gallbladder is less infected."
(4) "They will try to dissolve the stones before they do the surgery."

9 The client is admitted to the hospital with acute pancreatitis. The nurse taking a history should question the client about which of these risks for developing pancreatitis?

(1) Inflammatory bowel disease
(2) Alcoholism
(3) Diabetes mellitus
(4) High-fiber diet

10 The client with chronic pancreatitis is being discharged. The nurse should anticipate teaching the client about which of these medications?

(1) Pancrelipase (Pancrease)
(2) Morphine sulfate
(3) Biotin
(4) Lactulose (Cephulac)

See pages 297–298 for Answers and Rationales.

Answers and Rationales

Pretest

1 Answer: 1 *Rationale:* The liver produces between 700 and 1,000 mL of bile a day. The gallbladder stores and concentrates bile and then releases it when stimulated, but is not an essential structure.
Cognitive Level: Application
Nursing Process: Analysis; *Test Plan:* PHYS

2 Answer: 3 *Rationale:* Hyperbilirubinemia (total serum bilirubin greater than 2.5 mg/dL) manifests in jaundice, a yellow discoloration of the body tissues. Ascites (option 1) may accompany liver disease in later stages, but there is no evidence in the question to indicate this. Options 2 and 4 are unrelated to the question as stated.
Cognitive Level: Application
Nursing Process: Assessment; *Test Plan:* PHYS

3 Answer: 2 *Rationale:* Clay-colored stools indicate that no bile is reaching the intestine and suggests obstructive jaundice. Options 1 and 3 are unrelated to the question. Option 4 could be present due to cardiovascular disease or as an indirect consequence of portal hypertension with impaired venous return, but

there is insufficient information in the question to support this option.
Cognitive Level: Application
Nursing Process: Assessment; *Test Plan:* PHYS

4 **Answer: 3** *Rationale:* Jaundice frequently causes pruritis. Comfort measures include keeping the air temperature cool (68° to 70°F) and the humidity at 30 to 40 percent. Tepid baths (not hot) with colloidal agents decrease itching (option 2). Use of an emollient lotion is also helpful, but anything drying should be avoided (option 4). Hot beverages (option 1) are of no benefit as a comfort measure for pruritus due to jaundice.
Cognitive Level: Application
Nursing Process: Implementation; *Test Plan:* PHYS

5 **Answer: 2** *Rationale:* The incubation period for hepatitis A is 4 to 6 weeks in length with viral shedding highest 10 to 14 days before the onset of symptoms and during the first week of symptoms. The other options do not fall within this time frame.
Cognitive Level: Application
Nursing Process: Implementation; *Test Plan:* SECE

6 **Answer: 1** *Rationale:* The liver is responsible for the production of albumin, which in turn is responsible for maintaining colloidal osmotic pressure. With less production of albumin, osmotic pressure decreases and edema develops. Options 2, 3, and 4 are false statements that do not explain the relationship between cirrhosis and edema.
Cognitive Level: Application
Nursing Process: Implementation; *Test Plan:* PHYS

7 **Answer: 1** *Rationale:* Complications of liver biopsy include hemorrhage or accidental penetration of biliary canniculi. The nurse should assess for signs of hemorrhage (increased pulse, decreased blood pressure) every 30 minutes for the first few hours and then hourly for 24 hours. The client should be monitored for fever every 4 hours and remain on bedrest for 24 hours.
Cognitive Level: Application
Nursing Process: Implementation; *Test Plan:* SECE

8 **Answer: 2** *Rationale:* Lactulose (Cephulac) is a disaccharide laxative used to decrease the absorption of ammonia in the intestines, thereby lowering the serum ammonia and resulting in improvement in hepatic encephalopathy.
Cognitive Level: Application
Nursing Process: Evaluation; *Test Plan:* PHYS

9 **Answer: 4** *Rationale:* Factors that increase the risk of gallstone formation include female gender, aging, use of oral contraceptives, pregnancy, rapid weight loss, high cholesterol level, and diseases of the ileum.
Cognitive Level: Application
Nursing Process: Assessment; *Test Plan:* PHYS

10 **Answer: 1** *Rationale:* Pancrelipase (Lipancreatin) aids in the digestion of starches and fats and should be taken with meals. It should not be crushed since hydrochloric acid destroys the drug, and it should not be mixed with alkaline foods (milk, ice cream).
Cognitive Level: Application
Nursing Process: Implementation; *Test Plan:* PHYS

Posttest

1 **Answer: 1** *Rationale:* In cirrhosis, the liver becomes fibrotic, which obstructs the venous blood flow through the liver. This increases the vascular pressure in the portal system, and causes congestion in the spleen and development of varicosities in the esophagus. Bleeding esophageal varices are a complication of portal hypertension and result in vomiting of blood and possible hemorrhage and death.
Cognitive Level: Application
Nursing Process: Assessment, *Test Plan:* PHYS

2 **Answer: 4** *Rationale:* Any medication that is metabolized by the liver should be avoided, such as acetaminophen, sedatives, and barbiturates. Ranitidine is a histamine$_2$ receptor antagonist, psyllium is a laxative, and ascorbic acid is vitamin C.
Cognitive Level: Application
Nursing Process: Implementation; *Test Plan:* PHYS

3 **Answer: 3** *Rationale:* A low-sodium diet is recommended for clients that have cirrhosis and ascites. Potato chips are high in sodium. Cookies and hard candy are high in sugar, while bread is high in complex carbohydrates.
Cognitive Level: Application
Nursing Process: Implementation; *Test Plan:* PHYS

4 **Answer: 1** *Rationale:* The liver synthesizes clotting factors I, II, VII, IX, and X as well as prothrombin and fibrinogen. These substances are needed for adequate clotting, so their reduction leads to increased risk of bleeding. The other responses do not address this concern.
Cognitive Level: Application
Nursing Process: Implementation; *Test Plan:* PHYS

5 **Answer: 2** *Rationale:* HBsAg is hepatitis surface antigen and is usually present before symptoms mani-

fest. It indicates acute disease. The other options are incorrect conclusions regarding this test result.
Cognitive Level: Application
Nursing Process: Analysis; *Test Plan:* PHYS

6 **Answer: 1** *Rationale:* Vasopressin causes vasoconstriction and may precipitate an acute anginal attack or myocardial infarction, especially in those with known cardiovascular disease. The other options are unrelated to the question.
Cognitive Level: Application
Nursing Process: Assessment; *Test Plan:* PHYS

7 **Answer: 1** *Rationale:* After the extracorporeal shock wave lithotripsy, the nurse should monitor for biliary colic and nausea. The colicky pain is caused by passage of stone fragments through the biliary tree into the small intestine. Headache, diarrhea, and hiccups are unrelated manifestations.
Cognitive Level: Application
Nursing Process: Implementation; *Test Plan:* PHYS

8 **Answer: 3** *Rationale:* With the advent of laparoscopic surgical technique, the only absolute con-

traindication for surgery is acute infection. The other options do not address this concern.
Cognitive Level: Application
Nursing Process: Implementation; *Test Plan:* PHYS

9 **Answer: 2** *Rationale:* Pancreatitis is associated with alcoholism in men and gallstones in women. The disorders in options 1 and 3 are not associated with increased risk of pancreatitis, while option 4 promotes health.
Cognitive Level: Application
Nursing Process: Assessment; *Test Plan:* PHYS

10 **Answer: 1** *Rationale:* The client with chronic pancreatitis may require pancreatic enzyme supplements such as pancrelipase (Lipancreatin). These will promote proper digestion of foods. The other medications do not address this need.
Cognitive Level: Application
Nursing Process: Planning; *Test Plan:* PHYS

References

Brozenec, S. (2003). Assessment of the hepatic system. In W. Phipps, J. Sands, & J. Marek (Eds.), *Medical-surgical nursing: Concepts and clinical practice* (7th ed.). St. Louis, MO: Mosby, pp. 1136–1146.

Brozenec, S. (2003). Hepatic problems. In W. Phipps, J. Sands, & J. Marek (Eds.), *Medical-surgical nursing: Concepts and clinical practice* (7th ed.). St. Louis, MO: Mosby, pp. 1147–1185.

Heuther, S. (2002). Structure and function of the digestive system. In K. McCance & S. Heuther (Eds.), *Pathophysiology: The biologic basis for disease in adults and children* (4th ed.). St. Louis, MO: Mosby, pp. 1288–1321.

Heuther, S. (2002). Alterations of digestive function. In K. McCance & S. Heuther (Eds.), *Pathophysiology: The biologic basis for disease in adults and children* (4th ed.). St. Louis, MO: Mosby, pp. 1322–1379.

Johnson, A. (2002). Interventions for clients with liver problems. In D. Ignatavicius & M. Workman, (Eds.), *Medical-surgical nursing: Critical thinking for collaborative care* (3rd ed.). Philadelphia: W. B. Saunders, pp. 1463–1491.

LeMone, P. & Burke, K. (2000). *Medical surgical nursing: Critical thinking in client care.* Upper Saddle River, NJ: Prentice Hall Health, pp. 511–552.

Pagana, K. & Pagana, T. (2001). *Manual of diagnostic and laboratory tests* (5th ed.). St. Louis, MO: Mosby, p. 109.

Sands, J. (2003). Gallbladder and exocrine pancreatic problems. In W. Phipps, J. Sands, & J. Marek (Eds.), *Medical-surgical nursing: Concepts and clinical practice* (7th ed.). St. Louis, MO: Mosby, pp. 1373–1393.

CHAPTER 8

Gastrointestinal Disorders

Debera Jane Thomas, DNS, FNP/ANP, RN-CS

CHAPTER OUTLINE

OBJECTIVES

▮ Identify basic structures and functions of the gastrointesinal system.

▮ Describe the pathophysiology and etiology of common gastrointestinal disorders.

▮ Discuss expected assessment data and diagnostic test findings for selected gastrointestinal disorders.

▮ Identify priority nursing diagnoses for selected gastrointestinal disorders.

▮ Discuss therapeutic management of selected gastrointestinal disorders.

▮ Discuss nursing management of a client experiencing a gastrointestinal disorder.

▮ Identify expected outcomes for a client experiencing a gastrointestinal disorder.

[**Media Link**]

Use the CD-ROM enclosed with this text, or log onto the address given to access the free, interactive Companion Website created for this series. The CD-ROM and Companion Website accompanying this book offer additional practice opportunities and information—NCLEX Review, Case Studies, Glossary, In Depth with NCLEX, and more.

www.prenhall.com/hogan

REVIEW AT A GLANCE

Barrett's epithelium *esophageal epithelial tissue that has undergone change as a result of repeated exposure to gastric juice and is more resistant to erosion, but is premalignant*

body mass index (BMI) *estimates total body fat stores in relation to height and weight*

bulk-forming agents *high-fiber supplements that increase fecal bulk*

chyme *stomach contents—partially digested food mixed with gastric juice*

colostomy *surgical diversion of large intestine fecal contents to an external collection device*

diarrhea *increase in frequency, amount or liquidity of stool that is a change from the individual's normal pattern*

dumping syndrome *complication of gastric resections where there is rapid emptying of stomach contents into the jejunum causing physiologic manifestations*

esophagogastroduodenoscopy (EGD) *direct visualization of esophagus, stomach, and duodenum through a fiberoptic endoscope and used to diagnose disorders of aforementioned structures*

esophagogastric tube *also known as the Sengstaken-Blakemore and Minnesota tube, consisting of a tube with several lumens used to inflate a gastric balloon, esophageal balloon and drain stomach contents*

fistula *abnormal pathway between structures or from an internal organ to an outside surface*

gastroesophageal reflux disease (GERD) *disorder characterized by the backward flow of gastric contents into the lower portion of the esophagus*

gavage *referring to intermittent feeding through a tube in the stomach or jejunum*

hernia *referring to a protrusion of an organ through a weakness in muscle*

ileostomy *surgical diversion of fecal contents at the level of the ileum to an external collection device*

intestinal tube *long tube, 6 to 10 feet in length, used to decompress the intestines*

lavage *irrigation of the stomach using a tube inserted into the stomach*

lower esophageal sphincter (LES) *the sphinchter located at the esophageal gastric junction*

nasogastric tube (NG) *a tube inserted through the nose and into the stomach and used to drain contents or for feeding*

non-steroidal anti-inflammatory drugs (NSAIDs) *medications usually used for analgesia and to reduce inflammation*

Zollinger-Ellison syndrome *disorder in which a pancreatic tumor secretes gastrin, which then stimulates secretion of acid and pepsin*

Pretest

1 Which of the following assessments is essential for the nurse to make when caring for a client who has just had an esophagogastroduodenoscopy (EGD)?

(1) Auscultate bowel sounds
(2) Check gag reflex
(3) Monitor salivary pH
(4) Measure abdominal girth

2 A client has a nasogastric (NG) tube in place for gastric decompression and complains of increasing nausea. Which action should the nurse take first?

(1) Advance the tube 2 cm
(2) Place client in a recumbent position
(3) Instill 20 mL of saline
(4) Obtain abdominal x-ray to assess placement

3 A client with a subtotal gastrectomy is scheduled for discharge. Which of these instructions should the nurse give the client to reduce the possibility of dumping syndrome?

(1) "Be sure to eat foods high in complex carbohydrates."
(2) "It is helpful to take a walk after eating."
(3) "Avoid drinking fluids with your meal."
(4) "Don't lie down for at least 2 hours after eating."

4 A 32-year-old client is admitted to the hospital with a body mass index (BMI) of 25. The nurse interprets this to mean:

(1) The client is undernourished.
(2) The client has an optimal amount of body fat.
(3) The client is 10 percent overweight.
(4) The client is morbidly obese.

5 The nurse teaches the client with gastroesophageal reflux disease (GERD) about ways to minimize symptoms. Which of the following statements made by the client indicates that more teaching is needed?

(1) "I will be sure to drink tea instead of coffee."
(2) "I will take a walk after I eat."
(3) "I will try to eat smaller meals more frequently."
(4) "I will sleep with the head of the bed elevated about 12 inches."

6 The client with a gastric ulcer is admitted to the hospital. The nurse should assess the client for intake of which of these substances that increases the risk of developing a gastric ulcer?

(1) Aspirin
(2) Spicy foods
(3) Acetaminophen (Tylenol)
(4) Coffee

7 The client with gastroesophageal reflux disease (GERD) is prescribed famotidine (Pepcid). In order to provide effective teaching, the nurse must have which of these understandings about the action of the drug?

(1) The drug improves gastric motility.
(2) The drug coats the distal portion of the esophagus.
(3) The drug increases LES tone.
(4) The drug decreases the secretion of gastric acid.

8 The client is admitted to the hospital with ulcerative colitis. The nurse should assess the client for which complication of the disease?

(1) Anemia
(2) Steatorrhea
(3) Cholelithiasis
(4) Thrombocytopenia

9 The nurse is developing a health promotion program for intestinal health. Which of the following pieces of information should the nurse include in the program?

(1) The addition of dietary fiber can reduce the risk of diverticulosis.
(2) A diet high in fat increases the risk of developing Crohn's disease.
(3) Irritable bowel syndrome is caused by a deficiency in soluble fiber.
(4) Laxatives can improve motility and bowel health.

10 A client is admitted to the hospital with a bowel obstruction. Which of these findings by the nurse would indicate that the obstruction is in the early stages?

(1) High-pitched tinkling bowel sounds
(2) Low rumbling bowel sounds
(3) No bowel sounds auscultated
(4) Normal bowel sounds heard in all four quadrants

See pages 332–333 for Answers and Rationales.

I. Overview of Anatomy and Physiology

A. Oral cavity/pharynx

1. Mouth, also referred to as oral or buccal cavity

    a. Lined with mucous membranes

    b. Bordered by lips, cheeks, hard and soft palate, and tongue

        1) Lips and cheeks: keep food in the mouth during chewing

        2) Hard palate: hard surface at the roof of the mouth against which the tongue pushes food during chewing and swallowing

        3) Soft palate: distal to the hard palate and rises during swallowing (reflex) to close the oropharynx

        4) Tongue: mostly skeletal muscle and contains mucous and serous glands, papillae and taste buds; mixes food and saliva to form bolus and initiates swallowing

    c. Salivary glands: drain into mouth; secrete saliva to moisten food and provide amylase to initially break down carbohydrates

    d. Teeth: 32 permanent in adults; tear and grind food into smaller pieces providing more surface area for the action of saliva

2. Pharynx: composed of oropharynx and laryngopharynx

    a. Passageway for food, fluids, and air; moves food into esophagus by peristalsis

    b. Lined with mucous membranes and mucous-secreting glands to ease the passage of food

B. Esophagus: muscular tube 10 in. (25 cm) extending from pharynx to stomach

    1. Lined with squamous epithelium except where it joins stomach where it is lined with columnar epithelium

    2. Enters stomach through cardiac orifice that is surrounded by the gastroesophageal sphincter (also called lower esophageal sphincter or LES), which keeps orifice closed when no food is swallowed; keeps gastric contents (acid) out of esophagus

C. Stomach: distensible food reservoir located high on left side of abdomen; can hold as much as 4 L of food and fluid; empty it is about 10 in (25 cm) in size; continues mechanical breakdown of food and mixes food with gastric juice forming a mixture called **chyme**

    1. Divided into four regions (see Figure 8-1)

        a. Cardiac region; surrounds the cardiac orifice

        b. Fundus; upper portion (high concentration of gastric glands)

        c. Body; includes the greater and lesser curvatures (high concentration of gastric glands)

        d. Pyloric region; surrounds the pyloric sphincter

Figure 8-1

Regions of the stomach.

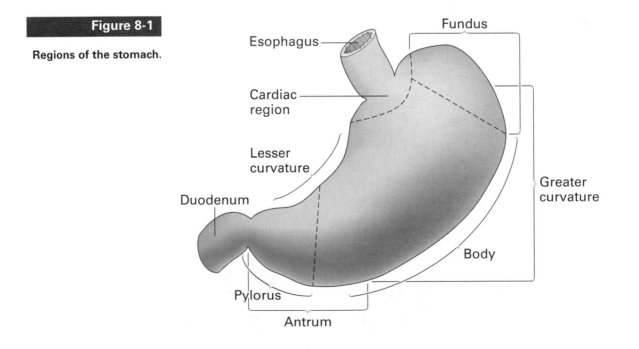

2. Lined with columnar epithelial cells that contain secretory cells

   a. Mucous cells: secrete alkaline mucus to protect stomach lining from acidic gastric juice

   b. Zymogenic cells: produce pepsinogen, a precursor to pepsin, which digests proteins

   c. Parietal cells: produce hydrochloric acid and intrinsic factor

      1) Hydrochloric acid: converts pepsinogen to pepsin for protein digestion and acts as a bactericidal agent

      2) Intrinsic factor: needed for absorption of vitamin B_{12} in small intestine

   d. Enteroendocrine cells: secrete the hormones gastrin, histamine, endorphins, serotonin, and somatostatin

3. Gastric secretion is under neural (sympathetic, parasympathetic) and hormonal control and is divided into three phases

   a. Cephalic phase: preparation for digestion; stimulated by sight, odor, taste, or thought of food

   b. Gastric phase: starts when food enters stomach and is initiated by stimulation of gastric stretch receptors and chemically by partially digested proteins; gastrin is secreted and stimulates production of more gastric juice

   c. Intestinal phase: initiated when chyme enters the small intestine

4. Mechanical churning of gastric contents via peristalsis aids digestion and is influenced by gastric distention and gastrin; normal gastric emptying takes 4 to 6 hours

D. **Small intestine:** begins at the pyloric sphincter and ends at the ileocecal valve; is about 20 ft (6 m) long and 1 in (2.5 cm) in diameter

   1. Divided into three regions

      a. Duodenum: begins at the pyloric sphincter around the head of the pancreas; pancreatic enzymes (trypsin, chymotrypsin, lipase, and amylase) and bile enter in response to secretin and cholecystokinin (produced by intestinal mucosa cells in response to presence of chyme)

      b. Jejunum: middle section

      c. Ileum: terminal section

   2. Digestion is completed and most absorption occurs in small intestine through microvilli, villi, and circular folds that increase the absorptive surface area

E. **Large intestine:** also known as colon; is 5 ft (1.5 m) long and extends from ileocecal valve to the anus

   1. Divided into five areas

      a. Cecum

      b. Appendix: small outpouching attached to cecum where bacteria accumulate and may cause inflammation

      c. Colon: ascending, transverse, and descending segments

      d. Rectum: mucosa-lined reservoir for feces; 12 cm in length

      e. Anus: terminal end of digestive tract with internal and external sphincters that control defecation through the defecation reflex (spinal cord reflex)

    2. Major function is to absorb water, salts, and vitamins formed by bacteria in large intestine and eliminate undigestible food and residue from the body

F. Digestion: the breakdown of food to molecules that can be absorbed and used by the cells of the body

    1. Begins in mouth by the action of chewing and the addition of salivary amylase from salivary glands, which initiates carbohydrate digestion

    2. Continues in the stomach where food is mixed by the muscular action of the stomach and gastric juice is added; gastric juice contains acid, enzymes, hormones, intrinsic factor, and mucus

      a. Hydrochloric acid is secreted by the parietal cells in the gastric mucosa; acts to dissolve food fibers

      b. Pepsinogen, enzyme precursor to pepsin, is secreted by the zymogenic (chief) cells; converted to pepsin in an acid environment; breaks down protein

      c. Hormones: gastrin to stimulate secretion of HCl and pepsinogen

      d. Intrinsic factor: necessary for absorption of vitamin B_{12}

      e. Mucus: protects gastric mucosa from digestive action of acid and enzymes

    3. Digestion continues in proximal portion of small intestine; pancreatic enzymes, intestinal enzymes, and bile salts are added

      a. Pancreatic enzymes: trypsin, chymotrypsin, and carboxypeptidase break down proteins; pancreatic lipase breaks down fats

      b. Intestinal enzymes: lactase, maltase, and sucrase break down carbohydrates; aminopeptidases and dipeptidase break down proteins

      c. Bile salts: emulsify fats and make them ready for action by pancreatic lipase

    4. Absorption of nutrients takes place in capillaries in the villae of the small intestine; nutrients are then transported to the liver by way of the portal vein

G. Elimination: end process of digestion where food residue, unabsorbed GI secretions, shed epithelial cells, and bacteria are removed from the body

    1. Accomplished by segmental contractions in the colon that propel fecal material toward the rectum

    2. Once in the rectum, the defecation reflex is triggered by stretch receptors in the rectal wall; evacuation is accomplished by the Valsalva maneuver

II. Diagnostic Tests and Measurements

A. Upper GI series: series of x-rays with contrast medium (barium sulfate or Gastrografin)

    1. Lower esophagus, stomach, and duodenum are examined for tumors, ulcerations, inflammation, varices, obstruction, and/or anatomic abnormalities (hiatal **hernia**)

2. After client drinks barium, a series of x-rays document the progression of the contrast as the client is placed in different positions

3. **Gastroesophageal reflux** (reflux from stomach into esophagus) can be assessed during the procedure with the client in a flat or head-down position

4. Contraindications: complete bowel obstruction, esophageal or gastric perforation (may use Gastrografin), or unstable vital signs

5. Possible complications: aspiration of contrast medium, constipation (if barium used), or partial bowel obstruction; if Gastrografin is used there may be significant diarrhea

B. **Lower GI series:** series of x-rays utilizing contrast medium (barium enema)

1. Colon, including the appendix, is visualized for anatomic abnormalities, polyps, ulcers, tumors, Crohn's disease, **fistulas,** and diverticula

2. Barium enema can also stop bleeding from diverticula

3. Contraindications: perforated colon or uncooperative clients

4. Possible complications: colonic perforation or barium impaction

5. Scheduling considerations: should be performed before an upper GI study to prevent residual barium from being in the colon, and colon should also be empty

   a. Clear liquid diet day before test

   b. Magnesium citrate or other bowel prep night before the test

   c. NPO after midnight and continue until test is complete

   d. Cleansing enemas may be ordered before the test

C. **Upper GI endoscopy: esophagogastroduodenoscopy (EGD),** gastroscopy

1. Direct visualization of esophagus, stomach, and duodenum through lighted endoscope; detects mucosal inflammations (gastroesophageal reflux, gastritis), tumors, varices, hiatal hernias, polyps, ulcers, and obstruction

2. Endoscopy can also be used to directly sample tissues and fluids, stop areas of active GI bleeding by injection of sclerosing agents or cautery, and to perform GI surgery using laser beams

3. Contraindications: uncooperative clients, esophageal diverticula, suspected perforation, recent upper GI surgery, and severe upper GI hemorrhage

4. Possible complications: pulmonary aspiration of GI contents; perforation of esophagus, stomach or duodenum; bleeding from biopsy site; and reactions to sedative medication given during the test

5. Special nursing considerations post-procedure: NPO until client is completely alert and swallowing/gag reflexes have returned (2 to 4 hours); general safety precautions because of sedation; monitor for signs of bleeding, dyspnea, or dysphagia

D. **Colonoscopy:** fiberoptic direct visualization of the colon from anus to cecum

1. Detects tumors (benign or malignant), polyps, inflammation, ulcerations, and bleeding; may biopsy any suspicious tissue

2. Contraindications: uncooperative or medically unstable clients, rectal hemorrhage, suspected colon perforation

3. Possible complications: perforation of colon, bleeding from biopsy sites, oversedation

4. Special nursing considerations: requires complete bowel prep; monitor vital signs post-procedure for signs of bleeding and colon perforation

E. **Sigmoidoscopy:** direct visualization of anus, rectum, and sigmoid colon with either a rigid or flexible sigmoidoscope; similar to colonoscopy in procedure, contraindications, complications, and nursing considerations, but is a less extensive study

F. **Ultrasonography:** visualization of abdominal organs through the use of high-frequency sound waves that penetrate the organ and are bounced back to a transducer where the sound waves are converted to an electronic pictorial image

1. Can detect organ size, cyst formation, tumors, and filling defects

2. No contrast medium or radiation is involved so there are no contraindications

3. Possible complications: none

G. **CAT scan:** radiologic procedure (with or without contrast medium) used to diagnose conditions such as tumors, cysts, abscesses, perforation, bleeding inflammation, aneurysms, and obstruction

1. X-rays are passed through the abdominal organs at many angles; because of the differing densities of the organs, the penetration of the x-rays varies, producing the image after digital computation into shades of gray

2. Contraindications: allergy to shellfish or iodinated dye, pregnancy, unstable vital signs, morbid obesity, and claustrophobia

3. Possible complications: allergic reaction to contrast medium (iodinated), and renal failure from contrast

4. Special nursing considerations: clients should be encouraged to drink fluids to promote contrast elimination and monitor client for delayed reaction to contrast medium

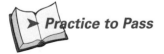

> **Practice to Pass**

A client is scheduled for a CAT scan of the abdomen. What questions should the nurse ask before the test can be done?

H. **Gastric analysis:** stomach contents are aspirated with an NG tube and pH is measured at a basal rate (BAO—basal acid output) and also during a stimulated state (MAO—maximal acid output); or tubeless gastric analysis where a resin dye (Diagnex Blue) is ingested and gastric acid displaces the dye from the resin and the dye is absorbed by the bowel and excreted by the kidneys

1. Used to differentiate causes of hypergastrinemia including **Zollinger-Ellison syndrome** (elevated levels of gastrin from pancreatic tumor), chronic antacid ingestion or atrophic gastritis; direct measurement of gastrin levels is used most often for this purpose

2. Most often used to assess the effect of antiulcer therapy, either surgical or medical

3. Precautions: anyone with heart failure, carcinoid syndrome, or hypertension may have an exacerbation of symptoms with this test since histamine is used to stimulate gastric acid

I. **Stool examination:** fecal specimen is examined for obvious and occult blood, and fat, as well as assayed for clostridial toxin, and cultured for bacterial, viral, and parasitic pathogens

  1. Stool culture: common bacterial pathogens include *Salmonella, Shigella, Campylobacter, Yersinia,* pathogenic *Escherichia coli, Clostridium,* and *Staphylococcus;* parasitic pathogens include *Ascaris* (hookworm), *Strongyloides* (tape worm), and *Giardia* (protozoans)

  NCLEX!

  2. Stool for occult blood: stool is tested with a reagent to detect blood that is not visible; causes of occult blood include: benign and malignant GI tumors, ulcers, inflammatory bowel disease, diverticulosis, and hemorrhoids; see Box 8-1 for substances that cause a false-positive test for blood

  3. Fecal fat: measures the fat content of the stool over a 24-hour period

     a. Conditions causing fat in stool: cystic fibrosis, celiac disease, sprue, Crohn's disease (regional enteritis), Whipple's disease, and maldigestion from pancreato-biliary tree obstruction

     b. Nursing considerations: client should be instructed to eat a diet that contains 100 g of fat per day for 3 days before and during the stool collection

  4. Stool for Clostridial toxin: *Clostridium difficile* bacteria release a toxin that causes necrosis of bowel epithelium; infection occurs in people who are immunocompromised or after taking broad-spectrum antibiotics

---

Box 8-1	
Stool for Occult Blood	**Common Substances Causing False-Positive Results**
	• Red meat
	• Fish
	• Oral iron supplements
	• Iodine
	• Boric acid
	• Colchicine
	• Drugs irritating to gastric mucosa
	Aspirin
	NSAIDs
	Corticosteroids
	Common Substances Causing False-Negative Results
	• Vitamin C
	• Turnips
	• Horseradish
	• Beets
	• Melons

III. Common Nursing Techniques and Procedures

A. Nasogastric (NG) tube: pliable plastic tube inserted through the nose and advanced to the stomach

1. Types of tubes include: double lumen gastric sump tube (most common), single lumen tube, nasogastric feeding tubes

   a. Gastric sump tube: two-lumen tube in various sizes (14 to 18 Fr) and 120 cm (48 in) long; the large lumen is used for suction and drainage of stomach contents while the small lumen (blue vent) acts as an air vent preventing the tube from being sucked up against the gastric mucosa when attached to a suction device; this tube can also be used for short-term gastric feeding and medication administration

   b. Single lumen gastric tube: larger lumen tube used to quickly drain stomach contents in cases of poisoning

   c. Feeding tubes: smaller diameter tubes (6 to 12 Fr) that often have a weighted tip and are placed using a stylet

2. Purpose: NG tubes are used for gastric decompression (drainage), gastric **lavage** (gastric irrigation), or gastric feeding (**gavage**)

3. Nursing interventions

   a. Insertion

   1) In order to assure proper placement, measure the tube from the tip of the nose to the ear and then to the xyphoid process; place adhesive tape at this measurement (approximate length of the esophagus from nose to stomach)

   2) Insert the tube in the nares with client in a high-Fowler's position and with the head forward (chin toward chest)

   3) Once the tube is in the posterior pharynx, ask the client to sip water through a straw to facilitate passage into the esophagus (rather than trachea) if able

   b. Check placement

   1) The placement of the tube is checked immediately after insertion and each time before placing anything into the tube

   2) Most accurately done by checking the pH of aspirated secretions (should be < 5.0); small bore tubes may collapse with aspiration, making this method unusable

   3) Still commonly done by using a syringe to instill 10 to 20 mL of air into the tube while auscultating with a stethoscope for a "burp" in the LUQ; initial placement should be verified by x-ray

   c. Suction should be maintained when the NG tube is used for gastric decompression and should be assessed every 1 to 4 hours

   d. Tube patency: should be assessed every 4 hours or according to agency policy; thick secretions and/or particles may obstruct the holes in the tube and drainage ceases; the tube can be irrigated with 20 mL of saline or water in small amounts to keep the tube clear

   e. Oral and nasal care is important since the presence of the tube is irritating to the mucosa

NCLEX!

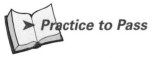

Practice to Pass

The client is to have an NG tube inserted. How should the nurse explain the procedure to the client?

B. Enteral feedings

1. Types

   a. Feeding can be given through an NG tube continuously or intermittently; can be given through a gastrostomy tube either continuously or intermittently; can be given through a jejunostomy tube or nasojejunal tube continuously but is controlled by an enteral feeding pump

   b. Numerous formulas are commercially available and vary in the proportions of nutrients, calories, and osmolarity; the physician usually orders the formula and the rate of administration

2. Purpose: enteral feedings bypass the mouth to deliver a balance of nutrients directly to the GI system; they are given to people who are unable to eat on their own for a variety of reasons (including coma, oropharyngeal surgery/cancer, anatomical abnormalities, inability to swallow, esophageal obstruction) and to clients who are able to eat but cannot ingest an adequate number of calories

3. Nursing interventions

   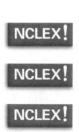

   a. Assess proper placement of the feeding tube before beginning enteral feedings

   b. Place the client in high-Fowler's position if the client can tolerate it to decrease the risk of aspiration

   c. Feeding formula should be at room temperature to prevent abdominal cramping, but must not be left at room temperature (continuous feeding) for more than 8 to 12 hours (or less according to product directions) to limit bacterial growth; equipment should be changed every 24 hours

   d. If the feeding is intermittent, clamp the feeding tube before the gavage bag or syringe is attached to prevent air from entering the stomach

   e. Give the intermittent feeding slowly (over 10 to 15 min) to prevent nausea, vomiting, flatus, and abdominal cramps

   f. When an intermittent feeding is finished, clamp the tube and flush with water to prevent blockage

   g. Recheck placement and residual every 4 hours (or according to agency policy) when giving continuous feedings

   h. Ensure that the head of bed remains elevated to at least 30 degrees at all times while continuous NG tube feedings are given

C. Intestinal tubes: long pliable tubes capable of advancing the length of the GI tract; double or single lumen; can be inserted nasally or orally

1. Types

   a. The single lumen tubes are the Harris tube (6 ft long) and Cantor tube (10 ft long); each is weighted with a mercury bag attached to the tip and assists movement of the tube through the GI tract

   b. The double lumen tube is the Miller-Abbot tube (10 ft long) with one lumen used to inflate the balloon at the end with mercury, and the second lumen decompresses the intestines

2. Purpose: to drain or decompress the intestine when a bowel obstruction is diagnosed

3. Nursing interventions

NCLEX!

NCLEX!

   a. Are inserted by a physician in the same way as NG tubes are; do not tape to the nose to allow the tube to advance further by gravity

   b. Place the client on his or her right side for a few hours to facilitate passage of the tube into the duodenum

   c. After the tube reaches the small intestine, encourage the client to ambulate, move in bed and change position, which encourages peristalsis and further movement of the tube

   d. A drainage device and/or suction can be used to aid in bowel decompression

   e. X-rays are used to verify the position of the tube

D. **Esophageal and gastric tubes (esophagogastric):** tubes with multiple lumens and two balloons; a large esophageal balloon to provide tamponade to bleeding in the esophagus and a smaller gastric balloon that provides tamponade to the cardiac region and distal esophagus (see Figure 8-2)

   1. Types

      a. Sengstaken-Blakemore tube: triple lumen tube; esophageal balloon lumen, gastric balloon lumen, and a distal lumen to the tip that drains stomach contents

      b. Minnesota tube: similar to Sengstaken-Blakemore tube but has four lumens; the additional lumen opens proximal to the esophageal balloon and is used to drain esophageal secretions

   2. Purpose: classic method to treat bleeding esophageal varices by applying direct pressure (tamponade) through the use of inflated balloons

Figure 8-2

Sengstaken-Blakemore tube.

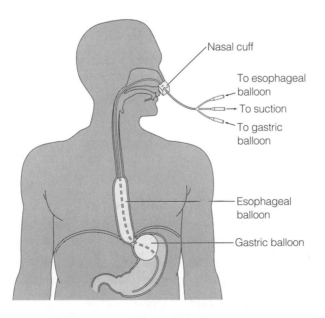

Nasal cuff

To esophageal balloon

To suction

To gastric balloon

Esophageal balloon

Gastric balloon

3. Nursing interventions

   a. Maintain pressure of the esophageal balloon between 20 to 25 mmHg and monitor for loss of pressure or overinflation, which can cause rupture of the esophagus

   b. Apply traction to the tube so the gastric balloon is tight against the lower esophageal (cardiac) sphincter to keep the tube in place

   c. Monitor the client for sudden respiratory distress caused by upward displacement of the esophageal balloon; if respiratory distress occurs, the nurse should cut the tube to deflate both balloons and remove the tube; keep scissors at the bedside for prn emergency use

E. **Gastric lavage:** irrigation of the stomach

   1. Purpose: remove toxic substances from the stomach or slow bleeding

      a. Lavage is performed in cases of accidental poisoning and drug overdose; a large diameter tube is used for rapid removal of stomach contents and irrigation is done to dilute toxins

      b. Lavage (with cool saline or sometimes with iced saline) and aspiration are performed in cases of upper GI bleeding to remove blood and slow the bleeding; use of iced saline poses risk of ischemia to hypothermic tissue and is controversial

   2. Nursing interventions

      a. Assess placement of the gastric tube before any fluid is instilled into the stomach

      b. Strictly measure the fluid instilled and removed to assess the quantity of bleeding

      c. In cases of poisoning, the fluid removed from the stomach may be sent to the laboratory for examination

IV. **Nursing Management of the Client Having Gastrointestinal Surgery**

   A. **Colostomy:** fecal diversion to an external collection device; named for the portion of the colon from which they are formed: ascending colostomy, transverse colostomy, descending colostomy, or sigmoid colostomy

      1. Preoperative period

         a. Provide preoperative teaching about the procedure and what to expect in the postoperative period, including pain relief, breathing exercises, and the appearance of the stoma; these will reduce client anxiety and promote postoperative participation in care

         b. Carry out bowel preparation orders, which usually include bowel cleansing with cathartics and enemas as well as oral or parenteral antibiotics

         c. Ensure that usual preoperative activities are completed: consent for procedure is signed; preanesthetic medications are given as prescribed

      2. Postoperative period

         a. Routine care for surgical client: monitor vital signs and bowel sounds; assess intake and output including wound drainage and drainage from tubes (NG, urinary drainage, etc.); evaluate incision(s), and perianal area; assess

NCLEX!

Practice to Pass

The client returns from the operating room following a colostomy. What should the nurse include in the initial assessment?

level of consciousness and encourage deep breathing, use of incentive spirometer, and splinting of incision

b. Assess appearance and drainage from stoma, identify any changes and notifying the surgeon if stoma becomes pale or cyanotic or bleeding increases

c. Monitor pain control and take appropriate actions if pain is not controlled (check patency of IV access, notify physician, provide comfort measures)

d. Encourage ambulation as ordered to stimulate peristalsis

e. Resume oral intake as ordered and monitor for nausea, abdominal distention, and adequacy of bowel sounds

f. Begin discharge teaching: possible postoperative complications and preventative measures (infection, bowel obstruction, abdominal abscess); colostomy care (irrigation depending on location of the stoma, pouch management, skin care)

B. Ileostomy: large intestine is completely removed and fecal diversion is created at the level of the ileum

   1. Preoperative period

   a. Allow client to verbalize fears and concerns regarding surgery and lifestyle changes that will result and provide appropriate referrals and support (United Ostomy Association, enterostomal therapy nurse referral as examples)

   b. Administer bowel preparation as prescribed (cathartics, enemas, and antibiotics)

   c. Document that all preoperative activities are completed

   2. Postoperative period

   a. Assess vital signs, stoma color and drainage, incision, intake and output, pain control, and signs of infection

   b. Apply ostomy appliance (pouch) over the stoma and teach client and family about the procedure and nature of effluent (initially dark green, more liquid, but will thicken over time and become yellow-brown)

NCLEX!

   c. Protect skin around stoma with a skin barrier from the irritating effects of effluent which contains digestive enzymes and bile salts

   d. Begin educating the client and family as soon as possible teaching them how to manage the stoma, appliance, and skin care, and when to report any abnormalities in the stoma, effluent, or abdomen

NCLEX!

   e. Emphasize the importance of good nutrition and the need for adequate fluid and electrolyte intake and the signs and symptoms of an imbalance

C. Gastrectomy: removal of the stomach with anastomosis of the esophagus to the jejunum (esophagojejunostomy); rarely performed, usually only for extensive gastric cancer or Zollinger-Ellison syndrome unresponsive to medical treatment

   1. Preoperative period

   a. Clarify procedure with the client and family so they understand the risks and benefits and obtain a signed consent form as per individual hospital policy

b. Prepare the client and family about what to expect postoperatively, including pain relief, breathing exercises, expected tubes (NG, drains, jejunostomy feeding tube), and ambulation

2. Postoperative period

a. Assess vital signs, lung and bowel sounds, intake and output including drainage from nasogastric tube, wound drainage (amount and character), effectiveness of pain control measures

NCLEX!

b. The nasogastric tube should not be repositioned, irrigated, or checked for placement because of the risk of disrupting the esophagojejunostomy sutures (depending on surgeon's orders)

c. Implement standard postoperative care (pain management, progressive activity to ambulation)

NCLEX!

d. Discuss limitations in oral intake and alternative methods to maintain nutrition; may require jejunostomy tube with an elemental (requires no digestion) enteral feeding

e. Teach the client about postoperative complications, including pernicious anemia, abdominal abscess or infection, and decreased nutrition

D. **Gastric resection:** portion of the stomach removed for diseases such as cancer and peptic ulcer disease refractory to medical management; in this case, the antrum, which contains most of the gastrin-producing cells, is removed

1. Preoperative period

a. Insert NG tube if ordered and connect to suction (may be inserted in operating room)

b. Provide standard preoperative interventions as mentioned previously for any client undergoing abdominal surgery

2. Postoperative period

a. Assess vital signs, lung and bowel sounds, intake and output including drainage from NG tube, wound drainage (amount and character), effectiveness of pain control measures

NCLEX!

b. The nasogastric tube should *not* be repositioned, irrigated, or checked for placement (unless the physician orders specifically indicate to do so) because of the risk of disrupting the sutures inside the stomach

c. Encourage ambulation to promote peristalsis and prevent postoperative complications such as paralytic ileus and obstruction

d. Implement standard postoperative care for clients with abdominal surgery (see above)

e. Be alert for development of acute gastric dilation as a postoperative complication; signs and symptoms include epigastric pain, fullness, hiccups, tachycardia, and hypotension; this complication results from a malfunctioning NG tube and rapidly improve after flushing the tube (physician order) or placement of a new one

3. **Dumping syndrome** is a common complication of gastric resection when the pylorus is bypassed and is a postprandial problem of rapid dumping of food into the jejunum without proper mixing and duodenal digestion

   a. Early manifestations: occur 15 to 30 minutes after eating and include vertigo, tachycardia, syncope, sweating, pallor, and palpitations; believed to be caused by a rapid shift of extracellular fluid into the bowel to dilute the hypertonic chyme thereby causing a decrease in blood volume

   b. Late manifestations occur 2 to 3 hours postprandial and include epigastric fullness, distention, diarrhea, abdominal cramping, nausea and high-pitched bowel sounds; these symptoms are caused by excessive release of insulin in response to a rapid rise in blood glucose due to the high-carbohydrate bolus entering the jejunum

   c. Dumping syndrome can be minimized by a low-carbohydrate, high-protein, high-fat diet; suggest also that the client avoid drinking fluids with meals and lie down after eating; antispasmodics or sedatives may be ordered to delay gastric emptying

E. **Billroth I (gastroduodenostomy):** a partial gastrectomy where the distal portion of the stomach (including the antrum) is removed and the remainder is anastomosed to the duodenum (see Figure 8-3); the gastrin-producing cells in the antrum are removed as well as some of the parietal cells (acid-pepsinogen secreting cells)

   1. Preoperative and postoperative care is the same as for any client having gastric surgery

   2. Dumping syndrome is a common complication of this procedure

F. **Billroth II (gastrojejunostomy):** a partial gastrectomy where the lower portion of the stomach is removed and the proximal remnant is anastomosed to the jejunum (see Figure 8-3); used to treat gastric and duodenal ulcers

   1. Preoperative and postoperative care is the same as for any client having gastric surgery

   2. Dumping syndrome is a common complication of this procedure

NCLEX!

Figure 8-3

**Partial gastrectomy.
A. Billroth I; B. Billroth II.**

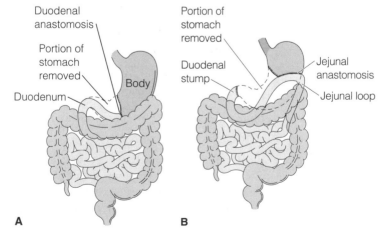

V. Malnutrition

A. Description

1. Insufficient amounts, improper proportions, malabsorbed, or improper distribution of food substances necessary to provide the body with energy for normal body functions such as temperature regulation, cardiac output, respiration, muscle function, protein synthesis, and energy storage

2. Can also result from increased loss of nutrients as in vomiting

B. Etiology and pathophysiology

1. When more energy is expended for body processes than is consumed in food, the body uses stored forms of energy in a certain order: first carbohydrates stored as glycogen are used; then fat stores are consumed; and lastly protein stores in the form of muscle tissue are used

2. Malnutrition can result from a variety of conditions and diseases

   a. Insufficient nutrients: liver failure (liver normally makes blood proteins), starvation, anorexia nervosa/bulimia, severe illness/trauma (increases protein and calorie requirements)

   b. Improper proportions: fad dieting, unavailability of variety of foods, maldigestion of certain foods because of a loss of enzymes, acid, or hormones

   c. Malabsorption: rapid GI transit time, gastric resection, partial gastrectomy, intestinal infections, absence of some enzymes as in celiac disease, decreased production or release of bile

   d. Improper distribution: in the absence of insulin glucose cannot enter the cell and be used for energy

   e. Loss of nutrients: vomiting and severe diarrhea

C. Assessment

1. **Body mass index (BMI)** estimates total body fat stores in relation to height and weight (weight in kg ÷ body surface area)

2. Clinical manifestations include: cheilosis, glossitis, stomatitis, muscle wasting, anemia, edema, alopecia, spongy bleeding gums, dry scaling skin, subcutaneous fat loss, bone pain, confusion, disorientation, paresthesia, heart failure, and decreased hair pigmentation

3. Diagnosed by history, physical exam, and laboratory evaluation of protein, iron stores, vitamin levels, serum cholesterol, and electrolytes

D. Priority nursing diagnoses: Imbalanced nutrition: less than body requirements; Risk for impaired skin integrity related to depleted protein; Risk for infection related to suppressed immune system

E. Planning and implementation

1. Ensure that the proper diet as ordered by the healthcare provider (high-calorie, high-protein) is delivered to the client and provide a pleasant environment in which to eat, removing sources of unpleasant odors (bedpans, urinals, soiled dressings)

2. Encourage the client to eat in a slow relaxed manner

3. Provide enteral nutrition following guidelines previously discussed in this chapter and as prescribed by healthcare provider

4. Provide skin care and encourage activity to prevent skin breakdown

5. Assess for signs of infection and instruct client about signs and symptoms of infection and to report them to the healthcare provider if they occur

F. Medication/pharmacological intervention

1. Indicated for treatment of malnutrition as a result of enzyme deficiency, diarrhea, vomiting, vitamin and mineral deficiency, and when the GI tract must be bypassed

2. Generally includes pancreatic enzymes, vitamins, minerals, antiemetics, antidiarrheals, antibiotics (for infectious diarrhea), insulin, and lastly, total parenteral nutrition (TPN)

G. Client education

1. Reinforce diet teaching provided by the dietitian and the importance of adhering to the diet prescription; safe weight gain is 1 to 2 lbs/wk

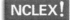

2. Help client choose high-calorie, high-protein foods

3. Teach client about the use of medications for digestion, vomiting, diarrhea, or intestinal infections if ordered

4. Teach client about proper administration of enteral or parenteral feedings if prescribed

H. Expected outcomes/evaluation: client gains weight; experiences no further weight loss, symptoms of vitamin or mineral deficiency decrease, and ingests a diet with proper proportions of nutrients

VI. Obesity

A. Description

1. More than 20 percent above ideal body weight; morbid obesity is generally more than 100 percent above the ideal body weight and having an adverse effect on a person's health

B. Etiology and pathophysiology

1. Caused by an excess of body fat; can exist in a person of normal weight

   a. Men: greater than 22 percent body fat in young men and greater than 25 percent body fat in older men

   b. Women: greater than 35 percent body fat

2. Causes of obesity include genetic factors (Prader-Willi syndrome), but these are uncommon

3. Neuroendocrine causes of obesity include Cushing's syndrome, polycystic ovarian syndrome, hypogonadism, insulinoma, and growth hormone insufficiency

NCLEX!

4. Most common cause is dietary; associated with high-fat diet and sedentary lifestyle

NCLEX!

5. Some drugs promote obesity, such as estrogens, corticosteroids, antidepressants, antiepileptics, antihypertensives, **nonsteroidal anti-inflammatory drugs (NSAIDs),** and phenothiazines

6. Social factors, such as loneliness, stress, depression, guilt, boredom, and cultures that view obesity as desirable and a sign of prosperity, influence eating habits and the development of obesity

7. About 34 percent of Americans are overweight (10 percent over ideal weight or BMI greater than 27)

8. Complications of obesity include hypertension, hiatal hernia, diabetes mellitus, hyperlipidemia, coronary artery disease, sleep apnea, cholelithiasis, osteoarthritis, back pain, and increased susceptibility to infection

C. **Assessment**

1. Measure height and weight and compare to Metropolitan Life™ tables

2. Diagnose by calculating BMI (see formula in section on malnutrition), percent of body fat as measured by skinfold thickness, underwater weight, or bioimpedance

3. Complications of obesity or comorbid conditions are determined by measuring serum glucose, serum cholesterol, lipid profile, and electrocardiogram (ECG)

4. Obtain history of eating habits, duration of obesity, medications, culture, 24-hour food recall, usual physical activity, situations that trigger eating and eating behavior

5. Assess methods used for previous attempts at weight loss

D. **Priority nursing diagnoses:** Imbalanced nutrition: more than body requirements; Disturbed self esteem

E. **Planning and implementation**

1. Assist the client in decision making about weight loss options appropriate for the individual's situation

   a. Diet therapy, developed collaboratively between client, healthcare provider, and dietitian

   b. Behavioral therapy is aimed at ways to assist the client to change daily eating habits and includes keeping a food diary, establishing exercise patterns, controlling external cues to eating behavior, and switching focus from physical appearance to health

   c. Surgery is an option for morbidly obese individuals who do not respond to other methods of weight loss, have a BMI that is > 35, and who have additional health risks or anyone with a BMI > 40; operative procedures include: gastroplasty (most common), intestinal bypass, maxillomandibular fixation, and esophageal banding; pre- and postoperative care is similar to that described earlier for gastric surgery

2. Reinforce explanations about various weight loss methods and the importance of maintaining calorie expenditure greater than intake; exercise recommendations for a healthy lifestyle include at least 30 minutes per day; walking is recommended; plan with the client an activity that is appropriate for the individual considering physical and environmental limitations

3. Provide information about support groups for obese individuals such as Overeaters Anonymous and Weight Watchers

F. Medication/pharmacological intervention

1. Drug treatment is controversial and is usually only suggested for clients with a BMI > 30 (or > 27 with comorbidities) and in conjunction with diet and exercise modifications

2. Anorexic medications are commonly used to suppress the appetite so the client eats less and loses weight slowly over time; but they are contraindicated in clients who are pregnant or lactating or in clients who have cardiac, hepatic, or renal disease

3. Amphetamines and antidepressants are controversial because of reported cases of toxicity and dependency

G. Client education

1. Reinforce information about prescribed diet therapy and exercise

2. Provide information about the food pyramid and portion sizes, e.g., a serving of meat is 3 oz and is about the size of a deck of cards; a serving of dry breakfast cereal is 1 oz or 1 cup

3. Clients taking medications to assist in weight loss should be instructed about symptoms of possible side effects, such as chest pain, shortness of breath, insomnia, and nervousness

H. Expected outcomes/evaluation: client identifies the importance of healthful lifestyle change to affect long-term weight loss and establishes a sustained pattern of change

VII. Gastroesophageal Reflux Disease (GERD)

A. Description: the backward movement of stomach contents into the esophagus without vomiting

B. Etiology and pathophysiology

1. Caused by relaxation of the lower esophageal sphincter (LES), decreased LES tone, increased intra-abdominal pressure, increased gastric volume, or a combination (see Box 8-2 for factors influencing LES tone)

2. Reflux of gastric contents is irritating to esophagus and causes breakdown of the mucosal barrier leading to inflammation and erosion

3. Healing of esophageal erosion involves the substitution of columnar epithelium (**Barrett's epithelium**) for the normal squamous epithelium in the lower esophagus

4. Barrett's epithelium resists acid (and thus supports healing) but is a premalignant tissue that is associated with an increased incidence of cancer of the esophagus

5. Occurs at any age, but increases in individuals over age 50; availability of H_2 receptor antagonists over-the-counter have decreased reported mild cases

C. Assessment

1. Heartburn or substernal burning pain is the most common symptom and is exacerbated by bending over, use of recumbent position, or straining

Box 8-2

Factors Decreasing Lower Esophageal Sphincter (LES) Tone

- Nicotine
- Caffeine (coffee, tea, cola)
- Chocolate
- Fatty foods
- Alcohol
- Peppermint, spearmint
- High levels of estrogen and progesterone
- Anticholinergic drugs
- Beta-adrenergic blockers
- Calcium channel blockers
- Nitrates
- Theophylline
- Diazepam
- Tight, restrictive clothing
- Bending, straining
- Hiatal hernia

2. Other clinical manifestations include: regurgitation not associated with vomiting or nausea, bad or sour taste upon awakening in the morning, coughing, hoarseness, or wheezing at night, belching, and flatulence

3. Adult onset asthma is most often caused by GERD

4. Chronic GERD may cause dysphagia indicating possible stricture or cancer

5. Diagnosis is most accurate through 24-hour pH monitoring

6. Esophagoscopy may be necessary in longstanding GERD to rule out malignancy

D. **Priority nursing diagnoses:** Pain related to pyrosis; Ineffective therapeutic regimen management

E. **Planning and implementation**

1. Avoid foods and medication that reduce LES tone (see Box 8-2)

2. Do not eat within 2 hours of bedtime or assume a recumbent position after eating

3. Avoid restrictive clothing that increases intra-abdominal pressure

4. Avoid large meals; eat smaller meals more frequently

5. Elevate the head of the bed for sleeping

6. Stop smoking

F. **Medication/pharmacological intervention**

1. Antacids neutralize stomach acid and are used to treat mild to moderate symptoms

2. Histamine receptor antagonists such as ranitidine (Zantac), famotidine (Pepcid), nizatidine (Axid), and cimetidine (Tagamet) are available over-the-counter and are advertised to the public widely for treatment of symptoms associated with GERD

3. Proton pump inhibitors: omeprazole (Prilosec) and lansoprazole (Prevacid) have been recently approved by the FDA for long-term treatment

G. Client education

1. Reinforce the importance of smoking cessation and avoidance of caffeine

2. Avoid bending over, especially after eating

3. Take medications as prescribed

4. Lose weight if overweight to decrease intra-abdominal pressure

5. Raise the head of the bed by using concrete or wooden blocks to reduce nighttime reflux

H. Expected outcomes/evaluation: identifies ways to reduce symptoms of reflux and incorporates them into lifestyle; experiences no GERD symptoms

VIII. Hiatal Hernia

A. Description

1. Diaphragmatic weakness through which a portion of the stomach protrudes into the thoracic cavity

2. Incidence may be as high as 40 percent of the general population but reaches 60 percent by the sixth decade of life

3. Affects women more than men

B. Etiology and pathophysiology

1. Caused by congenital weakness of diaphragm, trauma, obesity, aging, increased intra-abdominal pressure, or a combination of these factors

2. Two major types (see Figure 8-4)

    a. Sliding hernia (90% of hernias): esophagogastric junction and portion of fundus move into the thorax through the esophageal hiatus

    b. Rolling hernia (paraesophageal): only the fundus and (less frequently) part of greater curvature roll into thorax

Practice to Pass

The client with GERD is diagnosed with Barrett's epithelium. How should the nurse explain this condition?

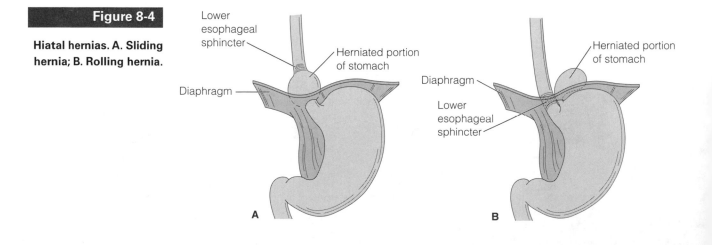

Figure 8-4

Hiatal hernias. A. Sliding hernia; B. Rolling hernia.

Lower esophageal sphincter

Herniated portion of stomach

Diaphragm

A

Herniated portion of stomach

Diaphragm

Lower esophageal sphincter

B

C. Assessment

1. Most cases are asymptomatic

2. Symptoms include heartburn (pyrosis), substernal burning or pain, feeling of fullness, dysphagia, belching; these are usually worse when reclining

3. Diagnosed by upper GI series and symptom history

D. Priority nursing diagnosis: Pain related to heartburn (pyrosis)

E. Planning and implementation

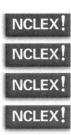

1. Conservative treatment: diet therapy and lifestyle modifications (same as discussed for GERD)

2. Avoid straining

3. Avoid excessive vigorous exercise

4. Sleep with head of bed elevated 8 to 12 inches

5. Assist client in decision-making about surgical procedure (only used when conservative treatment has failed)

6. Reinforce explanations about surgical procedures

   a. Nissen fundoplication (used for GERD as well) most common; fundus of stomach is wrapped 360 degrees around lower portion of the esophagus

   b. Hill repair: similar to Nissen repair but fundus is only wrapped around esophagus 180 degrees

7. Provide preoperative and postoperative care as discussed previously for the client undergoing gastric surgery

F. Medication/pharmacological intervention

1. Part of conservative treatment regimen

2. Generally includes antacids and histamine-2 receptor antagonists (see treatment for GERD)

G. Client education

1. Report any increase in symptoms

2. Do not take antacids within 2 hours of other medications

3. Avoid alcohol, caffeine, NSAIDs, and any medication that contains aspirin (such as Alka-Seltzer™)

4. Reinforce diet and lifestyle modifications

H. Expected outcomes/evaluation: identifies and maintains diet, lifestyle, and medication regimen and experiences a decrease in symptoms

IX. Peptic Ulcer Disease: generic term for ulcers or breaks in the mucosal lining in the GI tract that come in contact with gastric juice; can occur in the stomach (gastric ulcers), duodenum (duodenal ulcers), or rarely the lower esophagus (esophageal ulcers)

A. Gastric ulcer

1. Occurs most often on the lesser curvature near the pylorus

2. Results from a disruption in the normal protective mechanism that keeps the gastric epithelial pH normal

3. Prostaglandins in the gastric mucosa increase the resistance to acid so that substances (medications) that reduce prostaglandins will decrease gastric mucosal resistance (such as aspirin, NSAIDs, alcohol)

4. Gastric ulcers are associated with gastritis and an increased incidence of gastric cancer

B. Duodenal ulcer

1. A chronic break in the duodenal mucosa to the muscularis mucosae layer and is the most common type of ulcer

2. Results from increased gastric acid from: increased number of parietal cells, increased vagal activity, or increased secretion of gastrin

3. Not associated with an increase in gastric cancer

4. Associated with chronic *H. pylori* infection

C. Peptic ulcer disease (PUD)

1. Description (see above descriptions for gastric and duodenal ulcers)

2. Etiology and pathophysiology

    a. *H. pylori* is associated with 90 to 95 percent of clients with duodenal ulcers

    b. Chronic NSAID use (aspirin is the worst) is associated with a four-fold increased risk for gastric ulcers

    c. Factors that increase risk for PUD include: cigarette smoking, family history, blood group O (duodenal ulcer), alcohol use

    d. Incidence of ulcers increases steadily with age and peaks in the sixth decade

    e. Men and women are affected equally

3. Assessment

    a. Pain: gnawing, burning, aching, hungerlike, in the epigastrium

    b. Duodenal ulcers: pain relieved by eating

    c. Gastric ulcers: pain exacerbated by food

    d. Diagnosis is made most conclusively by EGD (see previous section for discussion)

    e. Upper GI series often done initially

    f. Tests for *H. pylori* usually positive

    g. Observe for complications: perforation (signaled by pain, signs of peritonitis, shock), hemorrhage (noted by hematemesis, tarry stool, stool positive for occult blood), or pyloric obstruction (noted by vomiting, feeling of fullness)

4. Priority nursing diagnosis: Pain related to mucosal injury

5. Planning and implementation

    a. Reinforce the importance of following treatment plan in reducing symptoms

b. Prepare client for upper GI or EGD diagnostic test (discussed earlier)

c. No foods have been determined to be ulcerogenic but some foods aggravate active PUD (coffee, cola, tea, chocolate, foods high in sodium and spicy food) and these should be avoided in the acute phase; even decaffeinated coffee stimulates gastrin release

d. Refer client to smoking cessation program

6. Medication/pharmacological intervention

   a. Antacids are used to neutralize acid

   b. Antisecretory agents: H_2 receptor antagonists block histamine stimulated gastric secretions; proton pump inhibitors suppress the production of hydrochloric acid

   c. Prostaglandin analogs: misoprostol (Cytotec) contributes to mucosal barrier preventing NSAID-induced ulcers

   d. Mucosal barrier fortifier: sucralfate (Carafate) forms protective barrier over ulcer crater and prevents further erosion by acid and pepsin

   e. Treatment for *H. pylori* changes frequently but generally includes: antibiotics, antisecretory agents, and bismuth subsalicylate (Pepto-Bismol™)

7. Client education

   a. Take medications as prescribed

   b. Learn signs of complications: blood in the stool, vomiting, increased pain

   c. Follow diet recommendations restricting caffeine, alcohol, and nicotine

8. Expected outcomes/evaluation: reduction or alleviation of pain following treatment

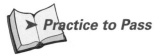

Practice to Pass

A client with peptic ulcer disease asks the nurse what the difference is between a gastric ulcer and a duodenal ulcer. How should the nurse respond?

X. Irritable Bowel Syndrome (IBS)

A. Description

1. Common noninflammatory functional bowel disorder also known as spastic bowel, functional colitis, and mucous colitis

2. Motility disorder of lower GI tract

B. Etiology and pathophysiology

1. Cause is unknown, but factors that aggravate the condition are: stress, anxiety, depression, certain foods and food additives in some clients, drugs, toxins, and hormones

2. There is no change in physical characteristics of intestinal mucosa

3. Usually manifests in three patterns: predominantly diarrhea, predominantly constipation, or combination of diarrhea and constipation; each pattern may or may not include abdominal pain

C. Assessment

1. Abdominal pain

   a. Relieved by defecation

    b. Intermittent and colicky

    c. Continuous and dull

  2. Change in bowel motility and character

    a. Diarrhea

    b. Constipation

    c. Presence of mucus

    d. Feeling of incomplete evacuation

  3. Other manifestations include: bloating, flatulence, urgency

  4. Diagnosis is made by excluding organic causes of the clinical manifestations

  5. Sigmoidoscopy may demonstrate spastic contractions that may be painful; mucosa is normal in appearance

D. Priority nursing diagnoses: Constipation; Diarrhea

E. Planning and implementation

  1. No specific treatment

  2. Dietary fiber 30 to 40 g may help in predominantly constipation type

  3. Assist the client to identify and eliminate foods that exacerbate problem

  4. Common offenders: fruit, berries, lettuce, lactose, caffeinated drinks, preservatives (sodium sulfite), alcohol

  5. Encourage a program of relaxation and stress reduction

  6. Regular exercise may help control symptoms

F. Medication/pharmacological intervention

  1. No standard pharmacologic treatment

  2. Bulk-forming agents (Metamucil, Fibercon) may help predominantly constipation-type IBS

  3. Antidiarrheal agents (Imodium, Lomotil) may be used for predominantly diarrhea-type IBS

  4. Antidepressants, anxiolytics, antispasmodics, or anticholinergics may be used

G. Client education

  1. Provide information about fiber content of various foods

  2. Follow prescribed regimen

  3. Encourage bathroom privacy and a regular time for defecation

  4. Provide information about programs of relaxation or support groups

H. Expected outcomes/evaluation: client identifies triggers for IBS symptoms and follows prescribed treatment plan

XI. Chronic Inflammatory Bowel Disease

A. Ulcerative colitis

  1. Description

    a. Area of chronic inflammation of the mucosa and submucosa in the colon and rectum

b. Peak incidence is between 15 and 35 years of age with a second peak in people aged 50 to 70 years

c. Characterized by periods of exacerbation and remission

2. Etiology and pathophysiology

   a. Cause is unknown

   b. May have relationship to stress, genetics, infection, dietary factors (low fiber intake), or antibody formation

   c. Inflammation (at the base of the crypts of Lieberkuhn usually in rectum) develops into abscesses that penetrate the mucosa and spread laterally

   d. Begins in rectum and can progress proximally, but is usually limited to sigmoid colon and rectum

   e. Can range in severity from mild to severe

3. Assessment

   a. Diarrhea; 10 to 20 liquid stools per day often containing blood and sometimes mucus; nocturnal diarrhea is common

   b. May complain of fatigue resulting from blood loss, lack of sleep, and/or fluid imbalance

   c. May affect quality of life; client may be afraid to leave the house because of severe diarrhea

   d. Complications include: hemorrhage, abscess formation, toxic megacolon, malabsorption, bowel obstruction, bowel perforation, increased risk of colon cancer, and extraintestinal symptoms (arthritis, uveitis)

   e. Diagnosed conclusively by sigmoidoscopy: characteristic edematous, friable mucosa with a granular appearance with evident crypt abscesses

4. Priority nursing diagnoses: Diarrhea related to bowel inflammation; Acute and chronic pain related to bowel mucosal inflammation

5. Planning and implementation

   a. Provide pre- and post-sigmoidoscopy care as outlined earlier in this chapter

   b. Rest is required to decrease intestinal activity

   c. Diet therapy may include a low-residue diet or in severe cases nothing by mouth to rest the bowel; TPN will be ordered in severe cases

   d. Surgery (ileostomy) may be necessary if the disease cannot be controlled by medical means; see section earlier in this chapter

   e. Provide an atmosphere in which the client feels free to talk about concerns related to the disease process and its effect on lifestyle

6. Medication/pharmacological intervention

   a. Corticosteroids during exacerbations to decrease bowel inflammation

   b. Salicylate compounds (sulfasalazine [Azulfidine], mesalamine [Asocol]) are used to decrease prostaglandin formation in bowel thus reducing inflammation

   c. Antidiarrheal drugs are used to provide symptom management

7. Client education

   a. Take medications as ordered

   b. Avoid foods that exacerbate symptoms: raw vegetables, raw fruits, whole-grain breads and cereals, seeds, nuts, popcorn, and any highly spiced or flavorful food

   c. Notify healthcare provider if symptoms increase or there is blood in the stool

   d. Instruct the postoperative client in the care of stoma and incision as described in earlier section

   e. Provide information about ulcerative colitis support groups in the area

   f. Teach client importance of good perianal skin care to prevent complications

   g. Educate client about exacerbation and remission nature of the disease and symptom management

8. Expected outcomes/evaluation: identifies measures to decrease diarrhea and pain; has less diarrhea and pain; identifies signs and symptoms of complications and notifies healthcare provider of these if they occur

B. Crohn's disease (regional enteritis)

1. Description

   a. Chronic inflammation of GI mucosa occurring anywhere from mouth to anus but occurring most often in the terminal ileum

   b. Characterized by exacerbations and remissions

   c. Peak onset is between ages 10 and 30

2. Etiology and pathophysiology

   a. Cause is unknown

   b. Possible factors are autoimmune, genetics, infectious agents, and environmental (stress)

   c. Lesions extend to all thicknesses of the bowel wall and are prone to fistula formation

   d. Lesion have a "cobblestone appearance" with sections on normal mucosa between lesions called "skip" lesions

   e. Over time the chronic inflammation causes fibrotic changes in the bowel wall leading to obstruction

   f. Depending on the severity and the location of the lesions, malabsorption may occur as well as losses of protein from the lesions themselves

3. Assessment

   a. Diarrhea (5 to 6 liquid to semiformed stools/day) is most common symptom (usually without blood); depending on location steatorrhea (fatty stool) may occur

   b. Abdominal pain in RLQ that is relieved by defecation

   c. Systemic manifestations include fever, fatigue, malaise, weight loss

  d. Complications include abscess and fistula formation, intestinal obstruction, malnutrition, and bowel perforation; hemorrhage is uncommon

  e. Barium enema and upper GI series are often diagnostic showing areas of ulceration, narrowing, strictures, and fistulas

  f. Diagnosed by colonoscopy; characteristic aphthoid ulcers, strictures, and segmental involvement is visualized; biopsy of lesion is done

  g. Other tests are ordered to assess for complications and to rule out other causes of diarrhea (serum albumin, folic acid, hemoglobin, and hematocrit)

 4. Priority nursing diagnoses: Diarrhea related to bowel inflammation; Acute and chronic pain related to bowel inflammation; Imbalanced nutrition: less than body requirements

 5. Planning and implementation

NCLEX!

  a. Provide prescribed diet: usually high-calorie, high-protein; involve client in making appropriate menu choices

  b. Encourage intake of prescribed nutritional supplements

  c. Weigh daily, maintain calorie count, and monitor intake and output

  d. Allow client to express fears and anxiety about course of illness and possibility of surgical intervention (not as common as for ulcerative colitis because it is not necessarily curative)

NCLEX!

 6. Medication/pharmacological intervention

  a. Medications are the same as those for ulcerative colitis (antidiarrheals, salicylate-containing compounds, corticosteroids)

  b. Metronidazole (Flagyl), a broad-spectrum antimicrobial, is also given

  c. Antispasmotics decrease abdominal cramping following eating

  d. Total parenteral nutrition (TPN) may be ordered during periods of severe exacerbation to totally rest the bowel

 7. Client education

  a. Reinforce information about disease process, prescribed medication regimen, and dietary needs

  b. Teach client and family signs and symptoms of complications: increased pain, rectal bleeding, fever, chills, lethargy

  c. If TPN is ordered, teach the client and family about proper catheter care and feeding techniques

  d. Encourage intake of nutritional supplements, such as Ensure™ to promote optimum nutrition

 8. Expected outcomes/evaluation: client has fewer episode of diarrhea and associated abdominal pain; identifies foods high in protein, low in fat and high in nutritional value, and follows prescribed nutrition regimen

XII. Diverticulitis

A. Description

 1. Inflammation of diverticula, which are outpouchings in the wall of the intestine (diverticulosis is the presence of diverticula)

2. Majority of diverticula occur in sigmoid colon (90 to 95 percent)

3. Incidence increases with age

4. Diverticular disease is unknown in countries where people eat a high fiber, un-refined diet

B. Etiology and pathophysiology

1. Caused by increased pressure in the intestinal lumen and herniation of mucosa through defects in the bowel wall; decreased fecal bulk (low-fiber diet) contribute to bowel wall hypertrophy and resultant increased intraluminal pressure

2. Diverticula become inflamed when undigested food or bacteria are trapped; abscess formation contributes to the disease and the diverticulum may rupture

C. Assessment

1. Pain, usually left-sided ranging in severity from mild to severe and can be constant or cramping; if perforation occurs, abdominal pain is generalized

2. Most cases of diverticular disease are asymptomatic

3. May note constipation alternating with increased frequency bowel elimination pattern

4. Fever, chills, and tachycardia along with generalized abdominal pain may indicate perforation of diverticulum and onset of peritonitis

5. Diverticular disease is diagnosed with barium enema; however, this is contraindicated when diverticulitis is present because of the risk of rupturing the diverticulum with instillation of barium

6. CT scan or ultrasonography can be used to diagnose acute diverticulitis

D. Priority nursing diagnoses: Pain related to inflamed diverticula; Impaired tissue integrity: gastrointestinal; Deficient knowledge related to dietary management

E. Planning and implementation

1. Reinforce dietary modifications to reduce complications of diverticulosis

   a. High-fiber diet after acute phase

   b. Bowel rest: NPO or low-residue diet during initial acute phase

   c. Addition of bran to everyday foods

   d. Avoid intake of seeds and foods with small seeds such as berries and figs

2. Assess for signs of bleeding: check stool for occult blood

3. Prepare for possible surgical intervention; colon resection is done in 25 percent of cases of diverticulitis

F. Medication/pharmacological intervention

1. Antibiotics decrease bowel flora and reduce infection

2. Opioid analgesics relieve pain

3. Stool softeners may be used but laxatives and enemas are contraindicated

G. Client education

1. Provide information about the fiber content of various foods

2. Instruct client about self-administration and side effects of medications ordered

3. Teach client about signs and symptoms of complications of diverticulitis

H. Expected outcomes/evaluation: client identifies ways to increase dietary fiber; demonstrates understanding of disease process and symptoms of complications; follows therapeutic regimen

XIII. Intestinal Obstruction

A. Description

1. Failure of bowel contents to be moved forward

2. Can be partial or complete

B. Etiology and pathophysiology

1. Mechanical obstruction results from forces outside of the intestines, (adhesions, hernia, fibrosis); or blockage in the lumen (fecal impaction, edema, tumor, stricture, volvulus, intussusception)

2. Nonmechanical obstruction or paralytic ileus results from impairment of muscle tone or nervous system innervation preventing forward movement of intestinal contents (anesthesia, abdominal surgery, spinal injuries, peritonitis, vascular insufficiency)

3. Obstructions occur most often in ileum where the intestinal diameter is the smallest

4. Peristalsis increases in the intestine above the blockage leading to increased secretions, edema, and increased capillary permeability and resulting in fluid and electrolyte imbalances and hypovolemia

NCLEX**!**

C. Assessment

NCLEX**!**

1. Early in bowel obstruction, bowel sounds may be high-pitched and tinkling proximal to the obstruction and silent distal to the obstruction

2. Late in bowel obstruction bowel sounds become absent

3. Abdominal pain can be colicky and increase in intensity as the obstruction progresses

4. Vomiting is common and may have a fecal odor

5. Abdominal distention is common and peristalsis may be visible in the early stages of the obstruction

6. Vital signs may be normal in early obstruction but client can demonstrate signs of shock as obstruction progresses (tachycardia, fever, tachypnea, hypotension)

7. Diagnosed by history, physical findings, and abdominal x-ray; dilated loops of bowel can be seen (barium studies are contraindicated)

D. Priority nursing diagnoses: Impaired tissue perfusion: gastrointestinal; Deficient fluid volume; Pain

E. Planning and implementation

1. Prepare client for possibility of surgery: exploratory laparotomy, colon resection, colostomy

2. Prepare client for insertion of NGT or intestinal tube (see earlier section)

3. Provide mouth care to minimize the fecal nature of secretions

4. Provide IV therapy as prescribed

5. Maintain NPO status until peristalsis returns

6. Provide comfort measures such as frequent position changes

7. Monitor vital signs including intake and output; early detection of hypovolemic shock can prevent complications (bowel ischemia and necrosis)

8. Monitor level of pain: sudden change in the nature of pain may indicate complications (ischemia and necrosis)

9. Monitor progression and drainage from intestinal tube

F. Medication/pharmacological intervention

1. Analgesic medication is generally limited because opioid analgesics decrease GI motility which will further compromise the bowel; meperidine (Demerol) may be given in small amounts

2. IV fluid with appropriate electrolyte replacement will be ordered to prevent hypovolemia and shock

G. Client education

1. Instruct client about the insertion and maintenance of NG tube or intestinal tube

2. Reinforce instructions for postoperative use of incentive spirometer, coughing and deep breathing exercises, ambulation, activity, and wound care

3. Provide support to the client and family in dealing with the possibility of a colostomy

4. Stress importance of maintaining a healthy lifestyle on discharge

H. Expected outcomes/evaluation: client identifies understanding of disease process and treatment options; verbalizes ways to prevent future bowel obstructions

---

Case Study

M. W., a 47-year-old female, is admitted to the hospital to rule out chronic gastroesophageal reflux disease (GERD) versus peptic ulcer disease (PUD). You are the nurse assigned to care for this client.

❶ What diagnostic tests should you anticipate being ordered to differentiate her diagnoses?

❷ What are the priorities of care after these tests?

❸ What instructions about lifestyle changes should you give M.W. if she has gastroesophageal reflux disease (GERD)?

❹ What instructions about signs and symptoms of complications of GERD and PUD should you provide to M. W.?

❺ If M. W. asks you about the possibility of developing cancer, how would you respond?

For suggested responses, see page 737.

Posttest

1 A client is to receive gavage feeding through an NG tube. Which of the following nursing actions should be instituted to prevent complications?

(1) Flush with 20 mL of air
(2) Place client in high-Fowler's position
(3) Advance tube 1 cm
(4) Plug the air vent during feeding

2 A client is to have an intestinal tube placed to decompress the bowel. Which of the following explanations should the nurse give to the client about what to expect?

(1) "You will need to remain on bedrest until the tube is removed."
(2) "While the tube is in place you will need to lie on your right side."
(3) "Walking in the hall will help move the tube forward."
(4) "Keeping the bed flat should make you more comfortable."

3 The nurse is caring for a client with a Sengstaken-Blakemore tube. Which of the following actions should the nurse take first if the client suddenly experiences difficulty breathing?

(1) Elevate the head of the bed
(2) Apply oxygen with a nasal cannula
(3) Listen to the client's lungs
(4) Cut and remove the tube

4 The client returns to the nursing unit postoperatively after a colostomy. Which of the following assessments would require immediate action by the nurse?

(1) Stoma is bright red.
(2) Stoma is bluish.
(3) Stoma is draining serous fluid.
(4) Stoma is draining no fluid.

5 A client who had a Billroth I procedure is beginning to eat solid foods. The nurse should assess the client for the development of dumping syndrome by determining the presence of which of the following?

(1) Bradycardia
(2) Diarrhea
(3) Dyspnea
(4) Coughing

6 A client is admitted to the hospital in a malnourished state. The nurse understands the client is at a high risk for which of the following conditions as a result of decreased nutrition?

(1) Infection
(2) Diarrhea
(3) Fever
(4) Tumor formation

7 The nurse is preparing a client with hiatal hernia for discharge. Which of the following statements made by the client would indicate that teaching has been effective?

(1) "I will join the gym and get in shape by lifting weights."
(2) "I know I need to eat a high-fat diet to slow down my digestion."
(3) "I will join a support group. "
(4) "I will take a walk after dinner each night."

8 The nurse should question the client with gastroesophageal reflux disease (GERD) about the use of which of these medications that decrease LES pressure?

(1) Antidepressants
(2) Calcium channel blockers
(3) Antiestrogen agents
(4) Alpha-adrenergic blocking agents

9 The client with irritable bowel syndrome (IBS) asks the nurse what causes the disease. Which of the following responses by the nurse would be most appropriate?

(1) "This is an inflammation of the bowel caused by eating too much roughage."
(2) "IBS is caused by a stressful lifestyle."
(3) "The cause of this condition is unknown."
(4) "There is thinning of the intestinal mucosa caused by ingestion of gluten."

10 A client with Crohn's disease (regional enteritis) who is taking sulfasalazine (Azulfidine) asks the nurse why this medication is necessary. Which information should the nurse include in the response?

(1) The drug decreases abdominal cramping by slowing peristalsis.
(2) The drug decreases prostaglandin production in the bowel so it decreases inflammation.
(3) The drug inhibits neurotransmission of pain impulses.
(4) The drug stimulates the release of endorphins so pain is relieved.

See page 333 for Answers and Rationales.

Answers and Rationales

Pretest

1 **Answer: 2** *Rationale:* The posterior pharynx is anesthetized for easy passage of the endoscope into the esophagus. The return of the gag reflex indicates that normal function is returning and the client is able to swallow.
Cognitive Level: Application
Nursing Process: Assessment; *Test Plan:* PHYS

2 **Answer: 3** *Rationale:* Thick secretions and particulate matter may obstruct the tube causing drainage to cease and the client may experience nausea and vomiting. The tube should be gently flushed to ensure patency and rule out obstruction as the cause of the client's symptoms.
Cognitive Level: Application
Nursing Process: Implementation; *Test Plan:* PHYS

3 **Answer: 3** *Rationale:* Dumping syndrome is the rapid dumping of food into the jejunum without proper mixing and digestion. Interventions that help to minimize dumping syndrome are lying down after eating, eating a diet high in fat and protein and low in carbohydrates, and no fluids with meals.
Cognitive Level: Application
Nursing Process: Implementation; *Test Plan:* PHYS

4 **Answer: 2** *Rationale:* BMI is an estimation of total body fat in relation to height and weight. An optimal BMI is 20 to 25 and increasing to 24 to 27 in the elderly.
Cognitive Level: Analysis
Nursing Process: Analysis; *Test Plan:* PHYS

5 **Answer: 1** *Rationale:* The client with GERD is encouraged to eat smaller, low-fat frequent meals and to avoid lying down after eating. Clients are instructed to not eat for at least 2 hours before bedtime and avoid foods that decrease lower esophageal sphincter pressure, such as anything containing caffeine (coffee, tea, cola, chocolate).
Cognitive Level: Analysis
Nursing Process: Evaluation; *Test Plan:* PHYS

6 **Answer: 1** *Rationale:* Gastric ulcers are usually a result of a disruption of the protective mechanism of the gastric epithelium. Substances that reduce prostaglandin secretion in the gastric mucosa (aspirin, NSAIDs, alcohol) are responsible for gastric ulcers. Although certain foods and fluids may aggravate an existing ulcer, they do not cause them.
Cognitive Level: Application
Nursing Process: Assessment; *Test Plan:* PHYS

7 **Answer: 4** *Rationale:* Famotidine (Pepcid) is a histamine-2 receptor antagonist and reduces the secretion of gastric acid. This class of drugs does not have a direct effect on reflux, LES tone, or GI motility.
Cognitive Level: Comprehension
Nursing Process: Planning; *Test Plan:* PHYS

8 **Answer: 1** *Rationale:* Hemorrhage and bleeding is a common feature of ulcerative colitis, and over time this can lead to significant loss of RBCs. The client should be assessed for possible anemia.
Cognitive Level: Application
Nursing Process: Assessment; *Test Plan:* PHYS

9 **Answer: 1** *Rationale:* Diverticular disease is virtually unknown in cultures where highly refined foods are not available (Africa, Asia) and was unknown in the U.S. prior to 1900. The other statements are false.
Cognitive Level: Analysis
Nursing Process: Planning; *Test Plan:* HPM

10 **Answer: 1** *Rationale:* Early in a bowel obstruction, the bowel attempts to move the contents past the obstruction, and this is heard as high-pitched tinkling

bowel sounds. As the obstruction progresses, bowel sounds will diminish and may finally become absent.
Cognitive Level: Analysis
Nursing Process: Assessment; *Test Plan:* PHYS

Posttest

1 **Answer: 2** *Rationale:* Keeping the client in a high Fowler's position minimizes the risk of aspiration. The other options do not address this priority issue of care.
Cognitive Level: Application
Nursing Process: Implementation; *Test Plan:* PHYS

2 **Answer: 3** *Rationale:* Activity, including position changes and ambulation, stimulate intestinal peristalsis and assist in the forward movement of the tube.
Cognitive Level: Application
Nursing Process: Implementation; *Test Plan:* PHYS

3 **Answer: 4** *Rationale:* Scissors should be kept at the bedside of all clients with an esophagogastric tube and the tube should be cut if the client experiences respiratory compromise. Maintaining the client's airway is the first priority of care.
Cognitive Level: Analysis
Nursing Process: Implementation; *Test Plan:* PHYS

4 **Answer: 2** *Rationale:* A healthy stoma is red to reddish-pink, moist, and shiny. A stoma that appears dark red, bluish, or black indicates ischemia or necrosis. This finding must be reported immediately because the viability of the tissue is at risk. Options 3 and 4 are of no concern immediately postop.
Cognitive Level: Application
Nursing Process: Implementation; *Test Plan:* PHYS

5 **Answer: 2** *Rationale:* Symptoms of dumping syndrome can occur within 5 minutes to 3 hours after eating and include nausea, vomiting, tachycardia, diaphoresis, abdominal pain, diarrhea, syncope, and hyperactive bowel sounds.
Cognitive Level: Application
Nursing Process: Assessment; *Test Plan:* PHYS

6 **Answer: 1** *Rationale:* Undernutrition affects many systems, causing decreases in metabolic function and cell-mediated and humoral immunity, thereby increasing the susceptibility to infection. The other responses are incorrect.
Cognitive Level: Analysis
Nursing Process: Analysis; *Test Plan:* PHYS

7 **Answer: 4** *Rationale:* Conservative treatment for hiatal hernia consists of lifestyle changes including remaining upright after eating; avoiding straining, tight clothing, and vigorous exercise; and eating small, frequent, low-fat meals.
Cognitive Level: Analysis
Nursing Process: Evaluation; *Test Plan:* PHYS

8 **Answer: 2** *Rationale:* Many common substances contribute to decreased LES pressure including fatty foods, caffeinated beverages, nicotine, beta-adrenergic blocking agents, calcium channel blockers, nitrates, theophylline, peppermint, alcohol, high levels of estrogen and progesterone, and anticholinergic drugs.
Cognitive Level: Application
Nursing Process: Assessment; *Test Plan:* PHYS

9 **Answer: 3** *Rationale:* There is no known cause of IBS, and diagnosis is made by excluding all the other diseases that cause the symptoms. There is no inflammation of the bowel. Some factors exacerbate the symptoms, including anxiety, fear, stress, depression, some foods and drugs, but these do not cause the disease.
Cognitive Level: Application
Nursing Process: Implementation; *Test Plan:* PHYS

10 **Answer: 2** *Rationale:* Sulfasalazine is a GI anti-inflammatory medication that exerts its action by decreasing prostaglandin production in the bowel. It does not have the other effects listed.
Cognitive Level: Application
Nursing Process: Implementation; *Test Plan:* PHYS

References

Beyea, S. (2002). Interventions for clients with stomach disorders. In D. Ignatavicius & M. Workman (Eds.), *Medical-surgical nursing: Critical thinking for collaborative care* (4th ed.). Philadelphia: W. B. Saunders, pp. 1379–1403.

Beyea, S. & Kazanowski, M. (2002). Interventions for clients with noninflammatory intestinal disorders. In D. Ignatavicius & M. Workman (Eds.), *Medical-surgical nursing: Critical thinking for collaborative care* (4th ed.). Philadelphia: W. B. Saunders, pp.1405–1431.

Craven, R. & Hirnle, C. (2000). *Fundamentals of nursing: Human health and function* (3rd ed.). Philadelphia: Lippincott, pp. 913–949; 1077–1114.

Huether, S. (2000). Structure and function of the digestive system. In S. Huether & K. McCance (Eds.), *Understanding pathophysiology.* St. Louis, MO: Mosby, pp. 917–941.

Huether, S. (2000). Alteration of digestive function. In S. Huether & K. McCance (Eds.), *Understanding pathophysiology.* St. Louis: Mosby. pp. 942-983.

Johnson, A. (2002). Assessment of the gastrointestinal system. In D. Ignatavicius & M. Workman (Eds.), *Medical-surgical nursing: Critical thinking for collaborative care* (4th ed.). Philadelphia: W. B. Saunders, pp. 1313–1332.

Kazanowski, M. & Beyea, S. (2002). Interventions for clients with inflammatory intestinal disorders. In D. Ignatavicius & M. Workman (Eds.), *Medical-surgical nursing: Critical thinking for collaborative care* (4th ed.). Philadelphia: W. B. Saunders, pp. 1433–1462.

Lemone, P. & Burke, K. (2000). *Medical-surgical nursing: Critical thinking in client care* (2nd ed.). Upper Saddle River, NJ: Prentice-Hall, Inc., pp. 422–509; 769–875.

Pagana, K. & Pagana, T. (1998). *Manual of diagnostic and laboratory tests.* St. Louis, MO: Mosby, pp. 509–578, 761–771, 900–906, 933–939, 999–1202.

Sands, J. (1999). Management of persons with problems of the intestines. In W. Phipps, J. Sands, & J. Marek (Eds.), *Medical-surgical nursing: Assessment and management of clinical problems* (6th ed.). St. Louis, MO: Mosby, pp. 1313–1371.

Sands, J. (1999). Management of persons with problems of the stomach and duodenum. In W. Phipps, J. Sands, & J. Marek (Eds.), *Medical-surgical nursing: Assessment and management of clinical problems* (6th ed.). St. Louis, MO: Mosby, p. 1277–1312.

Shelton, S. & Ignatavicius, D. (2002). Interventions for clients with malnutrition and obesity. In D. Ignatavicius & M. Workman (Eds.), *Medical-surgical nursing: Critical thinking for collaborative care* (4th ed.). Philadelphia: W. B. Saunders, pp. 1543–1569.

Thomas, D. (2002). Interventions for clients with esophageal problems. In D. Ignatavicius & M. Workman (Eds.), *Medical-surgical nursing: Critical thinking for collaborative care* (4th ed.). Philadelphia: W. B. Saunders, pp. 1355–1377.

Turkoski, B., Lance, B., & Bonfiglio, M. (1999). *Drug information handbook for nursing.* Hudson, OH: Lexi-Comp, Inc., p. 1079.

CHAPTER 9

Musculoskeletal Disorders

Ann Marie John, MS, RN

CHAPTER OUTLINE

OBJECTIVES

▎ Identify basic structures and functions of the musculoskeletal system.

▎ Describe the pathophysiology and etiology of common musculoskeletal disorders.

▎ Discuss expected assessment data and diagnostic test findings for selected musculoskeletal disorders.

▎ Identify priority nursing diagnoses for selected musculoskeletal disorders.

▎ Discuss therapeutic management of selected musculoskeletal disorders.

▎ Discuss nursing management of a client experiencing a musculoskeletal disorder.

▎ Identify expected outcomes for the client experiencing a musculoskeletal disorder.

[*Media Link*]

Use the CD-ROM enclosed with this text, or log onto the address given to access the free, interactive Companion Website created for this series. The CD-ROM and Companion Website accompanying this book offer additional practice opportunities and information—NCLEX Review, Case Studies, Glossary, In Depth with NCLEX, and more.

www.prenhall.com/hogan

REVIEW AT A GLANCE

arthrogram *the injection of contrast media into the joint cavity to examine joint structures through a series of x-rays*

arthrocentesis *a surgical procedure to remove fluid from the joint to reduce swelling and pain and/or to obtain fluid for examination using sterile technique*

arthroscopy *a surgical procedure used to examine the internal structure of a joint using an arthroscope*

Bouchard's nodes *raised bony growths over the proximal interphalangeal joint of the hand seen less frequently than Heberden's nodes in osteoarthritis*

cancellous bone *a spongy bone resulting from structural units fitting loosely together leaving many spaces between thin processes and labyrinth of the bone tissue*

compact bone *a dense structured bone resulting from structural units fitted closely together*

compartment syndrome *occurs when circulation to a compartment is impeded due to excessive pressure against the non-*

elastic fascia; compartment pressure exceeds 30 mmHg (normal 10 to 20 mmHg), resulting in tissue death and nerve injury

countertraction *a pulling force exerted in the opposite direction to prevent the client from sliding to the end of the bed*

crepitation *a grating or popping sound caused by the splinters of a fractured bone or rough joint surfaces rubbing against other structures or by air entering subcutaneous tissue in a compound fracture*

degenerative joint disease *a slowly progressive disorder of articulating joints, especially weight-bearing joints, primarily affecting middle-aged to older adults*

gout *a metabolic disorder characterized by elevated uric acid levels in the blood resulting in deposition of urate crystals in synovial fluid and joint tissues*

Heberden's nodes *raised bony growths over the distal interphalangeal joints that occur frequently in osteoarthritis and are a common manifestation of the disease in women*

internal fixation *a surgically implanted fracture immobilization device to realign a fracture*

laminectomy *a surgical incision of the lamina primarily done to relieve symptoms related to an intervertebral disc*

osteitis deformans *also known as Paget's disease, a chronic skeletal bone disease resulting in enlarged and deformed bones*

osteomyelitis *an acute or chronic infection of the bone usually caused by the Staphylococcus aureus organism*

osteoporosis *disease characterized by low bone mass and structural deterioration of bone tissue causing the bone to become fragile and susceptible to fractures*

sprain *a stretch and/or tear of a ligament*

strain *a stretching or tearing of muscle fibers*

traction *direct pulling force applied to a fractured extremity that results in realignment of the bone*

Pretest

1 The primary care provider determines that a 55-year-old female client is experiencing menopause and is also at risk for osteoporosis. What foods other than milk can the nurse suggest to this client to increase her calcium intake?

(1) Seafood, wheat, corn, green vegetables
(2) Chicken, green vegetables, sardines, broccoli
(3) Green vegetables, sardines, salmon with the bone, broccoli
(4) Eggs, cheese, sardines, fish

2 What risk factors identified by the nurse would put a client at risk for developing osteoporosis?

(1) Menopause, stress, sedentary lifestyle, smoking, excessive alcohol intake, and diet deficient in calcium and vitamin D
(2) Family history, age, history of falls, smoking, alcohol, and diet deficient in protein
(3) Diet deficient in protein and carbohydrates, smoking, excessive alcohol intake, stress, and sedentary lifestyle
(4) Inadequate sunlight exposure, obesity, depression, poor dietary intake of calcium, and excessive alcohol intake

3 Alendronate (Fosamax) is ordered for a client with osteoporosis. Which information should the nurse include in teaching the client about this drug?

(1) It is a selective estrogen receptor modulator.
(2) It increases bone mass.
(3) It may be obtained as a nasal spray.
(4) It prevents bone resorption and is taken orally.

4 The nurse is preparing a client who sustained a hip fracture for discharge. The nurse should teach the client to avoid which of the following groups of activities to prevent dislocation of the hip?

(1) Crossing legs, bending at hips, and sitting on low toilet seats
(2) Taking leisurely walks, low chair seats, and bending at hips
(3) Using reachers for applying shoes and socks, and sitting in chairs with arms
(4) All exercises, bedrest, and using raised toilet seats

5 A client with a total hip replacement is concerned about dislocation of the prosthesis. What can the nurse say to reassure this client?

(1) "Avoiding activities that cause adduction of the hip can prevent dislocation."
(2) "Use of elevated toilet seats alone will prevent dislocation."
(3) "Perform bending exercises as often as able to prevent dislocation."
(4) "Remove the foam abduction pillow as soon as possible postoperatively."

6 A client has undergone a lumbar laminectomy and has just returned to the nursing unit. It is essential for the nurse to perform which of the following activities during this period?

(1) Early ambulation
(2) Vital signs checks every half-hour
(3) Neurovascular checks
(4) Assessment of bladder function

7 A client in traction slides down in the bed so that the feet touch the foot of the bed. What should the nurse do to ensure that the pull of traction remains uninterrupted?

(1) Release the weights, pull the client up in bed, and then reapply weights
(2) Ask the physician for a change in the amount of weight ordered
(3) Move the client up in bed without releasing the pull of traction on the extremity
(4) Elevate the client's feet on a pillow

8 The nurse is caring for a client with skeletal traction. It is most important that the nurse monitors which of the following?

(1) The pin site for unusual redness, swelling, purulent drainage, and foul odor
(2) The distance between the client's hip and the traction
(3) The number of times the client exercises the affected limb
(4) How the client is coping with immobilization

9 A client in skeletal traction complains of unrelieved pain at rest and paresthesia in the affected extremity. The assessment by the nurse reveals diminished pulse, pallor, and increased pain on passive motion. What must the nurse do first?

(1) Administer oxygen
(2) Encourage deep-breathing and coughing exercises
(3) Administer pain medication as ordered
(4) Notify the physician immediately

10 The nurse is caring for a client who had open reduction and internal fixation (ORIF) of the right femur four days ago. The client complains of intense pain, swelling, tenderness and warmth at the site, chills, malaise, and has a temperature of 102.2°F (39°C). This data indicates which of the following?

(1) Fat embolism
(2) Compartment syndrome
(3) Osteomyelitis
(4) Malunion of the bone

See pages 369–370 for Answers and Rationales.

I. Overview of Anatomy and Physiology of the Musculoskeletal System

A. Skeleton

1. Supports the framework of the body and protects soft tissue and vital organs and is composed primarily of calcium phosphate and calcium carbonate

2. Bones, joints, and cartilage are the primary components of the skeleton

3. The skeleton serves as storage for calcium, playing a major role in calcium balance in the blood

4. The skeleton also serves as a stable point of attachment for muscles

B. Classification of bones

1. Two major classifications of bones are based on structure—**compact** (dense) or **cancellous** (spongy)

2. Structural units of compact bone fit closely together resulting in a dense bone composition

3. Structural units of cancellous bone fit loosely together, leaving many open spaces between thin processes and labyrinth of the bone tissue

4. A central shaft (diaphysis) and two end portions (epiphyseals) characterize long bones (examples: humerus and radius)

5. Short bones are characterized by cancellous bone covered by a thin layer of compact bone (examples: carpals and tarsals)

6. Flat bones are characterized by two layers of compact bone separated by a layer of cancellous bone (example skull, ribs, scapula, and sternum)

C. Bone marrow

1. Soft, spongy, highly cellular blood-forming tissue that fills the cavity of bones and is the site for hematopoiesis (red blood cell production) and storage of red blood cells

2. Responsible for production of white blood cells, red blood cells, and platelets

3. Becomes predominantly fatty with age, particularly in the long bones of the limb

D. Axial section

1. Each vertebra is constructed like a ring, piled one on top of the other with a padding of cartilage between; vertebral rings are studded with bony projections called processes, which function as attachments for muscles and points of articulation with bones

2. Twelve pairs of ribs attach to the thoracic vertebrae; the upper seven opposing pairs attach to the front to the sternum; three of the remaining five pairs attach to the rib immediately above by cartilage, and the last two pairs are unattached

E. Appendicular section

1. Connected to the axial skeleton by the bones of the upper and lower extremities

   a. The shoulder girdle supports the arms

b. The humerus is the bone of the upper arm; the ulna and the radius form the forearm

c. Each innominate bone (hip bone) consists of three parts—the ileum, the ischium, and the pubis; the innominate bones unite with the sacrum and the coccyx of the vertebral column to form the pelvic girdle, which supports the legs

F. Joint articulations

1. Result when two bones are joined together; categorized according to type of motion

2. Composed of fibrous connective tissue and cartilage (dense avascular connective tissue) that covers the ends of bones making movement smooth

3. Joint cavity secretes synovial fluid, which lubricates the joint and reduces friction

4. Other information about joints

   a. Some joint unions can be so close that no movement occurs, for example the skull

   b. The pivot joint permits the head to rotate from side to side around a single axis

   c. The hinge joint of the elbow, knee or jaw permits back and forth or up and down movement

   d. The wrist produces a gliding motion in which one bone glides a short distance over another

   e. The shoulder and hip joints are ball and socket joints; the ball-shaped end of one bone fits into the socket at the end of another bone

G. Joints and ligaments

1. Ligaments are bands of rigid connective tissue that hold joints together allowing for movement and stability

2. Ligaments have a relatively poor blood supply which significantly prolongs the healing process after injury

H. Muscles

1. Muscle is the tissue of the body that primarily functions as a source of power and pull against bones to make the body move

2. There are three primary types of muscle: skeletal muscle (striated, voluntary) moves extremities and external areas of the body; cardiac muscle (striated, involuntary) is found in the heart; smooth muscle (nonstriated, involuntary) is found in the walls of the arteries and the bowel

II. Diagnostic Tests and Assessments

A. Radiologic tests

NCLEX!

1. Are diagnostic studies performed using x-rays, with or without injection of contrast media, to detect musculoskeletal problems and monitor effectiveness of treatment

2. X-ray (radiograph): most common and widely used radiologic test for assessment of musculoskeletal problems and effectiveness of treatment

B. EMG (electromyogram or myogram): records and evaluates the electrical activity of muscles during contraction

1. Detects abnormal electrical activity in muscle

2. There are two different types of EMG: intramuscular (IM) EMG (more commonly used) and surface EMG (SEMG)

3. Long, small-gauge needles are inserted through the skin into muscle

4. Needles detect electrical activity of the muscle and transmit information into electromyogram machine; electrical activity is displayed visually on an oscilloscope or heard audibly through an audiotransmitter (microphone)

5. SEMG: electrodes are placed above muscle to detect the electrical activity

C. Arthroscopy: a surgical procedure used to examine the internal structure of a joint using an arthroscope (a pencil-sized device with optical fibers and lenses), which is inserted into very small skin incisions; device is connected to a video camera to allow for visualization of the interior of the joint

1. Procedure may be used for diagnosis or treatment of musculoskeletal disorders such as osteoarthritis, rheumatoid arthritis, infectious types of arthritis, and internal joint injuries like meniscus tears, ligament strains or tears and cartilage deterioration

2. Arthroscopic surgery can be done during procedure to repair joint tissue; arthroscopic surgery creates less tissue trauma, less pain, and allows for a rapid recovery

NCLEX!

3. Client education: postprocedure

   a. Encourage client to take analgesics for comfort and limit activity as directed

   b. Instruct client to observe site for hematoma or bleeding

   c. Teach client how to perform neurovascular assessment (temperature, color, capillary refill, movement, and sensation) on affected extremity

   d. Teach client about signs and symptoms of infection to report: elevated temperature, warmth at injection site, purulent discharge, and redness

D. Arthrogram: contrast media or air is injected into the joint cavity to allow for visualization of joint structures; client moves joint through a series of movements while a series of x-rays are taken; assess for allergy to contrast media

NCLEX!

1. Client education preprocedure: if injected contrast dye is used, inform client that once the dye is injected there may be a feeling of warmth, nausea, headache, salty taste in the mouth, itching, hives, and rash throughout the body (symptoms are usually temporary and will be treated if necessary)

NCLEX!

2. Client education postprocedure

   a. Inform client that temporary discoloration of the skin and urine is normal after injection of dye

   b. Teach client to perform neurovascular assessment on affected extremity

E. **CT scan (computerized axial tomography):** combines x-rays with computer technology to produce a highly detailed, cross-sectional image of internal organs and structures of the body; also known as CAT scan

1. Body is visualized from skin to central part of the body being examined; recorded image is called a "tomogram"

2. Client education

   a. If ingested contrast dye is used, instruct client to increase fluid intake to assist in elimination of dye

   b. Monitor for evacuation of contrast media and possible constipation

   c. Initial stools may be white in color, which is normal until all contrast media is evacuated

F. **MRI (magnetic resonance imaging):** radiologic technique (without radiation) that uses magnetism, radio waves, and a computer to produce cross-sectional images of the body structures

1. Machine is extremely noisy and may cause or exacerbate a claustrophobic sensation

2. Client education

   a. Explain procedure to the client; a mild sedative may be given preprocedure to help decrease any anxiety associated with a claustrophobic feeling

   b. Instruct client to notify healthcare providers of any metallic body parts such as implants, pacemakers, artificial joints, metallic bone plates, prosthetic devices, surgical clips, bullet fragments, metallic clips, or other metal objects within the body that can distort the MRI image or affect the magnetic field

G. **Bone scan:** technique used to create images of bones on a computer screen or on a film using a small amount of radioactive material that travels through the bloodstream

1. Radioactive material is especially absorbed in abnormal areas of a bone; degree of dye absorption is related to the amount of blood flow to the bone

2. A camera scans the entire body and a recording is made on a special film

3. Increased dye absorption is seen with osteomyelitis, osteoporosis, fractures, Paget's disease and cancer of the bone

H. **Arthrocentesis (joint aspiration) and analysis:** fluid is removed from joint to reduce swelling and pain and/or obtain fluid for examination using a sterile needle and syringe

1. Post-procedure complications are uncommon but may include localized bruising, minor bleeding into the joint cavity, and loss of pigment at injection site (septic arthritis is a rare but serious complication)

2. Client education

   a. If cortisone medication was injected into the joint, teach client to monitor for inflammation of the injected area, atrophy or loss of pigment at the injection site, and increased blood glucose

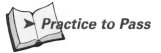

Practice to Pass

The nurse is preparing a client for a CT scan. What information should the nurse include in client teaching about this procedure?

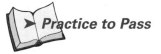

Practice to Pass

It is important that the nurse know that the MRI procedure is contraindicated for which clients?

      b. Instruct client to follow post-procedure activity restrictions as directed by healthcare provider

      c. Instruct client to monitor for post-procedure complications and check dressing for excessive bleeding

III. Laboratory Studies

  A. Antinuclear antibodies (ANA): sensitive screening blood test used to detect autoimmune disease

    1. ANAs destroy the nucleus (innermost core of the cell that contains the DNA) of the cells

    2. Test not definitive but suggests presence of auto-antibodies (antibodies directed against the body's own tissue)

    3. Present in clients with a number of autoimmune diseases such as rheumatoid arthritis, systemic lupus erythematosus, scleroderma, and others

NCLEX!

  B. Calcium (Ca^{++}): one of the most abundant electrolytes in the body that causes neuromuscular irritability and contractions; adult normal reference value is 9 to 11 mg/dL

    1. Stored in bone and gives bone stability

    2. Blood specimen is obtained to monitor calcium level

    3. Normal ranges vary slightly among healthcare institutions

    4. Decreased calcium levels may be found in osteomalacia, inadequate dietary intake of calcium, renal disease, and hypoparathyroidism

NCLEX!

NCLEX!

    5. Increased calcium levels may be seen in bone neoplasm, multiple fractures, immobilization, renal calculi, and hyperparathyroidism

  C. Phosphorus (2.5 to 4.5 mg/dL is normal reference range): blood sample is obtained to monitor level and compare phosphorus level with other electrolytes in the body (such as calcium)

    1. A high percentage of total phosphorus in the body is combined with calcium in teeth and bones

    2. Decreased levels can be seen with hypercalcemia, starvation, malabsorption syndrome, osteomalacia, and vitamin D deficiency

    3. Increased levels can be seen with healing fractures, metastatic bone tumors, and hypocalcemia

  D. Rheumatoid factor (RF) (Normal—negative or <1:20): screening blood test used to detect antibodies (IgM, IgG, or IgA) found in clients with rheumatoid arthritis; elevated RF level may indicate diseases other than rheumatoid arthritis

  E. Erythrocyte sedimentation rate (ESR); normal is < 20 mm/hr; gender variations exist; nonspecific serologic test that measures the rate at which red blood cells settle out of unclotted blood in millimeters/hour; elevated levels indicate inflammatory process in diseases such as rheumatoid arthritis and osteomyelitis

  F. Uric acid (Normal male 4.5 to 6.5 mg/dL, female 2.5 to 5.5 mg/dL): test generally used to monitor serum uric acid levels during the treatment of gout and may be used to diagnose other health problems

    1. Uric acid is the end product of purine metabolism; the kidneys normally excrete excess uric acid

NCLEX!

2. Hyperuricemia (elevated urine or serum uric acid levels) occurs because of poor renal function, excessive purine metabolism, and/or excessive dietary intake of purine foods

3. Elevated uric acid level is seen in gout

IV. Common Nursing Techniques and Procedures

A. Instructing the client on the use of crutches

1. Crutch gaits: safe method of walking using crutches, alternating body weight on one or both legs and the crutches; see Box 9-1 for crutch walking techniques, Box 9-2 for transfer techniques (getting in and out of a chair) using crutches, and Box 9-3 for negotiating stairs while using crutches

B. Traction: direct pulling force applied to a fractured extremity that results in realignment of bone; see Figure 9-1

NCLEX!

1. Reduces fracture, lessens muscle spasms, relieves pain, corrects deformities, promotes rest, and allows for exercise

---

Box 9-1

Instructions for the Client on the Use of Crutches

Four-Point Gait
- Slow gait
- Requires good coordination
- Weight-bearing is on both legs
- Move each foot and crutch forward separately (right crutch, left foot; left crutch, right foot)

Two-Point Gait
- Faster than four-point gait
- Requires more balance
- There is partial weight-bearing on each foot
- Arm movements simulate arm movement when walking
- Move left crutch and right foot forward together; move right crutch and left foot forward together

Three-Point Gait
- Fast gait
- Two crutches and unaffected leg bear weight alternately
- Weaker leg and both crutches move together followed by stronger leg

Swing-To Gait
- Fast gait
- Used by clients with paralysis of legs and hips
- Prolonged use may lead to atrophy of unused muscles
- Advance crutches forward together, lift body using arms, then swing to meet crutches

Swing-Through Gait
- Fast gait
- Good balance, skill, coordination and strength required
- Move both crutches forward together
- Lift body using arms, then swing through and beyond crutches

Box 9-2

**Transfer Techniques for
Clients with Crutches**

Getting Into a Chair

1. Use chair with armrests and support back of chair against a wall for stability.
2. Center the back of the unaffected leg against the chair.
3. Transfer crutches to the hand on the affected side.
4. Hold crutches by horizontal hand bars.
5. Grasp the arm of the chair with the hand on the unaffected side.
6. Lean forward, flex the knees and hips, and lower into the chair.

Getting Out of a Chair

1. Move forward to the edge of the chair.
2. Place unaffected leg slightly under or at the edge of the chair (this position helps the client to stand up from the chair and achieve balance, since the unaffected leg is supported against the edge of the chair).
3. Grasp the crutches by the horizontal hand bars using the hand on the affected side.
4. Grasp the arm of the chair using the hand on the unaffected side (the body weight is placed on the crutches and the hand on the armrest to support the unaffected leg when the client rises to stand).
5. Push down on the crutches and the chair armrest while raising the body out of the chair.
6. Assume a *tripod position* (crutches out laterally in front of feet, approximately 6 inches, with feet slightly apart creating a wide base of support) for balance before moving.

2. Skin and skeletal traction are most commonly used; manual traction is only used briefly under physician direction

NCLEX!

  a. Skin traction (using tape, boots, splints)

  1) Assists in reduction of a fracture (does not primarily achieve reduction) and helps decrease muscle spasms

  2) Generally used for short-term treatment (48 to 72 hours) and is applied directly to the skin

  3) Weights range from 5 to 10 pounds

Box 9-3

**Instructions for Clients
with Crutches:
Negotiating Stairs**

Going Up Stairs (stand behind client slightly to the affected side for support if needed)

1. Assume the tripod position.
2. Transfer the weight to crutches and move the unaffected leg onto the step.
3. Transfer weight to the unaffected leg on the step and move crutches and the affected leg up to the step.
4. Repeat steps 2 and 3 until client reaches the top of the stairs.

Going Down Stairs (stand one step below client on the affected side for support if needed)

1. Assume tripod position at the top of the stairs.
2. Shift weight to the unaffected leg.
3. Move crutches and the affected leg down onto the next step.
4. Transfer weight to the crutches and move the unaffected leg to that step.
5. Repeat steps 2 and 3 until the client reaches bottom step.

Figure 9-1 Traction is the application of a pulling force to maintain bone alignment during fracture healing. Different fractures require different types of traction. A. Skin traction (also called straight traction) such as Buck's traction shown here, is often used for hip fractures. B. Balanced suspension traction is commonly used for fractures of the femur. C. Skeletal traction, in which the pulling force is applied directly to the bone, may be used to treat fractures of the humerus.

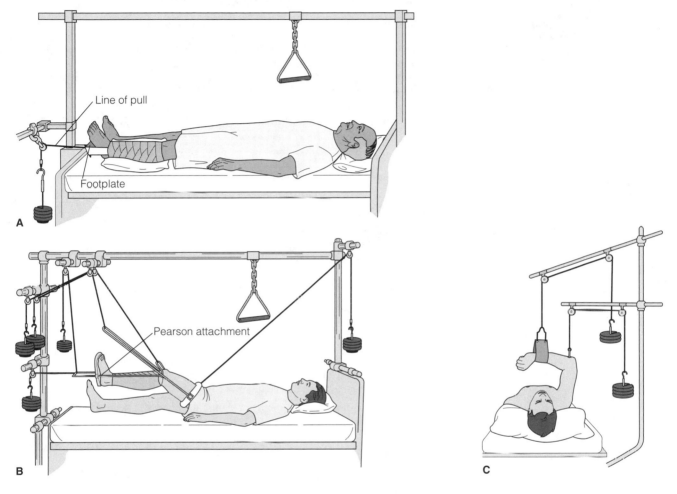

NCLEX!

    b. Skeletal traction (using pins or wires inserted into bones)

        1) Indicated for long-term use

        2) Used to align injured bones and joints or to treat joint contractures and congenital hip dysplasia

        3) Weights range from 5 to 45 pounds and amounts of weight may be adjusted initially until full fracture reduction is achieved by x-ray results

NCLEX!

    c. Balanced suspension (traction that is a hanging support to immobilize body part in a desired position)

        1) Used with skeletal traction to improve mobility while maintaining alignment of fracture

        2) Body part is suspended using splints, ropes, and weights

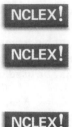

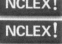

3) Client able to perform activities such as toileting and personal hygiene; bed linen can be changed without disturbing traction alignment

d. **Countertraction:** pulling force exerted in the opposite direction to prevent the client from sliding to the end of the bed; examples of countertraction include the client's weight, elevating the foot of the bed (Trendelenburg), and elevating the head of the bed with cervical traction

e. See Box 9-4 for nursing care of the client in traction

C. **Cast care:** a cast is applied for immobilization to ensure stability of a fracture; see Box 9-5 for associated nursing care

D. **Splinting and immobilization:** like casts, splints are used to immobilize a fractured extremity to ensure stability after closed reduction and external fixation; teach client how to perform neurovascular assessment (color, temperature, capillary refill, and pulses)

Box 9-4
Nursing Care of the Client in Traction

- Ensure that all ropes, weights, and pulleys are hanging freely, not shredded or torn, in a straight line.
- Bed linen should be kept off traction ropes.
- Teach client that weights should not be lifted for any reason (lifting of weights alters the line of pull and could potentially interfere with bone healing).
- Ensure that the ordered amount of weight is maintained at all times.
- Avoid jarring bed or equipment.
- Ensure that knots are not lying on or near the pulley.
- Perform neurovascular assessment to monitor for superficial nerve damage (radial, median, ulnar, femoral, sciatic, peroneal nerves).
- Teach client how to perform circulatory assessment on unaffected and affected limb, comparing observations (color, temperature, capillary refill, pulses)
- Teach client how to perform skin assessment to monitor and prevent skin breakdown on bony prominence and pressure areas.
- Ensure that body is always kept in proper alignment to prevent complications such as external rotation of the joint, increased pain, and poor healing of the fracture.
- Teach client how to monitor for infection at pin sites (fever, localized warmth, redness, swelling, abnormal drainage, and odor).
- Inform client to avoid massaging calves or reddened areas to prevent clot dislodgment caused by venous stasis.
- Encourage client to increase fluid intake (2500 mL/day unless contraindicated) and roughage (fresh fruits and vegetables) in diet to prevent constipation, urinary tract infection, and renal calculi.
- Teach client how to perform deep-breathing and coughing exercises to prevent respiratory complications.
- Encourage client to use the overhead trapeze (and unaffected leg if possible) to reposition for comfort, shift weight to prevent skin breakdown, perform exercises, and assist with personal care, toileting, and bed linen changes.
- Encourage client to adhere to exercise regimen to maintain muscle tone, endurance, and prevent bone demineralization.
- Provide diversional activities and encourage social interaction with family and friends to prevent potential isolation.

Box 9-5
Nursing Care of the Client in a Cast

- Teach client that cast made from plaster of Paris should not get wet and that cast padding should not be removed; if cast becomes soiled with feces, clean with a damp cloth or rub baking soda on soiled area to limit odor.
- Teach client that no foreign objects should be inserted into the cast (sticks, food crumbs, etc.) to prevent skin breakdown; teach client how to smooth rough edges.
- Instruct client to avoid covering a new cast with blanket or plastic for extended periods (air cannot circulate, and heat builds up in the cast).
- Turn client from side to side (using palms not fingertips) every 2 hours to facilitate drying for the first 24 to72 hours (use of fingertips causes indentation and pressure areas when cast is dry).
- Instruct client to apply ice for the first 24 hours over fracture site to control edema, ensuring that ice is securely contained so cast does not become wet.
- Instruct client to elevate extremity above the level of the heart to promote venous return for the first 24 hours after application.
- Instruct client to perform active range of motion (AROM) to joints above and below immobilized extremity.
- Teach client about signs and symptoms to report to healthcare provider: increasing pain in immobilized extremity, excessive swelling and discoloration of exposed limb, burning or tingling under cast, sores, or foul odor under cast.

V. Nursing Management of Client Undergoing Musculoskeletal Surgery

A. Laminectomy: surgical incision of the lamina done primarily to relieve symptoms related to herniated intervertebral disc

1. Assess effectiveness of pain management

NCLEX!

2. Perform neurological and neurovascular assessment; monitor bowel and bladder function

NCLEX!

3. Assess client for complaints of severe headache or leakage of cerebrospinal fluid (CSF), nausea, abdominal discomfort, incontinence, amount and character of drainage on dressing

NCLEX!

4. Use the *logroll* technique (turning a client as a unit) to turn and reposition client; maintain proper alignment of the spine at all times

5. Inform client that bedrest may be maintained for the first 24 to 48 hours after procedure; pillows may be used for comfort under the thighs in the supine position and between the legs in the side-lying position

6. Assist client to "rise as a unit" when getting out of bed (especially for the first time)

7. Instruct client that paresthesias (numbness and tingling of extremities) may not be relieved immediately after procedure

B. Internal fixation: fracture immobilization with a metal device (made of screws, pins, and/or plates) that is surgically inserted to realign and maintain a fracture

1. Inform client that x-rays will be taken at regular intervals to ensure proper alignment of the fixation device

2. Instruct client about signs and symptoms to report related to infection: elevated temperature, localized pain and warmth, tenderness, chills, malaise, and changes in neurovascular status of affected extremity

C. **Joint replacement, total hip replacement (THR)**

1. THR is frequently performed for client with conditions such as rheumatoid arthritis, malignant bone tumors, arthritis associated with Paget's disease, juvenile rheumatoid arthritis, and hip fractures

2. Advantages of THR: substantial relief of pain, improved function and quality of life

3. Teach client about plan for effective pain management and side effects/adverse effects of pain medications

4. Teach client about dislocation precautions

NCLEX!
   a. Avoid extremes of internal rotation, adduction, and 90-degree flexion of affected hip for at least 4 to 6 weeks after procedure

NCLEX!
   b. Prevent adduction: use an abduction pillow, avoid crossing the legs, avoid twisting to reach for objects behind, and avoid driving a car and taking tub baths for at least 4 to 6 weeks

NCLEX!
   c. Modify equipment to avoid 90-degree hip flexion (raised toilet seats, platform under chair, use of reaches, long-handled shoe horns, and sock pullers)

NCLEX!
5. Teach client about signs and symptoms to report to healthcare provider

   a. Infection—redness, swelling, abnormal drainage, foul odor, and elevated temperature

   b. Deep vein thrombosis (pain, sudden swelling in affected extremity, enlargement of superficial veins, skin discoloration, and localized warmth)

6. Inform client that physical therapy exercises will begin on the first postoperative day to restore and maintain range of motion, muscle strength, and mobility, and to prevent complications such as DVT

7. Instruct client that homecare management program will include:

   a. Ongoing nursing assessment of pain management

   b. Periodic dressing changes and monitoring for infection

NCLEX!
   c. Monitoring and adjustment of coagulation status weekly if taking warfarin (Coumadin) and less often if taking enoxaparin (Lovenox), a low-molecular-weight heparin

   d. An exercise program assisted by a physical therapist to assess and restore muscle strength and range of motion

8. Instruct client to inform all healthcare providers (dentists, etc.) of history of joint replacement surgery so that prophylactic antibiotics can be prescribed as necessary

9. Inform client that periodic x-rays will be required as followup throughout lifetime

D. Amputation

1. Provide client teaching about effective pain management techniques; signs and symptoms to report: redness, elevated temperature, and/or unusual, foul-smelling drainage; abrasions; and any other signs of skin breakdown

NCLEX!

2. Teach client how to care for residual limb: wash daily using warm water and bacteriostatic soap, rinse and gently pat dry thoroughly, expose to air for at least 20 minutes after washing; avoid use of lotions, alcohol, powder, or oils unless prescribed by healthcare provider; change limb sock daily, wash sock using mild soap and dry flat, and discard sock that is in poor condition

3. Instruct client to perform upper extremity active range of motion (AROM) exercises daily

NCLEX!

4. Instruct client to lay prone for 30 minutes 3 to 4 times/day (if client is able and if part of standard of care) and avoid elevating or sitting with residual limb on pillows to prevent flexion contractures

NCLEX!

5. Tell client that pain may persist in the amputated extremity and that this is normal and real; the discomfort will be treated with analgesics or other interventions

VI. Disorders of the Musculoskeletal System

A. Osteoporosis (porous bone)

1. Description

   a. Disease characterized by low bone mass and structural deterioration of bone tissue, causing the bone (especially weight-bearing bones such as the hip, spine, and wrist) to become fragile and more susceptible to fractures

   b. Affects both women and men; however, women are at greater risk

2. Etiology and pathophysiology

   a. As people age, bone resorption happens faster than bone formation, which causes the bone to lose Ca^{++} and bone density; since most of the body's calcium is stored in bones and teeth, this rapid bone resorption leads to porous bone or osteoporosis

   b. When serum Ca^{++} decreases, the body takes stored Ca^{++} from bone

3. Assessment

   a. Risk factors include female gender; increasing age; thin, small body frame; Caucasian or Asian-American ethnicity; family history; inadequate dietary intake of calcium; sedentary lifestyle; smoking; excessive alcohol intake; steroid medications; postmenopausal state; chronic liver disease; anorexia; and malabsorption

   b. Females are at a higher risk for osteoporosis than men

      1) Women have smaller body frames, which contribute to less bone density

      2) Bone resorption begins at an earlier age in women and is accelerated in menopause

3) Breast-feeding and pregnancy deplete skeletal reserves unless calcium intake is increased to match demands

4) Since currently women often live longer than men, longevity increases the likelihood of osteoporosis

4. Priority nursing diagnoses: Pain; Impaired physical mobility; Risk for injury; Imbalanced nutrition: less than body requirements

5. Planning and implementation

a. Provide client teaching about prevention: take adequate amounts of Ca^{++} throughout lifetime to decrease the incidence of osteoporosis; proper nutrition for adequate calcium intake; weight-bearing exercises to force Ca^{++} back into the bone; safety measures to prevent falls that can result in fractures; bone mineral density (BMD) tests to measure bone mass in clients at risk for developing osteoporosis

b. Provide clients with information about recommended daily dietary intake of calcium: Ca^{++} 1,000 mg/day for premenopausal and postmenopausal women taking estrogen replacement therapy (ERT), and 1,500 mg/day for postmenopausal women who are not taking ERT

c. Provide information about foods high in Ca^{++} and the importance of calcium intake with vitamin D: dark, green leafy vegetables (such as broccoli, bok choy, collard greens, spinach), sardines, salmon with the bone, dairy products (such as milk, cottage cheese, cheese, yogurt, and ice cream); Ca^{++} supplements can also be used to supplement dietary intake

6. Medication therapy

a. Estrogen replacement therapy (ERT) is generally used for prevention of osteoporosis after menopause

1) Usually given in the form of a pill or skin patch

2) Decreases bone demineralization and symptoms of menopause

3) Can increase risk for endometrial cancer (progesterone may be given with estrogen, called hormone replacement therapy or HRT, to decrease risk)

4) Client is at risk for developing deep vein thrombosis (DVT)

b. Calcitonin (Micalcin, Calcimar): naturally occurring hormone secreted by the thyroid gland

1) Currently available as a nasal spray or injection

2) Regulates calcium and bone metabolism

3) Slows bone loss, increases spinal bone density, relieves pain from bone fractures, and reduces risk for spinal and hip fractures

4) Side effects: flushing of face and hands, urinary frequency, nausea, skin rash (injectable), and nasal discharge/rhinorrhea (nasal spray)

c. Alendronate (Fosamax): prevents bone resorption; used to treat both men and women with glucocorticoid-induced osteoporosis

d. Raloxifene (Evista): used for prevention and treatment of osteoporosis; selective receptor modulator (SERM) that prevents bone loss; side effects are rare but may include hot flashes or DVT

NCLEX!

    e. Risedronate sodium (Actonel): biphosphonate, used for prevention and treatment of osteoporosis in postmenopausal women and for prevention and treatment of glucocorticoid-induced osteoporosis in both men and women

        1) Slows and stops bone loss, increases mineral density and reduces the risk of fractures

        2) Instruct client to take drug with a glass of water at least 30 minutes before the first food or beverage of the day and avoid eating for at least 30 minutes after taking the medication

        3) Remain in an upright position for at least 30 minutes after taking the medication

7. Client education

    a. Reinforce the importance of weight-bearing exercises (jogging, walking, hiking, stair climbing, tennis, dancing, and weight training)

    b. Encourage client to stop smoking

    c. Encourage client to avoid excessive intake of alcohol

8. Expected outcomes/evaluation

    a. Client will verbalize decrease in pain

    b. Client will stop smoking

    c. Client maintains optimal physical activity

    d. Client increases vitamin D and calcium intake

B. Osteomyelitis

1. Description: acute or chronic infection of the bone usually caused by the *staphylococcus aureus* organism

2. Etiology and pathophysiology

    a. Infection can occur from direct or indirect invasion of infectious organisms; see Figure 9-2

    b. Direct invasion generally occurs from invasive procedures such as surgery (joint prosthesis, arthroplasty) and injuries such as fractures

    c. Infection can also be caused by indirect invasion (also referred to as hematogenous dissemination), where the infection of the bone tissue or joint is caused by spread of the infectious organism through the bloodstream from a preexisting infectious focus; course and virulence of infection is influenced by blood circulation to the affected bone

    d. Long bones are common sites of infection in children, and spine, hip, and foot are common sites of infection in adults

    e. At-risk populations include children, elderly, and individuals with weakened immune systems

    f. Osteomyelitis warrants aggressive immediate treatment with antibiotics or surgery (wound debridement) if infection of bone is extensive

---

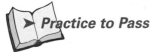

NCLEX!

➤ *Practice to Pass*

What information should you include when teaching a 38-year-old female client about risk factors associated with osteoporosis and its prevention?

Figure 9-2   **Osteomyelitis. A. Site of initial infection. Bacteria enter and multiply in the bone and the inflammatory response is initiated. B. Acute phase, in which infection spreads to other parts of the bone. Pus forms, edema occurs, and the vascular supply is compromised. If the infection reaches the outer margin of the bone, the periosteum is lifted, and ischemia and necrosis eventually occur. C. Chronic phase. Necrotic bone separates, a new layer of bone forms around the necrotic bone, and a sinus develops to allow the wound to drain.**

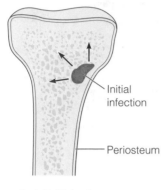

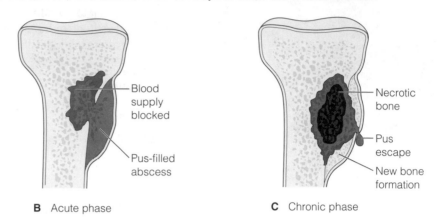

A   Initial infection   **B**   Acute phase   **C**   Chronic phase

3. Assessment

   a. Observe for symptoms of local and/or systemic infection: elevated temperature, chills, restlessness, severe bone pain unrelieved by analgesics or rest and aggravated by movement, swelling, redness, and warmth at the infection site

   b. Wound culture, bone scan, CT scan, and MRI provide information for diagnosis and assessment of the extent of infection

4. Priority nursing diagnoses: Pain, Hyperthermia, Impaired physical mobility, Ineffective therapeutic regimen management, Risk for impaired skin integrity

5. Planning and implementation

   a. Explain all therapies and interventions to client and family to decrease anxiety and enhance cooperation with plan of care

   b. Use a rating scale to assess pain and evaluate effectiveness of pain management measures

   c. Provide ongoing education and emotional support since the seriousness of the infectious process, duration and uncertainty surrounding time for recuperation, potential complications, and associated risk can be a very fearful experience for client and family

   d. Teach client about risk factors for osteomyelitis, which include previous joint replacement surgery and implants

   e. Use sterile technique for all dressing changes and manipulation of affected limb; handle extremity very gently

   f. Avoid activities that increase circulation to affected area or cause edema, pain, and pathologic fractures, such as exercise, application of heat, or keeping extremity in dependent position

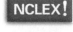

g. Immobilize affected extremity as prescribed by physician and keep body in proper alignment

    h. Monitor temperature at least every 2 hours

    i. Provide cool environment, light clothing, antipyretic medication, antibiotics, and other therapies as prescribed and/or appropriate to keep temperature within the client's baseline

    j. Keep client well hydrated to prevent dehydration from insensible water loss

    k. If long-term management is required, provide client with instructions about wound care using sterile technique, medication regimen (including instruction on venous access devices if needed), antibiotic administration, proper diet, rest, followup visits, and laboratory tests

    l. Provide information about adverse effects of antibiotic therapy such as ototoxicity and nephrotoxicity (aminoglycosides) and hepatotoxicity (cephalosporins)

    m. Instruct and assist client with interventions to prevent complications associated with immobility (turn and reposition every two hours, coughing and deep breathing exercises, etc.)

6. Medication therapy

    a. Indicated with or without surgical intervention

    b. Generally includes antibiotics and analgesics

    c. Reinforce information about adverse effects of antibiotic therapy as outlined in previous section

7. Client education

    a. Teach client about the importance of taking antibiotic medications as prescribed (for the full duration) and to report adverse effects of the medication to prescriber

    b. Review medication regimen and have client verbalize an understanding of teaching

    c. Reinforce the importance of rest and proper diet to facilitate healing, and prevent constipation and dehydration

    d. Reinforce the importance of limb immobilization during treatment

8. Expected outcomes/evaluation

    a. Client experiences satisfaction with pain management plan

    b. Client's temperature remains within normal range

    c. Physical mobility gradually returns to client's functional baseline

    d. Client verbalizes understanding of care plan and confidence with ability to effectively carry out homecare program

C. Muscular dystrophy (MD)

1. Description

    a. Group of genetic childhood disorders characterized by progressive muscle weakness, muscle wasting of symmetrical groups of muscles, and increasing disability and deformity

    b. Types of muscular dystrophy include Duchenne, myotonic, Becker's, facioscapulohumeral, and limb girdle

    c. Most common form is Duchenne muscular dystrophy

2. Etiology and pathophysiology

    a. Inherited sex-linked group of disorders

    b. Significant risk factor is family history

    c. Each type differs in regard to muscle groups affected, age at onset, rate of progression, and pattern of inheritance

    d. Each type of MD affects specific muscle groups

3. Assessment

    a. Muscle biopsy is the primary test to confirm diagnosis (test shows degeneration of muscle fibers)

    b. EMG is also used as a diagnostic test that identifies origin of muscle weakness (destruction of muscle or nerve damage)

    c. Progressive muscle weakness, hypotonia (loss of muscle mass), and delayed development of motor skills such as walking may be observed and reported by parent or caregiver

    d. Ptosis (drooping of the eyelid), impaired chewing and swallowing, abnormal gait, fatigue with minimal activity, frequent falls may all be observed and reported by parent or caregiver

    e. Delayed intellectual development is seen with some forms of MD

    f. Muscle contractures and deformities common

    g. Abnormal curvature of the spine (scoliosis or lordosis)

    h. Enlargement of the calf muscle (pseudohypertrophy) caused by fatty infiltration causing muscular enlargement

    i. Cardiomyopathy or arrhythmia may be present with some forms of MD

4. Priority nursing diagnoses: Risk for aspiration; Risk for ineffective breathing pattern; Risk for injury; Risk for infection; Impaired physical mobility; Risk for constipation; Risk for impaired skin integrity; Self care deficit: feeding, bathing, dressing, toileting; Impaired transfer ability; Imbalanced nutrition: less than body requirements; and Disuse syndrome

5. Planning and implementation

    a. Provide support and assist family with decision-making process surrounding:

       1) Development of a homecare plan to support as much independence as possible

       2) Modifications in home environment to support the client's maximal functional ability

    b. Encourage family to actively involve client in care

    c. Family members may experience a myriad of emotions including fear, guilt, anger and blame; support family to enhance coping with client's progressively worsening disease; refer to local support groups including the Muscular Dystrophy Association of America

d. Assist client and family to cope with the progressive, incapacitating, and fatal nature of the disease

e. Encourage family to interact with the client based on developmental and not chronological age

f. Teach family strategies to prevent skin breakdown (frequent skin care and linen changes if incontinent, turn and reposition at least every 2 hours, use of protective skin barrier ointments, and adequate fluid intake)

g. Perform passive range of motion exercises to maintain function in unaffected extremities and prevent/delay contractures in affected extremities

6. Medication therapy

a. There is no effective pharmacological or other treatment

b. Corticosteroids are often used to increase muscle strength

7. Client education

a. Provide information about healthcare team members and roles, including those involved in homecare program for client

b. Instruct family to offer client soft foods and to cut into small pieces to prevent aspiration and choking

c. Encourage family members to seek genetic counseling (parents, female siblings, maternal aunts, and female offspring)

d. Assist family in decision-making about appropriate clothing and footwear because of contractures and wheelchair-bound status

e. Provide family with information on community support groups and agencies with respite services to prevent role strain

8. Expected outcomes/evaluation

a. Client is free from infection

b. Client does not experience aspiration

c. Client maintains as much independence with activities as possible

d. Client experiences minimal or no complications of immobility (constipation, respiratory infection, contractures, preventable muscle wasting)

e. Family verbalizes understanding of and confidence with homecare program for client

f. Family experiences minimal or no role strain in caring for client

D. Paget's disease (osteitis deformans)

1. Description

a. Chronic skeletal bone disease with insidious onset

b. Diagnosed around the fourth decade of life

c. Results in enlarged, deformed bones but does not affect normal bones

d. Generally affects skull, long bones, spine, and ribs

2. Etiology and pathophysiology

   a. Cause of disease unknown; however, viral infection has been hypothesized as a probable etiology

   b. Hereditary factor: may be seen in more than one family member

   c. Early diagnosis and treatment is important to prevent disease progression and deformity

   d. Excessive bone resorption followed by bone formation leads to weakened bone, bone pain, arthritis, deformity, and potential pathologic fractures

   e. Normal bone marrow is replaced by vascular, fibrous, connective tissue that leads to formation of larger, disorganized, and weaker bone tissue

3. Assessment

   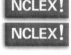

   a. X-ray is the most definitive diagnostic test

   b. Initial diagnostic tests include serum alkaline phosphatase (elevated level is a positive indicator for the disease)

   c. Bone scan may be done after positive serum alkaline phosphatase test (positive result will show characteristic abnormal appearance of bone for Paget's disease such as curved contours and thickened cortex)

   d. Positive bone scan prompts x-ray for definitive diagnosis

   e. Mild form of disease may be undetected because there may be no symptoms

   f. Symptoms include bone pain (most common complaint) and other symptoms depending on which bones are affected with the disease

      1) For example, if the skull is affected, headache and hearing loss may be reported as well as increasing head size

      2) Hip pain may be present if the pelvis or femur is involved

      3) Bowing of the lower extremities producing a waddling gait and curvature of the spine may be seen in advanced stages of the disease

   g. Arthritis may result because of damage to joint cartilage

   h. Complications are pathologic fractures (may be the first indicator of disease) and osteogenic sarcoma (form of bone cancer)

4. Priority nursing diagnoses: Disturbed body image; Chronic sorrow; Deficient knowledge; Risk for trauma: fractures

5. Planning and implementation

   a. Prognosis is good especially if treatment is started before major deformity occurs

   b. Provide analgesics and muscle relaxants for comfort

   c. Administer medications as directed to control progression of disease (see medication section)

   d. Encourage client to take medication as directed by healthcare provider since deformity and loss of bone strength will continue without prescribed medications

       e. If skull is affected, assist with diet modification, dentures, and eating utensils since teeth may become weak from the disease

       f. Hearing aid may be recommended if hearing loss results from the disease

       g. Refer client and family to support group

    6. Medication therapy

       a. The goal of treatment is to control progression of the disease

       b. The following medications are approved by the Federal Drug Administration (FDA): biphosphonates, etidronate disodium (Didronel), pamidronate disodium (Aredia), alandronate sodium (Fosamax), tiludronate disodium (Skelid), risedronate sodium (Actonel), and calcitonin (Miacalcin)

    7. Client education

       a. Ensure that client has a good understanding of plan for pain management

       b. Encourage client to take analgesics as prescribed to enhance comfort

       c. Teach client about the importance of a balanced diet, high in calcium (1,000 mg to 1,500 mg/day) and vitamin D (at least 400 units/day); vitamin D can be obtained from exposure to sunlight

       d. Instruct client to inform healthcare provider of any history of kidney stones or disease before taking calcium

       e. Encourage client to participate in an exercise program to maintain skeletal muscle health, ideal body weight, and joint mobility

       f. Instruct client to sleep on a firm mattress if back discomfort is present; if back brace is needed, instruct client on the prevention of skin breakdown under brace (undershirt) and safety measures (no driving with brace)

       g. Encourage client to modify environment at home to prevent falls that may lead to subsequent fractures

       h. Encourage client to participate in community support group

    8. Expected outcomes/evaluation

       a. Client is free of bone pain associated with the disease

       b. Client maintains ideal body weight

       c. Client verbalizes the importance of and adheres to a balanced diet including adequate intake of calcium, vitamin D, and protein

       d. Client verbalizes the importance of adhering to medication regimen to control progression of disease

       e. Client verbalizes an understanding of disease progression and ways to prevent progression

E. Musculoskeletal trauma

    1. Fractures

       a. Description

          1) A fracture is a break in the continuity of a bone

2) Fractures may be classified as:

   a) Closed (simple fracture): the bone breaks but the skin remains intact

   b) Open (compound fracture): broken ends of the bone penetrate the skin

3) Fractures may also be classified as:

   a) Avulsion: a fracture resulting from the tearing of supporting tendons and ligaments

   b) Comminuted: the broken bone fragments into more than two pieces

   c) Compressed: the bone is crushed

   d) Impacted: ends of the broken bone are driven into each other

   e) Depressed: such as in skull fracture, where the bone structure is broken and pressed inward

   f) Spiral: the break spreads in a spiral fashion along the bone shaft; is usually caused by sports injuries

   g) Greenstick: an incomplete break in the bone where one side splinters leaving the other side bent or intact; more common in children

b. Etiology and pathophysiology

1) Fractures occur in all age groups, although the elderly are more prone to fractures resulting from falls

2) When a bone breaks, the healing process occurs in three phases

   a) A fracture initiates an inflammatory response (inflammatory phase)

   b) Calcium eventually is deposited in the area and osteoblasts promote new bone formation (reparative phase)

   c) Eventually the ends of the fracture reunite (remodeling phase)

NCLEX!

c. Assessment

1) Deformity: the deformity may be caused by the break in the continuity of the bone itself and the pull of muscles on the fragmented bones

2) Edema and swelling caused by bleeding into surrounding tissues may be present

3) Pain may be caused by muscle spasms and nerve pressure

4) Crepitus may also be present on palpation; **crepitation** is a popping or grating sound created by the movement of broken bone fragments

5) Muscle spasms may be noted near the fractured bone

6) Ecchymosis or a bluish discoloration of the area caused by blood extravasation into the surrounding subcutaneous tissues

7) Pain that may be intense and possibly shock if blood loss is severe

d. Priority nursing diagnoses: Risk for impaired tissue perfusion; Pain; Impaired physical mobility; Risk for infection; Activity intolerance; Risk for impaired skin integrity

e. Planning and implementation

1) Perform frequent neurovascular assessment, which includes the five Ps: pain, pallor, paresthesias, pulses, and paralysis

2) Immobilize the joints above and below the fracture; movement of the affected area may cause a closed fracture to become open; immobilization may be accomplished by the application of splints

3) Cover open wounds with sterile dressings

4) Manage the pain associated with the fracture with prescribed analgesics

5) Elevate the fractured extremity to reduce swelling and pain

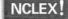

6) Apply ice to the affected extremity

7) Assist in fracture reduction

   a) Closed: involves external manipulation to realign the bones

   b) Open: involves a surgical procedure to realign the bones

8) Maintain traction as prescribed; see section on nursing care of the client in traction

9) See also section on nursing care of a client in a cast

10) Monitor for complications

   a) **Compartment syndrome:** impairment of circulation within inelastic fascia caused by external pressure (> 30 mmHg) that results in tissue death and nerve injury; external pressure can be created by casts, splints, or dressings; manifestations include unrelieved pain, diminished or absent pulses distal to the injury, cyanosis of the extremity, tingling or diminished sensation (paresthesia), loss of sensation, pallor, coolness of the extremity, and weakness; bivalving may be necessary if the cast is too tight

   b) Infection: wound drainage, fever, pain, and odor

   c) Fat embolism: chest pain, dyspnea, tachycardia, decreased O_2 saturation, apprehension, changes in level of consciousness, petechiae on upper trunk and axilla

   d) Deep vein thrombosis: calf pain and tenderness, swelling or edema

f. Medication therapy: includes analgesics and antibiotics

g. Client education

1) Teach the client to exercise the extremities not immobilized to prevent muscle atrophy

2) Teach client regarding cast care, splint, and/or traction (see previous discussions)

3) Teach the client about neurovascular assessments that need to be done

4) Teach client regarding pin care procedure and methods of preventing wound infection

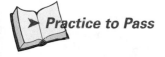

Practice to Pass

You are caring for a client in the Emergency Department who presents with an open fracture of the right tibia. What are your priority interventions for this client?

  h. Expected outcomes/evaluation

   1) Client verbalizes tolerable or decreased intensity of pain

   2) There is no evidence of infection

   3) Client has normal neurovascular findings

   4) Client has resumption of activities of daily living

   5) There is no evidence of skin breakdown under casts

2. Hip fracture

  a. Description: the hip can be fractured at different sites, namely, the head, neck, and trochanteric areas; see Figure 9-3

  b. Etiology and pathophysiology: incidence of hip fracture increases with age; 90 percent of hip fractures are caused by falls

  c. Assessment

   1) A hip fracture is a medical emergency

   2) Hip fractures are generally sustained from falls; monitor level of consciousness and assess for other injuries

   3) Perform neurovascular assessment on affected extremity

   4) Extremity of affected hip will be shorter than unaffected extremity

   5) Fractured hip will generally externally rotate

  d. Priority nursing diagnoses: Risk for peripheral neurovascular dysfunction, Pain, Risk for infection, Impaired physical mobility, Risk for impaired skin integrity, and Risk for ineffective therapeutic regimen management

Figure 9-3 A. Hip fractures can occur in the head, neck, or trochanteric regions of the femur. B. An intracapsular fracture affects the femur head or neck. C. An extracapsular fracture occurs across a trochanteric region. All fractures disrupt blood supply to the bone.

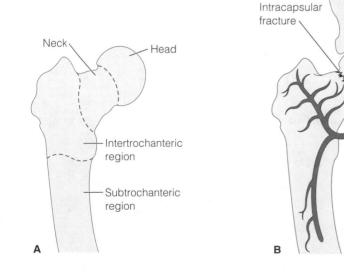
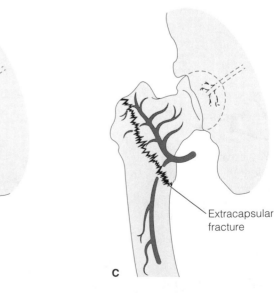

e. Planning and implementation

1) Prepare client for surgical intervention (verify allergies, informed consent, etc.)

NCLEX!

2) Instruct client that an abductor pillow or splint may be necessary to prevent disarticulation of the femur

NCLEX!

3) Inform client that sandbags may be used along the external border of the affected limb to prevent external rotation

4) Inform client that pain medication will be available for comfort postoperatively (generally patient controlled analgesia [PCA] is used)

5) Teach client about the pain rating scale to be used postoperatively and encourage client to report any discomfort

6) Teach client deep-breathing and coughing exercises preoperatively

NCLEX!

7) Use aseptic technique for dressing changes and wound drainage

8) Provide information on therapies and equipment to expect postoperatively (indwelling urinary catheter, PCA, IV therapy, possible traction, etc.)

NCLEX!

9) Monitor preoperative use of skin traction to immobilize the limb until surgery is ordered

f. Medication therapy: analgesics to manage pain

g. Client education

1) Reinforce deep-breathing and coughing exercises postoperatively

NCLEX!

2) Preoperatively teach client about postoperative precautions to prevent hip dislocation (no hip flexion greater that 90 degrees, internal rotation of affected hip, or adduction of affected hip); these include such activities as avoiding low chairs, using raised toilet seat, no excessive bending

3) Reinforce teaching about postoperative course

h. Expected outcomes/evaluation

1) Client experiences effective pain management

2) Client cooperates with mobilization precautions

3. Sprains and strains

a. Description

1) A **sprain** is a stretch and/or tear of a ligament

2) A **strain** is a twist, pull, and/or tear that may involve both muscles and tendons

b. Etiology

1) Direct or indirect trauma (caused by fall, blow to the body, muscle exhaustion)

2) Overuse or prolonged repetitive motion of muscles and tendons

      3) Inadequate rest periods during intensive training

      4) Ankles, knees, and wrist are most vulnerable

      5) Frequently seen in athletes and individuals with poor physical conditioning or who are overweight

c. Assessment

      1) Sprains are classified based on the degree of ligament injury

      2) Pain is aggravated by continuous use and influenced by the degree of injury

      3) Assess for bruising, edema, joint swelling, muscle spasms, and inflammation at the affected site

      4) Assess for changes in neurovascular status (pulse, temperature, capillary refill, and movement) of affected extremity

      5) Decreased mobility in affected extremity

d. Priority nursing diagnoses: Pain, Impaired physical mobility

e. Planning and implementation

      1) Teach client about the R.I.C.E. approach to recovery

          a) *R*est affected extremity

          b) *I*ce for 15 to 30 minutes at a time for 2 to 3 days

          c) *C*ompression elastic support bandages or adhesive tape

          d) *E*levation

      2) Perform neurovascular assessment on affected extremity

      3) Encourage client to wrap affected extremity with elastic support bandages before strenuous activities

      4) Inform client that x-rays of injured extremity may be necessary

      5) Administer analgesics as needed

      6) Teach client about the importance of stretching and warm-up exercises before athletic activities

      7) Encourage client to adhere to exercise program to regain muscle tone and strength in collaboration with the physical therapist

f. Medication therapy: analgesics, muscle relaxants, and anti-inflammatory agents as necessary

g. Client education: reinforce information covered above in planning and implementation section

h. Expected outcomes/evaluation

      1) The client has restored function of affected muscle and tendon

      2) The client verbalizes relief of pain

      3) The client verbalizes understanding of precipitating factors to the development of sprains or strains

F. Gout

1. Description

   a. Primary form of disease is hereditary; secondary form is acquired

   b. Laboratory findings show elevated serum uric acid (hyperuricemia)

   c. Characterized by recurring attacks of acute joint inflammation

2. Etiology and pathophysiology

   a. Inherited abnormality in the body's ability to process uric acid

   b. Hyperuricemia is caused by increased purine synthesis and/or decreased renal excretion of uric acid

   c. Elevated serum uric acid level can also be caused by prolonged fasting and excessive alcohol intake

3. Assessment

   a. Risk factors: obesity, excessive weight gain, excessive alcohol intake, impaired renal function, hypertension, chemotherapy for leukemia and certain lymphomas, certain thiazide diuretics, aspirin, and tuberculosis medications

   b. Diagnosis of the disease includes analysis of synovial fluid, serum uric acid, and 24-hour urine

   c. Joint inflammation is extremely painful and is caused by deposits of uric acid crystals in the synovial lining and fluid

   d. Assess for elevated temperature (may not always be present), tenderness and cyanosis of affected extremity, inflammation of small joints (commonly seen in great toe), and multiple joint involvement

   e. Precipitating factors generally include dehydration, fever, injury to joint, and excessive ingestion of alcohol

4. Priority nursing diagnoses: Pain, Impaired physical mobility, Ineffective health maintenance

5. Planning and implementation

   a. Prevent any bed linen from touching affected extremity because of extreme tenderness (bed cradle and/or footboard can be used)

   b. Instruct client to adhere to activity restriction such as bedrest and immobilization of affected extremity during periods of exacerbation

   c. Monitor uric acid levels to prevent exacerbation and evaluate effectiveness of treatment

   d. Instruct client about precipitating factors for the disease

   e. Encourage diet low in purines

6. Medication therapy: usually includes anti-inflammatory agents (such as colchicine, NSAIDs or corticosteroids), an antihyperuricemic (such as allopurinol [Zyloprim]) and uricosurics (such as probenecid [Probalan])

7. Client education

    a. Reinforce teaching covered in planning and implementation sections above

    b. Teach client about action, side/adverse effects of medication

    c. Teach client that medications should be taken with meals to avoid gastric irritation

    d. Instruct client to avoid use of alcoholic beverages when taking medication

    e. Instruct client to drink at least 2.5 to 3 liters of fluid/day when taking medication

8. Expected outcomes/evaluation

    a. Client and family verbalize an understanding of medication regimen

    b. Client reports satisfaction with pain management

    c. Serum uric levels remain within therapeutic range

    d. Client verbalizes an understanding of precipitating factors that exacerbate attacks

G. Degenerative joint disease (DJD) or osteoarthritis (OA)

1. Description

    a. Slowly progressive disorder of articulating joints especially weight-bearing joints

    b. Commonly affects hand and weight-bearing joints (knees, hips, feet, and back)

    c. Breakdown of articular cartilage occurs

    d. Injury is usually limited to joint and surrounding tissue

    e. Disease ranges from very mild to very severe

2. Etiology and pathophysiology

    a. Cartilage degeneration causes bones to rub against each other, causing pain and decreasing function of the joint

    b. Risk factors

        1) Age (most significant): primarily affects middle-age to older adults

        2) Obesity (generally causes arthritis of the knees)

        3) Repetitive joint injuries caused by sports, accidents, or work-related injuries

        4) Genetics (especially seen with OA of the hands): client may be born with defective cartilage or slight defect in the way the joint fits together, and as the client ages, the joint cartilage continues to progressively degenerate and enzymes (hyaluronidase) are released, which cause further breakdown

3. Assessment

    a. Disease is diagnosed with physical exam and a history of symptoms

    b. X-ray confirms the disease

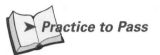

NCLEX!

► *Practice to Pass*

You are caring for a client diagnosed with gout. The client is being treated with probenecid (Probalan). The client asks, "How will this drug help decrease the pain from my gout?" How would you respond?

NCLEX!

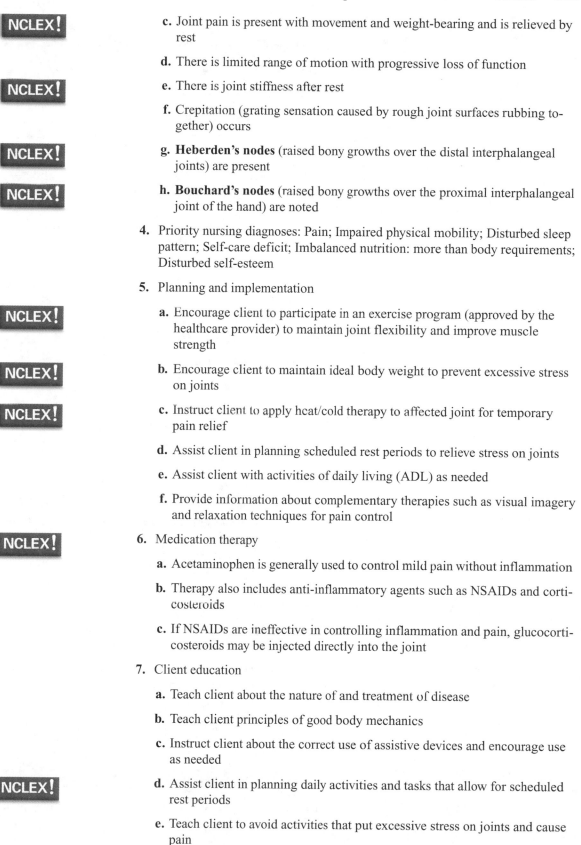

c. Joint pain is present with movement and weight-bearing and is relieved by rest

d. There is limited range of motion with progressive loss of function

e. There is joint stiffness after rest

f. Crepitation (grating sensation caused by rough joint surfaces rubbing together) occurs

g. Heberden's nodes (raised bony growths over the distal interphalangeal joints) are present

h. Bouchard's nodes (raised bony growths over the proximal interphalangeal joint of the hand) are noted

4. Priority nursing diagnoses: Pain; Impaired physical mobility; Disturbed sleep pattern; Self-care deficit; Imbalanced nutrition: more than body requirements; Disturbed self-esteem

5. Planning and implementation

   a. Encourage client to participate in an exercise program (approved by the healthcare provider) to maintain joint flexibility and improve muscle strength

   b. Encourage client to maintain ideal body weight to prevent excessive stress on joints

   c. Instruct client to apply heat/cold therapy to affected joint for temporary pain relief

   d. Assist client in planning scheduled rest periods to relieve stress on joints

   e. Assist client with activities of daily living (ADL) as needed

   f. Provide information about complementary therapies such as visual imagery and relaxation techniques for pain control

6. Medication therapy

   a. Acetaminophen is generally used to control mild pain without inflammation

   b. Therapy also includes anti-inflammatory agents such as NSAIDs and corticosteroids

   c. If NSAIDs are ineffective in controlling inflammation and pain, glucocorticosteroids may be injected directly into the joint

7. Client education

   a. Teach client about the nature of and treatment of disease

   b. Teach client principles of good body mechanics

   c. Instruct client about the correct use of assistive devices and encourage use as needed

   d. Assist client in planning daily activities and tasks that allow for scheduled rest periods

   e. Teach client to avoid activities that put excessive stress on joints and cause pain

8. Expected outcomes/evaluation

   a. Client experiences satisfaction with pain management

   b. Client successfully balances rest periods with activity

   c. Client uses joint protection and energy conservation measures

   d. Client maintains joint function

H. Low back pain

1. Description

   a. Pain may be a result of acute or repeated stress on the lower back over a period of years

   b. Pain occurs because of degeneration and/or acute injury to the tissue of the lower back

      1) Caused by sprain or strain of ligaments and muscles

      2) Pain may be felt at the site of the injury or referred

   c. Overall health of muscles of the lower back determines the degree of risk for injury as well as the speed of recovery

2. Etiology and pathophysiology

   a. Low back pain occurs because of repeated injury and progressive degeneration of the spine

   b. The two most common causes of low back pain are mechanical strain (irritation or injury to the disc causing degeneration) and herniation of the nucleus pulposus (putting pressure on the nerve roots)

3. Assessment

   a. Risk factors include but are not limited to: degenerative disc disease, poor muscle tone of the lower back, sedentary lifestyle, obesity, poor body mechanics, smoking, and stress

   b. Client will report pain caused by a shift of one vertebra on another or pinching and irritation of the nerve root

   c. Muscle spasms are a common symptom

   d. Pain does not appear at time of injury but is related to the gradual increase of muscle spasms of the paravertebral tissue

   e. The straight leg raise test may not be positive with acute injury but pain is present with radiation to the buttock and leg along the path of the sciatic nerve with chronic injury

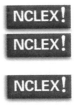

4. Priority nursing diagnoses: Pain, Disturbed sleep pattern, Ineffective individual coping, Ineffective therapeutic regimen management, Disturbed body image

5. Planning and implementation

   a. The goal of treatment is to improve symptoms and slow progression of the degenerative process

    b. Include client and family in plan of care

    c. Provide emotional support

6. Medication therapy

    a. Medication therapy includes but is not limited to analgesics, NSAIDs, and muscle relaxants

    b. Epidural corticosteroid injections may be used if conservative treatment is ineffective

7. Client education

    a. Teach client about expected therapeutic effects, side/adverse effects, and contraindications with medication use

    b. Teach client about the pain rating scale

    c. Teach client the importance of adhering to activity restrictions such as bedrest as indicated

    d. Teach client the importance of adhering to gradual increase in activity and adherence with exercise plan

    e. Teach client the importance of maintaining ideal body weight

    f. Inform client that physical therapy will be part of the rehabilitation process to assist in maintaining muscle strength and flexibility as well as improving muscle tone

    g. Teach client the use of heat/cold therapy for comfort

    h. Teach client about the importance of adhering to the principles of body mechanics to avoid excessive strain on the lower back

    i. Encourage client to sleep on a firm mattress

    j. Have client demonstrate correct sleeping position using the principles of body mechanics (side lying or supine with knees and hips flexed)

    k. Encourage client to avoid or stop smoking

    l. Teach client about use of prescribed brace or corset (if needed) to prevent flexion and extension motions of lower back

8. Expected outcomes/evaluation

    a. Client experiences satisfaction with pain management

    b. Client demonstrates use of the pain rating scale

    c. Client adheres to exercise regimen

    d. Client uses proper body mechanics with all activities

    e. Client experiences progressive muscle strengthening and flexibility

    f. Client maintains ideal body weight

    g. Client performs at optimal level of function

    h. Client adapts to lifestyle changes

Case Study

P. J. is a 67-year-old retired nurse who had an open reduction with internal fixation (ORIF) of the right hip yesterday. Vital signs remain stable within the client's baseline. The client is receiving hydromorphone (Dilaudid) via PCA for pain. The client uses the incentive spirometer every hour as instructed. An abduction pillow is positioned between the client's legs.

❶ What assessments would you perform on the client at this time?

❷ What position constraints must be observed when turning and repositioning this client?

❸ What is the purpose of the abduction pillow between the client's legs?

❹ What activities would put this client at risk for dislocation of the affected hip?

❺ Why is it important to get this client out of bed by postoperative day one?

For suggested responses, see page 737.

Posttest

1 The nurse prepares a client for an arthrogram with contrast dye. What priority nursing assessment should be performed for this client?

(1) History of claustrophobia
(2) History of allergic reaction to contrast dye
(3) Vital signs
(4) Presence of metallic implants such as a pacemaker or aneurysm clips

2 A retired 66-year-old female client is being evaluated for osteoporosis as part of a yearly physical. The client tells the nurse that she is a smoker, watches television for most of the day, and has been hospitalized with three different fractures within the last year. Based on the information given by the client, the nurse suspects which of the following?

(1) Low bone mass leading to increased bone fragility
(2) Degeneration of the articular cartilage
(3) Recurrent attacks of acute arthritis
(4) Personality changes caused by the chronic nature of the illness

3 Following laminectomy surgery, the nurse should turn and reposition the client by doing which of the following?

(1) Having the client use the side rails of the bed
(2) Elevating the head of the bed 45 degrees, then turning the legs together towards the floor, bending at the waist
(3) Logrolling the client as a unit, keeping the body in proper alignment
(4) Turning the client's head and shoulders then hips

4 The nurse receives a client with a hip spica cast that is not completely dry. When turning the client the nurse uses the palms and not the fingertips. The nurse chooses this technique for which of the following purposes?

(1) To speed-dry the cast
(2) To decrease pain from moving
(3) To prevent damage to the cast
(4) To prevent swelling

5 The nurse is assigned to a 70-pound client in skin traction. The nurse plans care to maintain effective countertraction by doing which of the following?

(1) Elevating the head of the bed
(2) Adding weights to the existing traction
(3) Placing the bed in slight Trendelenburg position
(4) Keeping the bed flat

6   A client underwent hip replacement yesterday. Which nursing diagnosis is of highest priority to be included in the client's plan of care?

(1) Deficient self-care
(2) Chronic pain
(3) Disturbed body image
(4) Impaired physical mobility

7   The nurse observes that a female client has asymmetry of the shoulder, hips, and the tail/hem of her dress. The nurse suspects that the client may be presenting with which of the following disorders?

(1) Congenital hip dislocation
(2) Scoliosis
(3) A fractured tibia
(4) Degenerative disc disease

8   The nurse is caring for a client in Russell's traction. The nurse observes the client's son playing with the weights attached to the traction. The nurse takes immediate action for which of the following reasons?

(1) Manipulation of the weights will affect healing of the client's fracture
(2) Traction should only be released once a day
(3) The spasms of the extremity might increase
(4) The client's hip may dislocate and create pain

9   The nurse encourages a 68-year-old client to discuss estrogen replacement therapy with the physician after explaining that estrogen has which of the following benefits?

(1) Enhances the storage of vitamin D
(2) Helps prevent progression of osteoporosis
(3) Increases longevity in postmenopausal women
(4) Cures osteoporosis

10   A client is ready for discharge from the hospital following hip surgery. The nurse would ensure that which of the following is available for the client at the time of discharge?

(1) Raised toilet seat
(2) Portable Buck's traction
(3) Soft cushion to use on chairs
(4) Crutches

See pages 370–371 for Answers and Rationales.

Answers and Rationales

Pretest

1   **Answer: 3** *Rationale:* Women of menopausal age are at risk for osteoporosis, and foods high in calcium should be encouraged. All the foods in option 3 are high in calcium. Chicken and eggs are high in protein; wheat and corn are high in carbohydrates.
Cognitive Level: Analysis
Nursing Process: Analysis; *Test Plan:* HPM

2   **Answer: 1** *Rationale:* The factors presented in option 1 put the client at risk for osteoporosis. Smoking, alcohol intake and dietary deficiency of calcium and vitamin D are major factors in the development of osteoporosis. Deficient protein and carbohydrate intake, obesity, depression, and history of falls do not contribute to the development of osteoporosis.
Cognitive Level: Application
Nursing Process: Analysis; *Test Plan:* HPM

3   **Answer: 4** *Rationale:* Fosamax is the drug that prevents bone resorption. Calcitonin (Micalcin) in-

creases bone mass and is dispensed as a nasal spray; raloxifene (Evista) is a selective receptor modulator.
Cognitive Level: Analysis
Nursing Process: Planning; *Test Plan:* PHYS

4   **Answer: 1** *Rationale:* The client with hip surgery should avoid all activities that will cause hip adduction, internal rotation, and flexion beyond 90 degrees. The focus of the teaching on clients with hip surgery is to avoid dislocation and the risk for further injury.
Cognitive Level: Application
Nursing Process: Implementation; *Test Plan:* HPM

5   **Answer: 1** *Rationale:* Extremes of internal rotation, adduction and 90 degree flexion of the hip should be avoided 4 to 6 weeks after surgery to prevent dislocation. Although use of elevated seats prevents excess flexion of the hip, it alone does not suffice in preventing dislocation. Bending activities (such as putting on shoes) places the client at risk for dislocation. Abduc-

tion pillows are used to prevent external rotation and must be used postoperatively.
Cognitive Level: Application
Nursing Process: Implementation; *Test Plan:* SECE

6 **Answer: 3** *Rationale:* Musculoskeletal injuries and subsequent treatment have the potential to cause complications. Bleeding and swelling from the surgery may cause compression of nerves that can lead to permanent neurological damage and paralysis. Frequent assessment of the neurovascular status of the client is essential following laminectomy. Neurovascular assessment includes assessing for pain, pulses, pallor, paresthesia, and paralysis. The physician usually orders ambulation. Vital signs are not done every 30 minutes unless the client is in the post-anesthesia care unit. Although loss of bladder tone may indicate nerve damage, it may also be a residual effect of the anesthesia. Assessing ability to void becomes of prime importance if the client is due to void, usually 6 to 8 hours after last voiding.
Cognitive Level: Analysis
Nursing Process: Assessment: *Test Plan:* PHYS

7 **Answer: 3** *Rationale:* The pull of traction on the affected limb should never be disturbed to ensure healing and union of the bone in proper alignment. This intervention is an independent nursing activity and does not require a physician's order. A change in weight is not indicated. Elevating the client's feet will not correct the situation.
Cognitive Level: Application
Nursing Process: Implementation; *Test Plan:* SECE

8 **Answer: 1** *Rationale:* A major complication of skeletal traction is infection. The nurse must provide pin site care using aseptic technique to prevent infection. Although the other options might be appropriate, option 1 is an essential nursing intervention.
Cognitive Level: Application
Nursing Process: Planning; *Test Plan:* SECE

9 **Answer: 4** *Rationale:* Unrelieved pain, diminished pulses, pallor, paresthesias, and pain on passive motion are all symptoms of compartment syndrome. This is a medical emergency because the pressure must be relieved in the affected limb. Otherwise, the swelling in the closed compartment may lead to further permanent complications, such as loss of the limb. Options 2 and 3, although appropriate, are not the priority interventions in this case. The administration of oxygen is an inappropriate initial action in this situation.
Cognitive Level: Analysis
Nursing Process: Analysis; *Test Plan:* PHYS

10 **Answer: 3** *Rationale:* The elevated temperature, chills, malaise, and pain are all clinical manifestations of osteomyelitis. Symptoms of fat embolism include acute respiratory distress. Symptoms of compartment syndrome include progressively worsening pain distal to the affected site unrelieved by analgesics. Malunion of the bone will not cause an elevated temperature.
Cognitive Level: Analysis
Nursing Process: Analysis; *Test Plan:* PHYS

Posttest

1 **Answer: 2** *Rationale:* An arthrogram involves injecting dye into a joint for diagnostic purposes. It is critical that the nurse evaluate the client for history of allergic reaction to contrast dye before the procedure since this can lead to a life-threatening response such as anaphylactic shock. The other options are not priority assessments or are irrelevant.
Cognitive Level: Analysis
Nursing Process: Assessment; *Test Plan:* SECE

2 **Answer: 1** *Rationale:* Low bone mass, structural deterioration of bone tissue leading to bone fragility, and increased susceptibility to fractures is seen with osteoporosis. The client also has risk factors associated with osteoporosis: smoking, sedentary lifestyle, and being female and postmenopausal.
Cognitive Level: Application
Nursing Process: Analysis; *Test Plan:* PHYS

3 **Answer: 3** *Rationale:* After laminectomy it is critical that proper body alignment is maintained to prevent postoperative complications such as neurological damage. Logrolling technique ensures that the client turns as a unit. All the other options put stress on the spine.
Cognitive Level: Application
Nursing Process: Implementation; *Test Plan:* PHYS

4 **Answer: 3** *Rationale:* Handling a cast that is not completely dry with the fingertips creates indentations in the cast. These indented areas are thinner and are prone to cracks when the cast is completely dry. A wet cast should be handled with the flat part of the hands and exposed to air to assist in drying.
Cognitive Level: Application
Nursing Process: Implementation; *Test Plan:* SECE

5 **Answer: 3** *Rationale:* Countertraction will prevent the client from sliding to the foot of the bed. This can be achieved with Trendelenburg position of the bed or raising the foot of the bed slightly if the client's body

weight is not sufficient. The other options do not add to countertraction.
Cognitive Level: Application
Nursing Process: Planning; *Test Plan:* SECE

6 Answer: 4 *Rationale:* Clients with joint replacement require aggressive physical therapy postoperatively to regain range of motion in the joint caused by pain and swelling. The other nursing diagnoses are not a priority at this time.
Cognitive Level: Analysis
Nursing Process: Analysis; *Test Plan:* PHYS

7 Answer: 2 *Rationale:* A classic sign of scoliosis is asymmetrical dress or skirt tail/hem caused by unevenness of the affected shoulder and hip. The lateral curvature resulting from the spinal deformity causes the asymmetry. The other options do not necessarily cause all the manifestations listed in the question.
Cognitive Level: Application
Nursing Process: Assessment; *Test Plan:* HPM

8 Answer: 1 *Rationale:* Weights help to keep the fractured extremity in proper alignment to facilitate healing and therefore should not be manipulated. Nursing interventions for clients in traction should include ensuring that the weights hang freely at all times to

maintain the line of pull. Traction is not released because there should be a steady pull (option 2). Options 3 and 4 do not address the issue of the question.
Cognitive Level: Analysis
Nursing Process: Analysis; *Test Plan:* SECE

9 Answer: 2 *Rationale:* Estrogen therapy decreases bone demineralization preventing progression of osteoporosis. It also increases bone density in the spine and hip and therefore reduces the risk of fractures. The other options do not appropriately describe the action of estrogen in the preventive and therapeutic management of osteoporosis.
Cognitive Level: Application
Nursing Process: Analysis; *Test Plan:* PHYS

10 Answer: 1 *Rationale:* A client who undergoes surgery to the hip must be careful to avoid flexing the joint to greater than 90 degrees postoperatively to prevent dislocating the hip. There is no portable Buck's traction, although traction may be used preoperatively to immobilize the limb. A soft cushion is not essential. The client may need to use a walker for assistance, but does not need crutches.
Cognitive Level: Application
Nursing Process: Implementation; *Test Plan:* HPM

References

Ackley, J. B. & Ackley, L. G. (1999). *Nursing diagnosis handbook* (4th ed.). St. Louis, MO: Mosby Inc., pp. 52, 56, 73–74, 78–79.

American Academy of Orthopedic Surgeons. (2000, March). *Musculoskeletal conditions in the U.S.* (2nd ed.). Retrieved January 06, 2001, from the World Wide Web: http://orthoinfor.aaos.org.

Kee, L. J. (1999). *Laboratory diagnostic tests with nursing implications.* Stamford, CT: Appleton & Lange, pp. 89–94, 333–335.

Kozier, B., Erb, G., Berman, A., & Burke, K. (2000). *Fundamentals of nursing: Concepts, process, and practice* (6th ed.). Upper Saddle River, NJ: Prentice Hall, Inc., pp. 1051–1057.

Lewis, M. S., Heitkemper, M. M., & Dirksen, R. S. (2000). *Medical surgical nursing: Assessment and management of clinical problems* (5th ed.). St. Louis, MO: Mosby, Inc. pp. 1745–1859.

LeMone, P. & Burke, K. (2000). *Medical surgical nursing: Critical thinking in client care* (2nd ed.). Upper Saddle River, NJ: Prentice Hall, Inc., pp. 1514–1623.

Lilley, L., & Aucker, S. R. (1999). *Pharmacology and the nursing process* (2nd ed.). St. Louis, MO: Mosby, Inc., pp. 579–585.

MedicineNet.com. (2000, July, 14). Arthritis disease and conditions. Retrieved January 06, 2001, from the World Wide Web: http://www.medicinenet.com.

National Institutes of Health. (2001, January 06). National resource center: Osteoporosis and related bone disease. Washington, DC: Author. Retrieved January 06, 2001, from the World Wide Web: http://www.osteo.org/pdisbone.html.

Pagana, D. K., & Pagana, J. T. (2001). *Mosby's diagnostic and laboratory test reference* (5th ed.). St. Louis, MO: Mosby Inc., pp. 67–68, 87–89, 376–377, 876–879.

Wilkinson M. J. (2000). *Nursing diagnosis handbook with NIC interventions and NOC outcomes* (7th ed.). Upper Saddle River, NJ: Prentice Hall, Inc., pp. 561–562, 605–606.

Wong, L. D., & Eaton, H. M. (2001). *Wong's essentials of pediatric nursing* (6th ed.). St. Louis, MO., p. 1261.

CHAPTER 10

Integumentary Disorders

Jill C. Cash, RN-CS, MSN, FNP
Julie A. Adkins, RN, MSN, FNP

CHAPTER OUTLINE

OBJECTIVES

▋ Identify basic structures and functions of the integumentary system.

▋ Describe the pathophysiology and etiology of common integumentary disorders.

▋ Discuss expected assessment data and diagnostic test findings for selected integumentary disorders.

▋ Identify priority nursing diagnoses for selected integumentary disorders.

▋ Discuss nursing management of a client experiencing an integumentary disorder.

▋ Identify expected outcomes for the client experiencing an integumentary disorder.

[Media Link]

Use the CD-ROM enclosed with this text, or log onto the address given to access the free, interactive Companion Website created for this series. The CD-ROM and Companion Website accompanying this book offer additional practice opportunities and Information—NCLEX Review, Case Studies, Glossary, In Depth with NCLEX, and more.

www.prenhall.com/hogan

REVIEW AT A GLANCE

acne *androgenically stimulated inflam-matory disorder of the sebaceous glands resulting in comedones, papules, pustules, and occasional scarring*

actinic keratosis *pre-malignant macules found on the skin surface of fair-skinned people often after age 50 but may be present at any age*

basal cell carcinoma *abnormal cell growth of the basal layer of the epidermal skin*

candidiasis *infection caused by Candida albicans, a yeast-like fungus that most often causes superficial cutaneous infection*

contact dermatitis *an eruption of the skin related to contact with an irritating substance or allergen*

eczema *inflammatory response in which the skin appears erythemic, scaly, dry, and thickened*

macule *non-palpable, flat lesion with color measuring <1 cm*

nodule *elevated firm lesion with a circumscribed border measuring 1 to 2 cm*

papule *elevated, palpable mass measuring < 0.5 cm*

pediculosis *an infestation of the skin or hair by the species of blood-sucking lice capable of living as external parasites on the human host, such as Pediculosis capitis (head) and Pediculosis pubis (pubic)*

plaque *elevated group of papules that have convalesced into one lesion measuring > 0.5 cm*

pressure ulcers *ischemic lesions of the skin and underlying tissues caused by external pressure that impairs the flow of blood and lymph*

psoriasis *a genetically determined chronic epidermal proliferative disease characterized by erythematous, dry scaling patches*

pustule *elevated, serous (pus) filled vesicle that can measure any size*

scabies *a contagious disease caused by the infestation of the skin by the mite Sarcoptes scabiei var. hominis*

squamous cell carcinoma *a cutaneous malignancy that arises from keratinocytes*

Tinea corporis *commonly known as ringworm; a fungal infection affecting the face, trunk and extremities with exclusion of the palms of the hands, soles of the feet, and groin*

Tinea pedis *commonly known as athlete's foot; a fungal infection affecting the plantar surface of the feet*

urticaria *an itchy rash*

vesicle *fluid-filled, elevated mass which measures < 0.5 cm; if greater than 0.5 cm, it is a bulla*

vitiligo *totally white macules where there is absence of melanocytes*

wheal *elevated erythemic lesion that contains fluid in the tissue of the skin with an irregular border and variable in size*

Pretest

1 The nurse notes that a client has an elevated lesion that contains clear fluid and measures >1 cm in diameter. This finding is best documented by the nurse as which of the following?

(1) Papule
(2) Vesicle
(3) Bulla
(4) Pustule

2 The nurse alerts the primary care practitioner about a mole. Which of these characteristics indicates the need for intervention?

(1) A dark brown, irregular-bordered mole with a black-appearing center that has grown approximately 2 cm in the past 2 months.
(2) A 2 cm waxy papule that has a "stuck on" appearance.
(3) A small, flat mole that has been on the client's back since birth.
(4) Multiple small, flat, nonpruritic moles that have been on the client's elbow for 10 years.

3 A client with herpes simplex virus 1 makes the remark that she hopes she never gets another lesion on her lip "like this one." What is the nurse's best response?

(1) "The chances of getting another lesion on your lip are very low."
(2) "Herpes simplex virus 1 can be reactivated at any time."
(3) "The lesions will also appear on other parts of the body."
(4) "A red, pinpoint painless rash will continue to develop for the next two weeks."

4   The nurse would include which of the following priority interventions in the plan of care for a client diagnosed with herpes zoster?

(1) Monitor daily dietary intake and daily weights.
(2) Encourage daily activity routines to keep the client mobile.
(3) Monitor skin integrity for secondary bacterial infections.
(4) Maintain a warm environment to decrease the intensity of the pruritus.

5   The client telephones that she wants to come to the office for evaluation of a painful wart. The nurse anticipates that the client will present with which of the following cutaneous lesions that is commonly painful?

(1) Common wart
(2) Flat wart
(3) Plantar wart
(4) Filiform wart

6   The client presents with an increase in the number of white patches across his chest and back. Multiple creams and lotions were not helpful. The nurse concludes that this client's clinical picture is consistent with which of the following conditions?

(1) Vitiligo
(2) Eczema
(3) Psoriasis
(4) Contact dermatitis

7   When counseling clients regarding first-line burn prevention, the nurse should plan to include which of the following items?

(1) Discuss the temperature setting of the water heater.
(2) Demonstrate the use of a fire extinguisher.
(3) Assist the planning of an escape route.
(4) Stress the need for smoke detectors.

8   When caring for a client with a burn in the emergent stage, which of the following has lowest priority as part of an accurate burn assessment?

(1) Where it occurred
(2) Cause of the burn
(3) First-aid treatment given
(4) Gender

9   The client presents with a pruritic rash. Questions about which of the following would help differentiate the cause?

(1) Location of the rash
(2) Age of the client
(3) Gender
(4) Recent travel

10   In obtaining a health history on a client with psoriasis, which recent infection is significant?

(1) Escherichia coli
(2) Streptococcus
(3) Staphylococcus
(4) Pneumonia

See pages 411–412 for Answers and Rationales.

I. Basic Structures of the Integumentary System

A. Epidermis

1. The outer layer of the skin structure made up of epithelial cells

2. The epidermis is broken down into four layers throughout the body, with the exception of the palms of the hands and the soles of the feet that contain five layers of cells within the epidermal layer

   a. Stratum basale

   b. Stratus spinosum

      c. Stratum granulosum

      d. Stratum lucidum

      e. Stratum corneum

B. Dermis

  1. The second layer of the skin is made up of lymph vessels, blood vessels, and nerve fibers

  2. The dermis is broken down into two layers, the papillary layer and the reticular layer

      a. Papillary layer: contains capillaries and receptor sites for touch and pain

      b. Reticular layer: contains receptors for deep touch as well as sweat and sebaceous glands

C. Subcutaneous tissue

  1. Is the layer that lies beneath the dermis

  2. Is made up of adipose (fat) tissue

D. Appendages

  1. Structures of the integumentary system that grow beyond the epidermal structure; include hair, nails, and glands

  2. Hair: composed of primarily dead cells; hair root begins in the bulb of the hair follicle and grows from the dermis outward; the hair root is located under the dermis and becomes the hair shaft after the hair exits the dermal layer

  3. Nails: primarily made up of dead cells that cover the nail bed; the nail structure begins in the epidermis and extends across the nail bed

  4. Glands

      a. Apocrine: sweat glands located in the axilla, anus, and genital area

      b. Eccrine: sweat glands located on the forehead, hands, and soles of the feet

      c. Sebaceous: glands located throughout the body that secrete sebum and that are highly influenced by increased hormones, especially androgens (see Figure 10-1)

II. Basic Functions of the Integumentary System

NCLEX!

A. Epidermis

  1. Outer layer of the skin that protects the body and internal structures from harm by providing a barrier to the external environment

  2. Phagocytes, which also protect the body from invading bacteria, are located in the epidermal layer

  3. This layer stores melanin to protect the body from harmful ultraviolet rays

  4. When sunlight reaches the skin, the cholesterol molecules located in this layer are converted to vitamin D

  5. The epidermis maintains the body's hydration status

Figure 10-1   **Anatomy of the skin.**

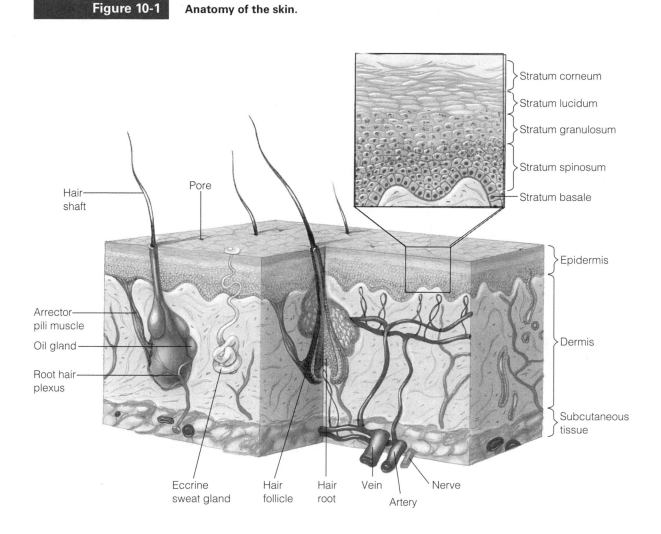

Stratum corneum

Stratum lucidum

Stratum granulosum

Stratum spinosum

Stratum basale

Epidermis

Dermis

Subcutaneous tissue

Hair shaft

Pore

Arrector pili muscle

Oil gland

Root hair plexus

Eccrine sweat gland

Hair follicle

Hair root

Vein

Artery

Nerve

B. Dermis

   1. This layer regulates the body temperature

   2. It also serves as a conducting agent to transmit messages from the nerve endings to the central nervous system (CNS)

C. Subcutaneous tissue

   1. Is the tissue below the dermis

   2. Assists in connecting the skin to the structures below the subcutaneous tissue

D. Appendages

   1. Hair: protects and pads the scalp from external objects as well as serves as a mechanism to maintain body temperature

   2. Nails: cover the dorsum of each digit on the hands and feet to protect the nail bed of each digit

3. Glands

   a. Apocrine: function unknown

   b. Eccrine: maintain a stable temperature for the body through perspiration when the body is overheated

   c. Sebaceous: oil glands that secrete sebum to lubricate the skin and hair as well as aid in killing bacteria on the surface of the skin

III. Assessment of the Integumentary System

A. Subjective data

1. Past medical history

   a. Note previous problems with skin, hair, scalp, or nails; discuss duration of symptoms, associated symptoms, treatments used and results

   NCLEX!

   b. Medical disorders: discuss all systems of the body (cardiovascular, respiratory, endocrine/metabolic, hepatic, and hematology) that may manifest as a skin disorder; be sure to note any allergies to medications, foods, environment, etc.; note allergies to tape, povidone iodine (Betadine), alcohol, and other substances

   c. Nutrition: note dietary changes, new foods introduced, and fluid intake

   NCLEX!

   d. External exposure: note new products exposed to the skin, such as soaps, lotions, sun, and chemicals

   e. Activity: note daily physical activity and exercise routine

   f. Sleep-rest: note number of hours of sleep each night and any rest periods

   g. Coping: discuss skin disorders and how skin is affected when stress is experienced; note coping behaviors used and results

2. Current medications: list current medications, onset and dose of medications

3. Recent surgeries or treatments: note any recent surgeries or treatment that may affect the skin, e.g., phototherapy, radiation therapy

   NCLEX!

4. Current problem: elicit information regarding current problem; for skin rash, obtain detailed information such as the date rash began, how it has changed, medications or ointments used and results of treatment

B. Objective data/physical examination

1. Inspection

   a. Note color (pink, yellow, white, purple, bruising, etc.)

   NCLEX!

   b. For lesions, document color, size, shape, symmetry, and border (see Box 10-1)

   c. Inspect hair for color, amount, distribution, lesions, and hygiene

   d. Inspect nails for color, growth pattern, and thickness; inspect nail bed for inflammation or trauma

2. Palpation

   a. Note texture, temperature and moisture of skin

   b. Palpate skin turgor for hydration status

   c. Palpate lower extremities (tibia and ankle) for edema

Box 10-1

Characteristics of Skin Lesions

Clients should be informed about how to monitor skin lesions. The "ABCD" rule is useful in teaching clients how to monitor changes in skin lesions and will assist clients to know when to seek further assessment from the practitioner. The following is the "ABCD" rule of thumb for monitoring skin lesions:

A = Asymmetry: Note any asymmetrical changes of the skin lesion. Lesions are normally symmetrical in shape. Any changes in the symmetry of the lesion need to be evaluated for possible removal.

B = Border: The border of the lesion should appear smooth. Note changes in the border that appear rough and jagged and have the lesion evaluated for possible removal.

C = Color: The color of a lesion should stay the same. Lesions that get darker (brown or black) or have more than one color need to be evaluated for possible removal.

D = Diameter: The diameter or size of the lesion should be measured and documented. Lesions that change in size and enlarge need to be monitored and evaluated for possible removal.

    d. For lesions, note location and palpate texture, consistency, and mobility

    e. Palpate hair for texture (coarse, fine); palpate nails for texture and check capillary refill

IV. Disorders of the Integumentary System

  A. Problems caused by vascularity

    1. Spider angioma: a flat, bright red spot with radiating blood vessels at the edges, commonly found on the upper body; it varies in size from a tiny dot up to 1.5 to 2 cm; spider angiomas are caused by vascular dilation of the vessels commonly seen with high estrogen levels, pregnancy, liver disease, and/or vitamin B deficiency

    2. Petechiae: flat red spots, approximately 1 to 2 mm in diameter that do not change in color when blanched; these are caused by tiny capillaries that have broken, possibly caused by thinning of the blood (anticoagulant effect), liver disease, vitamin K deficiency, or septicemia

    3. Purpura: purple/blue-appearing patch, varies in size and shape, caused by a bleeding disorder or broken blood vessels and may appear throughout the body

  B. Primary skin lesions (see Figure 10-2)

    1. Macule: nonpalpable, flat lesion that has color and measures < 1 cm; examples: freckles, chloasma

    2. Nodule: an elevated firm lesion with a circumscribed border that measures approximately 1 to 2 cm

    3. Papule: elevated, palpable mass, measuring less than 0.5 cm; examples include warts and moles

      a. Management of papules depends on the diagnosis, such as cryotherapy for wart removal

      b. Mole removal may be recommended if the mole is considered premalignant; different methods of mole removal are available

      c. Excision of the mole is one treatment that may be done in the office setting; nursing care prior to treatment would be to explain the procedure to the client and obtain history of allergies (betadine, alcohol)

Figure 10-2

Primary skin lesions.

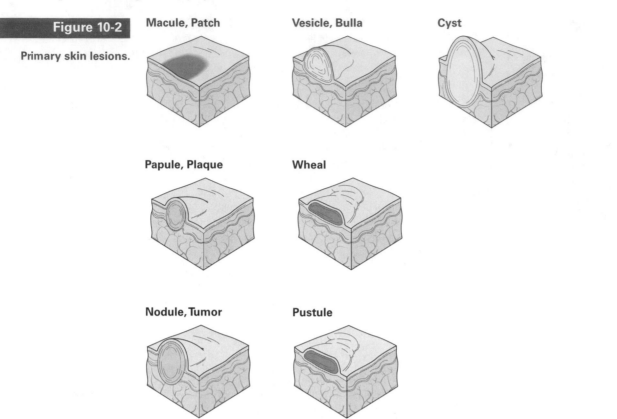

Macule, Patch

Vesicle, Bulla

Cyst

Papule, Plaque

Wheal

Nodule, Tumor

Pustule

4. **Plaque:** elevated group of papules that have convalesced into one lesion measuring greater than 0.5 cm; examples are actinic keratosis and psoriasis

5. **Pustule:** elevated, serous (pus)–filled vesicle that can measure any size; examples include acne and boils

6. **Vesicle:** fluid-filled, elevated mass that measures less than 0.5 cm; if the fluid mass measures greater than 0.5 cm, the mass is termed a bulla; examples of vesicles include chickenpox, small burns, and herpes virus lesion

7. **Wheal:** variable-sized, elevated erythemic lesion with an irregular border that contains fluid in the tissue of the skin; examples include insect bites and hives

C. Secondary skin lesions

1. Atrophy: dry, thin, taut skin that appears wasted from loss of collagen; an example is aged skin; hydration with fluids and keeping skin well-moisturized with emollients such as Eucerin™ cream are helpful for this condition

2. Crusts: dried pus or blood on the skin surface resulting from a vesicle that has ruptured; examples of crusts include the final stages of chickenpox lesions or impetigo lesions

3. Erosion: superficial indentation of the skin that results from a previous lesion; an example of erosion is a scratch mark that has not healed over time; therapeutic management includes warm, moist compresses to the site for comfort; keep site clean and dry, cleaning with antibacterial soaps at least three to four

NCLEX!

times a day; may need to apply topical antibiotics if site gets secondary bacterial infection

4. Fissure: linear break in the skin with sharp edges, extending into the dermis; examples include athlete's foot or cracks in the corner of the mouth from chapped lips; therapeutic management for athlcte's foot includes antifungal medications along with keeping the feet cool and dry; encourage use of white, cool socks and avoid allowing the feet to sweat; fissures of the lips may bc treated with topical ointments such as petroleum jelly or Blistex™ ointment

5. Scales: dry, dead skin that sloughs off the skin surface and that may be dry or greasy; examples include dandruff or psoriasis

6. Scar: the flat connective tissue resulting from healing over the site of previous injury, which may vary in size, color, and shape; examples include healed surgery incisions or acne scars

7. Ulcers: deep excavations in the skin; they may vary in size and shape and extend into the dermis or subcutaneous tissue; examples include chancres and pressure ulcers

D. Chronic dermatologic problems

1. Eczema

    a. Description: inflammatory response in which the skin appears erythemic, scaly, dry and thickened; eczema may appear in various stages, depending on the type (e.g., infantile eczema vs. adult eczema); the etiology is unknown; eczema is characterized by lymphohistiocytic infiltration of the vessels of the skin

    b. Clinical manifestations: are generally secondary to scratching of the skin; dry, pruritic skin that appears thickened and discolored, may even cause a break in the skin in which bleeding or oozing occurs; lesions may appear as papules or pustules that can lead to excoriation

    c. Therapeutic management

        1) Bath: advise the client not to use harsh soaps; avoid frequent bathing

        2) Wet dressings of Burow's solution may be used in severe cases

        3) Emollients: frequent use of emollients (Eucerin™, Aquaphor™) is recommended

        4) Allergens: remove all triggers and/or allergens; avoid skin contact with all wool products and lanolin preparations

    d. Priority nursing diagnoses: Impaired skin integrity, Altered comfort

    e. Medication thcrapy: antihistamines such as diphenhydramine hydrochloride (Benadryl™); severe cases may require topical or oral steroids for brief periods

2. Psoriasis

    a. Description: a chronic, inflammatory skin disorder in which lesions appear as whitish, scaly plaques on the scalp, knees, and/or elbows; psoriasis has no known etiology; it is thought to be a multifactorial disease in which a

T-lymphocyte mediated dermal immune response occurs; most clients with psoriasis have a family history of the disease

NCLEX!

b. Clinical manifestations: dry, scaly rash that may appear as silvery scales or plaques usually found on the scalp, knees, or elbows

NCLEX!

c. Therapeutic management: direct sun exposure to the skin site may be beneficial for some clients; emollients: frequent use of emollients and keratolytic agents are beneficial for scalp psoriasis; topical steroids may also be prescribed; antihistamines may be used for pruritus

d. Priority nursing diagnoses: Impaired skin integrity, Altered comfort

3. Seborrheic dermatitis

a. Description: a common chronic skin condition occurring in areas of active sebaceous glands, such as the face, scalp, body folds, sternal area, and axilla; this dermatitis appears as an erythematous scaling lesion that may appear dry or greasy; etiology is unknown but possible causes are believed to be hormonal influence, nutritional deficiency, neurogenic influence, dysfunction of the sebaceous glands, and/or fungal infection

b. Clinical manifestations: erythemic, scaly lesions that appear in varying degrees (oily or flaky dry skin), are pruritic, and may cause secondary bacterial infections; common sites include scalp, eyebrows, nose, ears, sternal area, and axilla; seborrheic dermatitis is seen more frequently in colder weather periods, and it is thought to be caused by decreased humidification and decreased exposure to sunlight

NCLEX!

c. Therapeutic management: scalp treatment: selenium sulfide 2.5 percent suspension or coal tar shampoos and topical steroid creams

d. Priority nursing diagnoses: Impaired skin integrity, Altered comfort, Risk for infection

E. Malignant neoplasms

1. Actinic keratosis

a. Description: pre-malignant macules found on the skin surface of fair-skinned individuals who are 50 years of age or older, but can be seen in high-risk individuals at any age; development of these lesions occurs because of chronic sun exposure to the skin; persons with light-skin complexion are at the highest risk for actinic keratosis; these lesions are considered pre-malignant lesions; approximately 1 percent of these lesions will progress to squamous cell carcinoma

b. Clinical manifestations: erythematous, rough, and shiny-textured macules that may appear as a single macule or in groups; they are commonly seen on the face, ears, scalp, lips, neck, and hands

c. Therapeutic management

1) Prophylactic treatment is recommended to prevent development of these lesions

2) Protection from ultraviolet rays of the sun with the use of clothing and sunscreens are recommended when exposed to sunlight

3) Biopsy and removal of the lesion is recommended if changes in the lesion occur; these changes include the color, border, size, and shape of the lesions; refer back to Box 10-1 if needed

2. Basal cell carcinoma

   a. Description: an abnormal cell growth of the basal layer of the epidermal skin; the most common contributor to this growth is ultraviolet rays from sunlight exposure; the basal cells do not mature appropriately into keratinocytes, which results in neoplastic growth of the cells; the surrounding tissue is also destroyed; basal cell carcinoma is the least aggressive type of skin cancer and rarely metastasizes to other organs

   b. Clinical manifestations: types and characteristics of the five types of basal cell carcinoma are:

     1) Nodular basal cell carcinoma: small, firm papule, which appears as pearly, white, pink, or flesh-colored, and is commonly seen on the face, neck, and/or head

     2) Superficial basal cell carcinoma: this papule or plaque is the second most common lesion and is commonly seen on the trunk and extremities

     3) Pigmented basal cell carcinoma: this tumor is less common and usually found on the head, neck, or face; it has the ability to concentrate melanin, which causes deeper pigmentation of the center of the tumor

     4) Morpheaform basal cell carcinoma: this is the least common form; this tumor is found on the head and neck, appearing like a tumor with finger-like projections (usually ivory- or flesh-colored) and typically resembles a scar; it has the ability to invade and destroy adjacent tissue and structures

     5) Keratotic basal cell carcinoma: this tumor is found on the preauricular or postauricular area; it contains both basal cells and squamous cells that keratinize; if removed, this tumor is likely to recur; it also has a high risk of metastasizing to other structures

   c. Therapeutic management

     1) Monitor progress of growth of all lesions; lesions that measure >2 cm have a high reoccurrence rate; suspicious lesions are excised and sent for pathological examination

     2) Educate clients regarding importance of monitoring lesions and early identification of new lesions; suggest monthly assessment of the skin by the client and periodic screening based on symptoms by healthcare provider

     3) Encourage protection from ultraviolet light exposure by using sunscreen products with SPF > 15 and wearing clothing such as hats and clothing to protect the skin

   d. Priority nursing diagnoses: Impaired skin integrity, Risk for disturbed body image, Fear or anxiety

   e. Medication therapy: none

Practice to Pass

A client tells you that she has a mole that she has noticed for the past year, and she is concerned that it is cancer. What is your immediate response to teach her how to evaluate the mole?

NCLEX!

NCLEX!

3. Cutaneous T-cell lymphoma

   a. Description: a type of lymphoma involving the skin that rarely invades the lymph nodes; it is a thymus-derived helper cell cancer

   b. Clinical manifestations: three stages of this disease exist; however, the stages may occur either in sequence or at the same time

      1) Stage 1—erythematous stage: erythemic, well-defined border patch that is pruritic and may resemble psoriasis or eczema; the patch may become diffuse with severe itching

      2) Stage 2—plaque stage: erythemic scaly patches that become indurated and/or elevated; the center of the plaque may appear healed, with rough ring-shaped borders; this stage may resemble tertiary syphilis or erythema multiforme perstans

      3) Stage 3—tumor stage: the terminal stage in which tumor growth of the plaques occur, often seen with secondary bacterial infection

   c. Therapeutic management: initial stages may only require a tar cream and treatment with ultraviolet B therapy; PUVA has also been effective in this treatment; nitrogen mustard treatment has also been beneficial when used in earlier stages

   d. Priority nursing diagnoses: Impaired skin integrity, Fear or anxiety, Risk for disturbed body image

   e. Medication therapy: systemic corticosteroids are used for the first two stages; radiation therapy and electron-beam radiation may be used at any point in the disease; systemic chemotherapy has been used during the plaque and tumor stage, but may not always be successful

4. Kaposi's sarcoma

   a. Description: a rare skin cancer of the endothelial lining of the small blood vessels, seen most commonly on the face, nose, and ears; the etiology is unknown; Kaposi's sarcoma is a cancer speculated to be related to an infective agent such as a retrovirus, such as the virus that causes acquired immunodeficiency syndrome (AIDS)

   b. Clinical manifestations

      1) Vascular lesions (macules, papules, nodules) that can affect the skin and viscera

      2) Over time the lesions enlarge and become confluent, forming large masses; as these masses enlarge, the tissue below the mass becomes involved and the tumor then invades the lymphatic tissue, which may then result in varying degrees of lymphedema, primarily affecting the genitalia and lower extremities

      3) As the disease progresses, this tumor may interfere with internal organ function and may even cause bleeding to the point of hemorrhage (commonly seen as a late sign)

      4) Initially Kaposi's sarcoma may be symptom-free; however, pain maybe experienced in the later stages

NCLEX!

NCLEX!

c. Therapeutic management: isolated lesions may be removed by excision, cryotherapy, and/or local radiation for comfort and/or cosmetic treatment

d. Priority nursing diagnoses: Impaired skin integrity, Fear or anxiety, Risk for disturbed body image

e. Medication therapy: chemotherapy treatment can be used as a single agent or a combination treatment

F. Nonmelanoma: *Squamous cell carcinoma*

1. Description

a. The most common type of skin cancer; fair-skinned males tend to have a higher incidence of nonmelanoma skin cancer, with the majority of these cancers occurring from 30 to 60 years of age

b. Squamous cell carcinoma occurs on areas of the skin that are frequently exposed to ultraviolet light, such as the face, ears, nose, lips, and hands; of two nonmelanoma types of carcinoma, squamous cell carcinoma grows quicker, is more aggressive, and is more likely to metastasize than basal cell carcinoma

2. Etiology and pathophysiology

a. The etiology of squamous cell carcinoma is multifactorial

b. Environmental causes include ultraviolet radiation, chemicals, physical trauma, and pollution

c. With exposure of ultraviolet light to the skin, the rays penetrate the tissue and alter normal DNA and suppress the body's T-cell and B-cell immunity, producing tumors of the squamous epithelial or mucous membranes

d. As the tumor grows, the cells increase in size and an irregular shape is formed

e. Tumors may proliferate and invade the dermal layer of the skin

f. Squamous cell carcinoma may also present from preexisting skin lesions, such as old scars; these tumors may proliferate into the dermal structure and can cause metastasis by the lymphatic tissue

3. Clinical manifestations

a. Squamous cell carcinoma may present as a small fleshy colored papule that is firm to touch

b. As the tumor grows, the color may change and appear erythemic, sore, and/or even bleed if touched

4. Therapeutic management

a. Recommended management of squamous cell tumors is removal of the tumors by a variety of methods, including cryotherapy, surgical excision, electrodesiccation, or radiotherapy

b. The cure rate with these methods is approximately 90 percent

c. It is recommended to remove these tumors as soon as identified to prevent the person's risk of metastasis

➤ *Practice to Pass*

A 20-year-old client who comes in to the ambulatory clinic for treatment mentions that her father was just diagnosed with skin cancer. She asks you what she can do to protect herself from developing skin cancer later in life. What strategies would you suggest to reduce her risk of developing skin cancer?

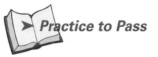

d. Nursing management for these clients includes teaching methods to prevent further tumors from arising, by minimizing sun exposure, wear protective clothing, wear sunscreen with a SPF of 15 or greater and to avoid tanning booths

5. Priority nursing diagnoses: Impaired skin integrity, Ineffective health maintenance, Fear or anxiety, Risk for disturbed body image

6. Medication therapy: none

G. Bacterial infections

1. Impetigo

a. Description: A superficial skin infection that initially appears as an erythemic vesicle and later changes to a honey-colored crusted lesion

1) Is most commonly seen in children but occasionally affects adults

2) An alteration in skin integrity occurs, and bacteria invade the epidermis and cause an infection

3) The most common organisms are *Staphylococcus aureas* and *group-A beta-hemolytic streptococcus*

b. Clinical manifestations

1) These skin lesions are commonly found on the face, arms, legs, and buttocks

2) The lesions appear as thin erythemic vesicles, which then becomes honey-colored crusts or erosions

3) They may occur as a single lesion or several lesions that have convalesced and appear as a group of lesions

c. Therapeutic management: encourage good handwashing with hot soapy water to prevent spreading the bacteria to others; for recurrent lesions, a culture of the site is obtained to isolate the pathogens

d. Priority nursing diagnosis: Ineffective health maintenance

e. Medication therapy: topical antibiotics, or for severe cases, systemic antibiotics are recommended

2. Folliculitis

a. Description

1) A superficial bacterial infection of the hair follicle

2) Folliculitis can occur at any age and is seen more frequently in males

3) It can be aggravated by shaving, particularly the skin on the face (beard), legs, and axilla

4) The most common pathogens responsible for folliculitis are *Staphyloccus aureus* and *Pseudomonas aeruginosa*

b. Clinical manifestations

1) Lesion appears as an erythemic, pruritic, mildly tender pustule located at the hair follicle; various stages of folliculitis may occur, including a simple pustule, progressing to a furuncle or carbuncle

2) In severe cases, fever and chills may be present

Practice to Pass

You see a young adult in the office whose mother thinks that he has impetigo. How could you teach the client to prevent spreading the infection to others?

NCLEX!

c. Therapeutic management

1) Topical treatment includes cleaning the site with warm soapy water two to three times a day

2) Warm compresses may be used for comfort as needed

3) If razors are being used, encourage the client to use clean, sharp razors, and to throw away old razors

4) Do not use irritating lotions or creams at the site

d. Priority nursing diagnosis: Impaired skin integrity

e. Medication therapy: for simple folliculitis, topical mupirocon (Bactroban) applied to the site three times a day is effective; for more severe cases, oral antibiotics are recommended

3. Furuncle

a. Description: an erythemic, warm, tender nodule of the skin; commonly seen in children, teens, and young adults; common sites are the nares, neck, axilla, and genital area; *Staphylococcus* is the most common infective organism and may be chronic in some cases

b. Clinical manifestations: warm, erythemic tender nodule of the hair follicle

NCLEX!

c. Therapeutic management: warm moist heat may be applied to the site for comfort; occasionally, incision and drainage of the site may be needed in which Gram stain, culture, and sensitivity is obtained

d. Priority nursing diagnosis: Impaired skin integrity

e. Medication therapy: oral antibiotics are not recommended except for immunocompromised clients

4. Furunculosis

a. Description: an infection of an inflammatory nodule most commonly seen in children, adolescents, and young adults; the hair follicle becomes inflamed, tender to touch, and warm at the site

b. Clinical manifestations: an erythemic hard, tender-to-touch nodule, frequently found at the site of a hair follicle

c. Therapeutic management: warm moist soaks to the site; incision and drainage of the site may be required; keep lesions clean with washing the site with warm soapy water several times a day

d. Priority nursing diagnosis: Impaired skin integrity

e. Medication therapy: simple furunculosis does not require systemic antibiotics; topical antibiotics may be used; however, complicated furunculosis with cellulitis requires systemic antibiotics; recurrent furunculosis may be controlled with prophylactic antibiotic therapy

5. Carbuncle

a. Description

1) An inflammatory lesion that is formed when several furuncles convalesce to form one larger infected lesion of the skin

2) Carbuncles are frequently seen in children, teens, and young adults, with males being affected more frequently; common sites are hair follicles in the nose, neck, face, buttocks, and axilla; *Staphylococcus* is a common causative organism

   b. Clinical manifestations: erythemic, tender nodule that develops at a hair follicle area with possible malaise and low-grade fever

NCLEX!

   c. Therapeutic management: warm moist heat may be applied to the site; incision and drainage of the site is recommended; frequent use of antibacterial soaps and frequent showers are recommended for preventative therapy

   d. Priority nursing diagnosis: Impaired skin integrity

   e. Medication therapy: antibiotic therapy

6. Cellulitis

   a. Description

      1) A bacterial infection of the dermal and subcutaneous tissues with lesions appearing in various stages, ranging from vesicles, bullae, abscesses, and plaques

      2) Cellulitis is most commonly seen in adults, with group-A beta-hemolytic *Streptococcus pyogenes* and *Staphylococcus aureus* being the most frequent organisms

      3) Cellulitis occurs because of a break in the integrity of the skin (abrasion, laceration, etc.); this bacterial infection may also occur secondary to a skin lesion

   b. Clinical manifestations: cellulitis is characterized by an erythemic, swollen, tender-to-touch area of the skin at the site of entry of the bacteria; associated symptoms include fever, chills, malaise, and anorexia with associated regional lymphadenopathy

NCLEX!

   c. Therapeutic management: rest, elevation of the extremity, moist heat to the site for comfort; consider culture and sensitivity of tissue site for severe cases; for necrotic tissue, surgical excision and debridement are recommended along with antibiotic therapy

   d. Priority nursing diagnosis: Impaired skin integrity

   e. Medication therapy: antibiotic therapy

H. Viral infections

1. Herpes simplex virus (Type 1, Type 2)

   a. Description

      1) A viral infection that is manifested by vesicles on the oral mucosa—mouth or lips, which is HSV Type I, or in the genital mucosa (HSV Type II)

      2) Herpes simplex virus (HSV) can occur at any age

      3) The virus is spread by direct contact of contaminated body fluids and has an incubation period range of 2 to 14 days

      4) The virus occurs in three stages

a) Primary—the initial outbreak in which blisters occur on the mucosa or lips; malaise and fever are also common symptoms

b) Recurrent infections—outbreaks of the virus may occur at any time and are commonly precipitated by stress and illness; symptoms of recurrent infections are usually milder than the primary outbreak; recurrent infection is commonly present with a prodrome of tingling, itching, or a burning sensation at the site prior to the outbreak of lesions

c) Latency period—the virus remains dormant in the body during this time

b. Clinical manifestations

1) The primary symptoms include malaise, fever, and vesicles appearing on the mucosa

2) Secondary symptoms include prodrome of tingling, burning sensation prior to the outbreak of vesicles on the mucosa; the latency period is asymptomatic

c. Therapeutic management: advise rest; encourage good handwashing technique to prevent spreading the virus; comfort measures such as petroleum jelly or lip balm may be used for oral lesions; to prevent spreading the virus, avoid close contact with others while lesions are present; to prevent HSV Type 2, advise the use of latex condoms to prevent spreading genital lesions

d. Priority nursing diagnosis: Impaired tissue integrity, Altered comfort

e. Medication therapy: over-the-counter medications, such as acetaminophen (Tylenol) or camphophenique may be used for comfort as needed; antiviral medications such as acyclovir (Zovirax), famciclovir (Famvir), or valacyclovir (Valtrex) may be used to check further replication of the virus and diminish symptoms if started within 24 to 48 hours after initial onset of lesions

2. Herpes zoster

a. Description

1) A viral infection manifested by vesicles on the skin and commonly seen in older adults and the elderly; it is estimated to occur in approximately 20 percent of the U.S. population

2) Herpes zoster is a reactivation of the varicella virus, which has been dormant for many years, in the dorsal root ganglia

b. Clinical manifestations: it presents as a vesicular rash on the skin that usually follows one dermatome; clusters of vesicles are common along with symptoms of tingling, itching, burning, and even pain at the site of the lesions; the client may also experience fatigue, malaise, fever, and headache in addition to the local discomfort of the rash

c. Therapeutic management: comfort measures include wet dressings or soaks (Burow's solution) at the lesion sites two to three times a day; oatmeal baths (Aveeno™) are soothing and help to dry up lesions; rest is recommended; the virus may be transmitted to others; therefore care should be

NCLEX!

NCLEX!

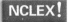

Practice to Pass

A 25-year-old female comes into the office for evaluation of a lesion on her labia. While interviewing the client, you ask if she has a history of genital herpes. She responds that she was diagnosed with genital herpes when she was 18 years old but states, "I took the medication and got rid of the genital herpes." She is certain that this lesion is not genital herpes because she got rid of the infection years ago. What is your response to her regarding the nature of the virus?

NCLEX!

taken to avoid persons at risk; lesions should be monitored for secondary bacterial infections

d. Priority nursing diagnoses: Impaired skin integrity, Altered comfort

e. Medication therapy: antiviral medications may be used if therapy is started within 24 to 48 hours after the outbreak of vesicles; current medications include acyclovir (Zovirax), famciclovir (Famvir), and valacyclovir (Valtrex); acetaminophen (Tylenol) and ibuprofen (Motrin) may be used for discomfort

3. Warts

a. Description

1) An elevation in the epidermal skin layer, commonly seen in children and young adults; frequently seen more commonly in women than in men

2) Warts are caused by the papillomavirus

3) A tumor develops on the skin, within the epidermal layer

4) The virus may be transmitted from person to person by touch and is commonly seen on the hands and feet

b. Clinical manifestations: a painless nodule on the skin surface, which is flesh-colored, and appears to have a rough surface with an irregular border; there are several types of warts

1) Common wart—flesh-colored nodule commonly seen on the hands or extremities, but can occur anywhere on the body; it commonly appears to have a "black seed" in the center of the lesion; these warts may come and go, usually lasting approximately 6 to 12 months without treatment

2) Flat wart—a tiny flesh-colored node, 1 to 3 mm in diameter, that may appear in clusters on the dorsum of the hand or forehead

3) Filiform wart—a tiny, thin, projected nodule that is commonly seen on the face, nose, or eyelids

4) Plantar wart—a hard nodule that is found on the bottom of the foot; it commonly projects into the foot from the constant pressure applied while walking on the nodule; it measures approximately 2 to 3 cm and is frequently associated with discomfort or pain at the site of the wart

c. Therapeutic management: no treatment is necessary for warts; since these lesions are viral in nature, eventually they will resolve on their own; even if a wart is successfully removed, it may reappear in the same site or on other areas of the skin

d. Priority nursing diagnosis: Impaired skin integrity

e. Medication therapy: over-the-counter therapy for wart removal includes salicylic acid (17 percent) and retinoic acid

I. Fungal infections

1. Candidiasis

a. Description

1) Infection caused by *candida albicans,* a yeast-like fungus that most often causes superficial cutaneous infections

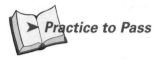

► Practice to Pass

A client comes into the office today for removal of a wart. He tells you that he has tried over-the-counter medications for removal; however, approximately 1 to 2 months later the wart reappears in the same spot. Now he wants the wart frozen and removed because he is tired of the wart coming back. What is your response to him?

NCLEX!

NCLEX!

2) Symptomatic infections occur on moist cutaneous sites and mucosal surfaces if local immunity is disturbed

3) Candida infections can affect all ages, but are most often seen as a cause of diaper rash in infants, summertime inframammary rash in women, vaginitis in premenopausal women, oral candidiasis in immunocompromised clients, and buttock and perineal rash in incontinent clients

4) Risk factors include moist, warm, or altered skin integrity, systemic antibiotics, pregnancy, birth control use, poor nutrition, diabetes or chronic illnesses, and immunosuppression

b. Clinical manifestations: the lesions are bright red, smooth macules with a macerated appearance and a scaling, elevated border; characteristic "satellite" lesions are small, similar-appearing macules outside the main lesion

1) Oral candidiasis is also known as thrush and is characterized by white, milky removable plaques on the oral mucosa; associated symptoms may include a burning sensation or decreased taste

2) Vulovaginitis is found on the vaginal mucosa and can spread to the perineum and groin; satellite lesions are usually present; other signs and symptoms include excessive itching and a thick, white, curd-like vaginal discharge

3) Perineal/diaper and skin-fold rash occurs on the perigenital and perianal areas and can extend to the inner thighs and buttocks; other areas affected include axilla, umbilical area, and under the breasts; erythema, papules, pustules, and a scaling border are characteristic

4) Balanitis is an inflammation of the glans and the prepuce of the penis that typically present as flattened pustules with edema, scaling, erosion, burning, and tenderness

5) Paronychial infection presents as erythema, edema, and tenderness of the nail folds; a creamy, purulent discharge may be expressed with pressure on the nail; the nails usually become discolored and have ridging

6) Candida organisms may also be a causative agent in otitis externa and scalp disorders

c. Therapeutic management: diagnosis is made by culture of scrapings or by microscopic examination of scaling with potassium hydrochloride (KOH) preparation

1) Avoid sharing linens or personal items

2) Use clean towel and washcloth daily

3) Dry all skin folds, avoid frequent immersion of hands in water

4) Wear clean cotton underwear daily

5) For vaginal candida, avoid tight clothing and pantyhose, bathe more frequently and dry genital area thoroughly; may need to treat sexual partner at the same time to avoid reinfection or have the partner use condoms until resolved; avoid douching and change perineal pads frequently

6) For balanitis, carefully retract the foreskin and perform careful cleaning and drying of the glans penis

7) Encourage weight loss for obese clients and maintenance of normal serum glucose levels in diabetics to decrease infection risk

d. Priority nursing diagnosis: Impaired tissue integrity, Acute pain

e. Medication therapy

1) Oral candidiasis: nystatin, clotrimazole, and in recurrent cases, ketoconazole, fluconazole, or itraconazole; liver function tests must be monitored because of risk of hepatotoxicity

2) Perineal: topical treatment with nystatin ointments BID

3) Balantitis: topical treatment with imidazole crease or nystatin powder BID

4) Paronychial: topical imidazole cream or application of 2 percent gentian violet; for nonresponsive cases, systemic ketoconazole or fluconazole; systemic medications require monitoring of liver function tests because of risk of hepatotoxicity

5) Hair/scalp: antifungal shampoo

6) Vulvovaginitis: vaginal creams/suppositories or treatment with Diflucan™

2. Tinea corporis

a. Description

1) A fungal infection of the face, trunk, and extremities with exclusion of the palms of the hands, soles of the feet, and groin; also known as ringworm of the body

2) All species of dermatophytes can be the causative agent; generally more prevalent in hot and humid climates

3) It can affect all age groups, but children are more often affected

4) It can be spread human-to-human, animal-to-human, and soil-to-human by direct contact; other risk factors include prolonged use of topical steroids or immunosuppression

b. Clinical manifestations

1) Classic lesions are annular (ringlike) plaques with an elevated border, sharp margins, and a clearing center

2) May occur singly or in groups of 3 to 4

3) KOH preparation from these lesions is usually positive; woods lamp fluoresces yellow; dermatophyte test media changes the medium from yellow to red

4) For most clinical purposes, classification by anatomic site is preferred

c. Therapeutic management

1) Avoid contact with suspected lesions

2) Topical creams are the treatment of choice

3) Clean environment to remove fungal scales

4) Avoid sharing towels or other items that can transmit fungal scales

5) Search out infected animals/pets and treat appropriately

6) Apply creams after bathing and reapply after swimming and exercising

7) Keep skin dry

8) Monitor for superimposed bacterial infections

d. Priority nursing diagnoses: Impaired tissue integrity, Altered comfort

e. Medication therapy

1) Topical drugs to treat superficial fungal infections include amphotericin B, ciclopirox, clotrimazole (Lotrimin) and econazole (Spectrazole); eradication is slow and treatment may take 2 to 8 weeks

2) For added benefit, the client should wash with an antifungal shampoo such as ketoconazole (Nizoral) prior to using a cream

3) Before an oral antifungal agent such as terbinafine (Lamisil) or Nizoral is prescribed, baseline liver function tests and complete blood count (CBC) should be obtained; repeat liver function tests and CBC are recommended at 4 to 6 weeks and then every 6 months

3. Tinea pedis

a. Description

1) Also known as athlete's foot, it is the most common of all fungal infections; it affects the plantar surface of the feet with mild to moderate erythema and scaly skin between the toes

2) This is caused by an infection by a dermatophyte (fungus that grows in nonliving, keratinized portions of the skin)

3) These dermatophytes are commonly termed tinea and are named by the affected location

4) Pustules may be present in severe cases with a foul odor, possibly indicating a secondary bacterial or yeast infection

5) Risk factors include: communal showers and pools, occlusive footwear, excessive sweating, sharing of footwear and hot, humid weather, immunocompromised status, and prolonged applications of topical steroids; both feet often are involved

b. Clinical manifestations

1) Interdigital scaling, crusting, and maceration; pruritis may or may not be present

2) Plantar/lateral surfaces of feet may also be affected

3) Vesicles/pustules and interdigital blisters may provide an entry of secondary bacteria such as *Streptococcus* organisms

c. Therapeutic management

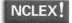

1) Keep involved areas clean, dry, and exposed to air when possible

2) Wear light cotton socks and change frequently throughout the day

3) Wear sandals or open-toed shoes when possible; avoid plastic footwear and occlusive shoes

NCLEX!

4) Careful drying between toes after showering or bathing

5) Apply drying or dusting powers, topical antiperspirants

6) Put socks on before underwear to avoid spreading to the groin

7) Instruct on signs and symptoms of bacterial infection such as pain, increased inflammation, pustules, or purulent exudates

d. Priority nursing diagnoses: Impaired skin integrity, Altered comfort

e. Medication therapy

1) Antifungal creams

2) Antifungal powders may be used as an adjunct treatment and aid in keeping areas dry

3) For severe cases: Burow's solution soak for lesions that are oozing, oral grieseofulvin, fluconazole, itraconazole, and tervinafine

J. Infestations and insect bites

1. Bees and wasps

a. Arthropods affect many by being pests, inoculating poison, invading tissue, or transmitting disease; inoculation of poison may occur as either a bite or sting

b. IgE-mediated hypersensitivity to the insect venom may be confirmed by skin testing with suitable dilutions of available venom, usually done by an allergist

c. Local tissue inflammation and destruction results from poison, allergic reaction from previous sensitization or toxic reaction from large inoculation of poison; stings by yellow jackets, hornets, honeybees, and wasps result in generalized allergic reactions of varying severity in approximately 0.4 percent of the population

d. Clinical manifestations

NCLEX!

1) Local reactions include erythema, pain, heat, swelling, itching, blisters, secondary infection, necrosis, ulceration, and drainage

2) Toxic reactions include nausea, vomiting, headache, fever, diarrhea, lightheadedness, syncope, drowsiness, muscle spasms, edema, and/or convulsions

NCLEX!

3) Systemic reactions include allergic/itching eyes, facial flushing, generalized urticaria, dry cough, chest/throat constriction, wheezing, dyspnea, cyanosis, abdominal cramps, diarrhea, nausea, vomiting, vertigo, chills/fever, stridor, shock, loss of consciousness, involuntary bowel/bladder action, frothy sputum, respiratory failure, cardiovascular collapse, and death

4) Delayed reactions include serum sickness-like reactions, fever, malaise, headache, urticaria, lymphadenopathy, polyarthritis

5) Unusual reactions include encephalopathy, neuritis, vasculitis, nephrosis, extreme fear/anxiety

    e. Therapeutic management

        1) Outpatient or inpatient depending on individual response

        2) First-aid measures, local treatment, activate emergency services in severe reactions

        3) Over-the-counter antihistamine unless contraindicated

NCLEX!

        4) Remove stinger by scraping—do not squeeze with a tweezer—then cleanse the wound

        5) Ice packs to bite or sting—alternate 10 minutes on and 10 minutes off

        6) Elevate and rest affected part

        7) Maintain adequate airway

        8) Persons with known sensitivity should wear medical ID tag

        9) Prevent reexposure in known hypersensitive persons

NCLEX!

        10) Educate on risks of increasing severity of responses in the future

        11) Instruct to use insect repellants when outdoors or in infested areas

        12) Instruct on Epi Pen use if prescribed

    f. Priority nursing diagnoses: Pain, Risk for injury

NCLEX!

    g. Medication therapy

        1) Local analgesics, diphenhydramine (Benadryl), or other antihistamines

        2) Topical or oral steroids

        3) Systemic (depending on severity and reaction type) include Epinephrine 1:1000 subcutaneous to combat urticaria, wheezing, angioedema (adult 0.3 to 0.5 ml/kg); treat shock, if present; diphenhydramine may be prescribed to combat urticaria, wheezing, angioedema; aminophylline for bronchospasm; hydrocortisone if needed for severe urticaria or spider bite; tetanus prophylaxis and antibiotics are also administered if needed; Valium 5 to 10 mg if needed for severe muscle spasms; morphine or meperidine (Demerol) if needed for pain may also be prescribed

        4) Anti-venom for black widow spider or scorpion

        5) Consider desensitization with immunotherapy in severe cases

        6) Epi-pen or anaphylactic kit

2. Pediculosis

    a. Description

        1) An infestation of the skin or hair by the species of blood-sucking lice capable of living as external parasites on the human host

        2) *Pediculosis capitis* is the head louse, the size of a sesame seed, clear in color when hatched but becomes grayish-white to red/brown after maturing

3) Head lice infestation is very common among schoolage children of all socioeconomic backgrounds and spread by sharing combs, hats, and scarves

4) *Pediculosis pubis,* also known as "crabs," infests the genital area and is one of the most common sexually transmitted diseases

5) Pubic lice can spread by sexual contact

6) Nits/eggs attach to the hair shaft by a cement-like/cocoon-like structure and are difficult to remove

7) Lice live up to 30 days and a female can lay up to 100 eggs

b. Clinical manifestations

1) Intensive pruritis is the most common symptom that may result in excoriations

2) Head lice may resemble dandruff flakes; however, they are not easily brushed off

3) Papular urticaria may be found at the neck or pubic area

c. Therapeutic management

1) Nits must be mechanically removed; a 50/50 white vinegar/water solution may loosen the nits; olive oil may also be used; a nit comb is used to remove nits from the hair shafts; lice may also be removed by fingers or tweezers; nits remove more easily by back-combing the hair

2) To treat eyelashes apply petrolatum to lashes b.i.d. for 10 days; lice will either suffocate or slide off

3) Educate children and parents about mode of transmission (person to person) and preventative measures, such as not sharing combs, brushes, hats, scarves, helmets, headphones, bedding, or sleeping bags

4) Coats and hats should be hung separately and not touching each other

5) Sleeping material should be labeled and kept separately in plastic bags, not stacked

6) All family members need to be examined and treated at the same time

7) Soak personal hair items in 2 percent Lysol or pediculocide for 1 hour

8) Shaving hair is not found to be helpful

9) Machine-wash all washable clothing used in the last 48 hours and dry in the dryer for at least 20 minutes

10) Place unwashable items in airtight plastic bags for a period of 1 week to kill lice

11) Upholstered furniture or pillows may be ironed with a hot iron

12) Clean any item in contact with hair with 2 percent Lysol or pediculocide

13) Vacuum mattresses, rugs, upholstered furniture, and stuffed animals regularly

d. Medication therapy

1) For *pediculosis capitis:* permethrin (Nix), pyrethrin shampoo (Rid), or lindane (Kwell) shampoo left on 5 to 10 minutes and then washed off; lindane can be repeated in 1 week; due to neurotoxicity of lindane, it should not be used by children, nursing or pregnant women, individuals with known seizure disorders, or on open skin

2) For pediculosis pubis: treatment includes lindane, pyrethrin (Rid) or permethrin (Nix) as a shampoo left on for 10 minutes or as a lotion left on for several hours

3) Co-trimoxazole (Bactrim DS): b.i.d. for 3 days has been shown to be effective; a second therapy 10 days later may be necessary to kill emerging nits before they reproduce

3. Scabies

a. Description

1) A contagious disease caused by infestation of the skin by the mite *Sarcoptes scabiei var hominis;* the impregnated mite burrows into the skin and remains there for life (approximately 30 days), laying 2 to 3 eggs per day; the eggs hatch in 3 to 4 days and reach maturity in 4 days, migrate to the skin surface, mate, and repeat the cycle

2) It is more common in people who don't have bathing facilities or access to clothes-washing facilities; mite can live in clothing fibers and can be transmitted by contact of infected clothing or bed linens

3) Pathological findings by skin biopsy of a nodule will reveal portions of the mite—although rarely performed; diagnosis is usually made by clinical presentation of burrows, vesicles, and nodules

b. Clinical manifestations

1) Presents as a generalized pruritic rash particularly of the hands, wrists, elbows, axillary areas, breasts, abdomen, or genitals

2) Itching may become intense; increased warmth of the skin and nocturnal itching is a classic symptom, since mites tend to have increased movment at night; exposure to hot water or steam also can increase pruritis

3) Lesions may be erythematous, crusted papules, or purplish nodules, which may be accompanied by flesh-colored, raised burrows (threadlike linear ridges a few millimeters in length with a minute black dot at one end); clients develop itch approximately 10 to 14 days after exposure

c. Therapeutic management

1) Close family members and personal contacts must be treated as well, even if there are no apparent signs or symptoms

2) All bed clothing, linens, unwashed worn clothing, and stuffed animals should be washed and dried in a hot dryer because the dryer kills the mite

3) Mites and eggs may be killed by placing items in airtight plastic bags for 7 days since the mite cannot live off the host more than 3 days;

mites can live 24 to 36 hours in room conditions and longer in humid environments

4) Relief from itching may not occur for 3 to 6 weeks after treatment because of hypersensitivity of the skin to debris left in the burrow

5) Lotions/creams should be applied from the neck down, using a toothbrush to get under fingernails and toenails; the lotion is showered off 8 to 12 hours later

d. Priority nursing diagnoses: Impaired skin integrity, Altered comfort

e. Medication therapy

1) Permethrin 5% cream (Elimite) is the treatment of choice; a second application in 48 hours is sometimes recommended

2) Crotamiton 10% (Eurax) is less toxic but is also slightly less effective; therefore application for 2 nights is advised

3) Lindane 1% cream or lotion (Kwell) is the least expensive but has the potential for neurotoxicity and should not be used by children, nursing or pregnant women, people with a known seizure disorder, or any widespread excoriations/open skin; treatment may be repeated after 1 week

4) Systemic antipruritics

5) May require emollients and midpotency corticosteroids after using scabicide to suppress hyperreactivity caused by the mites

K. Allergic reactions

1. Contact dermatitis

a. Description

1) An eruption of the skin related to contact with an irritating substance or allergen; primary irritant dermatitis affects individuals exposed to specific irritants and produces discomfort immediately

2) Common irritants include chemicals, dyes, metals, and latex gloves; allergic contact dermatitis affects only individuals previously sensitized to the contactant; it represents a delayed hypersensitivity reaction; most common are poison ivy, sumac, and oak

3) Contact dermatitis is an inflammation caused by an external irritant or allergic reaction mediated by IgE; the epidermal reaction is caused by T-lymphocytes; the location of the rash helps provide clues to the offending antigen; there is no specific age or sex affected, but black skin is less susceptible

b. Clinical manifestations

1) Acute: papules, vesicles, bullae with surrounding erythema; crusting, oozing, and pruritis may be present

2) Chronic: erythematous base, thickening with lichcnification, scaling, and fissuring

c. Therapeutic management

1) Identify and remove causative agents

2) Topical emollients in combination with mid- to high-potency corticosteroids

3) Drainage of large vesicles may be necessary without removing tops

4) Apply wet dressings to oozing, pruritic lesions to aid in drying and debridement; cool tap water, Burow's solution 1 to 40, saline 1 tsp/pint water and silver nitrate solution can be used

5) Suppress inflammation with antibacterial solution

6) May use topical steroid creams but do not use on the face

7) Aveeno (oatmeal) baths are helpful to decrease itching

8) Antihistamines of choice may be used to decrease itching and edema

9) Use calamine lotion to aid drying

d. Priority nursing diagnoses: Impaired skin integrity, Altered comfort

e. Medication therapy

1) Midpotency topical corticosteroids

2) High-potency topical corticosteroids such as amcinonide (Cyclocort) 0.1% or dexamethasone (Decaderm) 0.25%

3) Systemic medications including prednisone, antibiotics, and antihistamines

2. Urticaria

a. Description

1) An itchy rash; single or multiple superficial raised pale macules with red halo; subsides rapidly, no scars or change in pigmentation; this condition may be recurrent

2) Acute urticaria is a response to many stimuli; IgE-mediated histamine release from mast cells is sometimes seen in response to drug exposure and subsides over several hours

3) Chronic urticaria persists over 6 weeks; it is not mediated by IgE; it is also associated with fever, chills, arthralgia, myalgia, and headache

4) Urticaria is a response to massive release from mast cells in the superficial dermis; this can be caused by multiple agents such as drug reaction, food or food-additive allergy, inhalant, contact or ingestion allergy, transfusion reaction, insect bite or sting, bacterial, viral, fungal or helminthic infection, collagen vascular disease, lupus, heat, cold, sunlight, or emotional stress

5) True urticarial lesions do not remain in the same area of the skin longer than 24 hours; lesions that are present 72 hours or longer suggest cutaneous vasculitis as a possible cause

b. Clinical manifestations

1) Single or multiple raised, blanched, central wheals surrounded by red flare that is intensely pruritic

2) May occur anywhere on the body

3) Variable size of 1 to 2 mm to 15 to 20 cm or larger

4) Resolves spontaneously in less than 48 hours

c. Therapeutic management

1) Cool moist compresses help to control itching

2) Avoidance if etiology is known

3) Antihistamine if accidentally reexposed

4) Instruct client that there is risk of life-threatening reaction on reexposure

d. Priority nursing diagnoses: Impaired skin integrity, Risk for injury, Altered comfort

e. Medication therapy

1) Subcutaneous administration of epinephrine 1:1000 for intense itching

2) Antihistamines

3) Histamine (H_2) receptor antagonists may enhance effectiveness of conventional antihistamines

4) Cyprohepadine (Periactin) 4 mg every 6 hours for cold urticaria

5) Corticosteroids for pressure urticaria

6) Topical sunscreens and hydroxyzine (Vistaril) for solar urticaria

L. Benign conditions

1. Acne

a. Description

1) Androgenically stimulated, inflammatory disorder of the sebaceous glands resulting in comedones, papules, inflammatory pustules, cysts, and occasional scarring; acne cannot occur without a hair follicle

2) It has multifactorial causes that involve four principal factors

a) Increased sebum production

b) Abnormal keratinization of the follicular epithelium

c) Proliferation of proprioibacterium acnes

d) Inflammation

3) The rate of sebum production is determined genetically and is increased by the presence of androgens; the earliest changes in acne may be seen in prepubescent years

b. Clinical manifestations

1) Lesions may occur on the forehead, cheeks, nose, and may extend over the central back and chest

2) Closed comedones—whiteheads

3) Open comedones—blackheads

Box 10-2	
Stages and Grades of Acne	**Stages of Acne** Mild—few to several papules, no nodules, on face/neck only Moderate—several papules to many papules/pustules, few to several nodules on face, back, chest, or upper arms Severe—Numerous and/or extensive papules/pustules. Many nodules with acne-induced scarring **Grades of Acne** Grade 1—comedonal—closed and open Grade 2—papular—over 25 lesions on face and trunk Grade 3—pustular—over 25 lesions with mild scarring Grade 4—nodulocystic, inflammatory nodules and cysts with extensive scarring

        4) Nodules or papules, pustules, with or without redness and edema, scars

        5) Grades of acne (see Box 10-2)

    c. Therapeutic management

        1) Intended to control the disease and is not curative

        2) Use a gentle antibacterial soap and wash the affected areas with the fingertips

        3) Avoid cosmetics containing oil and confine moisturizing lotions to dry patches of skin

        4) Instruct not to pick lesions, which would increase scarring

        5) 6 to 8 weeks of treatment is usual before obvious improvement occurs

        6) Diet does not cause acne

        7) Stress-management if acne flares with stress

    d. Priority nursing diagnoses: Impaired skin integrity, Disturbed body image

    e. Medication therapy

        1) Topical retinoids are usually prescribed for all types of acne

        2) For mild acne, combination therapy of a topical retinoid plus one or more of the following: benzoyl peroxide, topical antibiotics, or azelaic acid

        3) For moderate acne, topical agents and oral antibiotics such as tetracycline for a specified period of time and then the antibiotic is discontinued

        4) For severe acne, isotretinoin (Accutane) 0.5 to 1.0 mg/kg daily

        5) Antiandrogens such as birth control pills and spironolactone inhibit sebum production

  2. Lentigo

    a. Description

        1) A brown macule resembling a freckle except that the border is usually irregular

2) Benign lentigo resembles a freckle; lentigo maligna (pre-melanoma) is a brown or black mottled, irregularly outlined, slowly enlarging lesion in which there are an increased number of scattered atypical melanocytes; it usually occurs on the face; one-third progress to melanoma but transition may take 10 to 15 years

3) Senile lentigo (liver spots) occurs on exposed skin of older white individuals

b. Clinical manifestations

1) Benign lentigo: freckle, pigmented, flat, or slightly elevated macule

2) Lentigo maligna: brown/black uneven macule with irregular border which slowly extends

3) Senile lentigo: pigmented flat areas usually on sun-exposed areas

c. Therapeutic management

1) Instruct on ABCD of skin lesions: asymmetry, border, color, and diameter

2) Teach to inspect skin routinely and seek professional advice for any noted changes

3) Instruct clients to use sunscreens, hats, or caps when out in the sun to avoid overexposure

d. Priority nursing diagnosis: Risk for ineffective health maintenance

e. Medication therapy

1) No medication needed for lentigo

2) Lentigo maligna: follow-up by a dermatologist is recommended

3. Psoriasis (see previous discussion under chronic dermatologic problems)

4. Seborrheic keratosis

a. Description

1) Benign plaques, beige to brown or even black in color, ranging in size from 3 to 20 mm in diameter with a velvety or warty surface

2) The pathophysiology of this condition involves the proliferation of immature keratinocytes and melanocytes totally within the dermis; it affects mainly males 30 years and older

b. Clinical manifestations

1) "Stuck-on" brown spots over the trunk which may bleed when irritated by clothing or picked

2) Size varies from 1 to 3 cm

3) May be skin-colored, tan, brown, or black and are usually oval-shaped with a warty, greasy feel

4) Usually present on the face, neck, scalp, back, and upper chest

    c. Therapeutic management

       1) Sunscreens, decrease sun exposure, and avoid tanning

       2) Wear hats when outdoors

       3) Teach the ABCD of skin lesions that indicate need for evaluation by a healthcare provider

    d. Medication therapy

NCLEX!

       1) No medications indicated for seborrheic keratosis

       2) May be removed by electrocautery or frozen with liquid nitrogen; the area may be hypopigmented after removal

5. Vitiligo

    a. Description

       1) Are totally white macules with an absence of melanocytes

NCLEX!

       2) An acquired, slowly progressive depigmentation in small or large areas of the skin caused by a decrease in active melanocytes

         a) Type A: nondermatomal and widespread involved in 75 percent of cases

         b) Type B: dermatomal and segmental; 50 percent of cases begin between ages 10 to 30

    b. Clinical manifestations

       1) Loss of pigment with increased sunburning of areas; more often occurs around the eyes, mouth, and anus

       2) May be pruritic and associated with premature graying

    c. Therapeutic management

       1) Avoid sun exposure, which may increase differentiation between normal and abnormal skin

       2) Skin dyes/cosmetics for blending purposes

    d. Priority nursing diagnosis: Risk for disturbed body image

    e. Medication therapy

       1) Localized with midpotency steroids

       2) Oral systemic steroids are effective in arresting disease progression

       3) Depigmenting of normal skin with hydroquinone cream (Melanex)

M. Pressure ulcers

    1. Description

       a. Ischemic lesions of the skin and underlying tissue caused by external pressure that impairs the flow of blood and lymph; also known as bedsores and decubitus ulcers

b. Pressure ulcers are a common and serious complication affecting the frail, disabled, acutely ill, or immobile client, usually in long-term care and rehabilitation settings

NCLEX!

c. Most common sites are over bony prominences, such as elbows, hips, heels, outer ankles, and base of spine; over 95 percent of ulcers develop on the lower part of the body

d. Causes include an uneven application of pressure over a bony hard site: high pressure applied for 2 hours (produces irreversible tissue ischemia and necrosis), shearing forces that develop when a seated person slides toward the floor or foot of the bed if supine, frictional forces that develop when pulling a client across a bed sheet, and moisture from incontinence or perspiration

NCLEX!

2. Clinical manifestations: pressure ulcers are staged according to their characteristics; see Box 10–3

NCLEX!

a. Assessment: risk factors include immobility, malnutrition, and low body weight, hypoalbuminemia, fecal and/or urinary incontinence, bone fracture, vitamin C deficiency, low diastolic blood pressure, age-related skin changes such as diminished pain perception, thinning of epidermis, loss of dermal vessels, altered barrier properties, reduced immunity and slowed wound healing, anemia, infections, peripheral vascular insufficiency, dementia, malignancies, diabetes, CVA, dry skin, and edema

b. Diagnostic and laboratory test findings: culture of the wound, WBC with differential and sedimentation rate to determine presence of primary or secondary infection; if no progression of ulcer, albumin levels may be obtained to determine dietary needs

3. Therapeutic management

a. Evaluate risk factors

NCLEX!

b. Improve overall nutritional status—adequate protein intake

c. Clean wound each time dressing is changed to remove dead tissue, excess fluid and debris

d. Maintain body temperature and acidic pH

e. Never use antiseptics and harsh skin cleansers that may harm tissue

f. Employ pressure reduction via specialized beds

NCLEX!

g. Reposition client every 2 hours

Box 10-3

Pressure Ulcer Stages

Stage 1: Non-blanching erythema, warmth, and tenderness
Stage 2: Skin breakdown limited to the dermis, excoriation, blistering, drainage, more sharply defined erythema, variable skin temperature, local swelling, and edema.
Stage 3: Ulcer formation into the subcutaneous tissues, crater formation, slough, eschar, and/or drainage.
Stage 4: Ulcers extend beyond the deep fascia into the muscle or bone, decayed area may be larger than visible apparent wound, osteomyelitis or sepsis may be present, granulation tissue and epithelialization may be present at wound margins.

h. Use support devices such as padding (gel pads), floatation pads, mattress overlays and specialized (such as air-fluidized, oscillating, or kinetic) beds

i. Avoid agents that delay wound healing such as topical corticosteroids, hydrogen peroxide, iodine, and hypochlorite

j. Control fecal and urine incontinence

k. Avoid massage over bony prominences

l. Use moisture barrier

m. Assess site every 8 to 12 hours; carefully document healing, e.g., state there is a "healing Stage III ulcer, rather than "Stage II ulcer" if ulcer was Stage III and exhibits healing

n. Use absorption dressing if wound has large amounts of exudate and change frequently

4. Priority nursing diagnoses: Impaired skin integrity; Disturbed body image; Risk for infection; Pain; Risk for imbalanced nutrition: less than body requirements; Risk for ineffective thermoregulation; Impaired tissue perfusion; Risk for impaired physical mobility; Anxiety

5. Planning and implementation

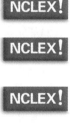

a. Provide relief of pressure on wound; perform passive range of motion and encourage active range of motion exercises

b. Encourage oral high-calorie and high-protein supplements

c. Encourage oral zinc, vitamins A and C, and iron to aid in tissue healing

d. Conduct systemic skin inspection at least once daily

e. Monitor weight and nutrition intake

f. Clean skin at time of soiling and routine intervals

g. Keep skin well-hydrated and lubricated

h. Avoid exposure to cold, dry environments

i. Document all risk factors and implement strategies

j. Ensure that proper positioning schedules are followed every 2 hours

k. Use pressure reduction aids

6. Medication therapy

a. Clindamycin (Cleocin) or gentamycin (Garamycin) may be ordered for complications such as cellulitis, osteomyelitis, or sepsis

b. Vitamin C 500 mg b.i.d. and zinc sulfate supplements aid healing

c. Antibiotic prophylaxis will eradicate bacterial component

d. A 2-week trial of topical antimicrobials should be used only for a clean superficial ulcer that is either not healing or producing a moderate amount of exudates—cultures are necessary to determine whether antifungal or specific antibacterial agents are indicated

e. Enzymatic debriding agents such as collagenase (Santyl, Granulex), fibinolysin-desoxyribonuclease (Elase), papin (Panafil), or sutilains (Travase) are used with a moisture barrier to protect surrounding tissue

f. Recommended dressings include polyurethane films (Op-Site™, Tegaderm™), absorbent hydrocolloid dressings (Duoderm™)

7. Client education

a. Need for frequent evaluation of all clients with a history of pressure sores, especially if they have limited mobility

b. Nutritional requirements and meal planning

c. Early identification of skin redness to prevent breakdowns

d. Skin cleansing routine

e. Underpads to absorb moisture

f. Repositioning techniques and frequency

g. Need to evaluate and ensure continence and facilities

h. Use of mattress overlays, seat cushions or special mattresses

i. Ways to avoid injuries

8. Evaluation: systematic staging of ulcers on a routine schedule documents healing; a schedule is maintained for mobility, nutritional assessment, and continence and is altered as necessary; client remains free of possible complications, such as growth of resistant organisms and possible development of gangrene secondary to poor healing

N. Burn injury

1. Description: a burn is an alteration in skin integrity resulting in tissue loss or injury caused by heat, chemicals, electricity, or radiation

2. There are several types of burn injury: thermal, chemical, electrical, and radiation

a. Thermal: results from dry heat (flames) or moist heat (steam or hot liquids); it is the most common type; it causes cellular destruction that results in vascular, bony, muscle, or nerve complications; thermal burns can also lead to inhalation injury if the head and neck area is affected

b. Chemical burns are caused by direct contact with either acidic or alkaline agents; they alter tissue perfusion leading to necrosis

c. Electrical burns: severity depends on type and duration of current and amount of voltage; it follows the path of least resistance (muscles, bone, blood vessels, and nerves); sources of electrical injury include direct current, alternating current, and lightning

d. Radiation burns: are usually associated with sunburn or radiation treatment for cancer; are usually superficial; extensive exposure to radiation may lead to tissue damage and multisystem injury

3. Emergent phase of burn management: the emergent/resuscitative stage lasts from the onset of injury through successful fluid resuscitation; during this

stage, it is determined whether the client is to be transported to a burn center for complex intervention depending on onset of injury, identification of burn source, and complicating factors

a. Classification of burn depth: done according to the depth of damaged tissue

1) Superficial thickness (formerly first-degree): involves the epidermis only and is recognized by characteristics of erythema, absence of blisters for 24 hours, local pain; healing occurs spontaneously in 3 to 5 days with no scar formation

2) Superficial partial thickness (formerly second-degree): involves the epidermis and dermis, characterized by moist areas that are red to ivory white in color, blisters form immediately; area is painful because touch and pain receptors are intact; area heals with greater or lesser amounts of scarring within 21 to 28 days

3) Deep partial thickness (formerly second-degree): involves possibly the entire layer of the dermis, and is more severe than a superficial partial thickness burn; skin appendages are left intact; area has a dry waxy whitish appearance and may be difficult to differentiate initially from full-thickness burns; may heal spontaneously in about 1 month although skin grafting is often done to close the wound, accelerate healing, reduce scarring, and reduce risk of infection

4) Full thickness (formerly third-degree): involves destruction of all skin elements with coagulation of subdermal plexus; muscle and tendons may be involved

b. An estimate of the burn size is calculated using the "Rule of Nines" (see Figure 10-3) or the Lund and Browder method; each chart accounts for 100 percent of the total body surface area (TBSA) although the Lund and Browder method takes into account the client's age when estimating body surface area

c. Severity of burn is classified using the American Burn Association criteria as minor burn, moderate uncomplicated burn, and major burn; these categories help determine treatment

d. Nursing assessment: history of injury, estimate burn extent and depth, obtain past medical history and medication history including date of last tetanus prophylaxis; assess for other concurrent injuries

e. Diagnostic and lab test findings: may have elevated hematocrit and decreased hemoglobin caused by fluid shift, decreased sodium and increased potassium caused by damage to capillary and cell membranes, elevated BUN and creatinine caused by dehydration, myoglobin in urinalysis, and possible deterioration of arterial blood gases and oxygen saturation readings depending on respiratory status

f. Priority nursing diagnoses: Risk for deficient fluid volume; Risk for infection; Impaired physical mobility; Imbalanced nutrition: less than body requirements; Ineffective breathing pattern; Impaired tissue perfusion; Risk for impaired gas exchange; Anxiety; Risk for ineffective thermoregulation; Pain; Impaired skin integrity

Figure 10-3 **Rules of nines.**

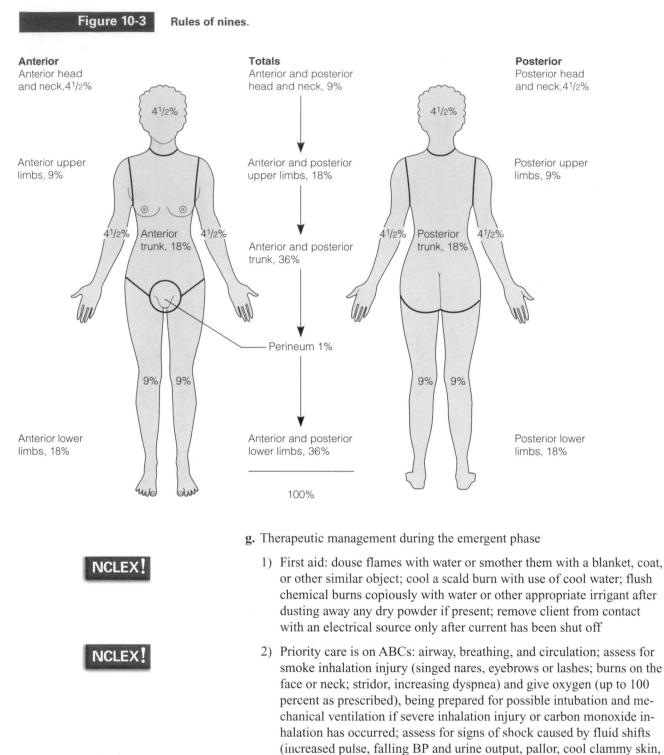

Anterior
Anterior head
and neck, 4½%

Anterior upper
limbs, 9%

4½% Anterior 4½%
trunk, 18%

Anterior lower
limbs, 18%

Totals
Anterior and posterior
head and neck, 9%

Anterior and posterior
upper limbs, 18%

Anterior and posterior
trunk, 36%

Perineum 1%

Anterior and posterior
lower limbs, 36%

100%

Posterior
Posterior head
and neck, 4½%

Posterior upper
limbs, 9%

4½% Posterior 4½%
trunk, 18%

Posterior lower
limbs, 18%

g. Therapeutic management during the emergent phase

1) First aid: douse flames with water or smother them with a blanket, coat, or other similar object; cool a scald burn with use of cool water; flush chemical burns copiously with water or other appropriate irrigant after dusting away any dry powder if present; remove client from contact with an electrical source only after current has been shut off

2) Priority care is on ABCs: airway, breathing, and circulation; assess for smoke inhalation injury (singed nares, eyebrows or lashes; burns on the face or neck; stridor, increasing dyspnea) and give oxygen (up to 100 percent as prescribed), being prepared for possible intubation and mechanical ventilation if severe inhalation injury or carbon monoxide inhalation has occurred; assess for signs of shock caused by fluid shifts (increased pulse, falling BP and urine output, pallor, cool clammy skin, deteriorating level of consciousness)

3) Fluid resuscitation: Brooke formula uses 2 mL/kg/% TBSA burned (¾ crystalloid plus ¼ colloid) plus maintenance fluid of 2,000 mL D_5W per 24 hours; Parkland (Baxter) formula uses 4 mL/kg/% TBSA burned

NCLEX!

NCLEX!

NCLEX!

per 24 hours (crystalloid only—lactated Ringer's); both formulas give half of 24 hour total in the first 8 hours, and the second half over the next 16 hours

4) Other considerations: remove all rings and jewelry to avoid tourniquet effect caused by swelling/edema of burn site; provide cardiac monitoring for the first 24 hours after an electrical burn

NCLEX!

    h. Medication therapy: pain therapy, tetanus prophylaxis, topical antimicrobial as well as systemic antibiotics

    i. Client education: focuses in this phase on brief explanations about the injury, treatments, and ongoing nursing care

2. Acute phase of burn management: this phase begins with the start of diuresis (usually 48 to 72 hours post-burn) and ends with closure of the burn wound

    a. Clinical manifestations: vary depending on cause, depth and TBSA of burn; associated symptoms arising from other organ systems may include nausea and vomiting, pain, skin redness, chills, respiratory distress, and hypovolemia

NCLEX!

    b. Therapeutic management: wound care management (debridement, dressing changes, hydrotherapy, possible escharotomy, wound grafting); nutritional therapies (high-calorie, high-protein diet with vitamins and minerals), infection control, pain management, psychosocial support, physical therapy, maintain fluid/hydration status, and maintain heated environment

    c. Medication therapy: topical and/or systemic antibiotic therapy; pain control with opioid analgesics is usually required

3. Rehabilitative phase of burn management: this phase begins with wound closure and ends when the client returns to the highest level of health restoration

    a. Clinical manifestations: depend on cause, body surface area affected and depth; may have immobility or restriction of mobility of affected area; scarring is possible

NCLEX!

    b. Therapeutic management: obtain psychosocial evaluation; provide support and management; arrange counseling if necessary; prevent immobility contractures with exercises or ongoing physical therapy; assist in returning to work, family and social life; use preventative measures for scar formation (such as burn garments); assess home environment for needs and accessibility; assess pain management needs

    c. Medication therapy: ongoing pain management and antibiotic therapy as necessary

    d. Client education

NCLEX!

    1) Environmental safety: use low temperature setting for hot water heater, ensure access to and adequate number of electrical cords/outlets, isolate household chemicals, avoid smoking in bed

NCLEX!

    2) Use of household smoke detectors with emphasis on maintenance

    3) Proper storage and use of flammable substances

    4) Evacuation plan for family

5) Care of burn at home

6) Signs and symptoms of infection

7) How to identify risk of skin changes

NCLEX!

8) Use of sunscreen to protect healing tissue and other protective skin care measures

4. Evaluation: client demonstrates knowledge and understanding of instruction and education about pain management, skin integrity and healing, need for counseling and family support, vocational and occupational interventions

---

Case Study

A 22-year-old client comes in for evaluation of a skin rash. She thinks she may have psoriasis. For several years, she has complained of a white scaly rash that comes and goes.

❶ When performing an initial work-up history, what questions would you ask the client regarding the skin rash?

❷ The client asks you to explain what kind of disease psoriasis is and would like you to discuss how the scaly patches develop. What is your response?

❸ The client is diagnosed with psoriasis and wants to know how to get rid of the rash and prevent it from coming back again. What methods do you suggest?

❹ She has been prescribed to use coal tar shampoo along with topical steroids as a first-line therapy on her skin. What other over-the-counter products would be useful for her psoriasis?

❺ The client would like to go golfing this weekend. What educational advice would you give to her regarding being outdoors?

For suggested responses, see pages 737–738.

Posttest

1 A client presents with silvery plaques on both elbows that are not itchy, but bleed when the scales are removed. The nurse concludes that the client most likely has which of the following conditions?

(1) Eczema
(2) Contact dermatitis
(3) Psoriasis
(4) Poison ivy

2 A client presents to the primary care clinic complaining of frequent scratching and itching of the skin that is worse at night. The nurse should suspect which of the following skin disorders?

(1) Scabies
(2) Hives
(3) Fleas
(4) Drug reaction

3 The nurse determines that which of the following reported by a client with acne would not contribute to the severity of the acne?

(1) Stress
(2) Oil-based cosmetics
(3) Diet
(4) Moisturizers

4 The nurse who is counseling a family about treatment for scabies would tell the family to avoid which of the following products, based on knowledge that the family has young children and the woman is pregnant?

(1) Elimite
(2) Lindane (Kwell)
(3) Permethrin (Nix)
(4) Pyrethrin shampoo (Rid)

5 Which of the following would not be included in the nurse's instructions to a client to prevent a recurrence of *Tinea pedis*?

(1) Wear rubber sandals in communal showers
(2) Wear light cotton socks
(3) Wear plastic shoes or sandals
(4) Carefully dry feet and toes after bathing

6 Which of the following clients that the nurse is scheduled to see this morning at the ambulatory care clinic is the least likely to be infected with herpes virus type 2?

(1) A smoker
(2) A client who has multiple sexual partners
(3) A client who consistently uses condoms during intercourse
(4) A 16-year-old client who uses a diaphragm

7 The client asks the nurse if a lesion on her hand could be a wart. The nurse would examine the area to determine the presence of which of the following characteristics?

(1) Firm, skin-colored papule
(2) Vesicle that is painful
(3) Oval erythemic lesion
(4) White round vesicle

8 The nurse would plan to include which of the following in the care of a client diagnosed with folliculitis?

(1) Warm compresses, good handwashing, and use of antibacterial soap
(2) Strict isolation of the site with sterile dressing changes four times a day
(3) Skin care is no different than routine skin care
(4) Keep skin site covered with clean bandage for 1 week

9 The nurse should plan to include which of the following statements in client teaching for impetigo?

(1) Poor hygiene is the only reason impetigo occurs.
(2) Good handwashing with antibacterial soap helps reduce spreading the infection to others.
(3) Impetigo is not contagious and cannot spread to other members of the family.
(4) Antibacterial medication is not useful in impetigo.

10 The nurse conducting health promotion about maintaining healthy skin in the community teaches clients that the epidermis has which of the following functions?

(1) To protect foreign objects from entering the eyes
(2) To regulate body heat by excretion of perspiration
(3) To produce androgens and regulate temperature
(4) To protect the tissues from physical damage and prevent water loss

See pages 412–413 for Answers and Rationales.

Answers and Rationales

Pretest

1 Answer: 3 *Rationale:* A bulla measures > 0.5 cm. A papule is solid; a vesicle measures < 0.5 cm; and a pustule contains purulent exudates.
Cognitive Level: Application
Nursing Process: Assessment; *Test Plan:* PHYS

2 Answer: 1 *Rationale:* The mole in option 1 meets the criteria of the "ABCD" rule: the size has increased in diameter over two months, the mole has two colors, the center is black, and the border is irregular.
Cognitive Level: Analysis
Nursing Process: Assessment; *Test Plan:* HPM

3 **Answer: 2** *Rationale:* Herpes simplex virus 1 may reappear in times of reactivation. The infection is described as a vesicular lesion that occurs on the oral mucosa (lips, mouth), making option 3 incorrect. Option 4 is false because herpes lesions are painful and because the description is incorrect.
Cognitive Level: Application
Nursing Process: Implementation; *Test Plan:* HPM

4 **Answer: 3** *Rationale:* The client with herpes zoster may experience impaired skin integrity and pruritis in which the client may frequently scratch the lesions, contributing to a secondary bacterial infection. Cool environments should be maintained because heat and scratching will make the pruritis worse (option 4). Options 1 and 2 are irrelevant to the client's case.
Cognitive Level: Application
Nursing Process: Planning; *Test Plan:* PHYS

5 **Answer: 3** *Rationale:* The common wart, flat wart, and filiform wart are not painful, whereas the plantar wart is often painful.
Cognitive Level: Comprehension
Nursing Process: Analysis; *Test Plan:* PHYS

6 **Answer: 1** *Rationale:* Vitiligo is a slowly progressive depigmentating condition of the skin caused by disappearance of melanocytes. Eczema is an inflammatory condition in which the skin appears erythemic, dry, and thickened. Psoriasis is a chronic inflammatory condition in which lesions appear whitish and scaly and commonly appear on the scalp, knees, and elbows. Contact dermatitis is an eruption of the skin related to contact with an irritating substance or allergen.
Cognitive Level: Application
Nursing Process: Assessment; *Test Plan:* PHYS

7 **Answer: 1** *Rationale:* Most burns occur at home caused by hot water or steam. All other aspects are important to general prevention but temperature setting of the water is a first-line prevention.
Cognitive Level: Analysis
Nursing Process: Planning; *Test Plan:* HPM

8 **Answer: 4** *Rationale:* In the emergent stage, the nurse assesses the cause and extent of the burn and determines first aid measures that were used. Gender is not a factor in burn assessment.
Cognitive Level: Application
Nursing Process: Assessment; *Test Plan:* PHYS

9 **Answer: 1** *Rationale:* The location of the rash helps identify the possible offending antigen. Age, gender, and recent travel are less helpful in identifying the etiology of the pruritic lesion.
Cognitive Level: Application
Nursing Process: Assessment; *Test Plan:* PHYS

10 **Answer: 2** *Rationale:* Psoriaris can often be brought on by a respiratory infection, particularly streptococcal pharyngitis. The other responses are insignificant findings as they relate to psoriasis.
Cognitive Level: Application
Nursing Process: Assessment; *Test Plan:* PHYS

Posttest

1 **Answer: 3** *Rationale:* Psoriasis is characterized by the presence of silvery plaques, particularly on the extensor prominences, that bleed when scales are removed. The other disorders listed are not characterized in this way.
Cognitive Level: Application
Nursing Process: Assessment; *Test Plan:* PHYS

2 **Answer: 1** *Rationale:* Even though all these problems may cause itching, a classical symptom of scabies is pruritus with worsening at night. The mites tend to have increased movement at night, which accounts for the worsening symptoms at that time.
Cognitive Level: Application
Nursing Process: Assessment; *Test Plan:* PHYS

3 **Answer: 3** *Rationale:* Dietary restrictions were once believed to be necessary to decrease acne, but this has not been clinically relevant or supported in research. Stress and the use of moisturizers and oil-based cosmetics do seem to affect the severity of the disorder.
Cognitive Level: Application
Nursing Process: Analysis; *Test Plan:* HPM

4 **Answer: 2** *Rationale:* Lindane (Kwell) can cause neurotoxicity in young children and nursing/pregnant women. This is not a concern with the other products listed.
Cognitive Level: Application
Nursing Process: Analysis; *Test Plan:* PHYS

5 **Answer: 3** *Rationale:* Plastic shoes or sandals increase moisture collection in the feet. This should be avoided as it increases the risk of recurrence. The other options describe helpful measures to prevent recurrence of *tinea pedis*.
Cognitive Level: Application
Nursing Process: Planning; *Test Plan:* HPM

6 **Answer: 3** *Rationale:* The consistent use of condoms helps protect from spreading herpes virus type 2 to other partners. The other options do not represent

circumstances that provide any protection against sexually transmitted diseases.
Cognitive Level: Application
Nursing Process: Analysis; *Test Plan:* PHYS

7   **Answer: 1** *Rationale:* A wart is described as being a round, raised, firm lesion of the skin that may have ragged borders. Warts do not contain fluid and generally have the color of normal flesh (options 3 and 4). Generally only plantar warts on the feet are associated with pain.
Cognitive Level: Application
Nursing Process: Assessment; *Test Plan:* PHYS

8   **Answer: 1** *Rationale:* To improve folliculitis, the use of antibacterial soap daily along with good hand-washing will control and prevent spread of the infection. Isolation is not needed. The site should also be

allowed to air dry and should not be covered with a bandage.
Cognitive Level: Application
Nursing Process: Planning; *Test Plan:* PHYS

9   **Answer: 2** *Rationale:* Good hygiene is recommended to help to prevent spreading the infection to other family members. Option 1 is false. Impetigo is contagious and antibiotic therapy is the recommended treatment (options 3 and 4).
Cognitive Level: Application
Nursing Process: Planning; *Test Plan:* PHYS

10   **Answer: 4** *Rationale:* The epidermis protects the tissues from damage and prevents fluid loss of the body. The dermis regulates body temperature (options 2 and 3). Option 1 is false.
Cognitive Level: Application
Nursing Process: Implementation; *Test Plan:* PHYS

References

Barker, L. (1999). *Principles of ambulatory care.* Baltimore, MD: Williams and Wilkins.

Cash, J. & Glass, C. (2000). *Family practice guidelines.* Philadelphia: Lippincott, Williams & Wilkins.

Dambro, M. (1999). *Griffith's 5 minute clinical consult.* Philadelphia: Lippincott.

Fauci, A. et al. (1998). *Harrison's principles of internal medicine* (14th ed.). New York: McGraw-Hill.

Lemone, P. & Burke, K. (2000). *Medical-surgical nursing: Critical thinking in client care* (2nd ed.). Upper Saddle River, NJ: Prentice-Hall, Inc.

Meredith, P. (2000). *Adult primary care.* Philadelphia: W.B. Saunders.

Robinson, D., Kidd, P., & Rogers, K. (2000). *Primary care across the lifespan.* St. Louis, MO: Mosby, Inc.

Singleton, J. (1999). *Primary care.* Philadelphia: Lippincott.

Weber, J. (2001). *Nurse's handbook of health assessment* (4th ed.). Philadelphia: Lippincott, Williams & Wilkins.

CHAPTER 11

Immunologic Disorders

Daryle Wane, APRN, BC, MSN, BSN

CHAPTER OUTLINE

OBJECTIVES

▌ Identify basic structures and functions of the immunologic system.

▌ Describe the pathophysiology and etiology of common immunologic disorders.

▌ Discuss expected assessment data and diagnostic test findings for selected immunologic disorders.

▌ Identify priority nursing diagnoses for selected immunologic disorders.

▌ Discuss therapeutic management of selected immunologic disorders.

▌ Discuss nursing management of a client experiencing an immunologic disorder.

▌ Identify expected outcomes for the client experiencing an immunologic disorder.

[Media Link]

Use the CD-ROM enclosed with this text, or log onto the address given to access the free, interactive Companion Website created for this series. The CD-ROM and Companion Website accompanying this book offer additional practice opportunities and information—NCLEX Review, Case Studies, Glossary, In Depth with NCLEX, and more.

www.prenhall.com/hogan

REVIEW AT A GLANCE

antibody *a specific substance produced by B lymphocytes in response to a specific antigen*

antigen *a protein substance that elicits a specific response that triggers an antibody response*

antigen-antibody complexes *a binding of antigen-antibody in the body to activate the immune response by either suppressing, amplifying or causing the activation of complement*

antihistamine *a substance that blocks the effects of histamine release in the body*

atopy *the incidence of increased allergic reactions as a result of hereditary disposition*

cell-mediated immunity *the recognition of T lymphocytes that are involved in the process of autoimmunity to afford protection*

colony-stimulating factors *a group of proteins that stimulate specific hematologic cell growth to help prevent bone marrow suppression or stimulate a client's response to it*

complement fixation *an antigen-antibody reaction whereby the complement*

system is activated, causing it to become "fixed"

human leukocyte antigens (HLA) *genetic markers found on chromosome 6 that are associated with specific diseases and used for tissue typing*

humoral immunity *a process in which B lymphocytes secrete circulating immunoglobulins that afford protection against specific antigens*

hypersensitivity *an exaggerated abnormal response to a specific indicator that leads to an overactive immune response*

immunoglobulins *a group of five structurally distinct humoral antibodies that are secreted in response to specific antigens*

major histocompatibility complex (MHC) *a group of proteins carrying specific genetic information that play an active role in autoimmune recognition and tissue rejection*

monoclonal antibodies *antibodies produced by a specific group of identical cells that are being used in the treatment of hematologic and oncologic disease, both to identify and treat tumors due to their specific targeting effect*

myelosuppression *the inhibition or destruction of blood cells in the bone marrow that can leads to immunosuppression*

neutropenic precautions *the institution of specific measures aimed at protecting an individual who is immunosuppressed from potential infection and injury during the course of treatment*

opportunistic infection *a nonpathogenic infection that becomes pathogenic as a result of an individual's baseline immunosuppressive state*

plasmapheresis *the process whereby plasma is removed from the body and sent through a machine membrane to remove immune complexes that are associated with disease processes*

tensilon *test the injection of cholinesterase substance (edrophonium), which is used as a diagnostic agent in the treatment of myasthenia gravis*

wasting syndrome *unexplained weight loss of > 10 percent ideal body weight (IBW) that is associated with a cycle of malnutrition and subsequent wasting that is an AIDS defining diagnosis*

Pretest

1 Which of the following atypical findings would the nurse look for in the older adult client who presents with an infection?

(1) Fever
(2) Erythema and edema
(3) Behavioral changes and confusion
(4) Leukocytosis

2 A client has an unexplained weight loss of more than 10 percent of ideal body weight (IBW) and voices nonspecific complaints of fatigue and nausea over the last 6-month period. The nurse should place the highest priority on further assessing the client when the client makes which of the following statements?

(1) "I have had a low-grade fever for the past week."
(2) "I had a blood transfusion several years ago after having surgery."
(3) "I have been taking vitamin supplements on a daily basis for the last 2 weeks."
(4) "I have been tested for HIV in the past, but the results were negative."

3 While obtaining a review of systems the client informs you that he is "highly allergic" to many food items and medications. You conclude that which hypersensitivity reaction would be responsible for this type of clinical presentation?

(1) Type 1, IgE mediated hypersensitivity
(2) Type 2, cytotoxic hypersensitivity
(3) Type 3. immune complex-mediated hypersensitivity
(4) Type 4, delayed hypersensitivity

4 A client who receives a positive antinuclear antibody (ANA) test result with a titer level > 1:40 does not understand what the test result means and asks the nurse for an explanation. Which of the following responses to the client would be most appropriate in this situation?

(1) "The test result is normal."
(2) "The test indicates that you may have an autoimmune disorder, and this result should be discussed in more detail with your physician."
(3) "You should have the test repeated to verify its specificity for autoimmune disorders."
(4) "Your test result is specific for the detection of systemic lupus, and this should be discussed further with your physician.

5 Which one of the following measures would be beneficial in helping a client with a past history of anaphylaxis to develop a plan for handling possible allergic reactions?

(1) Have acetaminophen (Tylenol) readily available.
(2) Have acetylsalicylic acid (ASA) readily available.
(3) Have diphenhydramine (Benadryl) readily available.
(4) Have epinephrine (EpiPen) readily available.

6 Hydroxychloroquine (Plaquenil) is prescribed for a client for the treatment of rheumatoid arthritis. The nurse would include which one of the following measures as part of client teaching with regard to this medication?

(1) Take this medication on an empty stomach to minimize gastric irritation.
(2) Have an initial baseline eye exam performed and adhere to scheduled follow-up exam to monitor for potential ocular changes.
(3) Monitor weight and vital signs as the medication can cause fluid retention and pulse elevations.
(4) Be aware that medication can cause drowsiness and do not take it if planning to drive a car.

7 The nurse has conducted discharge teaching for a client diagnosed with myasthenia gravis. The nurse evaluates that the client understood the instructions given with regard to the administration of anticholinesterase medication if the client takes the medication:

(1) On a full stomach.
(2) Only at night.
(3) With 8 ounces of milk.
(4) 30 minutes prior to meals.

8 The nurse would assess for which one of the following findings that is consistent with clinical manifestations of systemic sclerosis?

(1) Raynaud's phenomenon
(2) Conjunctivitis
(3) Photophobia
(4) Splenomegaly

9 Which one of the following statements indicates the client's understanding of measures used in the treatment of systemic lupus erythematosus?

(1) "I will be able to continue with my tanning bed appointments."
(2) "I can go visit this weekend with my grandmother who has been ill with a cold."
(3) "I can go for a walk on the beach after 3:00 P.M."
(4) "I have to apply SPF 10 sunscreen when I go to the beach."

10 Regardless of the type of isolation precautions that a client has been assigned, which of the following actions by the nurse should be given the highest priority in terms of infection control?

(1) Using strict aseptic technique
(2) Washing of hands before and after giving client care
(3) Checking sterile supplies for expiration date
(4) Changing intravenous tubing according to hospital policy

See pages 451–452 for Answers and Rationales.

I. Immunologic System

A. Basic structures of the immunologic system

1. Lymphoid system

   a. Lymphoid system consists of lymph nodes, spleen, thymus, tonsils, lymphoid tissues (in mucosa and connective tissues) and *bone marrow,* a myeloid tissue involved in blood cell formation (see Figure 11-1)

   b. Organs and tissues include lymphocytes as part of their basic structure

   c. Lymphoid organs consist of the lymph nodes, thymus, spleen and tonsils

   d. Lymphoid tissues consist of lymphocytes and plasma cells

   e. Lymphatic system consists of a communication network of vessels, lymph nodes, lymph node clusters, and circulating and resident lymphocytes that function as a primary component in the immune system response

2. Central lymphoid organs

   a. The *thymus gland,* which assists in T lymphocyte formation, is located in the superior mediastinum behind the sternum

   b. Bone marrow sources can be found in the iliac crest, the sternum and in bone cavities throughout the body

3. Peripheral organs

   a. Tonsils are a group of lymphoid tissue found in the palatine area of the oropharynx in the mouth

Figure 11-1

Components of the lymphoid system.

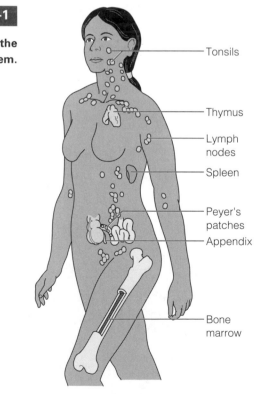

Tonsils

Thymus

Lymph nodes

Spleen

Peyer's patches

Appendix

Bone marrow

    b. Lymph nodes are found throughout the body and consist of a small rounded mass of tissue from which the lymph fluid drains

    c. Mucosa-associated lymph tissue (MALT) consists of a grouping of lymph tissue that is found in many organs of the body that work together to promote an immune response; specific locators identify the source of the tissue; for example: bronchial-associated lymph tissue (BALT), gut-associated lymph tissue (GALT), skin-associated lymph tissue (SALT)

    d. The spleen is located in the left upper quadrant of the abdomen and is composed of white and red pulp; the white pulp is composed of B and T lymphocytes; the red pulp is composed of erythrocytes

  4. Mononuclear phagocyte system (MPS)

    a. Monocytes are the largest component of the white blood cells (WBCs) and have one nucleus and very little cytoplasm; they are considered to be agranulocytes

    b. Macrophages are considered to be the mature cells of the MPS; they migrate to different areas of the body, becoming specialized cells to perform their function of defense

    c. The MPS functions to protect the body by participating in the immune response; it secretes chemical components and factors (enzymes, complement proteins, and interleukins)

B. Basic functions of the immunologic system

  1. Thymus gland

> NCLEX**!**

    a. In childhood, the gland is large; with aging, the gland atrophies because of fat infiltration

    b. The thymus gland gives rise to the differentiation and maturation of T lymphocytes, which are involved in **cell-mediated immunity,** a part of the process of autoimmunity

    c. It secretes thymic hormones such as thymosin; hormone level is stable from birth to age 25 and then gradually decreases thereafter

  2. Bone marrow

> NCLEX**!**

    a. Bone marrow serves as a diagnostic predictor for immunologic, hematologic, and oncologic disorders

    b. It provides for analysis of chemical markers leading to the identification of specific disease processes

    c. It is the source of primary lymphoid action that helps to initiate, maintain and provide for the immune response; marrow gives rise to cellular components of blood and stores stem cells

    d. Bone marrow gives rise to B lymphocytes and humorally mediated responses (**humoral immunity**) that involve the production of **antibodies,** specific substances produced in response to specific antigens

  3. Spleen

    a. The spleen is the site of destruction of RBCs as well as a storage site for blood

b. It acts as a reservoir for B lymphocytes

c. It filters and removes foreign material, worn-out cells, and forms of cellular debris

d. The spleen contains both red and white pulp tissues that help to perform functions of RBC removal and B lymphocyte development into mature plasma cells

C. Normal immune response

1. Defense

   a. The body provides for a communication network of protection that involves both nonspecific and specific forms of defense

   b. Nonspecific defense relates to external reactions that include anatomic and chemical barriers such as the skin and mucous membranes; they are considered non-selective, which means that they are activated against any foreign substance that the body would encounter

   c. Specific defense relates to internal physiological reactions of the body that include both cell mediated and humorally mediated antibodies; they are considered specific, which means that they are unique substances that require activation

   d. The body initiates its immune response in the presence of an **antigen,** a protein substance that triggers antibody production

2. Homeostasis

   a. The body seeks to maintain an immune balance where it can successfully remove damaged cells

   b. In homeostasis, there is a balanced response of circulating and resident lymphocytes to maintain adequate protection

3. Surveillance

   a. Surveillance is the ability of the body to use memory and recognition in order to maintain an immune response

   b. The body will remember the activation response even if the person doesn't remember the specific insult

D. Types of immunity

1. Acquired immunity

   a. Active acquired immunity is a long-term response in an organism that leads to the development of antibodies that offer protection

   NCLEX!

   1) This can be accomplished by the individual developing antibodies in response to having the disease process or by a response to artificial antigens as with the administration of vaccine or toxoid

   2) This immunization response can be boosted and maintained via repeated injections

   3) Titer serum levels can be monitored in the client to indicate whether or not immunity is present

    b. Passive acquired immunity requires that the antibody be introduced to the individual, either by maternal transfer (placenta and/or colostrum) or immune serum antibody injection, to promote a specific antigen response

  2. Natural immunity

    a. This type of immunity that exists in an individual is related to a species, race, or genetic trait

    b. An individual is born with natural immunity

  3. Humoral immunity

    a. This involves the recognition of antigens by the B lymphocytes

    b. B lymphocytes differentiate into plasma cells and memory cells

    c. Memory cells lead to a more rapid response by remembering the original insult

    d. Plasma cells secrete **immunoglobulins,** a group of glycoproteins, each of which has four polypeptide chains (two heavy and two light chains); the FAB fragment, which is different in each immunoglobulin, denotes specific antigen binding sites

    e. Immunoglobulins are identified as IgA, IgD, IgE, IgG, and IgM; see Table 11-1 for listing and characteristics of immunoglobulins

  4. Cell-mediated immunity

    a. T lymphocytes recognize a specific **major histocompatibility complex (MHC),** a group of proteins that play a role in autoimmune recognition and tissue rejection, and binds to them to elicit an immune response

    b. Protein markers on the surface of the T-cell help to define specific function receptor sites; these are called CD antigens or clusters of differentiation;

Table 11-1	**Class**	**Location**	**Characteristic**
Types of Immunoglobulins	**IgA**	Body secretions Tears, saliva Colostrum and breast milk	Lines mucous membranes Protects body surfaces
	IgD	Plasma	Present on lymphocytes
	IgE	Plasma Interstitial fluids Exocrine secretions	Allergic/anaphylaxis Bound to mast cells
	IgG	Plasma Interstitial fluid	Crosses placenta Complement fixation Secondary immune response
	IgM	Plasma	Complement fixation Primary immune response Involved in ABO antigens

CD markers serve as an important prognostic indicator of immune function and are used in the diagnosis and management of clients with human immunodeficiency virus (HIV) and acquired immunodeficiency syndrome (AIDS)

   c. Humoral immunity is considered a long-term process whereby the T lymphocytes help to protect the body against bacterial, viral, and fungal infections

   d. Cell mediated immunity is also responsible for the mediation of transplant rejection

5. A diagrammatic representation of T lymphocyte and B lymphocyte development from lymphoblasts is found in Figure 11-2

6. Other immune system participants

   a. Natural killer cell (Null cell, NK cell) activity is present at birth, increases as one reaches adulthood and decreases gradually in old age; null cells do not require prior sensitization and are not considered T- or B lymphocytes

   b. Cytokines (also referred to as lymphokines and monokines) are soluble protein mediators of the immune response; interleukins, tumor necrosis factor, and interferon are examples of these chemical messengers, which have been used as treatment options in boosting the immune response

NCLEX!

Figure 11-2

Development of T lymphocytes and B lymphocytes from lymphoblasts.

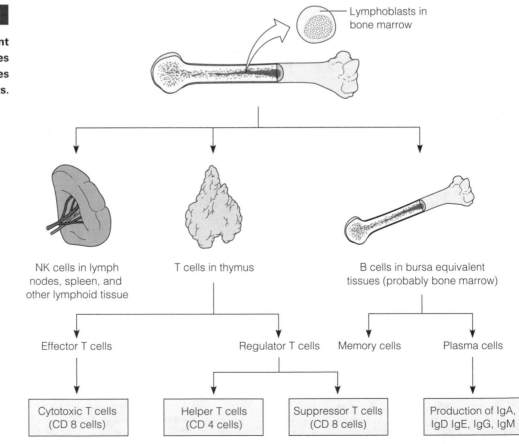

7. Complement system

   a. This is a group of glycoproteins that are activated in sequential order and provide a link to the humoral response

   b. IgG and IgM are responsible for activating the complement cascade; once this is activated, it is said that the complement has been fixed or **complement fixation** has taken place

   c. Complement assays are used in the diagnosis of immunodeficiencies and autoimmune diseases

   d. There is a classic pathway and an alternate pathway whereby the complement system can be activated

8. Biological response modifiers (BRMs)

   a. Are a group of substances that can elicit, modify, and restore the biological response between an inidvidual and a tumor cell

   b. This is an area of key research in which scientists are looking at developing better outcomes, thereby improving response and overall cure rates for immune disorders

   c. Examples include:

      1) **Monoclonal antibodies,** which are antibodies produced by a specific group of identical cells, that are then used to treat tumors because of their specific targeting effect

      2) **Colony-stimulating factors,** a group of proteins that stimulate growth of specific hematological cells (red blood cells or white blood cells) to prevent or help reduce a client's adverse response to disease; these types of BRMs are used as treatment measures in a variety of hematologic and immunologic diseases

II. Altered Immune Responses: Hypersensitivity Reactions

A. **Hypersensitivity** is an abnormal exaggerated response to a specific indicator that leads to an overactive immune response

B. **The Gell & Coombs Classification of Hypersensitivity Reactions** is widely accepted in clinical practice and categorizes a reaction according to type, class, and immunity (see Table 11-2)

1. Type 1: anaphylactoid reactions

   a. Type 1 involves an immediate response; however, the potential responses can be cumulative; for example, the initial or sensitizing dose may not elicit a strong response, but subsequent contacts, even if not long-term in nature, may cause a stronger response than the previous insult

---

Practice to Pass

A client's immunization schedule is up-to-date. What type of immunity does this provide to the client?

Table 11-2	Type	Class	Immunity
Gell & Coombs Classification	I	Immediate hypersensitivity	Humoral
	II	Cytotoxic reactions	Humoral
	III	Immune complex related	Humoral
	IV	Delayed hypersensitivity	Cell-mediated

    b. Etiology/pathophysiology: Type 1 involves the characteristic activation of IgE bound to mast cells, whereby histamine is released

    c. Clinical manifestations range from bronchospasm, wheezing, rhinorrhea, and urticaria to angioedema and finally anaphylaxis; there may be progression from local to systemic reactions; characteristic allergic "gape" and allergic "shiner" can be seen in individuals with **atopy** (allergic reactions stemming from hereditary disposition)

NCLEX!

    d. Diagnostic and laboratory test findings: immunoglobulin titers are predictive of potential allergen response; skin and patch testing are performed to determine potential allergens

NCLEX!

    e. Therapeutic management

        1) **Antihistamine** medications such as diphenhydramine (Benadryl) are used to block chemical release of mediators (histamines)

        2) Mast cell degradation inhibitors such as cromolyn sodium (Intal) also are used to block the chemical response

        3) Decongestants and corticosteroids can help to minimize the immune response; however, in potential anaphylactic reactions, the use of epinephrine is warranted; an Epipen may be prescribed as appropriate therapy for individuals who are at profound risk for hypersensitivity reactions; they are available in both adult and pediatric dosages

NCLEX!

    f. Nursing implications

        1) Immediately withdraw the offending allergen in presence of documented or suspected reaction

        2) Manage the client according to ABC protocol (airway, breathing, and circulation)

  2. Type II: cytotoxic and cytolytic reactions

    a. This type of immunity involves the activation of complement and is considered a form of humoral immunity

    b. Etiology and pathophysiology

        1) This involves the production of autoantibodies that result in destruction of one's own cells or tissues

        2) IgA and IgM are involved with this type of response and the complement system is activated

NCLEX!

    c. Clinical manifestations: a wide range of presentations occur ranging from hemolytic reactions (such as transfusion, erythroblastosis fetalis, hemolytic anemia and drug-induced hemolysis) to target cell destruction as seen in Goodpasture's syndrome (an autoimmune disease affecting pulmonary and renal systems) and other autoimmune disease processes such as myasthenia gravis and Graves' disease

    d. Diagnostic and laboratory test findings: Coombs blood test can define the presence of hemolytic anemia and identify potential ABO incompatibility

NCLEX!

    e. Therapeutic management: use of proper identification during blood product administration can help to prevent exposure and sensitization; recognition of certain blood types and an awareness that potential drug interactions can cause antigen complex activation can lead to early detection of reactions

NCLEX!

f. Nursing implications

1) Be sure to remain in the room during the first 15 minutes of any blood product administration since clients are more likely to experience a reaction during this time frame

2) Make sure to follow agency policy and procedure for the administration of any and all blood products; two RNs must verify the product before administration

3. Type III: immune complex reactions

a. A Type III reaction involves the formation of **antigen-antibody complexes** (a binding together of an antibody and an antigen)

1) This leads to the activation of serum factors, causing inflammation and leading to activation of the complement cascade

2) Rheumatoid arthritis and systemic lupus erythematosus are examples of Type III reactions

3) The deposition of the antigen-antibody complexes in body tissues is not localized and therefore can result in more extensive tissue or organ destruction

b. Etiology and pathophysiology: complement activation impacts vulnerable organs and leads to intravascular changes

c. Clinical manifestations

1) Arthrus reaction involves a localized inflammatory response with excess IgG causing edema and necrotic lesions

2) Serum sickness involves a systemic response leading to the deposit and activation of complement throughout the body that can be demonstrated as joint pain, pyrexia, and/or lymphadenopathy

3) Reactions can be acute or chronic in nature

d. Diagnostic and laboratory test findings: complement assays provide diagnostic and predictive indicators of the acute and/or chronic nature of the process; erythrocyte sedimentation rate (ESR) is elevated; proteinuria may be found on urinalysis

NCLEX!

e. Therapeutic management: analgesics, antihistamines and topical steroids may provide symptom relief; the disease process itself is usually self-limiting because of the use of human anti-tetanus serum and the availability of antibiotics

f. Nursing implications

1) Be aware that it is possible for localized inflammatory reactions to develop at the site of serum injections after 1 week; this can be followed by a more systemic response involving both regional as well as generalized lymphadenopathies

2) If symptoms arise, monitor client for potential complications; this is especially important because organ damage can occur and the kidneys can be compromised

4. Type IV: delayed hypersensitivity reactions

   a. Type IV is a form of cell-mediated immunity involving T lymphocytes; it is considered a delayed response

   b. Etiology and pathophysiology: delayed hypersensitivity reactions involve the recognition and response of T lymphocytes to foreign substances

   c. Clinical manifestations

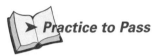

   1) There is a wide range of presentation from tuberculin response, poison ivy, and contact dermatitis to transplant or graft rejection; edema, ischemia and eventual tissue destruction may ensue

   2) Pyrexia, pain, edema, and failure of the transplanted organ characterize transplant rejection

   d. Diagnostic and laboratory test findings: purified protein derivative (PPD) test result of induration > 5 mm identifies Type IV hypersensitivity to the tubercle bacillus; abnormal test results indicating declining function of the transplanted organ are used to diagnose transplant rejection

   e. Therapeutic management

   1) Monitor client for evidence of potential transplant rejection

   2) Medicate the patient with immunosuppressive protocol drugs to prevent tissue rejection

   3) Identify potential irritants that can cause contact dermatitis and avoid exposure

   f. Nursing implications

   1) Make sure that the client avoids the offending irritant if a past exposure has been documented

   2) Use topical and oral medications as indicated to alleviate many of the symptom complaints and increase client comfort

III. Autoimmunity

A. Overview

1. Concept of autoimmunity

   a. Autoimmunity is an abnormal response of the body's immune system whereby it perceives "self" as a threat

   b. There are several mechanisms of action that can affect the autoimmune process, such as cell-mediated, antibody-mediated and immune complex reactions

2. Genetic component of the autoimmune response

   a. Genetic traits are associated with autoimmune diseases

   b. **Human leukocyte antigens (HLAs),** genetic markers found on chromosome 6, are involved with the diagnosis of many autoimmune diseases and are also used for tissue typing

> **Practice to Pass**
>
> A client becomes short of breath after eating strawberries. What are your immediate assessments and interventions?

3. Cell-mediated autoimmunity

   a. This type of autoimmunity is associated with an abnormal T-cell response

   b. There can be an overabundance of T-cytotoxic (killer) cells or there can be a deficiency of T-suppressor (helper) cells

4. Antibody-mediated autoimmunity

   a. This type of autoimmunity is associated with the development of autoantibodies that affect specific receptor sites causing tissue and organ damage

   b. Complement activation causes inflammatory reactions and leads to cell damage

   c. Graves' disease and myasthenia gravis are examples of antibody-mediated autoimmunity

5. Immune complex disease

   a. This type of autoimmunity is associated with the deposition of immune complexes at the serum level

   b. Complement activation causes inflammatory reactions and leads to further damage

6. Diagnostic testing for autoimmunity

   a. Autoantibody assays, complement fixation, and complement assays provide diagnostic information

   b. Identification of HLA antigens provides indication of genetic inheritance

7. Treatment for autoimmunity

   a. Immunosuppressive agents and corticosteroids are given to suppress the abnormal immune response

   b. Symptom management can be achieved through the use of anti-inflammatory agents to minimize pain that the client experiences from tissue damage caused by immune complex deposits

   c. **Plasmapheresis** is used to remove circulating immune complexes; in this treatment, plasma is removed from the body, sent through a machine membrane that traps immune complexes, and is returned to the client

8. Progression of disease

   a. Autoimmune diseases are characterized by acute exacerbation of a chronic condition

   b. They affect a large percentage of the average population and, depending on the specific disease, they can be seen across the lifespan, affecting both children and adults

   c. In many cases, splenectomy has been performed as part of the therapeutic management of many autoimmune diseases; while one can certainly live without a spleen, its removal is no longer always guaranteed as a form of therapeutic management; current therapeutic regimens are looking at different methods, such as chemotherapy and the use of biological response modifiers, instead of splenectomy

B. Systemic lupus erythematosus (SLE)

1. Description

   a. SLE is a multisystem autoimmune disease that is characterized by a fluctuating, chronic course

   b. Multiple organ involvement is seen in this disease process that results in eventual major organ system failure

   c. There are two forms of this disease: systemic and discoid; systemic involves the entire system response of the individual, whereas discoid involves the characteristic skin rash without systemic disease complaints

2. Etiology and pathophysiology

   a. Specific HLA antigens indicate this type of disease (HLA-B8, HLA-DR2, HLA-DR3)

   b. C_2 and C_4 complement deficiencies are also seen

   c. Estrogen inhibits suppressor T-cell function leading to an abnormal immune response

   d. The disease primarily affects women of childbearing age (30 to 50 years of age being most common)

   e. Ethnic presentations: it occurs more frequently in those of African American, Latino, Asian, and Native American descent

3. Assessment

   a. Clinical manifestations

      1) The American College of Rheumatology has developed a listing of 11 criteria that are used to define the classification of lupus

      2) Environmental triggers such as ultraviolet light, infection, and/or drugs can cause clinical responses

      3) Arthritis is the most common symptom presentation

      4) The butterfly rash (malar rash) is probably the most common dermatologic expression of this disease

      5) Drug-induced lupus can be found as a response to certain medications such as phenytoin (Dilantin), hydralazine (Apresoline), procainamide (Pronestyl), isoniazid (INH), and penicillamine (Depen); if a client exhibits any signs or symptoms of the disease and is on one of these medications, the medication should be stopped to see whether symptoms disappear

      6) Clients may present with pleural manifestations such as pleuritis and pleural cffusions

      7) Renal involvement is a serious consequence of disease progression; renal failure is the leading cause of death associated with this disease

      8) Cardiac involvement is another serious consequence of this disease progression; cardiac involvement is the second-leading cause of death

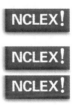

9) Central nervous system involvement is the third-leading cause of death from disease progression; manifestations can range from subtle behavioral changes to profound psychological disturbances and eventually result in stroke or seizure activity

10) Hematologic involvement can lead to altered immune responses, which result in increased risk of infection; clients can develop anemia, leukopenia, thrombocytopenia, and even hemolytic anemia

11) Pregnancy and the use of oral contraceptives can affect a client's estrogen level and therefore may pose an increased risk for disease flare-ups

b. Diagnostic and laboratory test findings

1) A positive ANA titer is present in clients who have this disease process; titers > 1:80 are seen in this disease state; a rim or speckled pattern to the antibody is more likely to be associated with SLE

2) During flare-ups of the disease process, complement (C_3 and C_4) may be decreased

3) During flare-ups of the disease process, erythrocyte sedimentation rate (ESR) and C reactive protein (CRP) may be elevated

4) A positive rheumatoid factor (+RF) may be seen in clients with a titer of > 1:40 who have this disease

5) Complete blood count (CBC) with differential may reveal a normochromic, normocytic anemia with leukopenia and thrombocytopenia

6) Positive Coombs result may be seen if the client develops hemolytic anemia as a consequence of the disease process

7) Lactic dehydrogenase (LDH) may also be elevated; LDH is usually elevated in many types of malignancies such as leukemias and high-grade lymphomas

8) Coagulation tests such as prothrombin time (PT) and activated partial thromboplastin time (APTT) may be elevated if circulating anticoagulants are present; a specific lupus anticoagulant can be tested to determine disease presence

9) Urinalysis may reveal presence of casts and sediment; creatinine levels may rise as renal involvement progresses

4. Therapeutic management

a. Management is aimed at recognizing flare-ups of the disease and preventing further complications of the disease process

b. The level of treatment is adjusted to the disease activity and the client receives individualized care

c. Treatment areas can be categorized as conservative and aggressive; conservative measures are aimed at promotion of rest and general support pharmacotherapy; aggressive measures include surgical interventions (splenectomy) and chemotherapy

d. Collaborate with dietician to support immune functions and maintain integrity of body systems during this chronic disease

5. Priority nursing diagnoses: Risk for infection; Ineffective protection; Impaired skin integrity; Ineffective health maintenance; Impaired tissue perfusion; Disturbed body image; Ineffective individual coping; Noncompliance; Social isolation; Pain, Chronic low self-esteem; Ineffective patterns of sexuality; Fatigue

6. Planning and implementation

   a. Plan for rest periods to avoid fatigue and lessen stress levels for the client

   b. Avoid environmental triggers such as prolonged ultraviolet light exposure that may cause client to develop skin eruptions; client can be photosensitive, so consider this when planning care

   c. Monitor client for symptom presentation and medicate as ordered to promote symptom relief

   d. Collaborate with other healthcare team members to institute a long-term treatment plan for the client that offers anticipatory guidance and emotional support

   e. Monitor the client for potential complications of the disease either due to treatment measures (glucocorticoids) or disease progression

   f. Clients with this disease should try to have a planned pregnancy; alternative birth control methods such as diaphragm and condoms should be utilized because oral contraceptives can affect a client's estrogen level

7. Medication therapy

   a. Nonsteroidal anti-inflammatory drugs (NSAIDs) and acetylsalicylic acid (aspirin, ASA) are used to control the common joint symptom presentations that the majority of clients experience during this disease

   b. Hydroxychloroquine (Plaquenil) is used to treat dermatologic symptoms of the disease

      1) This anti-malarial also helps decrease photosensitivity and prevent musculoskeletal flares

      2) It is critical to monitor the client for retinal toxicity

      3) A baseline ocular exam should be done along with periodic evaluations (monthly initially and then every 6 months) to determine ocular status

   c. Glucocorticoids are used to suppress disease activity and for symptom management; dosing can be adjusted in response to flare-ups; oral or IV route is preferred; tapered dose therapy (pulse dose) is usually initiated to achieve best results to arrive at the lowest possible dosage and to prevent side effects of steroid therapy

   d. Long-term steroid therapy can result in avascular necrosis that can affect the hips, knee, ankle, shoulder or elbow; surgical intervention may be necessary in order to correct and stabilize the joint to prevent further deterioration and/or injury

   e. Immunosuppressive agents such as cyclophosphamide (Cytoxan) and azathiopine (Imuran) can be given to effectively modulate an immune response; however, the client will be at increased risk for **myelosuppression**

(inhibition or destruction of bone marrow) because of this treatment regimen and therefore must be monitored accordingly

f. Gamma globulin can be given IV to the client to promote specific immune function

g. Plasmapheresis can be used to remove immune complexes to help to relieve client's symptoms

8. Client education

a. Assist the client to understand the occurrence of flare-ups and the chronic nature of the disease process

b. Establish a collaborative network for the client to maintain an optimum level of health

c. Promote client self-monitoring of condition to identify potential health problems more quickly

d. Discuss potential dynamic life changes such as pregnancy and childbearing that may influence disease activity

e. Discuss the interactions, potential consequences, and overall effects of medications so that the client is aware of followup measures and is an active participant in the health care team

9. Evaluation

a. The client will be able to identify potential environment risks and thereby prevent exposure to infection, dermatologic eruptions, and stress

b. The client will be able to monitor underlying disease process and complications that would heighten medical risks

c. The client will comply with treatment measures aimed at managing symptoms so that activities of daily living (ADLs) can be done at an optimal level

C. Rheumatoid arthritis (RA)

1. Description

a. RA is a systemic disorder involving symmetrical inflammation of synovial membranes and joints that leads to deformities and loss of joint function

b. The clinical course of RA has periods of remission and exacerbation but the underlying disease process is chronic in nature

c. There are four stages of classification with regard to this disease process

1) Stage 1: Disease present but no disability

2) Stage 2: Disease beginning to interfere with ADLs

3) Stage 3: Major compromise in function

4) Stage 4: Incapacitation

2. Etiology and pathophysiology

a. The exact etiology is still unknown, but it is suspected that RA is a form of autoimmune disease process

b. RA is thought to be associated with the deposition of antigen-antibody complexes and the development of rheumatoid nodules

c. Females are three times more likely than males to develop the disorder

d. RA has a bimodal appearance, as there is a juvenile form of the disease (JRA), as well as the more commonly seen adult form of the disease

e. American College of Rheumatology defines criteria that confirm the diagnosis of RA in an individual client

3. Assessment

   a. Clinical manifestations

     1) Client usually presents with complaints of fatigue, general malaise, and anorexia and weight loss

     2) Persistent joint pain lasting > 3 months is more evident on motion, but client will complain of pain also at rest; this is a significant finding

     3) Characteristic morning stiffness lasting > 1 hour is also an indication of the progression and severity of the disease; if present, note the onset, duration, and joints involved

     4) Early in the disease process, the client may experience tenderness, swelling, and restricted range of motion in the affected joints

     5) As the disease progresses and the joints become less stable, characteristic deformities appear ranging from contractures to subluxation; observe client for characteristic joint deformities such as swan neck deformity, Boutonniere deformity, subcutaneous nodules, and ulnar deviation or drift (see Figure 11-3)

     6) Systemic complaints range from fever to splenomegaly and reflect extraarticular findings

     7) Monitor client for occurrence of joint effusions

     8) Assess client's ability to perform ADLs

   b. Diagnostic and laboratory test findings

     1) Positive rheumatoid factor (RF) is seen in a majority of clients who have this disease process but it is also seen in a majority of the normal population, making it a nonspecific finding

     2) Elevated ESR, C-reactive protein, and serum complement are often seen in this disease process

     3) CBC with differential may reveal anemia as well as leukocytosis

     4) X-rays reveal a narrowing of joint spaces and erosive changes at bone margins as the disease progresses

     5) Aspiration of synovial fluid reveals characteristic findings such as turbidity, elevated cell counts, and formation of a poor mucin clot

4. Therapeutic management

   a. The major treatment goal is to help the client maintain the ability to function

   b. Treatment measures are aimed at decreasing joint pain and swelling

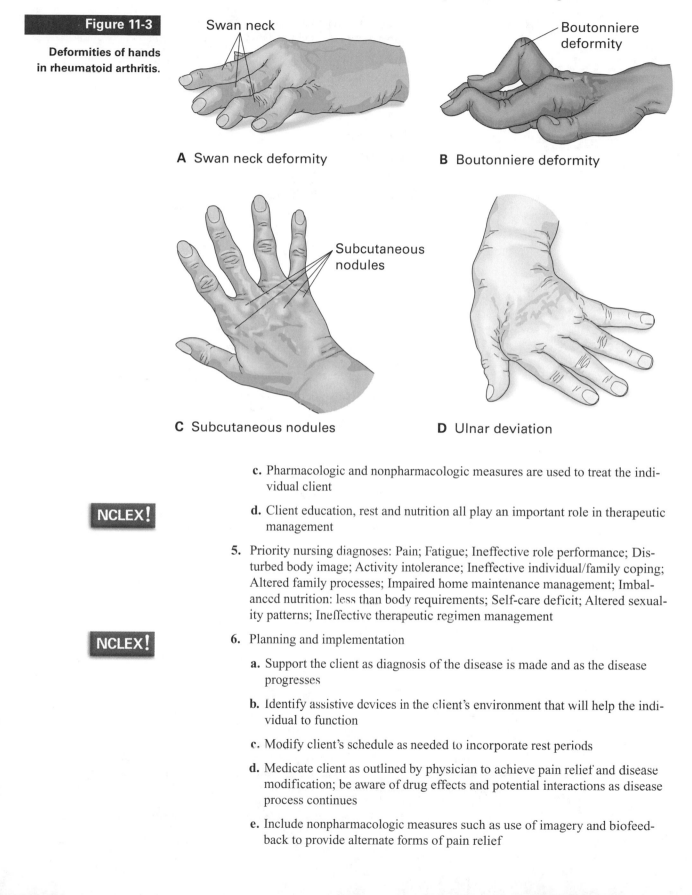

Figure 11-3

Deformities of hands in rheumatoid arthritis.

Swan neck

Boutonniere deformity

A Swan neck deformity

B Boutonniere deformity

Subcutaneous nodules

C Subcutaneous nodules

D Ulnar deviation

   c. Pharmacologic and nonpharmacologic measures are used to treat the individual client

   d. Client education, rest and nutrition all play an important role in therapeutic management

5. Priority nursing diagnoses: Pain; Fatigue; Ineffective role performance; Disturbed body image; Activity intolerance; Ineffective individual/family coping; Altered family processes; Impaired home maintenance management; Imbalanced nutrition: less than body requirements; Self-care deficit; Altered sexuality patterns; Ineffective therapeutic regimen management

6. Planning and implementation

   a. Support the client as diagnosis of the disease is made and as the disease progresses

   b. Identify assistive devices in the client's environment that will help the individual to function

   c. Modify client's schedule as needed to incorporate rest periods

   d. Medicate client as outlined by physician to achieve pain relief and disease modification; be aware of drug effects and potential interactions as disease process continues

   e. Include nonpharmacologic measures such as use of imagery and biofeedback to provide alternate forms of pain relief

NCLEX!

NCLEX!

    f. Use heat and cold applications to affected joints to provide relief; these measures should be individualized to afford maximum client comfort

    g. Include foods high in omega-3 fatty acids, since current research trends show that these are beneficial to clients who have RA as well as other diseases such as heart disease; suggested food items include fish oils and salmon

  7. Medication therapy

    a. ASA and NSAIDS are used to decrease joint inflammation and control symptoms

    b. Disease-modifying antirheumatic drugs (DMARDS) are used to alter the rate of disease progression; their onset of action is slower (> 8 weeks) and they are currently instituted when NSAIDS are considered to be ineffective; however, newer approaches to the treatment of RA suggest that this drug category should be utilized as a first-line approach, since they affect disease progression and not merely control symptoms; examples include gold salts, antimalarial agents (Plaquenil), sulfasalazine (Azulfidine), D-pencillamine (Cuprimine), and immunosuppressive agents (see Table 11-3 for DMARD classification)

    c. Immunosuppressive agents such as azathioprine (Imuran), cyclophosphamide (Cytoxan), and methotrexate (Rheumatrex) are used; these agents are used in clients who are experiencing severe disabling RA or who have been refractory to other forms of treatment

    d. Methotrexate is widely used in the treatment of RA; onset of action is similar to other DMARDs; dosage is adjusted to get the maximum response at the lowest dose; relief effect continues during the course of treatment

    e. The FDA has approved etanercept (Enbrel), a tumor necrosis factor, in combination with methotrexate to treat RA

NCLEX!

    f. It is critical to note that if the client is taking any form of immunosuppressive agent, he or she must be monitored for signs of clinical improvement, as well as myelosuppression and drug toxicity

  8. Client education

    a. Client should be referred to a rheumatologist to coordinate management of care

NCLEX!

    b. Assist the client to understand occurrence of flare-ups and chronic nature of disease process

Table 11-3 Disease-Modifying Antirheumatic Drug Classification	Class	Nursing Concerns
	Gold salts	Monitor for adverse effects Nitritoid reactions are likely
	Antimalarial	Monitor for adverse effects Instruct client to get eye exam as baseline and every 6 months
	Immunosuppressive agents	Monitor for myelosuppression Maximize effect at lowest dose Monitor for methotrexate interactions with ETOH and other drugs to avoid toxic levels

c. Discuss the importance of adequate symptom management to achieve an optimal level of function

NCLEX!

d. Discuss the importance of client self-monitoring and compliance with treatment and medication therapy

e. Discuss potential dynamic life changes that might occur as a result of progression of deformity and loss of function

9. Evaluation

    a. The client will maintain and preserve function to the best of personal ability as the disease progresses; assistive devices and alternate environment patterns will assist the client in meeting these goals

    b. The client will comply with treatment measures aimed at managing symptoms so that client can perform ADLs at an optimal level

D. Scleroderma: progressive systemic sclerosis (PSS)

1. Description

    a. A multisystem disease that presents with fibrosis (hardening) of visceral organs and the skin

    b. The resultant fibrosis leads to inability of involved organs to function with normal motility

NCLEX!

    c. CREST syndrome is a specific more limited form of the disease called Thibierge Weissenbach syndrome
        C = Calcium deposits
        R = Raynaud's syndrome
        E = Esophageal dysmotility
        S = Sclerodactyly (scleroderma digits)
        T = Teleangiectasia (spider nevi)

    d. Systemic sclerosis morphea is a specific form of the disease that affects only the skin

    e. Some clients have mild forms of the disease that may even go unrecognized unless disease activity progresses or other medical issues bring the disease to the forefront

2. Etiology and pathophysiology

    a. This is a systemic illness of unknown etiology; there are associated underlying common factors such as inflammation, vasoconstriction, and the presence of abnormal immune function and connective tissue that may eventually lead to defining an etiology

    b. Disease usually presents during the third to fifth decade of life

    c. Females are affected more often than males

3. Assessment

    a. Clinical manifestations

        1) Skin changes exist in two phases; edematous changes occur first and are usually painless and symmetrical; then indurative changes occur that involve hardening and thickening of skin

    2) GI tract changes can lead to dysphagia, esophageal reflux, malabsorption, and bowel obstruction

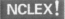

    3) Cardiac changes can present in the form of Raynaud's phenomenon (vasospastic disease), secondary bacterial endocarditits, myocardial fibrosis, left ventricular (LV) dysfunction, and heart failure

    4) Raynaud's phenomenon: vasospasm of small arteries in hands or feet, characterized by color changes (pallor and cyanosis) leading to a reactive hyperemia (redness) of affected extremity

    5) Respiratory changes can result from lung restriction caused by fibrosis

    6) Renal changes lead to development of uremia, malignant hypertension, and eventually renal failure

    7) This disease is often seen in conjunction with *Sjogren's syndrome,* an autoimmune disease affecting lacrimal and salivary glands, causing dryness of mucous membranes

  b. Diagnostic and laboratory test findings

    1) Biopsy of organs may reveal specific involvement

    2) Low ANA titers are found in a majority of the clients; nucleolar pattern is associated specifically with the disease

    3) SCL-70 antibody is highly specific for the disease

    4) Anticentromere antibodies are highly sensitive and specific; a positive presence indicates a good prognosis, as it is associated with a more limited form of the disease

    5) ESR is usually elevated; positive RF is usually seen

    6) Mild hypochromic, microcytic anemia can be seen in some clients

    7) Imaging and other studies may be indicated to detect specific organ sytem involvement, such as GI, pulmonary, heart, kidney, and skin

4. Therapeutic management

  a. Treatment is aimed at supportive and palliative measures

  b. Long-term follow up of diagnosed clients is indicated in order to monitor for potential disease progression

  c. Dialysis may be indicated if renal function deteriorates

  d. If end organ failure develops, renal or lung transplant may be indicated

5. Priority nursing diagnoses: Impaired skin integrity; Imbalanced nutrition; Impaired physical mobility; Low self-esteem; Disturbed body image; Ineffective individual coping; Fear; Hopelessness; Social isolation; Risk for peripheral neurovascular dysfunction

6. Planning and implementation

  a. Monitor client for symptom complaints and medicate as ordered

  b. Develop a support system for client and family members to help them cope with the stressors of chronic disease

c. Identify potential complications as they affect the client and coordinate healthcare team approach to manage developing risk situations

d. Monitor specific laboratory and diagnostic test results

e. Protect client's extremities from temperature changes that can exacerbate Raynaud's syndrome; encourage client to use gloves during activities that can affect temperature changes (such as washing dishes)

7. Medication therapy

a. Calcium channel blockers and peripheral alpha$_1$-adrenergic blocking agents are used to treat symptoms of Raynaud's

b. Anti-inflammatory agents are used to treat joint pain

c. H$_2$ receptor antagonists and proton pump inhibitors are used to treat esophageal reflux

d. Angiotensin converting enzyme (ACE) inhibitors are used to treat hypertension and prevent development of resultant renal crisis

e. Antibiotics are used to treat potential secondary infections of the bowel caused by decreased motility

f. Oxygen therapy is used to support pulmonary function

8. Client education

a. Discuss the importance of adequate symptom management to achieve an optimal level of health

b. Assist the client with understanding the chronic nature of the disease process

c. Support the client with the diagnosis and the impact that no known cause exists; recognize that the disease has an impact on both individual and family members; provide anticipatory guidance to support the client and family

d. Client may be referred to a rheumatologist to coordinate management of care

9. Evaluation

a. The client will be able to manage the symptoms of the disease and live more comfortably

b. The client will be an active participant in the healthcare team and contribute to decision making on his or her behalf

E. Myasthenia gravis (MG)

1. Description

a. MG is characterized as an autoimmune neuromuscular disease that causes extreme muscle weakness

b. A gamma globulin antibody is present that acts with T-cells on the receptor sites to interfere with nerve transmission

c. This disease process can also be cross-referenced and reviewed in Chapter 5, Neurologic Disorders

2. Etiology and pathophysiology

   a. MG is considered to be an autoimmune disease involving neuromuscular transmission of acetylcholine (ATCH) receptors at the post-synaptic membrane junction

   b. The receptor site involved in the autoimmune response is the nicotinic acetylcholine or AchR site

   c. The thymus gland is involved in the buildup of antibodies that are directed against the ATCH receptors

   d. The disease occurs more frequently in females than males in adults but this equalizes in the elderly population

   e. There is a genetic component identified with the disease process citing specific HLA antigens (HLA-B8, DR3); congenital MG and neonatal MG can occur

3. Assessment

   a. Clinical manifestations

      1) Clients present with extreme muscle weakness

      2) Ptosis (drooping of eyelids) is often seen in the early stages of this disease process; this can be seen in conjunction with diplopia (double vision) as well as generalized ocular weakness

      3) A sleepy, mask-like expression affects facial muscles

      4) The client experiences problems with chewing and swallowing (dysphagia) and is at risk for aspiration

      5) The client experiences problems with voice articulation (dysarthria)

   b. Diagnostic and laboratory test findings

      1) Detection of antibodies (AchR) in serum identifies autoimmune disease process

      2) **Tensilon test** is used in the identification of clients who have myasthenic crisis; this involves injecting a cholinesterase substance (edrophonium, Tensilon) to determine if it improves symptoms; improvement is compatible with a diagnosis of MG

      3) Thyroid studies and vitamin B_{12} levels are measured to rule out other disease processes that can result in muscular weakness

4. Therapeutic management

   a. Avoid and/or treat promptly factors that can lead to disease exacerbation, such as infection, stress, and temperature extremes

   b. Avoid certain medications such as novocaine, aminoglycosides, tetracyclines, and class I antiarrthythmics that can cause exacerbation of the disease process

   c. Pharmacologic therapy is directed at modulating the immune response at the receptor site

   d. Surgical removal of the thymus may be indicated if the client has a thymoma

e. Plasmapheresis may be indicated to effectively remove antireceptor antibodies

5. Priority nursing diagnoses: Ineffective airway clearance; Impaired swallowing; Fatigue; Activity intolerance; Ineffective role performance; Impaired social interaction; Disturbed body image; Self-care deficit; Risk for injury

6. Planning and implementation

   a. Closely monitor clients for associated respiratory problems that could result in potential life-threatening situations

   b. Institute aspiration precautions for clients at risk; cut food into small pieces

   c. Monitor clients for complications specifically related to disease process

      1) *Myasthenic crisis* can occur when the client is being undermedicated or not taking medication at all; onset is sudden, leading to a quick progression of disease symptoms with respiratory distress

      2) *Cholinergic crisis* is the result of overmedication; client experiences profound muscular weakness and respiratory paralysis

7. Medication therapy

   a. Anticholinesterase medications are used to modulate the immune response by increasing the relative concentration of ATCH at the myoneural junction, increasing the response of the muscles to nerve impulses and thereby improving strength; these medications can cause major side effects, such as GI upset and increased sweating and salivation

   b. Corticosteroids are used in a tapered dose approach to manage symptoms; effort must be made to avoid potential side effects associated with steroid therapy

   c. Immunosuppressive agents are given to clients who are experiencing profound weakness to decrease the production of antireceptor antibodies; this form of treatment may be lifelong in nature

8. Client education

   a. Teach client about the variable course of the disease and that it is critical to take medication therapy as directed; anticholinesterase agents should be given before meals to be most effective in assisting clients to chew and swallow properly

   b. Teach client about possible precipitating factors and potential stressors that might lead to further exacerbations

   c. Instruct client as to nature of crisis management; have available support network ready to manage potential crises; instruct to wear a Medic-Alert identification

   d. Educate client as to possible drug interactions that could arise and exacerbate the condition (see therapeutic management, section 4 above)

9. Evaluation

   a. Client is able to identify potential stressors and avoid them to maintain optimal health level

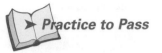

Practice to Pass

A client is diagnosed with an autoimmune disease and wants to know whether this will become a chronic occurrence. What information can you provide to the client that would explain the concept of autoimmune disease?

b. Client is able to identify specific medications, their side effects, and how they are to be taken as part of the treatment plan

c. Client is able to adapt his or her environment in order to maintain optimal health function

IV. Primary Immunodeficiency Disorders

A. Etiology and pathophysiology

1. Primary immunodeficiency disorders are caused by a primary defect or deficiency involving B lymphocytes, T lymphocytes, complement or phagocytic cells that results in severe infection that can be recurrent or chronic in nature (refer to Table 11-4 for a listing of selected primary immunodeficiency diseases)

2. These involve specific genetic alterations in the immune response that are seen in infants and young children

B. Assessment

1. Clinical manifestations

   a. The client's overall immune response is abnormal, leading to infections that may be caused by opportunistic agents and result in the development of **opportunistic infection**

   b. Recurrent infections can lead to subsequent tissue and organ damage of the heart and lungs, as the immune response cannot be supported

   c. Monitor for signs and symptoms of infection and inflammation: fever, chills, cough (nonproductive or productive), respiratory complaints associated with difficulty swallowing or breathing, erythema, edema, or drainage

   d. Diarrhea can be present in a wide variety of these disorders either due to overwhelming infection caused by offending agents or as a response to antimicrobial therapy.

2. Diagnostic and laboratory test findings

   a. CBC with differential, ESR, antibody titers, ANA, ANC (absolute neutrophil count) and culture and sensitivity of pertinent areas may all provide a baseline and allow for identification of potential source(s) of infection; if infections persist in a child or an adult, then further hematologic studies may be warranted

   b. Testing for immunoglobulins and complement assay levels provide an overview of immune system function

C. Therapeutic management

1. Therapy is most effective when aimed at infection prophylaxis, early treatment of infections, and replacement of immunologic factors

Table 11-4		
	Disorder	**Immune cell problem**
Selected Primary Immunodeficiency Disorders	Bruton's X-linked disorder	B lymphocytes
	DiGeorge's syndrome	T lymphocytes
	Graft-versus-host disease	B, T lymphocytes
	Wiskott-Aldrich syndrome	B, T lymphocytes

2. Bone marrow transplant (BMT) and/or thymus transplant may be indicated depending on the severity of presentation

D. Priority nursing diagnoses: Risk for infection; Fatigue; Fear; Imbalanced nutrition; Knowledge deficit; Risk for ineffective individual or family coping; Diarrhea; Caregiver role strain; Anticipatory grieving; Disturbed body image

E. Planning and implementation

   1. Identify clients who present with repeated infections

   2. Support family members with impending diagnosis of chronic medical condition

   3. Offer assistance in obtaining collaborative healthcare team management to establish treatment goals

   4. Assist client and family members in decisions regarding lifestyle changes to reduce infection and ADLs

   5. Refer clients of childbearing families for genetic counseling

   6. Collaborate with healthcare team members to support the client's ADLs and lifestyle changes during this hospitalization and after discharge

F. Medication therapy

   1. Antimicrobial therapy may be initiated to prevent infection or treat current infection

   2. Depending on the nature of the organism, antifungals may be warranted

   3. Gamma globulins may be needed to support and maintain deficient immunoglobulin levels

   4. Use of colony-stimulating factors may be warranted to boost the immune response

G. Client education

   1. Genetic counseling may be considered at this time

   2. Discuss antimicrobial therapy, including treatment, response and need for long-term compliance

   3. Teach the importance of prevention and protection from high-risk environments that could lead to further infection

H. Evaluation

   1. The client maximizes immunoglobulin levels in order to support immune response

   2. The client and family unit indicates an understanding of the recurrent nature of the disorder

   3. The client implements measures to prevent infection

V. Secondary Immunodeficiency Disorders

A. Etiology and pathophysiology

   1. Disease processes cause a secondary immunosuppressive response

   2. Diabetes, burns, malnutrition, some autoimmune diseases, and acquired immunodeficiency syndrome (AIDS) are examples of precipitating disease processes

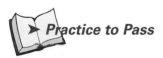

Practice to Pass

What information would genetic counseling provide to a client who has been diagnosed with a primary immunodeficiency disorder?

B. Assessment

1. Clinical manifestations

   a. The client presents with classic signs of immunosuppression and is unable to mount an immune defense

   b. A wide range of presentations reflect the client's current immune status

   c. Overwhelming infection and increased response to opportunistic organisms are characteristic

2. Diagnostic and laboratory test findings

   a. Client's WBC count and ANC count are abnormally low

   b. Culture and sensitivity tests will determine source of infection

C. Therapeutic management

1. Identify, treat and stabilize the client's underlying disease process

2. Institute **neutropenic precautions** (measures to protect the immunosuppressed client) if warranted to prevent further risk for infection and maintain protective isolation as indicated

3. Identify potential infectious sources and establish baseline immune level

4. Collaborate with dietician in order to provide nutrition that supports immune functions and maintains integrity of body systems

D. Priority nursing diagnoses: Risk for infection; Imbalanced nutrition; Activity intolerance; Anxiety; Fatigue; Knowledge deficit; Hopelessness; Risk for ineffective individual coping

E. Planning and implementation

1. Maintain protective isolation as warranted; monitor ANC, blood work, and pending cultures

2. Assist the client during times of stress and isolation caused by the chronic nature of disease process

3. Collaborate with healthcare team members to support the client's activities of daily living and lifestyle changes during this hospitalization and after discharge

4. Monitor client's nutritional status and hydration level

F. Medication therapy

1. Antimicrobial therapies provide support against infectious processes

2. Colony-stimulating factors boost immune response

3. Medications specific to underlying disease processes are used to maintain immune balance

G. Client education

1. Assist the client to understand the chronic nature of the disease process

2. Teach the client to avoid others with communicable diseases or other infections

3. Establish a collaborative network for the client to maintain contact during the discharge process

4. Promote client self-monitoring of condition to identify potential health problems more quickly

H. Evaluation

1. The client is able to identify environmental risks and thereby prevent exposure to infection

2. The client is able to monitor underlying disease process and complications that would increase medical risk

3. The client verbalizes how underlying disease process and the immune system are interrelated

VI. Human Immunodeficiency Virus (HIV)

A. Etiology and pathophysiology

1. An RNA retrovirus attacks the immune system at the CD_4 antigen, causing cell mutation that leads to eventual disease progression

2. HIV infection involves a process whereby the course of the disease progresses

3. Primary infection is followed by a clinical latency period during which time the individual may appear asymptomatic

4. The infected virus is transmitted through contact with blood and/or body fluids

B. Assessment

1. Clinical manifestations

   a. Primary HIV can manifest with flu-like symptoms

   b. Symptomatic HIV presentation leads to decreased CD_4 cell counts and progressive weight loss

   c. Systemic constitutional symptoms such as fatigue, fever, night sweats, and skin lesions may become apparent with further viral progression; once the latency period ends, HIV infection progresses to acquired immunodeficiency syndrome (AIDS)

   d. Take a health history, especially noting any "high-risk" exposures (IV drug use, sexual contact, contaminated blood products, and perinatal transmission—in utero, during delivery and/or breastfeeding)

2. Diagnostic and laboratory test findings

   a. Enzyme-linked immunosorbent assay (ELISA) is the screening test used to detect the development of antibodies to HIV; this test is described as positive or negative

   b. Western blot is used to confirm HIV infection because it detects both HIV antibodies and individual viral components that cause reactive bands; this test is described as positive or negative

   c. Polymerase chain reaction (PCR) is used to detect proviral DNA by identifying specific gene sequences of the HIV proviral DNA molecule

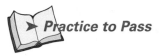

Practice to Pass

A client has an absolute neutrophil count (ANC) of 500. What are your immediate interventions?

     d. Nonspecific markers of disease progression include blood counts, albumin levels and ESR

NCLEX!

     e. Specific markers include CD_4 and viral load (VL) levels to indicate client's current status and response to treatment

     f. Other lab and diagnostic tests, such as skin biopsy, serum chemistries and imaging studies, may be indicated depending on organ/system involvement and disease progression

C. Priority nursing diagnoses: Risk for infection; Activity intolerance; Anxiety; Fear; Disturbed body image; Risk for ineffective individual coping; Anticipatory grieving; Hopelessness; Knowledge deficit; Imbalanced nutrition: less than body requirements

NCLEX!

D. Planning and implementation

     1. Periodic clinical reevaluation of client involves both physical examination and laboratory testing

NCLEX!

     2. The individual client is vaccinated against preventable illnesses

     3. The healthcare team coordinates their activities to assist the client in managing life issues that will be affected by the disease process

     4. Educate the client, family, and other support members about the disease progression

     5. Maintain awareness of current CDC recommendations, as they will affect the client during the course of treatment

     6. Establish an early working relationship with a dietician to deal with client's altered taste perception and prevent or delay **wasting syndrome** [unexplained weight loss of > 10 percent ideal body weight (IBW) that is associated with a cycle of malnutrition and subsequent wasting]

     7. Monitor client for potential fluid and electrolyte imbalances that might occur during course of disease process or in response to therapy

NCLEX!

E. Medication therapy

     1. Antiretroviral therapy is used to attack the virus at a basic level

     2. Nucleoside analogue reverse transcriptase inhibitors are aimed at specific processes to prevent the replication process

     3. Protease inhibitors are aimed at specific processes to prevent the replication process

     4. Nonnucleoside analogues are used to treat the emerging viral mutations

     5. Prophylactic medications are recommended based on CDC guidelines to provide primary and secondary prophylaxis of opportunistic infections

     6. Polypharmacy issues frequently arise

     7. Antiretroviral resistance and gene mutation lead to new treatment recommendations over time

     8. Oral progesterones (Megace, Winstrol) stimulate appetite thereby assisting with the treatment of weight loss and loss of taste perception

NCLEX!

F. Client education

1. Teach the client the importance of compliance with long-term treatment regimen and adherence to drug regimen; noncompliance could lead to drug resistance over time

2. Stress the need for follow-up physical examination and diagnostic tests to monitor response to treatment and disease progression

3. Teach the client to identify areas of concern, such as the possibility of increased infection caused by disease-related immunodeficiency

4. Discuss confidentiality and release of information concerning health matters in the areas of business and personal relationships

5. Discuss the importance of nutritional support and maintaining ideal body weight at an early phase of treatment

6. Explain the use of specific nutrition-related measures, such as having small frequent meals, fluids between meals, and dry crackers to help with mealtime issues of nausea; client may need to premedicate with antiemetics to reduce risk of nausea; the use of sorbets as palate cleansers, zinc supplementation, and the use of plastic utensils instead of metal ones may help clients who are experiencing altered taste perception

G. Evaluation

1. The client maintains health care follow-up visits as prescribed

2. The client is actively involved in monitoring for therapeutic response

3. The client is involved in prevention of infection and symptom management in order to limit hospitalizations

VII. Acquired Immunodeficiency Syndrome (AIDS)

A. Etiology and pathophysiology

1. AIDS is a progression of HIV disease

2. It is diagnosed when there is a CD_4 count of $< 200/mm^3$ in the presence of an AIDS-defining disease, such as opportunistic infections, malignancies and/or neurologic diseases; pulmonary TB, recurrent pneumonia, and invasive cervical cancer are also considered AIDS-defining diseases (see Table 11-5 for a listing of AIDS infections and malignancies)

3. Since AIDS affects the total individual, all body organs and tissues are affected

4. Refer to Table 11-5 again for testing for opportunistic infections

B. Assessment

1. Clinical manifestations

   a. Depending on organ and system that is affected, there can be a wide range of presentations

   b. Non-Hodgkin's lymphoma, Kaposi's sarcoma, and invasive cervical cancer are secondary malignancies often associated with AIDS

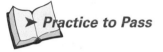

Practice to Pass

A male client who is HIV-positive wants to know why oral progesterone (Megace) has been prescribed. What information can you provide related to this medication?

NCLEX!

	Classification	Type
Table 11-5	Bacterial infection	Mycobacterium avium complex (MAC)
AIDS Infections and Malignancies	Fungal infection	Candidiasis
		Cryptococcus neoformans
		Histoplasmosis
	Protozoan infection	Pneumocystic carinii
		Toxoplasmosis
		Cryptosporidium
	Viral infection	Cytomegalovirus (CMV)
	Dementia	HIV encephalopathy
	Nutritional/malnutrition	Wasting syndrome
	Cancer	Kaposi's sarcoma
		Associated lymphomas

c. Wasting syndrome is seen in all individuals who have AIDS; aggressive nutritional support at the time of HIV-positive status assessment may prevent or deter possible effects of wasting and malnutrition

d. Continued observation of client's skin and mucous membranes reveals early signs and symptoms of infection

   1) Clients with HIV are at risk for oropharyngeal candida infections, leading to stomatitis

NCLEX!

   2) These clients can experience pain when eating, and benefit from soft foods and beverages that are neither too warm nor too cold

e. Assess client's nutritional status and hydration level, carefully noting baseline weight changes and alterations in taste perceptions

NCLEX!

   1) Because zinc deficiency is associated with altered taste, the client may benefit from zinc supplements

NCLEX!

   2) Dairy products, fish, and poultry are tolerated better than red meat in clients with altered taste

NCLEX!

   3) Use of plastic utensils instead of metal ones may reduce unpleasant taste also

f. Monitor for potential fluid and electrolyte imbalances

   1) Nausea and diarrhea are common problems

   2) Principles of treatment for these symptoms are similar to those used for clients receiving chemotherapy for cancer

NCLEX!

   3) Small frequent meals and low-fat foods help reduce the risk of nausea and vomiting

2. Diagnostic and laboratory test findings

   a. Obtain CD_4, VL, and PCR levels

   b. Obtain pertinent imaging studies as determined by client's presentation

    c. Biopsies and other invasive procedures are done to diagnose secondary malignancies

    d. Client will experience fluid and electrolyte imbalances as a consequence of disease progression, onset of opportunistic infection and in response to medical treatment; a common finding is hyponatremia

C. Priority nursing diagnoses: Risk for infection; Activity intolerance; Anxiety; Fear; Disturbed body image; Caregiver role strain; Risk for ineffective coping; Anticipatory grieving; Hopelessness; Knowledge deficit; Imbalanced nutrition: less than body requirements

D. Planning and implementation

    1. Provide ongoing coordination of healthcare team to afford the client the best possible assistance during this time of stress and crisis

    2. Have dietician analyze the client's nutritional requirements and make recommendations to maintain ideal body weight

    3. Provide for counseling and guidance for both the client and immediate support systems

    4. Assess the total impact of the disease on the client and the family support group

    5. Allow for ventilation of feelings relative to life situation

    6. Maintain client advocacy

E. Medication therapy

    1. Continue with current Centers for Disease Control (CDC) recommendations as they apply to primary and secondary prophylactic measures

    2. Antibiotic therapy may be warranted if the client develops an infection

    3. Chemotherapy treatment along with surgical intervention may be warranted if secondary malignancies are identified

    4. Pain management may be required as the disease progresses

    5. Antiemetics and appetite stimulants may be warranted to assist with nutritional problems such as nausea and vomiting and loss of appetite

    6. Antifungal medications may be indicated to treat active or chronic opportunistic infections; topical medications may be used for palliative care

F. Client education

    1. Continue to emphasize how new symptom progression will be managed and how the client is an active member of the healthcare team

    2. Discuss life issues with the client and support system members as disease progresses and prognosis worsens

G. Evaluation

    1. The client maintains comfort and privacy during hospitalizations

    2. The client participates in decisions regarding self-care and designation of a healthcare surrogate should the need arise

NCLEX!

NCLEX!

NCLEX!

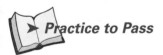

Practice to Pass

A client is concerned about the number of medications that have been prescribed for the treatment of AIDS and states that "there is no way to comply" with this regimen. What information could you provide to the client to support the importance of compliance with the treatment regimen?

VIII. Isolation Precautions

A. The CDC has developed and refined various categories of isolation precautions over time

B. Category-specific

1. Category-specific isolation precautions were outlined by the CDC in 1983 into the following categories: strict isolation, contact isolation, enteric precautions, drainage/secretion precautions, and blood/body fluid precautions

2. These categories identified specific measures that should be used to prevent the spread of infection in each of the identified areas

   a. Strict isolation involves the total separation of the individual client from all areas of contact

   b. Contact precautions isolate clients who have identified or suspected disease through which contact can cause the transmission of disease

   c. Enteric precautions isolate clients who have intestinal diseases that can be transmitted via contact with body fluids

   d. Drainage/secretion precautions isolate clients who could spread infection through contact with drainage/secretions

   e. Blood/body fluid precautions are used to isolate clients from spreading infection through body/body fluid contact

C. Disease-specific

1. Disease-specific isolation precautions were outlined by the CDC in 1983 and provided information relative to specific disease processes

2. This category of isolation looked at the use of private rooms for clients with specific diseases to prevent the possible spread of infection; if there was another client with the same disease process, then the two could share a room (cohorting)

3. The isolation rooms used in this category had laminar air flow to prevent the spread of infection throughout the rest of the hospital

4. Gowning and self-protection are considered to be a part of this precaution level to prevent the spread of certain infectious diseases

D. Hospital infection control guidelines

1. Tier 1 refers to the use of Standard Precautions (formerly Universal Precautions) as they relate to any client who is hospitalized regardless of diagnosis or potential infection; clients who are immunosuppressed fall under the category of standard precautions

2. Reverse isolation (protective isolation) is used to protect clients from risk of exposure from a compromised immune system

3. Neutropenic precautions can be employed to prevent risk of infection; the client is not allowed to have fresh flowers or raw foods, nor use black pepper because they may contain potential Gram-negative bacteria; invasive procedures and visitors are limited to prevent further exposures; the client's ANC determines whether or not the client will be placed or remain in this form of isolation

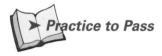

▶ *Practice to Pass*

A client is placed on contact precautions because of diarrhea. What are your immediate assessments and interventions?

NCLEX!

NCLEX!

NCLEX!

4. Tier 2 includes the use of Standard Precautions (as outlined in Tier 1) and further includes the specific application of isolation precautions such as airborne, droplet, and contact precautions for clients who have defined disease processes

E. OSHA infection control guidelines

1. Occupational Safety and Health Administration (OSHA) is concerned with protecting and limiting exposure of healthcare workers to infectious disease

2. This agency formulates guidelines for healthcare providers, agencies, and facilities that employ individual healthcare workers

3. Inspection of healthcare environments is an ongoing practice for this agency

NCLEX!

F. Isolation and other infection control practices

1. Wash hands

2. Maintain strict aseptic technique with regard to invasive procedures; maintain aseptic integrity of indwelling systems

3. Employ Standard Precautions when providing client care

4. Maintain skin integrity by turning and repositioning the client; promote respiratory expansion by encouraging coughing and deep breathing, unless coughing is contraindicated for some other reason

5. Monitor client's ANC count as necessary on clients who are on neutropenic precautions

NCLEX!

6. Use personal protective equipment such as gloves, gown, and face masks; as indicated, pay attention to the risk of latex allergy for both the client and the care provider; agencies generally have carts available that carry "latex-free" gloves and other client care supplies (e.g., tourniquets, IV tubing, etc.)

NCLEX!

7. Dispose of biohazardous equipment according to agency policy

NCLEX!

G. Nursing responsibilities

1. Post isolation signs and maintain communication among healthcare team members, the client, and family/visitors

2. Follow isolation procedures to determine appropriate client placement

3. Transport clients according to isolation procedures

4. Use dedicated equipment for clients on isolation precautions

5. Monitor client's lab values and diagnostic tests

6. Follow up with agency/facility infection control department

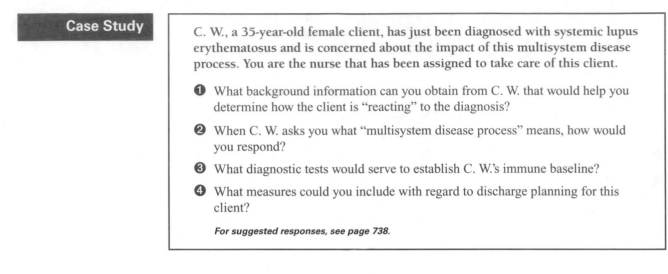

Case Study

C. W., a 35-year-old female client, has just been diagnosed with systemic lupus erythematosus and is concerned about the impact of this multisystem disease process. You are the nurse that has been assigned to take care of this client.

❶ What background information can you obtain from C. W. that would help you determine how the client is "reacting" to the diagnosis?

❷ When C. W. asks you what "multisystem disease process" means, how would you respond?

❸ What diagnostic tests would serve to establish C. W.'s immune baseline?

❹ What measures could you include with regard to discharge planning for this client?

For suggested responses, see page 738.

Posttest

1 A HIV-positive client now presents with a CD_4 count of < 200/μl and invasive cervical cancer. How would the nurse evaluate these findings in terms of current CDC definitions?

(1) The client has seroconverted.
(2) The client is HIV-positive.
(3) The client is in the latent period of the disease process.
(4) The client has acquired immunodeficiency syndrome.

2 A client who has been diagnosed with an autoimmune disorder questions the nurse as to what impact this may have on activities of daily living in the years to come. The best explanation that you, as the nurse, can give is:

(1) "The changes will be subtle at first so it won't be noticeable to others."
(2) "It is hard to predict what the disease process has in store for any one individual."
(3) "I can hear the concern in your voice. Perhaps we can talk for awhile and discuss some of your concerns."
(4) "I would suggest the use of any available remedy that might give you some comfort."

3 Which of the following nursing diagnoses has the highest priority for a client who has rheumatoid arthritis?

(1) Fatigue
(2) Pain
(3) Ineffective role performance
(4) Disturbed body image

4 A client who has been diagnosed with scleroderma is complaining of pain in his fingertips and pallor followed by blanching of the extremities and redness. The nurse communicates in intershift report that the client reports symptoms of which of the following disorders?

(1) Joint swelling and effusion
(2) Symmetric polyarthritis
(3) Swan-neck deformity
(4) Raynaud's phenomenon

5 A client who is HIV positive and is taking antiretroviral medications asks why he was told that a change in medication might be expected during the course of treatment. The best explanation to give the client is:

(1) "Antiretroviral medication regimens must be changed to prevent expected toxicity to major organs."
(2) "Antiretroviral resistance is a major challenge to long-term management of HIV infection, and drug therapy may change based on research results."
(3) "Monotherapy is recommended for the treatment of HIV and must be adjusted."
(4) "Your treatment regimen will remain in place and is unlikely to change."

6 A client receives a polio vaccine during a clinic visit. The nurse explains that this will provide what type of immunity to the client?

(1) Active natural immunity
(2) Active artificial immunity
(3) Passive natural immunity
(4) Passive artificial immunity

7 A client who is diagnosed with myasthenia gravis (MG) had not been compliant with his medication regimen and has missed several doses of pyridostigmine (Mestinon). For which complication would the nurse monitor?

(1) Gastrointestinal symptoms
(2) Vertigo
(3) Bradycardia
(4) Respiratory distress

8 A client with tuberculosis is being admitted to the medical-surgical unit. Which type of precautions should the nurse institute to protect the client and staff from possible exposure?

(1) Standard precautions
(2) Contact precautions
(3) Airborne precautions
(4) Droplet precautions

9 You have been asked to perform a home assessment on a client who has longstanding rheumatoid arthritis. Which one of the following findings should receive the highest priority for followup teaching?

(1) The client lives in an apartment building that has an elevator.
(2) The client has an installed handrail support in the bathroom.
(3) The client has area rugs scattered throughout the apartment.
(4) The client keeps her medications in a plastic case on the kitchen counter.

10 The nurse is performing an abdominal examination and is able to palpate the spleen. What information does this alert the nurse to suspect?

(1) That the client has an allergic reaction.
(2) That the client is dehydrated.
(3) That the client may be at risk for immune dysfunction.
(4) That deep palpation is warranted to verify the size of the organ.

See pages 452–453 for Answers and Rationales.

Answers and Rationales

Pretest

1 Answer: 3 Rationale: Mental status changes ranging from restlessness to confusion is one of the most frequent "atypical" signs of infection in older adults. Fever, erythema, edema, and leukocytosis may be present in varying degrees; however, these presentations are considered typical responses. Coexisting chronic conditions along with the use of prescribed medications may cause typical responses to be minimized or absent altogether in the elderly client.
Cognitive Level: Application
Nursing Process: Assessment; *Test Plan:* PHYS

2 Answer: 4 Rationale: Any client who presents with unexplained weight loss and persistent nonspecific complaints of fatigue and nausea should be evaluated with regard to HIV status. Testing measures are not always conclusive and it is not apparent from the client's statement exactly what specific tests were administered. Low-grade fever does not correlate directly with the presence of HIV. Vitamin supplements could be considered to be supportive and protective. A history of blood transfusion may prove to warrant further assessment but it is not the highest priority at the present time.
Cognitive Level: Analysis
Nursing Process: Analysis; *Test Plan:* PHYS

3 Answer: 1 Rationale: Type 1 hypersensitivity involves humorally mediated antigen-antibody reactions. Food allergies and medications can provide a localized as well as systemic response. Clients who have a history of multiple allergies usually have high IgE levels that are a characteristic measure of this

type of reaction. The other hypersensitivity reactions do not apply to this characteristic presentation.
Cognitive Level: Application
Nursing Process: Analysis; *Test Plan:* PHYS

4 **Answer: 2** *Rationale:* Antinuclear antibodies indicate the presence of an autoimmune disorder. They are not considered specific for systemic lupus, because many other autoimmune disorders have significant numbers of these antibodies. This reported titer is suggestive of the presence of ANA antibodies, and therefore it is an abnormal response.
Cognitive Level: Analysis
Nursing Process: Analysis; *Test Plan:* PHYS

5 **Answer: 4** *Rationale:* Clients with a past medical history of anaphylaxis should have epinephrine readily available for emergencies because it is the drug of choice for treatment. Tylenol and ASA will not mediate the chemical response to prevent anaphylaxis. Benadryl, although an antihistamine, may not be effective enough to prevent a full-blown anaphylactic response.
Cognitive Level: Application
Nursing Process: Planning; *Test Plan:* PHYS

6 **Answer: 2** *Rationale:* Plaquenil is an antimalarial agent used in the treatment of rheumatoid arthritis. This medication can cause retinal toxicity, and therefore the client should be closely monitored for this possibility with specified visual exams. Gastric irritation, fluid retention, pulse elevations, and drowsiness are not routinely seen with this type of medication.
Cognitive Level: Application
Nursing Process: Implementation; *Test Plan:* PHYS

7 **Answer: 4** *Rationale:* Anticholinesterase medications are aimed at symptom management. These medications should be taken prior to eating to help the client chew and swallow and to minimize gastric upset. Taking this medication at night may not provide symptom relief and since absorption is variable, the client may not be assured of receiving the correct dose. The medication does not have to be taken with milk in order to minimize gastric upset. Taking the medication on a full stomach (which would constitute after eating) would not allow for the primary effect of aiding with swallowing and chewing that is needed in clients who have this disease process.
Cognitive Level: Application
Nursing Process: Evaluation; *Test Plan:* PHYS

8 **Answer: 1** *Rationale:* Raynaud's phenomenon is one of the most common findings associated with systemic sclerosis. Conjunctivitis, photophobia and splenomegaly can all be seen in clients who experience the effects of systemic lupus erythematosus.
Cognitive Level: Application
Nursing Process: Assessment; *Test Plan:* PHYS

9 **Answer: 3** *Rationale:* The client's understanding is demonstrated by acknowledging the fact that sun exposure should be limited to times other than 10:00 A.M. to 3:00 P. M., (when the sun is at its highest intensity). Tanning bed exposure can be considered to be an ultraviolet light trigger and could exacerbate dermatologic presentations. Initial use of SPF 15 sunscreen (or higher value) is indicated, as is the reapplication of sunscreen during exposure periods. Clients should avoid exposure to potential infection.
Cognitive Level: Application
Nursing Process: Evaluation; *Test Plan:* HPM

10 **Answer: 2** *Rationale:* Regardless of isolation precautions, the basic action by the nurse to prevent infection is hand washing. All of the other options should also be followed but hand washing establishes the first line of defense and is therefore of highest importance.
Cognitive Level: Analysis
Nursing Process: Analysis; *Test Plan:* PHYS

Posttest

1 **Answer: 4** *Rationale:* CDC case definition of AIDS for adults states that the two factors described in the question are diagnostic of progression to AIDS. Seroconversion and positive HIV status has already occurred. The latent period is considered to be one in which the individual is asymptomatic.
Cognitive Level: Application
Nursing Process: Analysis; *Test Plan:* PHYS

2 **Answer: 3** *Rationale:* A client diagnosed with an autoimmune disease is faced with a lifetime of chronic illness and yet may not appear acutely ill because of the episodic nature of remissions and exacerbations. The nurse promotes a therapeutic relationship by allowing the client to ventilate feelings. It is inappropriate to minimize any changes that a client may experience that are unnoticeable to others as they may be quite unsettling to the individual. It is not the role of the nurse to speculate how a disease process will progress. Suggesting that the client use any "available remedy" may lead the client to potential harm or medical quackery.
Cognitive Level: Application
Nursing Process: Implementation; *Test Plan:* PSYC

3 **Answer: 2** *Rationale:* Pain and pain control are the most important elements of care for a client who has rheumatoid arthritis. Interventions aimed at pain management will allow the client to function at a more optimal level. While the other diagnoses are important, pain management remains the critical factor.
Cognitive Level: Analysis
Nursing Process: Analysis; *Test Plan:* PHYS

4 **Answer: 4** *Rationale:* Raynaud's phenomenon is a common presentation in clients who have scleroderma. It is characterized as a vasospastic disease of the periphery that causes color changes ranging from pallor to reactive hyperemia. Joint swelling, effusion, and symmetric polyarthritis can be seen in other autoimmune processes such as systemic lupus erythematosus and rheumatoid arthritis.
Cognitive Level: Analysis
Nursing Process: Analysis; *Test Plan:* PHYS

5 **Answer: 2** *Rationale:* One of the most critical problems with regard to antiretroviral therapy is the emergence of antiretroviral resistance as the HIV virus continues to mutate. Combination therapies have been proven to be more effective in treating disease progression. Antiretroviral therapies, in proper dosage, do not cause specific organ toxicity although they can cause myelosuppression.
Cognitive Level: Analysis
Nursing Process: Implementation; *Test Plan:* PHYS

6 **Answer: 2** *Rationale:* Vaccines are administered to client to promote the development of specific antibodies to afford protection. This is an example of active artificial immunity. Active natural immunity implies the development of antibodies in response to a client who had an actual active infection. Passive natural immunity implies the maternal and or placental transfer of antibodies. Passive artificial immunity implies the specific injection of an immune serum.
Cognitive Level: Application
Nursing Process: Analysis; *Test Plan:* PHYS

7 **Answer: 4** *Rationale:* The client should be monitored for myasthenic crisis, which is often a result of missed or under medication. The other options (gastrointestinal symptoms, vertigo, and bradycardia) are associated with cholinergic crisis. Cholinergic crisis is usually the result of overmedication. Both complications are viewed as acute in nature and may require airway assistance. The nurse must be acutely aware of the potential for clients with MG to have these types of complications.
Cognitive Level: Analysis
Nursing Process: Assessment; *Test Plan:* PHYS

8 **Answer: 3** *Rationale:* Airborne precautions should be instituted for all clients being admitted with a diagnosis of tuberculosis. Specific CDC guidelines may also be instituted to prevent TB transmission in healthcare facilities. Standard precautions should be maintained for all clients in the hospital setting. Contact and droplet precautions do not apply to this disease process.
Cognitive Level: Application
Nursing Process: Implementation; *Test Plan:* PHYS

9 **Answer: 3** *Rationale:* Scattered area rugs are a potential safety hazard for an individual who has longstanding RA because of possible joint deformities and contractures that could increase risk of falls. All of the other assessment findings are considered to be supportive of this client with RA because they enhance mobility, safety, and medication compliance.
Cognitive Level: Application
Nursing Process: Evaluation; *Test Plan:* PHYS

10 **Answer: 3** *Rationale:* The spleen is not usually palpated in an individual with normal immune function. Splenic enlargement (splenomegaly) is associated with a deviation from normal and bears further investigation. Deep palpation is not indicated when splenic congestion is noted as it may cause the spleen to rupture. Dehydration and allergic reaction are not consistent with enlargement of the spleen.
Cognitive Level: Application
Nursing Process: Analysis; *Test Plan:* PHYS

References

Bradley-Springer, L. (1999). Human immunodeficiency virus infection. In W. Phipps, J. Sands, & J. Marek (Eds.). *Medical-surgical nursing: Concepts & clinical practice* (6th ed.). St. Louis, MO: Mosby Inc., pp. 241–268.

Bush, M. (1999). Arthritis and other rheumatic disorders. In W. Phipps, J. Sands, & J. Marek (Eds.). *Medical-surgical nursing: Concepts & clinical practice* (6th ed.). St. Louis, MO: Mosby, Inc., pp. 1819–1836, 1841–1850.

DeLaune, S. C. & Ladner, P. K. (1998). *Fundamentals of nursing: Standards & practice.* Albany, NY: Delmar Publishers, pp. 734–738.

FayParpart, C., Perry, M. S., & Sawin, K. J. (1999). Immune system disorders: HIV/AIDS, mononucleosis and allergic responses. In E. Q. Youngkin, K. J. Sawin, J. F. Kissinger, & D. S. Israel (Eds.), *Pharmocotherapeutics: A primary care clinical guide.* Stamford, CT: Appleton & Lange, pp. 897–922.

Green-Nigro, C. (1999). Assessment of the immune system. In W. Phipps, J. Sands, & J. Marek (Eds.), *Medical-surgical nursing: Concepts & clinical practice* (6th ed.). St. Louis, MO: Mosby Inc., pp. 2147–2218.

Jarvis, C. (2000). *Physical examination and health assessment* (3rd ed.). Philadelphia: W.B. Saunders., pp. 624, 642.

Kozier, B., Erb, G., Berman, A., & Burke, K. (2000). *Fundamentals of nursing: Concepts, process, and practice* (6th ed.). Upper Saddle River, NJ: Prentice Hall, Inc., pp. 637–641, 658–670.

Lemone, P. & Burke, K. (2000). *Medical-surgical nursing: Critical thinking in client care* (2nd ed.). Upper Saddle River, NJ: Prentice-Hall, Inc., pp. 219–238, 247–252, 266–309, 1639–1663, 1853–1860.

Lewis, S. M. (1999). Altered immune responses. In W. Phipps, J. Sands, & J. Marek (Eds.), *Medical-surgical nursing. Concepts & clinical practice* (6th ed.). St. Louis, MO: Mosby Inc., pp. 212–234, 236–237.

Lilley, L. L., & Aucker, R. S. (1999). *Pharmacology and the nursing process* (2nd ed.). St. Louis, MO: Mosby Inc., pp. 229–244, 459–461, 523–534, 577–591, 595–612, 625–626, 645–657.

Metheny, N. M. (2000). *Fluid & electrolyte balance: Nursing considerations* (4th ed.). Philadelphia: Lippincott, Williams & Wilkins, p. 65.

Ozuna, J. M. (1999). Chronic neurologic problems. In W. Phipps, J. Sands, & J. Marek (Eds.), *Medical-surgical nursing: Concepts & clinical practice* (6th ed.). St. Louis, MO: Mosby Inc., pp. 1700–1702.

Porch, D. J. (1999, March). State of the art: Antiretroviral and prophylactic treatments in HIV/AIDS. *Nursing Clinics of North America, 34*(1): 95–112.

Rice, D. & Eckstein, E. (1999). Inflammation and infection. In W. Phipps, J. Sands, & J. Marek (Eds.), *Medical-surgical nursing: Concepts & clinical practice* (6th ed.). St. Louis, MO: Mosby Inc., pp. 207–252.

Silverthorn, D. S., Ober, W. C., Garrison, C. W., & Silverthorn, A. C. (1998). *Human physiology: An integrated approach.* Upper Saddle River, NJ: Prentice Hall, Inc., pp. 654–683.

Spratto, G. R. & Woods, A. L. (2000). *PDR nurses' drug handbook.* Montvale, NJ: Medical Economics Company, pp. 568–569, 868–869.

Whitney, E., Cataldo, C., DeBruyne, L. K., & Rolfes, S. (2001). *Nutrition for health and health care* (2nd ed.). Belmont, CA: Thompson Wadsworth, pp. 56–57, 294–295, 572–582.

Cataldo, C., DeBruyne, L. K., & Whitney, E. (2003). *Nutrition and diet therapy* (6th ed.). Belmont, CA: Thompson Wadsworth, pp. 948–956.

CHAPTER 12

Cellular Disorders (Oncology)

Joseann Helmes DeWitt, MSN, RN, C, CLNC

CHAPTER OUTLINE

*Overview of Anatomy
and Physiology*
Epidemiology of Cancer
*Risk factors for the Development
of Cancer*
*Recommendations of the American
Cancer Society for Early Cancer
Detection*

Diagnostic Tests and Assessments
*Common Nursing Techniques
and Procedures*
*Oncologic Emergencies: Diagnosis
and Management*

*Expected Outcomes of Clients
with Cellular Disorders*

OBJECTIVES

▮ Identify basic structures and functions of cells.

▮ Describe the pathophysiology and etiology of common cellular disorders.

▮ Discuss expected assessment data and diagnostic test findings for selected cellular disorders.

▮ Identify priority nursing diagnoses for selected cellular disorders.

▮ Discuss therapeutic management of selected cellular disorders.

▮ Discuss nursing management of a client experiencing a cellular disorder.

▮ Identify expected outcomes for the client experiencing a cellular disorder.

[Media Link]

Use the CD-ROM enclosed with this text, or log onto the address given to access the free, interactive Companion Website created for this series. The CD-ROM and Companion Website accompanying this book offer additional practice opportunities and information—NCLEX Review, Case Studies, Glossary, In Depth with NCLEX, and more.

www.prenhall.com/hogan

REVIEW AT A GLANCE

alopecia *hair loss that can occur secondary to chemotherapy or radiation*

benign neoplasm *localized growth, encapsulated, not malignant*

bone marrow suppression *decrease in the number of granulocytes, lymphocytes and thrombocytes, resulting in anemia, decreased ability to respond to infection, and decreased ability to form clots*

cancer *the mutation of normal cells into abnormal cells that proliferate*

carcinoma *tumor arising from epithelial tissue*

cell-kill hypothesis *chemotherapy kills a certain percentage of cells during each cell cycle, necessitating several courses of chemotherapy to adequately reduce the number of cancer cells*

chemotherapy *cytotoxic medications used to disrupt cell cycle of cancer cells, resulting in cell death*

differentiation *normal process by which cells specialize in order to perform certain tasks*

extravasation *leaking of chemotherapeutic agents into the surrounding tissues, occurs during intravenous administration invasion spreading of cancer cells into adjacent tissues*

malignant neoplasm *aggressively growing mass causing tissue death and possessing the ability to metastasize*

metastasis *spreading of malignant neoplasms through blood or lymph, forming a secondary tumor distant from the primary site*

sarcoma *tumor arising from supportive tissues*

stomatitis *painful mouth sores*

thrombocytopenia *decrease in platelet count*

tumor *also called neoplasm, a mass of new tissue functioning independently, serving no physiologic purpose*

tumor markers *proteins detected in serum or other body fluids, indicating the presence of malignancy*

vesicants *chemicals causing tissue damage on contact*

xerostomia *dry mouth*

Pretest

1 A 67-year-old female client refuses to be screened for cancer, stating, "I am too old to get cancer and if I don't have it by now, I will never get it." Which of the following would be the basis of your response to her?

(1) Unless symptomatic, screening the client for cancer is not necessary.
(2) Screening the elderly for cancer is essential.
(3) The incidence of cancer decreases with advancing age.
(4) Age is not a significant factor in the development of cancer.

2 A client just diagnosed with a benign neoplasm asks you if he is going to die. On which of the following items of information will you base your response?

(1) Benign neoplasms are localized, encapsulated growths that are easily removed and rarely cause death.
(2) Benign neoplasms are rapidly growing tumors that metastasize to other areas of the body.
(3) Benign neoplasms are associated with a high mortality rate.
(4) The client is experiencing an unusually high level of anxiety.

3 A client receiving intravenous chemotherapy is experiencing nausea. Which of the following would be the best intervention to lessen the severity of nausea?

(1) Administer antiemetics when client complains of nausea.
(2) Offer warm liquids during chemotherapy.
(3) Administer antiemetics before chemotherapy.
(4) Encourage the client to eat a full meal before receiving chemotherapy.

4 When teaching safety precautions to the client with an internal radiation implant, you would include which of the following in explanations to the client?

(1) No precautions are necessary for internal radiation implants.
(2) The client poses a risk of radiation exposure to others.
(3) The client must remain in solitary isolation for the entire hospitalization.
(4) Visitors should maintain a distance of 3 feet from the client at all times.

5 You are educating a client who will likely experience alopecia (hair loss) as a result of the current chemotherapy treatment. Further instructions are necessary when the client states which of the following?

(1) "I will wash my hair every day."
(2) "I will pat my hair dry and avoid the use of hairdryers."
(3) "My hair will begin to grow back after the chemotherapy is completed."
(4) "I will choose a wig or hairpiece before the loss of hair occurs."

6 A client receiving chemotherapy is experiencing a low white blood cell (WBC) count. The nurse should teach the client to avoid contact with which of the following family members?

(1) 34-year-old nephew with HIV infection
(2) 68-year-old husband with a history of exposure to tuberculosis as a youth
(3) 9-year-old grandchild with a recent exposure to chicken-pox (varicella)
(4) 31-year-old daughter who is 4 months pregnant

7 You are counseling a 22-year-old female in the health clinic. You determine that she understands your teaching instructions for the early detection and screening of breast cancer when she makes which of the following statements?

(1) "I should have a breast examination by a healthcare provider every 3 years."
(2) "I should have a breast examination by a healthcare provider yearly."
(3) "I should perform a breast self-examination every 3 months."
(4) "I should have a mammogram performed yearly."

8 A client is to receive intravenous chemotherapy via a peripherally inserted central catheter (PICC). The nurse should plan to take which of the following essential actions before beginning the administration?

(1) Make the client as comfortable as possible.
(2) Ensure patency of vein.
(3) Flush the catheter with the medication to test patency of the vein.
(4) Administer Tylenol (acetaminophen) prophylactically.

9 A client with a low platelet count demonstrates understanding of instructions to avoid potential complications by doing which of the following?

(1) Avoiding aspirin and aspirin (salicylate)–containing products
(2) Monitoring for fever every 4 hours
(3) Allowing for rest periods to avoid fatigue
(4) Brushing and flossing teeth daily to prevent infection

10 You are evaluating the nutritional status of a client who is receiving chemotherapy. On assessment, which finding could potentially affect the client's nutritional intake?

(1) Pale and moist mucous membranes
(2) Pale skin
(3) Ecchymotic areas on forearms
(4) Ulcerations of oral mucosa

See pages 480–481 for Answers and Rationales.

I. Overview of Anatomy and Physiology

A. Characteristics of normal cells

1. Normal cell growth (cell cycle) consists of five intervals or phases:

   a. G_0: the resting phase, not reproducing; some are normal while others are undergoing repair or are dying

   b. Interphase: contains three subphases that contribute to cell growth and prepare it for reproduction

   1) G_1: cellular production of RNA and protein

2) S: synthesis of DNA and proteins and new chromosomes appear

3) G$_2$: RNA synthesis

c. Mitosis (M): actual cell division

2. **Differentiation** refers to the process whereby cells develop specific structures and functions in order to specialize in certain tasks

3. Cellular adaptation

   a. *Hypertrophy* refers to an increase in size of normal cells

   b. *Atrophy* refers to the shrinkage of cell size

   d. *Hyperplasia* refers to an increase in the number of normal cells

   e. *Metaplasia* refers to a conversion from the normal pattern of differentiation of one type of cell into another type of cell not normal for that tissue

   f. *Dysplasia* refers to an alteration in the shape, size, appearance, and distribution of cells

   g. *Anaplasia* refers to disorganized, irregular cells that have no structure and have loss of differentiation; the result is almost always malignant

B. **Evolution of cancer cells**

1. **Cancer** refers to a disease whereby cells mutate into abnormal cells that proliferate abnormally; *neoplasia* refers to an abnormal cell growth or **tumor,** a mass of new tissue functioning independently and serving no useful purpose

   a. **Benign neoplasms** are slow-growing, localized, and encapsulated non-malignant growths with well-defined borders

      1) They are usually easily removed

      2) They generally do not cause tissue damage or other complications unless they interfere with tissue function or circulation

   b. **Malignant neoplasms** are aggressive growths that invade and destroy surrounding tissues; can lead to death unless interventions are taken

2. **Invasion** occurs when cancer cells infiltrate adjacent tissues surrounding the neoplasm

3. **Metastasis** occurs when malignant cells travel through the blood or lymph system and invade other tissues and organs to form a secondary tumor

C. **Characteristics of malignant cells**

1. Rapid cell division and growth: regulation of the rate of mitosis is lost

2. No contact inhibition: cells do not respect boundaries of other cells and invade their tissue areas

3. Loss of differentiation: cells lose specialized characteristics of function for that cell type and revert back to an earlier, more primitive cell type

4. Ability to migrate (metastasize): cells move to distant areas of the body and establish new site malignant lesions (tumors)

5. Alteration in cell structure: differences are evident between normal and malignant cells with respect to cell membrane, cytoplasm, and overall cell shape

6. Self-survival

   a. May develop ectopic sites to produce hormones needed for own growth

   b. Can develop a connective tissue stroma to support growth

   c. May develop own blood supply by secreting angiotensin growth factor to stimulate local blood vessels to grow into tumor

II. Epidemiology of Cancer

A. Incidence

1. Cancer affects every age group, though most cancer and cancer deaths occur in people older than 65 years of age

2. Cancer is attributable to 25 percent of all deaths; only cardiovascular diseases cause more deaths than cancer in the United States

3. Highest incidence of all cancer is prostate cancer

4. Highest cancer incidence in males in order of frequency: prostate cancer, lung cancer, and colorectal cancer

5. Highest cancer incidence in females in order of frequency: breast cancer, lung cancer, and colorectal cancer

B. Statistics

1. 8 million Americans today have a history of cancer

2. 1 in every 4 deaths in the United States is from cancer

3. Common sites of cancer and their sites of metastasis (see Table 12-1)

Table 12-1

Common Sites of Cancer and Their Sites of Metastasis

Cancer Type	Sites of Metastasis
Brain cancer	Central nervous system
Breast cancer	Brain Liver Regional lymph nodes Vertebrae
Colon cancer	Brain Liver Lung Lymph nodes Ovaries
Lung cancer	Bone Brain Liver Lymph nodes Pancreas Spinal cord
Malignant melanoma	Brain Liver Lung Regional lymph nodes Spleen
Prostate cancer	Bladder Bone Liver

III. Risk Factors for the Development of Cancer

A. Age

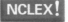

1. Increased risk for people over age of 65

2. Factors attributed to cancer in elderly include hormonal changes, altered immune responses, and the accumulation of free radicals

3. Age has been identified as the single most important factor related to the development of cancer

B. Gender

1. Certain cancers are more commonly seen in specific genders

2. For example, breast cancer occurs more commonly in females, colon cancer occurs more commonly in males

C. Geographic location

1. Risks for cancer vary according to environment and location

2. Rates for specific cancer sites, morbidity, and mortality vary from state to state, nation to nation, and in urban versus rural living

D. Genetics

1. 15 percent of cancers may be attributed to a hereditary component

2. Cancers demonstrating a familial relationship include breast, colon, lung, ovarian, and prostate

3. Clients with a genetic predisposition to cancer should be counseled and screened according to American Cancer Society (ACS) guidelines

E. Immune disturbance

1. Some viral infections tend to increase risk

2. Infections associated with cancer include Epstein-Barr, genital herpes, papillomavirus, hepatitis B, and human cytomegalovirus

F. Chemical agents

1. Over 1,000 chemicals are known to be carcinogenic

2. Exposure to chemicals in some occupations heightens this risk over decades

G. Race

1. Cancer can affect any population

2. Nonetheless African-Americans experience a higher rate of cancer than any other racial or ethnic group

H. Tobacco

1. A strong correlation between smoking and lung cancer exists

2. Other cancers associated with tobacco use include bladder, esophageal, gastric, laryngeal, oropharyngeal, and pancreatic

3. Smokeless tobacco (snuff and chewing tobacco) increases the risk of oral and esophageal cancers

4. Long-term exposure to secondhand smoke increases the risk for lung and bladder cancers

I. Alcohol

1. Serves as a promoter in cancers of the liver and esophagus

2. When combined with tobacco, the risks for other cancers are even higher

J. Diet

1. Diet has been demonstrated in research to correlate with some cancers

2. Diets high in fat, low in fiber, and those containing nitrosamines and nitrosin-doles found in preserved meats and pickled foods promote certain cancers such as colon, breast, esophageal, and gastric

K. Miscellaneous: stress, occupation, viruses also increase risk of cancer

IV. Recommendations of the American Cancer Society for Early Cancer Detection

A. For detection of breast cancer

1. Beginning at age 20, routinely perform monthly breast self-examinations (BSEs)

2. Women ages 20 to 39 should have breast examination by a healthcare provider every 3 years

3. Women age 40 and older should have a yearly mammogram and breast examination by a healthcare provider

B. For detection of colon and rectal cancer

1. All persons age 50 and older should have a yearly fecal occult blood test

2. Digital rectal examination and flexible sigmoidoscopy should be done every 5 years

3. Colonoscopy with barium enema should be done every 10 years

C. For detection of uterine cancer

1. Yearly papanicolaou (Pap) smear for sexually active females and any female over age 18

2. At menopause, high-risk women should have an endometrial tissue sample

D. For detection of prostate cancer

1. Beginning at age 50, have a yearly digital rectal examination

2. Beginning at age 50, have a yearly prostate-specific antigen (PSA) test

V. Diagnostic Tests and Assessments

A. Classification of cancer

1. **Carcinoma** refers to a tumor that arises from epithelial tissue; the name of the cancer identifies the location; example: basal cell carcinoma

2. **Sarcoma** refers to a tumor arising from supportive tissues; the name of the cancer identifies the specific tissue affected; example: osteosarcoma (see Table 12-2: Nomenclature for Selected Benign and Malignant Neoplasms, for comparison of tissue origins, benign and malignant neoplasms)

Table 12-2	Tissue of Origin	Benign Neoplasms	Malignant Neoplasms
Nomenclature for Selected Benign and Malignant Neoplasms	*Connective Tissue*		
	Bone	Osteoma	Osteosarcoma
	Fibrous tissue	Fibroma	Fibrosarcoma
	Adipose tissue	Lipoma	Liposarcoma
	Epithelial Tissue		
	Glandular	Adenoma	Adenocarcinoma
	Surface	Papilloma	Squamous cell carcinoma
	Hematopoietic		
	Erythrocytes		Erythroleukemia
	Granulocytes		Leukemia
	Lymphatic tissue		Hodgkin's disease, malignant lymphoma
	Lymphocytes		Lymphocytic leukemia
	Plasma cells		Multiple myeloma

B. Staging

1. The TNM tumor system is utilized for classifying tumors

   a. *T* indicates the tumor size

      1) *T0* indicates no evidence of tumor

      2) *Tis* indicates tumor in situ

      3) *T1, T2, T3, T4* indicate progressive degrees of tumor size and involvement

   b. *N* indicates lymph node involvement

      1) *N0* indicates no abnormal lymph nodes detected

      2) *N1a, N2a* indicate regional nodes involved with increasing degree from N1a to N2a, no metastases detected

      3) *N1b, N2b, N3b* indicate regional lymph nodes involvement with increasing degree from N1b to N3b, metastasis suspected

      4) *Nx* indicates inability to assess regional nodes

   c. *M* indicates distant metastases

      1) *M0* indicates no evidence of distant metastasis

      2) *M1, M2, M3* indicate ascending degrees of distant metastasis and includes distant lymph nodes

C. Tumor markers

1. **Tumor markers** are protein substances found in the blood or body fluids

2. Are released either by the tumor itself, or by the body as a defense in response to the tumor (called host response)

3. Tumor markers are derived from the tumor itself, and include the following:

   a. *Oncofetal antigens,* present normally in fetal tissue, may indicate an anaplastic process in tumor cells; carcinoembryonic antigen (CEA) and alpha-fetoprotein (AFP) are examples of oncofetal antigens

   b. *Hormones* are present in large quantities in the human body; however, high levels of hormones may indicate a hormone-secreting malignancy; hormones that may be utilized as tumor markers include the antidiuretic hormone (ADH), calcitonin, catecholamines, human chorionic gonadotropin (HCG), and parathyroid hormone (PTH)

    c. *Isoenzymes* that are normally present in a particular tissue may be released into the bloodstream if the tissue is experiencing rapid, excessive growth as the result of a tumor; examples include neuron-specific enolase (NSE) and prostatic acid phosphatase (PAP)

    d. *Tissue-specific proteins* identify the type of tissue affected by malignancy; an example of a tissue-specific protein is the prostatic-specific antigen (PSA) utilized to identify prostate cancer

  4. Host-response tumor markers include the following:

    a. C-reactive protein

    b. Interleukin-2

    c. Lactic dehydrogenase

    d. Serum ferritin

    e. Tumor necrosis factor

D. Biopsy/cytology

  1. Histologic and cytologic examination of specimens are performed by the pathologist on tissues collected by needle aspiration of solid tumors, exfoliation from epithelial surface, and aspiration of fluid from blood or body cavities

  2. Tissues may be obtained by excisional biopsy, incisional biopsy, and needle biopsy

  3. By examination of these tissues, the name, grade, and stage of the tumor can be identified

E. Laboratory tests: see Table 12-3

Table 12-3	Laboratory Tests Used in Diagnosing Cancer*	
Diagnostic Test	**Reference Value**	**Cancer-Related Abnormality Indicated**
Acid phosphatase (ACP)	0.0 to 0.8 U/L	Elevated in bone, breast, and prostate cancer, and multiple myeloma
Alanine aminotransferase (ALT)	5 to 35 U/ml	Elevated in liver cancer
Albumin	3.5 to 5.0 g/dl	Decreased in metastatic liver cancer and malnutrition
Alkaline phosphatase (ALP)	20 to 90 U/L	Elevated in cancer of bone, breast, liver, and prostate, and in leukemia and multiple myeloma
Alpha-fetoprotein (AFP)	<15 ng/ml in males and non-pregnant females	Elevated in testicular cancer and in germ cell tumors
Aspartate aminotransferase (AST)	5 to 40 U/ml	Elevated in liver cancer
Bilirubin	Total: 0.1 to 1.2 mg/dl Direct: 0.0 to 0.3 mg/dl	Elevated in liver and gallbladder cancer
Bleeding time	3 to 7 minutes (Ivy)	Prolonged in leukemia and metastatic liver cancer
Blood urea nitrogen (BUN)	5 to 25 mg/dl	Increased in renal cancer, decreased in malnutrition
Calcitonin	Male: <40 pg/ml Female: <20 pg/ml	Elevated in breast, lung, and thyroid medullary cancer

(continued)

Table 12-3	Laboratory Tests Used in Diagnosing Cancer (*Continued*)	
Diagnostic Test	**Reference Value**	**Cancer-Related Abnormality Indicated**
Calcium (Ca)	4.5 to 5.5 mEq/L 9.0 to 11.0 mg/dl	Elevated in bone cancer
C-reactive protein	>1:2 titer is positive	Elevated in metastatic cancer and Burkitts's lymphoma
Creatinine	0.5 to 1.5 mg/dL	Decreased in malnutrition, elevated in most cancers
Dexamethasone suppression test	> 50% reduction in plasma	Nonsuppression in adrenal cancer and ACTH producing tumors, severe stress
Estradiol-serum	Female: 20 to 300 pg/ml Menopausal female: <20 pg/ml Male: 15 to 50 pg/ml	Elevated in estrogen-producing tumors and testicular tumor
Gamma glutamyltransferase (GGT)	Male: 10 to 80 IU/L Female: 5 to 25 IU/L	Elevated in cancer of liver, pancreas, prostate, breast, kidney, lung, and brain
Haptoglobin	20 to 240 mg/dL	Elevated in Hodgkin's disease and cancer of lung, large intestine, stomach, breast, and liver
Hematocrit (Hct)	Male: 40% to 54% Female: 36% to 46%	Decreased in anemia, leukemia, Hodgkin's disease, lymphosarcoma, multiple myeloma, and malnutrition, and as a side effect of chemotherapy
Hemoglobin (Hgb)	Male: 13.5 to 18 g/dl Female: 12 to 16 g/dl 1:3 ratio of Hgb:Hct	Decreased in anemia, many cancers, Hodgkin's disease, leukemia, and malnutrition and as side effect of chemotherapy
Human chorionic gonadotropin (HCG)	Nonpregnant female <0.01 IU/L	Elevated in choriocarcinoma
Lactic dehydrogenase (LDH)	100 to 190 IU/L	Elevated in liver, brain, kidney, muscle cancers, acute leukemia, anemia
Occult blood	Negative	Positive in gastric and colon cancers
Parathyroid hormone (PTH)	400 to 900 pg/ml	Increased in PTH-secreting tumors
Platelet count (thrombocytes)	150,000/mm^3 to 400,000/mm^3	Decreased in bone, gastric, and brain cancer, in leukemia, and as a side effect of chemotherapy
Prostate-specific antigen (PSA)	0 to 4 ng/ml	Elevated from 10 to 120+ in prostate cancer
Red blood cells (RBCs)	Male: 4.6 to 6.0 million/mm^3 Female: 4.0 to 5.0 million/mm^3	Decreased in anemia, leukemia, infection, multiple myeloma
Uric acid	Male: 3.5 to 8.0 mg/dL Female: 2.8 to 6.8 mg/dL	Increased in leukemia, metastatic cancer, multiple myeloma, Burkitt's lymphoma, after vigorous chemotherapy
White blood cells (WBCs) Total leukocytes	4,500/mm^3 to 10,000/mm^3	Elevated in acute infection, leukemias, tissue necrosis; decreased as a side effect of chemotherapy
Neutrophils	50 to 70%	Elevated in bacterial infection, Hodgkin's disease; decreased in leukemia and malnutrition and as a side effect of chemotherapy
Eosinophils	1 to 3%	Elevated in cancer of bone, ovary, testes, and brain
Basophils	0.4 to 1.0%	Elevated in leukemia and healing stage of infection
Monocytes	4 to 6 %	Elevated in infection, monocytic leukemia and cancer; decreased in lymphocytic leukemia and as a side effect of chemotherapy
Lymphocytes	25 to 35%	Elevated in lymphocytic leukmemia, Hodgkin's disease, multiple myeloma; decreased in cancer and other leukemias, and as a side effect of chemotherapy

*Approximate lab values are provided, check your own agency's reference standards.
Source: LeMone, P. & Burke, K. (2000). *Medical-surgical nursing: Critical thinking in client care* (2nd ed.). Upper Saddle River, NJ: Prentice Hall.

F. American Cancer Society's seven warning signs of cancer (uses acronym CAUTION):

1. *C*hange in bowel or bladder habits

2. *A* sore that does not heal

3. *U*nusual bleeding or discharge

4. *T*hickening or lump in breast or elsewhere

5. *I*ndigestion or difficulty in swallowing

6. *O*bvious change in wart or mole

7. *N*agging cough or hoarseness

VI. Common Nursing Techniques and Procedures

A. Radiation therapy

1. Is used to kill a tumor, reduce the tumor size, relieve obstruction, or decrease pain

2. Causes lethal injury to DNA, so it can destroy rapidly multiplying cancer cells, as well as normal cells

3. Can be classified as internal radiation therapy (bachytherapy) or external radiation therapy (teletherapy)

B. The client undergoing brachytherapy (internal radiation)

1. Sources of internal radiation

   a. Implanted into affected tissue or body cavity

   b. Ingested as a solution

   c. Injected as a solution into the bloodstream or body cavity

   d. Introduced through a catheter into the tumor

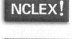

2. Side effects of internal radiation

   a. Fatigue

   b. Anorexia

   c. Immunosuppression

   d. Other side effects similar to external radiation (see section C2 below)

3. Priority nursing diagnoses: Impaired tissue integrity; Fatigue; Anxiety; Risk for infection; Social isolation; Imbalanced nutrition: less than body requirements

4. Client education

   a. Avoid close contact with others until treatment is completed

   b. Maintain daily activities unless contraindicated, allowing for extra rest periods as needed

   c. Maintain balanced diet; may tolerate food better if consumes small, frequent meals

   d. Maintain fluid intake to ensure adequate hydration (2–3 liters/day)

e. If implant is temporary, maintain bedrest to avoid dislodging the implant

f. Excreted body fluids may be radioactive; double-flush toilets after use

g. Radiation therapy may lead to bone marrow suppression (refer to precautions for anemia, thrombocytopenia, and immunosuppression later in chapter)

5. Nursing management of client receiving internal radiation

    a. Exposure to small amounts of radiation is possible during close contact with persons receiving internal radiation; understand the principles of protection from exposure to radiation: time, distance, and shielding

        1) Time: minimize time spent in close proximity to the radiation source; a common standard is to limit contact time to 30 minutes total per 8-hour shift; minimum distance of 6 feet used when possible

        2) Distance: maintain the maximum distance possible from the radiation source

        3) Shielding: use lead shields and other precautions to reduce exposure to radiation

    b. Place client in private room

    c. Instruct visitors to maintain at least a distance of 6 feet from the client and limit visits to 10 to 30 minutes

    d. Ensure proper handling and disposal of body fluids, assuring the containers are marked appropriately

    e. Ensure proper handling of bed linens and clothing

    f. In the event of a dislodged implant, use long-handled forceps and place the implant into a lead container; **never** directly touch the implant

    g. Do not allow pregnant women to come into any contact with radiation sources; screen visitors and staff for pregnancy

    h. If working routinely near radiation sources, wear a monitoring device to measure exposure

    i. Educate client in all safety measures

6. Evaluation: client demonstrates measures to protect others from exposure to radiation, identifies interventions to reduce risk of infection, remains free from infection, achieves adequate fluid and nutritional intake, and participates in activities of daily living (ADLs) at level of ability

C. The client undergoing external radiation therapy (teletherapy)

1. The radiation oncologist marks specific locations for radiation treatment using a semipermanent type of ink

    a. Treatment is usually given 15 to 30 minutes per day, 5 days per week, for 2 to 7 weeks

    b. The client does not pose a risk for radiation exposure to other people

2. Side effects of external radiation therapy

    a. Tissue damage to target area (erythema, sloughing, hemorrhage)

    b. Ulcerations of oral mucous membranes

    c. Gastrointestinal effects such as nausea, vomiting, and diarrhea

    d. Radiation pneumonia

    e. Fatigue

    f. Alopecia

    g. Immunosuppression

3. Priority nursing diagnoses: Risk for infection; Impaired skin integrity; Social isolation; Disturbed body image; Anxiety; Fatigue

4. Client education for external radiation

    a. Wash the marked area of the skin with plain water only and pat skin dry; do not use soaps, deodorants, lotions, perfumes, powders or medications on the site during the duration of the treatment; do not wash off the treatment site marks

    b. Avoid rubbing, scratching, or scrubbing the treatment site; do not apply extreme temperatures (heat or cold) to the treatment site; if shaving, use only an electric razor

    c. Wear soft, loose-fitting clothing over the treatment area

    d. Protect skin from sun exposure during the treatment and for at least 1 year after the treatment is completed; when going outdoors, use sun-blocking agents with sun protection factor (SPF) of at least 15

    e. Maintain proper rest, diet, and fluid intake as essential to promoting health and repair of normal tissues

    f. Hair loss may occur; choose a wig, hat, or scarf to cover and protect head (refer to care of client with alopecia later in chapter)

5. Nursing management of the client receiving external radiation

    a. Monitor for adverse side effects of radiation (see preceding section)

    b. Monitor for significant decreases in white blood cell counts and platelet counts

    c. Client teaching (refer to later sections for management of immunosuppression, thrombocytopenia, and anemia)

6. Evaluation: client identifies interventions to reduce risk of infection, remains free from infection, achieves adequate fluid and nutritional intake, participates in activities of daily living (ADLs) at level of ability, and maintains intact skin

D. The client undergoing chemotherapy

1. **Chemotherapy** involves the administration of cytotoxic medications and chemicals to promote tumor cell death; the intravenous route is the most preferred for administering chemotherapeutic agents, but they may also be administered by oral, intrathecal, topical, intra-arterial, intracavity, and intravesical routes

    a. Chemotherapy disrupts the cell cycle in various phases, interfering with cellular metabolism and reproduction

NCLEX!

NCLEX!

NCLEX!

NCLEX!

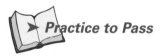

Practice to Pass

A 38-year-old male client undergoing external radiation for cancer refuses to allow his 5-year-old son to come in close contact with him because he fears exposing the son to radiation. How should you respond to the client?

> **b.** According to the **cell-kill hypothesis,** during each cell cycle a fixed percentage of cells are killed by chemotherapy, leaving some tumor cells remaining; this necessitates the repeated dosages of chemotherapy in order to reduce the number of cells, allowing the body's immune system to destroy any remaining tumor cells

> **2.** Chemotherapeutic agents are classified according to their mechanism of action (see Table 12-4 for listing of specific chemotherapeutic drugs by category)

>> **a.** *Alkylating agents* are non-phase-specific and act by interfering with DNA replication

>> **b.** *Antimetabolites* interfere with metabolites or nucleic acids necessary for RNA and DNA synthesis

Table 12-4	Chemotherapeutic Agents	
Drug Name	**Indications for Use**	**Side Effects**
Alkylating Agents		
Cyclophosphamide (Cytoxan)	Adenocarcinoma of breast and lung Leukemias Lymphomas Multiple myeloma	Alopecia Hemorrhagic cystitis Renal failure Stomatitis Pulmonary embolus or fibrosis
Busulfan (Myleran)	Chronic myelogenous leukemia (CML)	Leukopenia Pulmonary fibrosis Renal failure Thrombocytopenia
Mechlorethamine (Mustargen)	Chronic leukemia Hodgkin's disease Lung cancer Lymphosarcoma	Hyperuricemia Leukopenia Nausea and vomiting Thrombocytopenia
Antimetabolites		
5-Fluorouracil (5-FU)	Breast carcincoma Colon carcinoma Gastric carcinoma Pancreatic cancer Rectal carcinoma	Alopecia Anemia Diarrhea Enteritis Gastritis Leukopenia Nausea and vomiting Stomatitis Thrombocytopenia
Methotrexate	Acute lymphoblastic leukemia (ALL) Gestational trophoblastic carcinoma Possible osteosarcoma	Anorexia Leukopenia Nausea Oral and gastrointestinal ulcerations Pancytopenia Thrombocytopenia Headache Hepatotoxicity Hepatocirrhosis Pneumonitis Stomatitis

(continued)

Table 12-4   Chemotherapeutic Agents (*Continued*)

Drug Name	Indications for Use	Side Effects
Antitumor Antibiotics		
Bleomycin (Blenoxane)	Hodgkin's disease Lymphosarcoma Reticulum cell sarcoma Squamous cell carcinoma Testicular carcinoma	Alopecia Chills Fever Mucocutaneous ulcerations Nausea and vomiting Pneumonitis Pulmonary fibrosis/toxicity Headache Hyperpigmentation
Doxorubicin (Adriamycin)	Acute lymphoblastic leukemia (ALL) Acute myeloblastic leukemia (AML) Breast and ovarian cancer Lung cancer Neuroblastoma Thyroid cancer Wilms' tumor	Alopecia Anemia Cardiac toxicity: delayed congestive heart failure, ventricular arrhythmias, acute left ventricular failure Diarrhea Enteritis Gastritis Leukopenia Severe myelosuppression Nausea and vomiting Stomatitis Thrombocytopenia
Hormones and Hormone Antagonists		
Diethylstilbestrol (DES)	Advanced breast cancer Advanced prostate cancer	Nausea Feminization Fluid retention Uterine bleeding Thromboembolic disorders
Tamoxifen (Nolvadex)	Breast cancer	Hot flashes Nausea and vomiting Thrombosis
Prednisone	Leukemia Lymphoma Used in combination therapy for several tumors	Emotional lability/euphoria Fluid retention Hyperglycemia Hypertension Increased risk for infection Bleeding gastrointestinal ulcers
Plant Alkaloids		
Vinblastine (Velban)	Used in combination therapy for the following: Breast cancer Hodgkins' disease Kaposi's sarcoma Lymphocytic lymphoma Histocytic lymphoma Advanced testicular cancer	Alopecia Areflexia Bone marrow depression Nausea and vomiting Hemorrhagic enterocolitis Hyperuricemia
Vincristine (Oncovin)	Used in combination therapy for the following: Acute leukemia Hodgkin's lymphomas Non-Hodgkin's lymphomas Neuroblastoma Rhabdomyosarcoma Wilms' tumor	Areflexia Bone marrow depression Constipation Muscle weakness Parlytic ileus Peripheral neuritis Impaction Paresthesias, especially hands Hepatotoxicity

(*continued*)

Table 12-4	Chemotherapeutic Agents (*Continued*)	
Drug Name	**Indications for Use**	**Side Effects**
Miscellaneous Agents		
Etoposide (VP-16 or VePesid)	Nonresponsive testicular tumors Small-cell lung cancer	Alopecia Hypotension (during rapid infusion) Severe myelosuppression, leukopenia Bronchospasm
Cisplatin (CDDP) (Platinol)	Used in combination and single therapy for the following: Bladder cancer Tumors of head and neck Metastatic testicular cancer Metastatic ovarian cancer Non-small-cell lung carcinoma Neuroblastoma Osteogenic sarcoma	Deafness Leukopenia Renal tubular damage Thrombocytopenia Marked nausea/vomiting Hypomagnesemia

c. *Cytotoxic antibiotics* disrupt or inhibit DNA or RNA synthesis

d. *Hormones and hormone antagonists* are phase-specific (G1) and act by interfering with RNA synthesis

e. *Plant alkaloids*

1) Vinca alkaloids are phase-specific, inhibiting cell division

2) Etoposide acts during all cell-cycle phases, interfering with DNA and cell division at metaphase

f. *Miscellaneous agents* may be cell-cycle phase-specific or non-phase-specific and interfere with DNA replication

NCLEX!

3. Side effects of chemotherapeutic agents (see Figure 12-1)

a. **Bone marrow suppression** (see Figure 12-2)

1) Decreased WBC count (immunosuppression)

2) Decreased platelet count (**thrombocytopenia**)

3) Decreased hemoglobin and hematocrit (anemia)

b. Gastrointestinal effects: anorexia, nausea, vomiting, and diarrhea

c. **Stomatitis** (inflammation of the mouth) and mucositosis

d. **Alopecia** (hair loss)

e. Fatigue

f. **Xerostomia** (dry mouth)

g. Other side effects specific to chemotherapeutic agent (see Table 12-4)

4. Priority nursing diagnoses: Risk for infection; Fatigue; Anxiety; Risk for injury; Imbalanced nutrition: less than body requirements; Deficient fluid volume; Disturbed body image; Social isolation

Figure 12-1

**Multisystem effects
of chemotherapeutic
agents.**

Hair:
Alopecia

Heart:
Arrhythmias
Congestive heart failure
Cardiac toxicity

Mucous membranes:
Stomatitis

Lungs:
Pneumonitis
Pulmonary fibrosis

Liver:
Liver dysfunction

GI:
Mucositosis
Nausea
Vomiting
Diarrhea
Constipation
Gastrointestinal
  bleeding
Paralyticileus

Kidneys:
Renal failure

*Peripheral
nervous
system:*
Neuritis

Musculoskeletal:
Muscle weakness
Areflexia

Bone marrow suppression:
Leukopenia
Thrombocytopenia
Anemia

Figure 12-2

**Blood cells affected by
bone marrow
suppresion.**

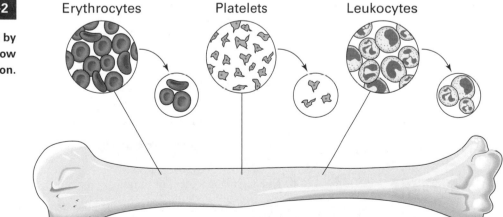

Erythrocytes   Platelets   Leukocytes

5. Immunosuppression

    a. Client education for immunosuppression

        1) Risk for infection is high when WBC count is low

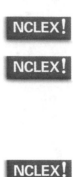

        2) Avoid crowds, people with infections, and small children when WBC is low

        3) Use meticulous personal hygiene to avoid infection

        4) Wash hands before and after eating, after toileting, and after contact with other people and pets

        5) Consume a low-bacteria diet; avoid undercooked meat and raw fruits and vegetables

        6) Be aware of signs and symptoms of infection and report them immediately to primary care provider

    b. Nursing management of immunosuppression

        1) Monitor laboratory values: CBC with differential, platelets, BUN, liver enzymes

        2) Assess for infection; monitor vital signs for early indication of infection: fever, tachycardia, and tachypnea

        3) WBC suppression, malnutrition and presence of disease increase the risk of infection

        4) Utilize neutropenic precautions (low-bacteria diet, no fresh plants or flowers in room, no pets, no visitors with infections) when WBC level falls below predetermined level (such as 2,000 mm^3)

    c. Evaluation of care for immunosuppression: client demonstrates techniques to reduce risk of infection, participates in activities that reduce risk of infection, and remains free from infection

6. Thrombocytopenia

    a. Client education for thrombocytopenia

        1) Monitor stools and urine for bleeding

        2) For shaving, use electric razor only

        3) Avoid contact sports and other activities that may cause trauma

        4) If trauma does occur, apply ice to area and seek medical assistance

        5) Avoid dental work or other invasive procedures

        6) Inform all healthcare providers of chemotherapy and/or radiation treatments

        7) Avoid aspirin and aspirin-containing products

        8) Safety precautions for oral hygiene: use soft toothbrushes and do not floss

    b. Nursing management of thrombocytopenia

        1) There is a high risk for spontaneous hemorrhage when platelet count is <20,000; precautions are necessary for platelet count <50,000

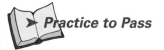

Practice to Pass

You are admitting a client to your hospital unit who is currently receiving chemotherapy for cancer at the outpatient oncology clinic. The client has a decreased platelet count and a decreased leukocyte count. What nursing interventions will you perform for this client?

NCLEX!

NCLEX!

NCLEX!

2) Assess for bleeding, monitor stools and urine for occult blood

3) Assess skin for ecchymoses, petechiae, and trauma

4) Educate client about bleeding safety precautions

5) Avoid intramuscular injections and limit venipunctures

c. Evaluation of care for thrombocytopenia: client demonstrates understanding of risks for hemorrhage, participates in activities that reduce the risk of hemorrhage, and client remains free from complications of bleeding

7. Stomatitis and mucositosis

a. Client education for stomatitis and mucositosis

1) Use a soft toothbrush; mouth swabs may be needed during acute episode

2) Avoid mouthwashes containing alcohol; do not use lemon glycerin swabs or dental floss

3) Consider using chlorhexidine mouthwash (Peridex) to decrease risk of hemorrhage and protect gums from trauma

4) Assess daily for lesions, infection, bleeding, or irritation

5) For xerostomia, apply lubricating and moisturizing agents to protect the mucous membranes from trauma and infection

6) May consider using "artificial saliva" and hard candy or mints to help with dryness

7) Avoid smoking and alcohol, which can further irritate oral mucosa

8) Teach signs and symptoms of oral infection and to report to primary healthcare provider

9) Drink cool liquids, and avoid hot and irritating foods

b. Nursing management of stomatitis

1) Assess oral mucous membranes every 4 hours

2) Teach and implement proper oral care (see client teaching above)

c. Evaluation of care for stomatitis: client participates in techniques to maintain integrity of oral mucosa; oral mucosa remains intact and free from ulcerations and inflammation

8. Inadequate nutrition and fluid and electrolyte imbalance

a. Client education for maintaining adequate nutrition, fluid and electrolyte balance

1) Eat frequent small, low-fat meals

2) Avoid spicy and fatty foods

3) Avoid extremely hot foods

4) Perform oral hygiene before and after meals

5) Maintain fluid intake as prescribed

6) Take nutritional supplements as prescribed (vitamins, liquid nutrition)

7) Maintain a daily journal of food and fluid intake

b. Nursing management of inadequate nutrition and fluid and electrolyte imbalances

1) Assess for adequate hydration; for duration of treatment, encourage daily fluid intake of 2 to 3 liters unless contraindicated

2) Administer antiemetics *prior* to chemotherapy

3) Weigh client routinely, monitor for weight loss

4) Monitor lab values indicative of nutritional status (hemoglobin, hematocrit, albumin, prealbumin)

5) Monitor for diarrhea or constipation, and nausea or vomiting

6) Encourage adequate nutritional intake with meals that are served attractively, and environment free of noxious stimuli (bedpan, urinal, odors)

c. Evaluation of nutrition, fluid and electrolyte balance: client participates in activities that maintain nutritional balance, exhibits stable weight, normal lab values, and shows no signs and symptoms of malnutrition

9. Fatigue

a. Nursing management of fatigue

1) Assure client that fatigue is a normal response to chemotherapy and that it does not indicate progression of disease

2) Encourage client to continue daily activities as much as possible, allowing for rest periods in between

3) Assist client in self-care needs when indicated

4) Allow for periods of rest; cluster activities

b. Evaluation of care for fatigue: client performs self-care and participates in activities at level of ability, and demonstrates techniques to conserve energy

10. Alopecia

a. Nursing management of client experiencing alopecia (hair loss)

1) Chemotherapy and radiation therapy may cause hair loss; the hair loss is temporary and will grow back, usually beginning about a month after completion of the chemotherapy; the client should know that the texture and color of the new hair growth may be different; hair loss during radiation therapy to the head may be permanent

2) Encourage the client to choose a wig *before* hair loss occurs in order to match texture and hair color

3) Care of hair and scalp includes washing hair two to three times a week with a mild shampoo; pat hair dry, and do not use a blow dryer

4) Allow client to express feelings concerning altered body image

b. Evaluation of care for alopecia: client demonstrates understanding and adaptation to body changes and participates in self-care activities

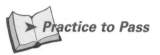

Practice to Pass

A client has lost 7 pounds since beginning chemotherapy. An assessment reveals ulcerations in the mouth, and the client states she experiences severe nausea and occasional diarrhea at home. She eats very little because of the pain, nausea, and diarrhea. What actions will you take?

NCLEX!

NCLEX!

NCLEX!

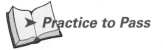

Practice to Pass

You are administering a chemotherapeutic agent intravenously. The client begins to complain of severe pain at the infusion site. What interventions do you perform?

11. Nursing implications for the administration of chemotherapy

a. Intravenous routes may be obtained by subclavian cathethers, implanted ports, or peripherally inserted catheters

b. **Extravasation,** the leaking of chemotherapeutic agents into the surrounding tissue, is the major complication of intravenous chemotherapy; extreme care must be used when administering **vesicant** agents (chemicals causing damage to tissue on contact)

c. Physicians and nurses should be specially trained to handle and administer chemotherapeutic agents

d. Vein patency must be assured before administering chemotherapeutic agents

e. Warning: never test vein patency with chemotherapeutic agents

f. If extravasation occurs, depending on the chemotherapeutic agent, interventions may include the injection of an antidote, the application of a cold compress, or the application of a warm compress

g. Assess respiratory and cardiac status; monitor EKG, assess for heart failure, and monitor vital signs

h. Monitor client closely for anaphylactic reactions or serious side effects; discontinue infusion according to protocol if reactions occur

i. Monitor intravenous site closely during administration; observe for pain and other symptoms of infiltration

j. Provide a calm, quiet environment for the client during administration

k. Use caution when preparing, administering, or disposing of chemotherapeutic agents; follow practice guidelines and protective standards for safe handling of chemotherapeutic agents provided by the Occupational Safety and Health Administration (OSHA) and Oncology Nursing Society

E. **The client undergoing a bone marrow transplant (BMT)**

1. BMT is used in the treatment of leukemias, usually in conjunction with radiation or chemotherapy

a. *Autologous BMT:* the client is infused with own bone marrow harvested during remission of disease

b. *Allogenic BMT:* the client is infused with donor bone marrow harvested from a healthy individual

2. The bone marrow is usually harvested from the iliac crests, then frozen and stored until transfusion

3. Before receiving the BMT, the client must first undergo a phase of immunosuppressive therapy to destroy the immune system; infection, bleeding, and death are major complications that can occur during this conditioning phase

4. After immunosuppression, the bone marrow is transfused intravenously through a central line

5. Side effects of bone marrow transplant:

a. Malnutrition

b. Infection related to immunosuppression

c. Bleeding related to thrombocytopenia

6. Priority nursing diagnoses: Risk for infection; Risk for hemorrhage; Risk for imbalanced nutrition; Social isolation; Anxiety

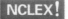

7. Client education: refer to previous sections on client education for altered nutrition, immunosuppression, and thrombocytopenia

8. Nursing management of client undergoing a bone marrow transplant (BMT)

   a. Monitor for graft-versus-host disease

   b. Provide private room for the hospitalized client; client will be hospitalized 6 to 8 weeks

   c. Encourage contact with significant others by using telephone, computer, and other means of communication to reduce feelings of isolation

   d. Refer to nursing management for imbalanced nutrition, immunosuppression, and thrombocytopenia

9. Evaluation: client demonstrates understanding of risks and participates in activities that reduce risk of infection, hemorrhage, and malnutrition; client demonstrates effective coping mechanisms

F. **The client undergoing other therapeutic interventions**

1. Immunotherapy/biologic response modifiers (BMR)

   a. Enhances the person's own immune responses in order to modify the biologic processes resulting in malignant cells

   b. Currently considered experimental in use

   c. *Monoclonal antibodies:* antibodies are recovered from an inoculated animal with a specific tumor antigen, then given to the person with that particular cancer type; the goal is destruction of the tumor

   d. *Cytokines:* normal growth-regulating molecules possessing antitumor abilities

      1) Interleukin-2 (IL-2) increases immune response effectiveness and destroys abnormal cells

      2) Interferons are substances produced by cells to protect them from viral infection and replication; interferon-alpha 2b is most commonly used

      3) *Hematopoietic growth factors,* such as granulocyte colony-stimulating factor (G-CSF) and erythropoietin, balance the suppression of granulocytes and erythrocytes resulting from chemotherapy

   e. *Natural killer cells* (NK cells): exert a spontaneous cytotoxic effect on specific cancer cells; they also secrete cytokines and provide a resistance to metastasis

2. Gene therapy

   a. Current use is investigational

   b. Increases susceptibility of cancer cells to the destruction by other treatments; insertion of specific genes enhances ability of client's own immune system to recognize and destroy cancer cells

3. Photodynamic therapy

   a. Used to treat specific superficial tumors such as those of the surface of bladder, bronchus, chest wall, head, neck, and peritoneal cavity

   b. Photofrin, a photosensitizing compound, is administered intravenously, where it is retained by malignant tissue

   c. Three days after injection, the drug is activated by a laser treatment, which continues for 3 more days

   d. The drug produces a cytotoxic oxygen molecule (singlet oxygen)

   e. During intravenous administration, monitor for chills, nausea, rash, local skin reactions, and temporary photosensitivity

   f. Drug remains in tissues 4 to 6 weeks after injection; direct or indirect exposure to sun activates drug, resulting in chemical sunburn; educate client to protect skin from sun exposure

VII. Oncologic Emergencies: Diagnosis and Management

A. Spinal cord compression

1. Occurs secondary to pressure from expanding tumors

2. Early symptoms include back and leg pain, coldness, numbness, tingling, paresthesias; progression leads to bowel and bladder dysfunction, weakness, and paralysis

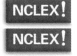

3. Early detection is essential: investigate all complaints of back pain or neurological changes

4. Treatment is aimed at reducing tumor size by radiation and/or surgery to relieve compression and prevent irreversible paraplegia; may receive corticosteroids to reduce cord edema

5. Nursing interventions include early recognition of symptoms, monitoring vital signs, neurological checks, and medication administration

B. Superior vena cava syndrome

1. Compression or obstruction of the superior vena cava (SVC)

2. Usually associated with cancer of lungs and lymphomas

3. Signs and symptoms are the result of blockage of venous circulation of head, neck, and upper trunk

4. Early signs and symptoms are periorbital edema and facial edema

5. Symptoms progress to edema of neck, arms, and hands; difficulty swallowing; shortness of breath

6. Late signs and symptoms are cyanosis, altered mental status, headache, and hypotension

7. Death may occur if compression is not relieved

8. Treatment includes high-dose radiation to shrink tumor and relieve symptoms

NCLEX!

9. Nursing interventions include monitoring vital signs, providing oxygen support, preparing for tracheostomy if necessary, initiating seizure precautions, and administering corticosteroids to reduce edema

C. Disseminated intravascular coagulopathy (DIC)

1. Severe disorder of coagulation, often triggered by sepsis, whereby abnormal clot formation occurs in the microvasculature; this process depletes the clotting factors and platelets, allowing extensive bleeding to occur; tissue hypoxia occurs as a result of the blockage of blood vessels from the clots

2. Signs and symptoms are related to decreased blood flow to major organs (tachycardia, oliguria, dyspnea) and depleted clotting factors (abnormal bleeding and hemorrhage)

NCLEX!

3. Treatment includes anticoagulants to decrease stimulation of coagulation and transfusion of one or more of the following: fresh frozen plasma (FFP), cryoprecipitate, platelets, and packed red blood cells (RBCs)

NCLEX!

4. Nursing interventions include assessing client, monitoring for bleeding, applying pressure dressings to venipuncture sites, and preventing risk of sepsis

5. Mortality for clients experiencing DIC is greater than 70 percent despite aggressive treatment

D. Cardiac tamponade

1. Pericardial effusion secondary to metastases or esophageal cancer can lead to compression of heart, restricting heart movement and resulting in cardiac tamponade

2. Signs and symptoms are related to cardiogenic shock or circulatory collapse: anxiety, cyanosis, dyspnea, hypotension, tachycardia, tachypnea, impaired level of consciousness, and increased central venous pressure

3. Pericardiocentesis is performed to remove fluid from pericardial sac

4. Nursing interventions include administering oxygen, maintaining intravenous line, monitoring vital signs, hemodynamic monitoring, and the administration of vasopressor agents

VIII. Expected Outcomes of Clients with Cellular Disorders

A. 5-year survival rate for all cancers is 59 percent; this rate decreases for African-Americans and underserved Americans

B. For cancers of the breast, colon, rectum, cervix, prostate, testis, oral cavity, and skin, the overall 5-year survival rate is approximately 80 percent; according to the American Cancer Society, this rate could increase to 95 percent if all Americans participated in regular cancer screenings

C. Survival rates for certain cancers are improving for cancers such as Hodgkin's disease, Wilms' tumor, testicular cancer, and ovarian cancer, while no significant improvement is noted in others such as lung cancer and colon cancer

D. Approximately 552,000 cancer-related deaths occurred in 2000

▶ Practice to Pass

A client with metastatic prostate cancer informs you that he has been experiencing back pain for 3 days and his legs are numb. What assessments should you make and what actions will you take?

Case Study

C. J., a 68-year-old female client on your nursing unit, has recently been diagnosed with cancer of the left breast.

❶ You enter C. J.'s room and find her crying. She states, "I can't believe I have cancer." What actions would you take?

❷ C. J. asks you what treatments and procedures she will most likely experience. How do you respond to her?

❸ Before beginning intravenous chemotherapy, what information and instructions will you give to C. J.?

❹ C. J. complains of experiencing severe nausea and vomiting during chemotherapy. What measures can be taken to lessen the severity or control the nausea and vomiting?

❺ C. J. expresses concern over the expected alopecia (hair loss) from the chemotherapy. How do you respond to her?

For suggested responses, see pages 738–739.

Posttest

1   A client undergoing radiation therapy has a severely depressed white blood cell (WBC) count. A priority nursing intervention would include which of the following?

(1) Place client in a private room and maintain strict aseptic technique with all procedures.
(2) Encourage client to include fresh fruits and vegetables in the diet.
(3) Educate client to avoid shaving with a razor.
(4) Encourage frequent visitors to reduce client's feelings of isolation.

2   You are the assessment nurse in a local clinic. Based on the history provided by the clients, which one of the following requires an immediate referral for screening and evaluation?

(1) The client who reports an unintended weight loss of 25 pounds over the past 3 months
(2) The client who smokes 2 packages of cigarettes a day
(3) The client who reports a history of long-term sun exposure
(4) The client who consumes a diet high in fat and low in fiber

3   You are counseling a client on risk factors associated with cancer. For which of the following will you assist the client in developing a plan to reduce the risk of cancer?

(1) Heredity
(2) Gender
(3) Age
(4) Diet

4   You are making a home visit to a client receiving external radiation therapy on an outpatient basis. Further teaching is necessary when you observe the client doing which of the following?

(1) Washing the radiation site with plain water and patting the skin dry
(2) Protecting the skin with soft, loose clothing
(3) Applying lotion to the irritated skin
(4) Inspecting the skin for damage

5 A hospitalized client with an internal radiation implant calls you to the room to report the implant is dislodged and is lying in the bed. Your actions would include which of the following?

(1) Apply gloves and place the implant in a biohazard bag
(2) Use long-handle forceps to pick up the implant and place it into a lead container
(3) Have the client pick up the implant and place it into a lead container
(4) Notify infection control personnel to dispose of the implant

6 A client with leukemia is undergoing the "conditioning phase" for a bone marrow transplant (BMT). The priority nursing diagnosis for this client is which of the following?

(1) Fatigue related to anemia
(2) Imbalanced Nutrition: less than body requirements
(3) Altered mucous membranes
(4) Risk for infection

7 You have counseled a male 52-year-old client about early detection and screening for prostate cancer. You evaluate that the client has understood your instructions when he states which of the following?

(1) "I should have a digital rectal examination and prostate-specific antigen (PSA) test done yearly."
(2) "I should have a prostate-specific antigen (PSA) test done yearly."
(3) "I should have a digital rectal examination done yearly."
(4) "I don't need a screening unless I develop symptoms."

8 A client who had a mastectomy yesterday refuses to look at the incision. You can best assist the client to cope with the disturbed body image by doing which of the following?

(1) Tell the client that eventually everyone accepts the loss of a body part.
(2) Encourage the client to express feelings about loss of body part.
(3) Delay wound care until client is prepared to look at the wound.
(4) Have the client assist you with the dressing change.

9 In assessing a client receiving chemotherapy, which of the following would require further evaluation?

(1) Dry mucous membranes
(2) Large areas of ecchymosis in various sites on body
(3) Complaints of fatigue
(4) Hair loss on scalp

10 A client receiving external radiation expresses concern to you about physical intimacy with spouse. When offering sexual counseling to the client and spouse, you tell them which of the following about intimate physical contact?

(1) It should be avoided during treatment to avoid radiation exposure to the spouse.
(2) It is safe during treatment; there is no risk of radiation exposure to the spouse.
(3) It should be avoided during treatment to conserve energy.
(4) It increases the risk of infection to the client with cancer.

Answers and Rationales

Pretest

1 Answer: 2 *Rationale:* Approximately 67 percent of all cancer occurs in people over age 65, necessitating early screening and detection. The incidence of cancer increases with age, making it a significant factor in the development of cancer.
Cognitive Level: Application
Nursing Process: Implementation; *Test Plan:* HPM

2 Answer: 1 *Rationale:* Benign neoplasms are localized, encapsulated growths. They are not malignant, and they do not metastasize. They are harmful only if they interfere with vital functions such as circulation. Malignant neoplasms have a high mortality rate unless therapeutic interventions are performed. The client's question is a normal, expected response.
Cognitive Level: Application
Nursing Process: Implementation; *Test Plan:* PSYC

3 **Answer: 3** *Rationale:* Administering antiemetics before chemotherapy helps reduce the severity of nausea. Waiting until the client is experiencing nausea demonstrates lack of planning. Cool foods and liquids are better tolerated and are less irritating than warm foods and liquids. Small, frequent meals are more easily tolerated and may reduce the incidence of nausea and vomiting.
Cognitive Level: Application
Nursing Process: Planning; *Test Plan:* PHYS

4 **Answer: 2** *Rationale:* The client is a risk to others as long as the radiation implant is present. Therefore, certain precautions to protect others must be taken. The client should have a private room, and visitors should maintain a distance of 6 feet and limit visits to 10 to 30 minutes. The client may not need isolation for the entire period of hospitalization, rather just for the time the implant is in place.
Cognitive Level: Application
Nursing Process: Implementation; *Test Plan:* PHYS

5 **Answer: 1** *Rationale:* Washing the hair daily will promote further hair loss. Hair washing should be limited to 2 to 3 times per week. Options 2, 3, and 4 are correct actions taken by the client.
Cognitive Level: Analysis
Nursing Process: Evaluation; *Test Plan:* PHYS

6 **Answer: 3** *Rationale:* The client with a low WBC count is at high risk for infection. The grandchild recently exposed to varicella could be contagious at this point. The nephew with HIV, unless currently infected with another communicable disease, does not pose a risk. There is no indication that the husband has tuberculosis. The pregnant daughter does not pose a risk.
Cognitive Level: Analysis
Nursing Process: Implementation; *Test Plan:* PHYS

7 **Answer: 1** *Rationale:* The American Cancer Society recommends a breast examination by a health care provider every 3 years for ages 20 to 39, then yearly from age 40 and older. Breast self-examinations should be performed monthly. Mammograms are recommended yearly beginning at age 40.
Cognitive Level: Analysis
Nursing Process: Evaluation; *Test Plan:* HPM

8 **Answer: 2** *Rationale:* Extravasation of the chemotherapeutic agent, especially if the agent is a vesicant, is a major complication of intravenous administration of chemotherapy. *Never* test vein patency with the medication. Making the client comfortable is

important, but assuring vein patency is the highest priority. There is no indication to administer acetaminophen.
Cognitive Level: Application
Nursing Process: Planning; *Test Plan:* PHYS

9 **Answer: 1** *Rationale:* The client with a low platelet count (thrombocytopenia) is at risk for bleeding. Aspirin further interferes with platelet functioning. Monitoring for fever (option 2) is necessary for low WBC count, and managing fatigue (option 3) is necessary for anemia. Flossing is contraindicated in the client with low platelet count (option 4).
Cognitive Level: Analysis
Nursing Process: Evaluation; *Test Plan:* PHYS

10 **Answer: 4** *Rationale:* Damage to the mucous membranes, especially oral mucous membranes (stomatitis), leads to painful ulcerations of the mouth, interfering with the client's desire to eat. The mucous membranes and mouth may be dry (xerostomia) as a side effect of the chemotherapy. Pale skin may be a sign of anemia, and ecchymosis may be indicative of a low platelet count.
Cognitive Level: Analysis
Nursing Process: Assessment; *Test Plan:* PHYS

Posttest

1 **Answer: 1** *Rationale:* The immunosuppressed client is at high risk for infection. A private room, maintaining aseptic technique, and limiting visitors will reduce exposure and risk. Fresh fruits and vegetables may harbor bacteria; serve cooked foods only. The client with a decreased platelet count should be counseled to avoid using razors.
Cognitive Level: Application
Nursing Process: Implementation; *Test Plan:* SECE

2 **Answer: 1** *Rationale:* Unexplained, rapid weight loss may be the first symptom associated with cancer, and immediate evaluation is required. Options 2, 3, and 4 are risk factors associated with cancer, and education and screening are important to reduce the risk of cancer.
Cognitive Level: Analysis
Nursing Process: Analysis; *Test Plan:* HPM

3 **Answer: 4** *Rationale:* Options 1, 2, and 3 are noncontrollable or nonmodifiable risk factors. Diet is the only listed risk factor that is controllable. Assisting the client to develop a diet plan low in fat and high in fiber will help reduce the risk of some types of cancer.
Cognitive Level: Application
Nursing Process: Implementation; *Test Plan:* HPM

4 **Answer: 3** *Rationale:* Lotion, deodorant, and powders should not be applied to the radiation site during the treatment period to avoid further irritation to the skin. Options 1, 2, and 4 are correct actions.
Cognitive Level: Application
Nursing Process: Assessment; *Test Plan:* PHYS

5 **Answer: 2** *Rationale:* Long-handle forceps should be used to pick up the implant. Lead containers are necessary to prevent exposure to radiation. Direct handling of the implant causes exposure to radiation; no one should directly touch the implant. Gloves and biohazard bags do not offer protection from radiation. Infection control personnel have no role in the disposal of the implant, which should be rturned to the radiation therapy department after properly being placed in the lead container.
Cognitive Level: Application
Nursing Process: Implementation; *Test Plan:* SECE

6 **Answer: 4** *Rationale:* The conditioning phase depresses bone marrow function, and infection is the major cause of death for clients with leukemia. Options 1, 2, and 3 are appropriate diagnoses for clients receiving chemotherapy and radiation, but the risk for infection is the highest priority during this phase.
Cognitive Level: Analysis
Nursing Process: Planning; *Test Plan:* PHYS

7 **Answer: 1** *Rationale:* The American Cancer Society recommends a digital rectal examination and PSA yearly for males beginning at age 50. Options 2 and 3 are only partly correct, and option 4 is incorrect.
Cognitive Level: Analysis
Nursing Process: Evaluation; *Test Plan:* HPM

8 **Answer: 2** *Rationale:* Denial is a protective mechanism, and during this time, the client needs a supportive environment. Allowing the client to express feelings will enable an effective adaptation to this change. Option 1 is not therapeutic. Wound care must be done in order to prevent complications (option 3), and the client is obviously not psychologically ready to participate in self-care (option 4).
Cognitive Level: Application
Nursing Process: Implementation; *Test Plan:* PSYC

9 **Answer: 2** *Rationale:* Options 1, 3, and 4 are common side effects of chemotherapy. Even though they do require intervention, ecchymotic areas may be a sign of decreased platelet count, making the risk of hemorrhage the priority.
Cognitive Level: Analysis
Nursing Process: Assessment; *Test Plan:* PHYS

10 **Answer: 2** *Rationale:* External radiation poses no risk of radiation exposure to contacts, even during intimate physical contact. Clients are encouraged to maintain their usual activities, as long as they are tolerated (option 3). There is no increase in risk of infection to the client with cancer during intimate physical contact unless that person has a current infection (then contact should be avoided until infection is treated).
Cognitive Level: Application
Nursing Process: Implementation; *Test Plan:* HPM

References

American Cancer Society. (2000). *Cancer facts and figures—2000*. Atlanta: Author.

Deters, G. (1999). Cancer. In W. Phipps, J. Sands, & J. Marek (Eds.), *Medical-surgical nursing: Concepts and clinical practice* (6th ed.). St. Louis: MO: Mosby, Inc. pp. 253–320.

Ignatavicius, D., Workman, M., & Mishler, M. (1999). *Medical surgical nursing across the health care continuum* (3rd ed.). Philadelphia: W. B. Saunders Company, pp. 475–492, 493–517.

Lemone, P. & Burke, K. (2000). *Medical surgical nursing: Critical thinking in client care* (2nd ed.). Upper Saddle River, NJ: Prentice-Hall, Inc., pp. 31–370, 1310–1316.

Lewis, S., Heitkemper, M., & Dirksen, S. (2000). *Medical-surgical nursing: Assessment and management of clinical problems* (5th ed.). St. Louis, MO: Mosby, Inc., pp. 407–444.

Smeltzer, S. C. & Bare, B. G. (2000). B*runner & Suddarth's textbook of medical surgical nursing* (9th ed.). Philadelphia: Lippincott, Williams & Wilkins, pp. 263–312.

CHAPTER 13

Endocrine and Metabolic Disorders

Carol Wolfensperger Bashford, MS, RN, CS

CHAPTER OUTLINE

*Overview of Anatomy
  and Physiology*
Diagnostic Tests and Assessments

*Disorders of the Posterior Pituitary
  Gland*
Disorders of the Thyroid Gland

Disorders of the Parathyroid Gland
Disorders of the Adrenal Cortex
Disorders of the Pancreas

OBJECTIVES

▋ Identify basic structures and functions of the endocrine system.

▋ Describe the pathophysiology and etiology of common endocrine disorders.

▋ Discuss expected assessment data and diagnostic test findings for selected endocrine disorders.

▋ Identify priority nursing diagnoses for selected endocrine disorders.

▋ Discuss therapeutic management of selected endocrine disorders.

▋ Discuss nursing management of a client experiencing an endocrine disorder.

▋ Identify expected outcomes for the client experiencing an endocrine disorder.

[*Media Link*]

Use the CD-ROM enclosed with this text, or log onto the address given to access the free, interactive Companion Website created for this series. The CD-ROM and Companion Website accompanying this book offer additional practice opportunities and information—NCLEX Review, Case Studies, Glossary, In Depth with NCLEX, and more.

www.prenhall.com/hogan

REVIEW AT A GLANCE

endocrine gland *ductless tissue secreting a hormone to regulate body functions*

exocrine gland *gland whose secretions reach a target via ducts*

glycosylated hemoglobin *saturation of the hemoglobin in the RBC with glucose; serum level >8% indicates poor serum glucose regulation in diabetes mellitus; reported as glycosylated hemoglobin or glycohemoglobin (GHB)*

hormone *chemical substance that is secreted by endocrine tissue and travels in body fluids (usually the bloodstream) to effect an action in specific target cells*

hyperkalemia *excess or elevated level of potassium in blood*

hyperglycemia *excess or elevated level of glucose in the blood*

hypersecretion *secretion of a chemical is above normal level; may be associated with increased (abnormal) function of an endocrine gland*

hypocalcemia *low level of calcium in the blood*

hyponatremia *low level of sodium in the blood*

hypophysectomy *surgical removal of the hypophysis (pituitary gland)*

hyposecretion *secretion of a chemical is below normal level; may be associated with abnormally low function of an endocrine gland*

ketosis *a state in which excessive ketones are produced in the body from incomplete fat metabolism; usually leads to elevated ketone levels in the urine and causes acidosis*

paresthesia *abnormal sensation described as tingling, burning, or prickling*

photophobia *unable to tolerate light*

polydipsia *excessive thirst*

polyphagia *eating an abnormally excessive amount of food*

polyuria *an abnormally large amount of urine output*

receptor *cell site that is sensitive to a specific stimulus or hormone*

sebum *lubricating secretion from the sebaceous glands of the skin*

thyroid crisis (thyroid storm) *occurrence of life-threatening extreme manifestations of hyperthyroidism: high fever, hypertension, tachycardia, restlessness, and delirium*

Pretest

1 A female client is being given 30 mCi sodium iodide-131 (Iodotope) to treat Graves' disease. Before giving the client her first dose you should do which of the following?

(1) Assess the client for hypersensitivity by asking if she is allergic to eggs.
(2) Instruct her that she must not sleep in the same room with another person for 8 days.
(3) Assess her temperature to use as a baseline to evaluate the medication effectiveness.
(4) Instruct the client not to drink the medication mixture with a straw in order to ensure she drinks the entire dose.

2 A client is 12 hours post-partial thyroidectomy. During the postoperative phase the nurse asks the client about any numbness or tingling of the face, mouth, or extremities for which of the following assessment purposes?

(1) Early identification of low thyroid hormone
(2) Detection of thyroid-induced hypoglycemia
(3) Early identification of hypocalcemia
(4) Detection of nerve damage related to surgery

3 The client is diagnosed with an allergy to iodine. In addition to client education about avoiding foods with iodine, the client should also be taught to report which of the following symptoms associated with endocrine malfunction related to low iodine intake?

(1) Diarrhea, weight loss, blurred vision
(2) Constipation, weight gain, muscle stiffness
(3) Fatigue, dry skin, increased BP
(4) Anorexia, dyspnea, weight loss

4 A client is 20 hours post-colon resection with end-to-end anastomosis for ruptured diverticulum. You have read in the medical record that he has an 8-year history of Addison's disease. After noting new onset of lethargy with the current assessment, you would do which of the following next?

(1) Review his patient-controlled analgesia (PCA) record for dose history
(2) Assess him for decreased urine output and blood pressure (BP)
(3) Check pupils for direct and consensual reaction
(4) Obtain a pulse oximeter to check his oxygen saturation level

5 A client has new onset type I diabetes mellitus (DM). He asks you why he needs to check his blood glucose level so frequently. You explain that frequent coverage with insulin to keep his blood glucose level between 80 and 155 mg/dL is important for which of the following reasons?

(1) Chronic elevated blood glucose levels damage cells and cause multiple organ damage.
(2) High glucose levels cause the body to use proteins for energy, causing lactic acidosis.
(3) Early identification of hypoglycemia before the onset of symptoms is easier to treat.
(4) Carbohydrates are constantly being converted to glucose and transported in the blood by insulin.

6 You have been teaching the client with new onset of syndrome of inappropriate antidiuretic hormone (SIADH) about the disorder. Which of the following statements by the client best indicates that he correctly understands how to manage this disease?

(1) "I should limit my sodium intake to 2 grams daily."
(2) "I should report constipation or fatigue to the doctor."
(3) "I should drink at least 3,000 cc or 10 glasses of water daily."
(4) "I should limit my fluid intake to approximately 800 cc or 4 glasses of water daily."

7 The client is admitted with decreased level of consciousness secondary to a closed head injury resulting from a fall while roller-skating. Urine output is 500 cc from 6:00 A.M. to 11:00 A.M., 1000 cc from 11:00 A.M. to 2:00 P.M. and 350 cc from 2:00 P.M. to 3:00 P.M. Which of the following actions by the nurse is appropriate?

(1) Realize that this is normal urine output and continue to monitor the client.
(2) Encourage the client to drink 8 to 10 glasses of fluid daily.
(3) Check the urine specific gravity and report any abnormality as well as the urine output.
(4) Decrease the IV rate from 100 cc/hr to 25 cc/hr, suspecting fluid excess.

8 The client with acromegaly secondary to excessive growth hormone (GH) states: "I'll be glad to have this surgery; after the pituitary gland is removed I will be cured—then no more lab tests and pills!" Which of the following statements should the nurse document to evaluate the client's understanding of preoperative teaching?

(1) Criteria met: Client correctly verbalized understanding of outcomes.
(2) Criteria not met: Client needs to know about routine postoperative lab tests done on first postoperative day to evaluate response to surgery.
(3) Criteria not met: Client needs to know surgery will slow down the disease process but client will need regular blood tests and x-rays for 1 year.
(4) Criteria not met: Client needs to know surgery will stop excess production of GH and probably other hormones, and thus will need daily replacement medications for life.

9 The client is admitted with metabolic acidosis secondary to diabetic ketoacidosis (DKA). Understanding metabolic acidosis, the nurse should choose which of the following as the priority nursing diagnosis?

(1) Decreased urinary elimination related to reduced output and muscle function.
(2) Decreased cardiac output related to fluid and electrolyte imbalance.
(3) Ineffective breathing pattern related to hyperventilation.
(4) Anxiety related to fears of long-term outcomes and discomfort.

10 An elderly female client with dry flaky skin and activity intolerance secondary to myxedema is admitted to the progressive care unit to improve her activity tolerance and gain independence in self-care. For hygiene care the nursing order is two total baths per week on Saturday and Wednesday with partial baths on the remaining days of the week. Which of the following would be the desired outcome of this intervention?

(1) Client is able to sleep through the night and stay awake most of the day
(2) Gradual increase in ambulation ability over the first month
(3) Increased energy by the end of the first week of paced rest and activity
(4) Intact elastic moist warm skin by the end of first week

I. Overview of Anatomy and Physiology

A. Basic structures of the endocrine system

1. Both exocrine and endocrine glands originate from glandular epithelial tissue

2. During development of the glands intracellular macromolecules are formed (which are the chemical substances secreted by the gland) and stored in vesicles called secretory granules

3. **Exocrine glands** secrete substances that reach their target tissue directly or by traveling through a duct; they include sebaceous, salivary, mammary and sweat glands

4. **Endocrine glands** secrete hormones directly into the blood stream; neuronal stimulation, chemical substances or hormones can control secretion of endocrine glands

5. A **hormone** is a biologically active substance secreted by an endocrine gland that circulates throughout the body, affecting the function of one or more target organs, tissues or bodily functions

6. Endocrine gland hormones control a variety of biologic functions

7. Various conditions can cause the endocrine gland to hypersecrete or hyposecrete, leading to altered body functions

8. **Hyposecretion** is a condition where an insufficient supply of the substance is secreted

9. **Hypersecretion** is a condition where an excessive amount of the substance is secreted

B. Basic functions of the endocrine system

1. Exocrine glands provide a vast variety of functions

   a. During lactation, milk is ejected from the mammary gland

   b. Salivary glands secrete saliva

      1) The mucus in saliva protects the oral mucous membranes, cleanses the oral mucosa, and contains the antibacterial-like enzyme lysozyme

      2) Saliva also contains two digestive enzymes, amylase and ptyalin, to initiate starch digestion before it enters the stomach

   c. Sweat glands secrete sweat onto the skin to regulate body temperature

   d. Sebaceous glands secrete **sebum,** composed of lipids and wax that insulate the skin to prevent excess evaporation and conserve body heat

2. Endocrine glands: coordinate and regulate long-term changes in function of all body organs and tissues to maintain homeostasis

3. Hormones: chemical messengers that travel in the circulatory system and alter cellular activities by changing enzymes and proteins in target cells

   a. **Receptor**: specially designed link on a target cell membrane or in the cytoplasm for a specific hormone to contact and initiate an action response

NCLEX**!**

   b. Regulation of secretion: the effects on the target tissue act as a negative feedback controlling mechanism to signal the initiating gland to slow or stop secretion

C. Major endocrine system glands

   1. Posterior pituitary gland: regulates fluid balance and facilitates childbirth and prostate gland function

   a. Releases antidiuretic hormone (ADH) and oxytocin, which are produced and stored in the hypothalamus

   b. ADH stimulates the kidneys to reabsorb water decreasing urine output, supporting BP and blood volume, and also stimulates peripheral blood vessels to constrict

   c. Oxytocin stimulates the uterus to contract for childbirth, the mammary glands for milk ejection, and the smooth muscles of the prostate gland to contract and eject secretions

   2. Anterior pituitary gland: the major role of this gland is to produce and release seven different hormones (most of which regulate the secretion of other hormones), which are: thyroid-stimulating hormone (TSH), adrenocorticotropic hormone (ACTH), follicle-stimulating hormone (FSH), luteinizing hormone (LH), prolactin (PRL), interstitial cell-stimulating hormone (ICSH), and growth hormone (GH), also called somatotropin

   3. Thyroid gland: determines the rate of cellular metabolism; in children, the hormones are responsible for normal development of the skeletal, muscular, and nervous systems

   a. Calcitonin targets bone and kidney cells to regulate calcium ion concentrations in body fluids

   b. Thyroxine (TX or tetraiodothyronine or T_4), and Triiodothyronine (T_3) bind to mitochondria and nucleus of cells to increase the rate of ATP production

   4. Parathyroid glands: monitor and maintain circulating concentration of calcium ions

   a. Secrete parathyroid hormone (PTH) to increase serum calcium level

   b. PTH stimulates osteoclasts, inhibits osteoblasts, promotes the absorption of calcium by the intestines, and decreases renal excretion of calcium

   5. Pancreas (islets of Langerhans): regulates blood glucose concentrations

   a. Alpha cells produce glucagon to break down stored fat and carbohydrate (CHO) into glucose in response to low glucose level

   b. Beta cells produce insulin that is needed by most cells to transport glucose across cell membranes

   c. Delta cells produce somatostatin that inhibits the production of glucagons and insulin

   6. Adrenal medulla: increases cellular energy use and muscular strength endurance, and mobilizes energy reserves

   a. Secretes epinephrine (adrenaline) and norepinephrine (noradrenaline); receptors are on skeletal muscle fibers, adipose tissues, and liver

        b. Mobilizes glycogen reserves, metabolizes glucose for ATP, and increases cardiac rate and force of contraction

  7. Adrenal cortex: hormones play a vital role for the body's survival and affect metabolism of many different tissues

NCLEX!

        a. Glucocorticoids: cortisol (hydrocortisone), corticosterone, and cortisone stimulate most cells to increase rate of glucose synthesis, glycogen formation, release of fatty acids, and break down fatty acids; exert an anti-inflammatory effect to suppress the immune system

NCLEX!

        b. Mineralocorticoids: aldosterone stimulates the kidneys to increase reabsorption of sodium and water, and reduces sodium and water loss by the sweat glands, salivary glands, and digestive tract

        c. Small amount of androgens

  8. Female gonads (ovaries): regulate secondary sexual characteristics and reproduction

        a. Estrogens stimulate most cells to develop secondary sex characteristics and behaviors, follicle maturation, and growth of uterine lining

        b. Provides negative feedback to the anterior pituitary gland to stop secretion of FSH

        c. Progestins stimulate the uterus to prepare for implantation and the mammary glands for lactation

  9. Male gonads (testes): regulate secondary sexual characteristics and reproduction

        a. Androgens, primarily testosterone, stimulate most cells for protein synthesis, maturation of sperm, secondary sexual characteristics and behaviors

        b. Inhibin secreted for negative feedback to the anterior pituitary gland to stop secretion of FSH

II. Diagnostic Tests and Assessments

A. Assessment of the endocrine system

  1. Dysfunction of any one of the endocrine glands or the receptor sites of the endocrine gland hormone causes an alteration of one or more body functions; obtain appropriate health information pertinent to the affected gland, such as signs and symptoms of hyper- or hypofunction

  2. Physical assessment: use an organized system approach, assessing the client's general appearance and proceeding with a head-to-toe assessment

B. Diagnostic studies of the endocrine system

  1. Computed tomography (CT) scan

        a. Description: a procedure that produces a detailed image of tissues from cross sectional beams of x-rays that are recorded as they pass through the body in 360-degree motion

NCLEX!

        b. Nursing implications include to:

           1) Assess for allergy to iodine, shellfish or other contrast medium

           2) For the female client, avoid x-ray until negative pregnancy status is confirmed, or counsel and shield abdomen and pelvis

3) Consider informed consent if contrast media is used

4) Encourage fluid intake after the scan if contrast was used to aid in excretion of contrast media via kidneys

2. Studies of the pituitary gland

   a. Serum studies include: GH or somatotropin, somatomedin C, GH release post-exercise, insulin-induced hypoglycemia, prolactin level, gonadotropin levels (FSH, LH) and water-deprivation test

   b. Radiologic studies include:

     1) Skull x-ray to detect the integrity of the bone and tumors of the bone

     2) CT scan

     3) Magnetic resonance imaging (MRI), which uses magnet and radio waves to produce visual image of an energy field; details organ structure, specific location and size of tumor(s), edema and infarcts, blood flow patterns and blood vessel integrity

     4) See Chapter 1 for further general information about diagnostic tests

3. Studies of the thyroid gland

   a. Serum studies include:

     1) L-thyroxine (total T_4): measures both free and protein-bound thyroxine; normal is 4.5 to 10.9 µg/dl in adults

     2) Free T_4 is the amount of thyroxine not bound to globulins; normal values are 0.8 to 2.7 ng/ml by actual assay or 4.6 to 11.2 by calculated method

     3) Triiodothyronine (T_3) (normal value 60 to 181 ng/dl), also called T_3 RIA, T_3 resin uptake (T_3RU)

     4) Additional tests are: TSH or thyrotropin (normal value 0.5 to 5.0 U/ml) and serum calcitonin

   b. Radiologic studies include: thyroid 131 (whole body scan to detect metastasis from a known malignant thyroid tumor) and thyroid scan or RAI uptake study to determine the amount of uptake by the thyroid gland

4. Studies of the parathyroid glands

   a. Serum studies include

     1) PTH (released by parathyroid glands to regulate serum calcium and phosphorus)

     2) Total calcium (including free calcium and calcium bound to plasma proteins)

     3) Phosphorus: reported as phosphorus (P) or phosphate (PO4) and 1,25 Dihydroxyvitamin D

   b. Radiologic studies include skeletal x-ray and CT scan

5. Studies of the adrenal glands

   a. Serum studies include cortisol (secreted by adrenal cortex, a larger amount in the morning then decreasing over the day), aldosterone (a mineral-ocorticoid hormone secreted by the adrenal cortex), ACTH stimulation (to confirm suspected disease of the adrenal cortex), dexamethasone suppression and metyrapone suppression

b. Urine studies

1) 17-Ketosteroids (17 KS): urine is collected for 24 hours to measure the amount of 17 KS or the metabolites of steroids produced by the adrenal cortex and testes; nursing implications for this test include the following points:

a) Check all medications taken by the client for drug interference with the test

b) Check to determine whether preservative was placed in the collection bottle by laboratory personnel

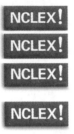

c) Begin collection by having client void and discard the specimen

d) Begin collecting all urine with next voiding

e) Exactly 24 hours after the client discarded the first specimen, have client void and save the specimen to end the collection process

f) It is imperative to collect all urine; if specimen discarded by accident then collection process needs to be restarted with a new container

g) Keep collection bottle or indwelling catheter bag on ice

h) Label the collection bottle with date and time started and ended

i) Instruct client about purpose and procedure of test

2) Aldosterone: mineralocorticoid hormone secreted by the adrenal cortex

3) Vanillylmandelic acid (VMA): a metabolite of catecholamines

a) Obtain collection bottle from lab containing HCL (a strong acid)

b) Warn client about the acid in the bottle, to keep face away from opening when removing cap to add urine and to avoid inhaling the odor from the bottle

c) Instruct client to avoid exposure to stress or exercise

d) Check with lab about specific foods to be avoided during testing period

e) If possible client should not take any medication for 7 days before the test and during the testing period

f) Record BP, height, and weight on lab slip

g) See 24-hour urine protocol as previously described

6. Studies of the pancreas

a. Serum studies (see also diagnostic tests section in Chapter 1)

1) Fasting blood glucose (FBG) levels or fasting plasma glucose

a) Fast for at least 8 hours, water is permitted

b) Withhold insulin for fasting period until specimen drawn

c) Adult reference value: 70 to 110 mg/dL (whole blood: 60 to 100 mg/dL), elderly 70 to 120 mg/dL

2) Oral glucose tolerance test (GTT): tests for transitional gestational glucose intolerance; medications, infection, trauma, bedrest and stress can alter results

a) Fast overnight, water permitted

b) Start test by drawing fasting glucose specimen and obtain urine specimen

c) Give client 75 or 100 g of glucose dissolved in water

d) Collect blood glucose specimen at 1, 2, and 3 hours after drinking glucose; some labs require blood specimens hourly up to 8 hours

e) Collect urine specimen(s) according to lab protocol; some labs do not collect urine

f) Fast during entire specimen collection period; water is encouraged

g) Reference values are measured in mg/dL for dose of 100 g of glucose

b. Capillary glucose monitoring

1) Warm extremity to encourage vasodilation; select digit to be used

2) Cleanse site with soap and water or 70 percent alcohol, dry with a gauze sponge

3) Avoid squeezing site to enhance blood flow since squeezing causes dilution with tissue fluid

4) Avoid touching skin with reagent strip; skin oils may affect results

5) Elevate digit and apply gentle pressure with dry sterile gauze to site until bleeding stops

c. **Glycosylated hemoglobin:** prolonged hyperglycemia causes hemoglobin (HGB) of the red blood cell to be saturated with glucose, called glycohemoglobin (GHB), for the remaining life of the RBC (up to 120 days)

1) Test determines diabetic control of blood glucose by measuring all three subunits of Hgb A

2) Value for GHB is 2 to 4 percent higher than the individual subunits of Hgb A; see Table 13-1 for interpretation of specific values

d. Urine studies

1) Glucose usually appears in urine once renal threshold for glucose is exceeded

2) Ketone: metabolic end product of fatty acid metabolism; body uses fatty acids for energy when there is insufficient supply of glucose; ketones should be absent in urine

3) Acetone: metabolite of fatty acid metabolism; should be absent in urine

Table 13-1	Reference Values	Interpretation
Laboratory Values for Glycosylated Hemoglobin	Up to 7.5%	Good diabetic control
	7.6%–8.9%	Fair diabetic control
	>8.9%	Poor diabetic control

III. Disorders of the Posterior Pituitary Gland

A. Syndrome of inappropriate antidiuretic hormone (SIADH)

1. Description: SIADH is an excessive amount of serum ADH resulting in water intoxication and hyponatremia

2. Etiology and pathophysiology

   a. The usual feedback mechanism does not function to decrease posterior pituitary secretion of ADH with decreased serum osmolality

   b. High levels of ADH leads to renal reabsorption of water and suppression of the renin-angiotensin mechanism, causing renal excretion of sodium

   c. This leads to water intoxication, cellular edema, and dilutional hyponatremia

   d. Causes of SIADH

      1) Malignant tumors (such as oat cell cancer of lung, pancreatic carcinoma, leukemia, and Hodgkin's lymphoma) secrete ADH independent of a normally functioning hypothalamus and feedback mechanisms

      2) Can also be caused by hypersecretion of ADH by the hypothalamus resulting from head injury, hydrocephalus, meningitis, encephalitis, pituitary surgery, cerebrovascular accident (CVA), brain hemorrhage, or some medications

      3) Positive pressure ventilation and other conditions causing increased intrathoracic pressure may stimulate the aortic baroreceptors and cardiopulmonary receptors that trigger the hypothalamus to secrete ADH

      4) Trauma, pain, stress, and acute psychosis may activate the limbic system that, in turn, stimulates the hypothalamus to secrete ADH

3. Assessment

   a. General manifestations of fluid volume excess, possibly including increased blood pressure, crackles auscultated in lung fields, distended jugular neck veins, taut skin, and intake greater than output

   b. Clinical manifestations: include headache, fatigue, anorexia, nausea, muscle aches, abdominal cramps, weight gain without edema, progressive altered level of consciousness, seizures, coma, and small amounts of concentrated amber colored urine

   c. Diagnostic and laboratory test findings: high urine osmolality (>1200 mOsm/kg H_2O) and specific gravity >1.032, low serum osmolality (<275 mOsm/kg), and decreased hematocrit, BUN and serum sodium (<135 mEq/l, also known as **hyponatremia**)

4. Therapeutic management

   a. Limit fluid intake; monitor urine osmolality, serum electrolytes, hematocrit, BUN, sodium and serum osmolality

   b. Supplement sodium intake orally or by hypertonic saline IV infusion

5. Priority nursing diagnoses: Altered thought processes; Acute pain; Imbalanced nutrition: less than body requirements; Fatigue; Deficient knowledge

NCLEX!
NCLEX!
NCLEX!
NCLEX!
NCLEX!
NCLEX!
NCLEX!
NCLEX!

6. Planning and implementation

NCLEX!

   a. Restrict oral fluids including ice chips to 80 ml/day to prevent further hemodilution

   b. Flush all enteral and gastric tubes with NS instead of water to replace sodium and prevent further hemodilution

   c. Monitor intake and output accurately

   d. Monitor serum sodium, and urine osmolality and specific gravity

   e. Weigh daily; a weight loss of 2 pounds indicates a loss of 1 L of fluid

NCLEX!

NCLEX!

   f. Assess for changes in level of consciousness (LOC), mentation, cognition, nutrition, muscle twitching and comfort

7. Medication therapy: IV hypertonic saline (3%) and demeclocycline (Declomycin) to replace electrolytes; diuretics to eliminate excessive fluid from the body

NCLEX!

8. Client education

   a. Instruct client about SIADH and symptoms to report

   b. Medication may be for life depending on the cause

   c. Identify hidden sources of water and fluids, such as ice and ice cream, to prevent accidental excessive intake

   d. Plan meal pattern and maintain fluid limitation and sodium prescription

NCLEX!

   e. Weigh daily on same scale and report gain of 2 pounds in 1 day

9. Evaluation

   a. Client cognition and mentation functions are intact

   b. Client verbalizes understanding of medications, fluid restriction, sources of water and sodium

   c. Client demonstrates ability to weigh self and verbalizes to report weight gain

   d. Excess fluid is eliminated; lab values normalize; client is free of seizures

B. Diabetes insipidus (DI)

1. Description: results from excessive loss of water caused by hyposecretion of ADH or the kidneys' inability to respond to ADH; the subsequent **polyuria** (excessive urine output ranging from 4 to 30 L in 24 hours) can lead to severe dehydration if the client does not replace the lost water

2. Etiology and pathophysiology

   a. Neurogenic DI: renal tubules excrete excessive amounts of water in the urine caused by insufficient ADH secretion by the posterior pituitary gland

   b. Nephrogenic DI: the inability of the kidney to respond to ADH

   c. Lithium carbonate and demeclocycline (Declomycin) can cause the kidneys to alter response to ADH

   d. Primary DI results from an inherited or idiopathic malfunction of the posterior pituitary gland

Practice to Pass

The client with SIADH is upset at not being able to drink fluids whenever she wants. How should you respond?

NCLEX!

  e. Secondary DI is caused by brain tumors, head trauma, infection, surgery on or near the pituitary gland, metastatic tumors from the lung or breast, cerebrovascular hemorrhage, granulomatous disease or cerebral aneurysm

 3. Assessment

  a. Assess for a history of head injury, brain surgery, infection, or tumor

  b. Obtain a list of current and past medications

NCLEX!

  c. Assess LOC, vital signs including orthostatic BP, skin turgor, intake and output, weight, skin integrity, **polydipsia** (excessive thirst), tenting or sagging skin, bowel sounds, constipation; see Figure 13-1 for full listing of multisystem effects of fluid volume deficit

NCLEX!

  d. Clinical manifestations: polyuria, excessive thirst, dry tented skin, dry mucous membranes, and severe hypotension leading to cardiovascular collapse (which can occur if the excessive water loss is not replaced)

NCLEX!

  e. Diagnostic and laboratory test findings: urine specific gravity <1.005, urine osmolality <300 mOsm/kg, positive water deprivation test, reduced serum ADH level in primary DI, serum sodium >145 mEq/L

 4. Therapeutic management

NCLEX!

  a. Water replacement orally is preferred or intravenous (IV) D_5W as needed to normalize lab values

NCLEX!

  b. For neurogenic DI, hormone replacement with desmopressin (DDAVP), a synthetic vasopressin; adjunctive medications (such as chlorpropamide (Diabinese), or carbamazepine (Tegretol) may act to increase ADH release or enhance the effect of ADH on the renal collecting duct

  c. For nephrogenic DI, correct the underlying disease or stop the causative medication; begin a low-salt, low-protein diet to decrease net excretion of solute

NCLEX!

 5. Priority nursing diagnoses: Deficient fluid volume; Risk for impaired skin integrity; Risk for constipation; and Knowledge deficit

NCLEX!

 6. Planning and implementation

  a. Monitor intake and output hourly; report urine output >200 ml/hour for 2 consecutive hours or 500 ml over 2 hours; assess for continence and provide easy access to restroom as appropriate

  b. Weigh daily; report weight loss

  c. Monitor urine specific gravity and report if it decreases; monitor serum osmolality and sodium for increases

  d. Encourage fluid intake greater than urine output; provide fluids within reach at all times

  e. Use skin protective barriers with incontinence

 7. Medication therapy: desmopressin (DDAVP) as supplemental ADH, chlorpropamide (Diabinese) or carbamazepine (Tegretol) to potentiate the renal effect of ADH, and replacement IV fluids as needed

Figure 13-1

Multi system effects
of fluid volume deficit.

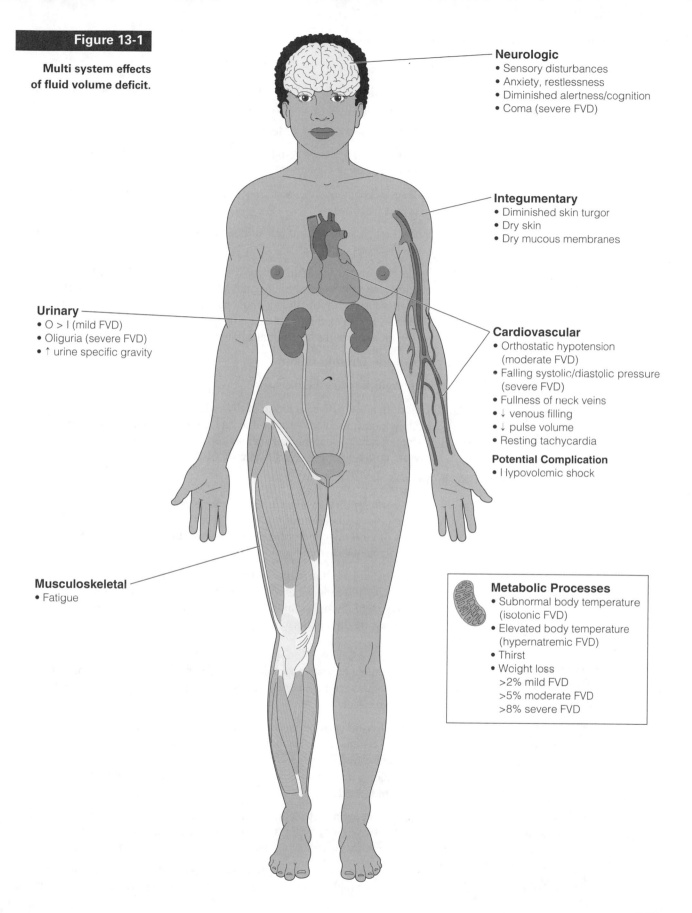

Neurologic
- Sensory disturbances
- Anxiety, restlessness
- Diminished alertness/cognition
- Coma (severe FVD)

Integumentary
- Diminished skin turgor
- Dry skin
- Dry mucous membranes

Urinary
- O > I (mild FVD)
- Oliguria (severe FVD)
- ↑ urine specific gravity

Cardiovascular
- Orthostatic hypotension
  (moderate FVD)
- Falling systolic/diastolic pressure
  (severe FVD)
- Fullness of neck veins
- ↓ venous filling
- ↓ pulse volume
- Resting tachycardia

Potential Complication
- Hypovolemic shock

Musculoskeletal
- Fatigue

Metabolic Processes
- Subnormal body temperature
  (isotonic FVD)
- Elevated body temperature
  (hypernatremic FVD)
- Thirst
- Weight loss
  >2% mild FVD
  >5% moderate FVD
  >8% severe FVD

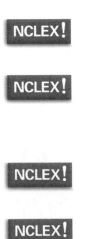

8. Client education

    a. Teach client about DI, self-administration of medication, and about possible need for lifelong medication

    b. Instruct client to wear a Medic-Alert bracelet listing DI and treatments

    c. Instruct to drink fluid equal to amount of urine output, keeping a log of intake and output

    d. Instruct client to weigh self daily, on same scale at same time of day, and to report weight loss

    e. Instruct client to consult practitioner before taking over-the-counter (OTC) medications

9. Evaluation: intake is within 500 ml of urine output; weight returns to client's baseline; lab values are within normal range, client wears Medic-Alert bracelet with appropriate information; skin is intact; bowel function is normal; client verbalizes understanding of medication and self administers medication correctly; monitors and records intake, output, and weight

IV. Disorders of the Thyroid Gland

A. Hyperthyroidism (Graves' disease)

1. Description: excessive secretion of thyroid hormone from the thyroid gland, leading to increased basal metabolic rate, cardiovascular function, gastrointestinal function, neuromuscular function, weight loss and heat intolerance; thyroid hormone affects metabolism of fats, carbohydrates and proteins

2. Etiology and pathophysiology

    a. Hyperthyroidism can be caused by excess secretion of TSH from the pituitary gland, autoimmune reaction (Graves' disease), thyroiditis (inflammation or viral infection of the thyroid gland), tumor, and excessive dose of supplemental thyroid hormone

    b. Graves' disease, the most common form, occurs 7 to 10 times more often in women <40 years old, and is caused by an autoimmune disorder triggering long acting thyroid stimulator (LATS) to stimulate the thyroid gland to oversecrete thyroid hormone

3. Assessment

    a. Clinical manifestations: range from very minimal to severe depending on the amount and time period of hypersecretion; see Figure 13-2 for multisystem effects of hyperthyroidism

        1) **Thyroid crisis** or **thyroid storm:** life-threatening emergency occurring in extreme hyperthyroidism; usually occurs in clients with long-term untreated hyperthyroidism or in clients with hyperthyroidism experiencing a stressor such as infection, trauma or manipulation of the thyroid gland

        2) Common manifestations of thyroid storm are: temperature >102° F (39° C), tachycardia, systolic hypertension, abdominal pain, nausea, vomiting, diarrhea, agitation, tremors, confusion and seizures

    b. Include in overall assessment: health history, vital signs, neck (for goiter), eyes (for exophthalmos), respiratory effort, peripheral pulses, energy level,

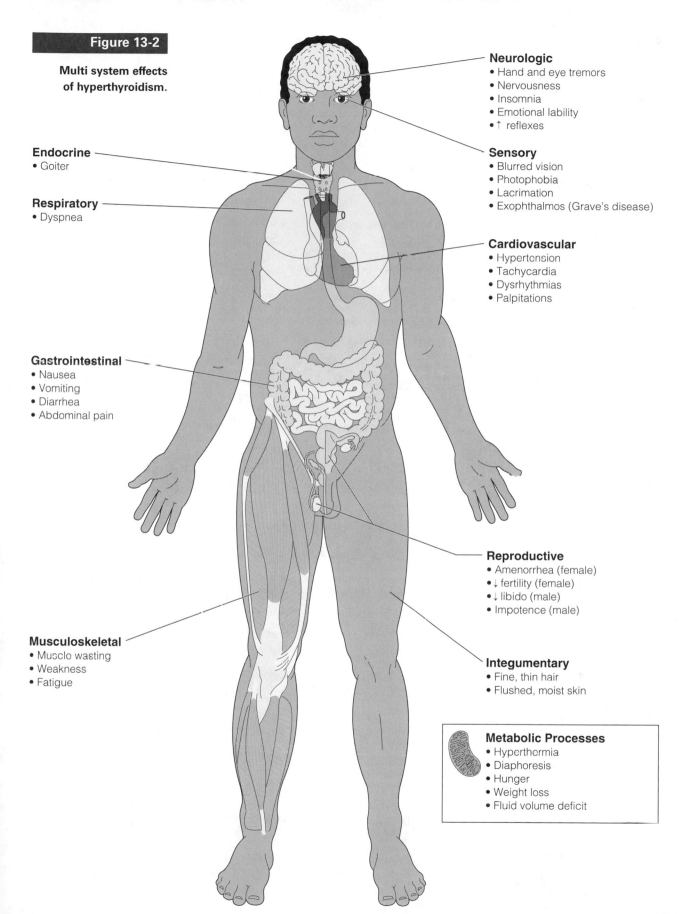

Figure 13-2

Multi system effects of hyperthyroidism.

Neurologic
• Hand and eye tremors
• Nervousness
• Insomnia
• Emotional lability
• ↑ reflexes

Sensory
• Blurred vision
• Photophobia
• Lacrimation
• Exophthalmos (Grave's disease)

Endocrine
• Goiter

Respiratory
• Dyspnea

Cardiovascular
• Hypertension
• Tachycardia
• Dysrhythmias
• Palpitations

Gastrointestinal
• Nausea
• Vomiting
• Diarrhea
• Abdominal pain

Reproductive
• Amenorrhea (female)
• ↓ fertility (female)
• ↓ libido (male)
• Impotence (male)

Musculoskeletal
• Muscle wasting
• Weakness
• Fatigue

Integumentary
• Fine, thin hair
• Flushed, moist skin

Metabolic Processes
• Hyperthermia
• Diaphoresis
• Hunger
• Weight loss
• Fluid volume deficit

activity tolerance, elimination pattern, oxygenation, weight pattern over weeks, fluid balance, nutritional status, sleep pattern and comfort

c. Diagnostic and laboratory test findings: elevated serum T_3, T_4, free T_4; decreased TSH; positive RAI uptake scan and thyroid scan (depending on the cause of the hyperthyroidism)

4. Therapeutic management: ethionamide drugs for life, ablative radioactive I-131, or surgical removal of part of the thyroid gland (partial or total thyroidectomy)

5. Priority nursing diagnoses: Risk for decreased cardiac output; Disturbed sensory perception: visual; Risk for ineffective airway clearance; Risk for imbalanced nutrition: less than body requirements; Disturbed body image; Hyperthermia; Activity intolerance; and Deficient knowledge

6. Planning and Implementation

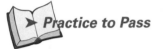

   a. Radioactive iodine 131: the thyroid gland absorbs the I-131, which destroys some of the thyroid cells over a period of 6 to 8 weeks

   1) Not recommended for pregnant women

   2) Radiation precautions are not required for small doses (<30mCi) of I-131

   3) Instruct client to drink solution with straw to minimize exposure to buccal cavity

   4) Monitor lab values, report weight gain, fatigue, decreased pulse and BP

   5) Total or subtotal (partial) thyroidectomy may be indicated based on situation

Practice to Pass

The client with Graves' disease and exophthalmos wants to know why he needs to perform special eye care after having the thyroid gland removed. What is your response?

   b. Preoperative preparation for thyroidectomy

   1) Teach deep breathing exercises and appropriate cough

   2) Instruct client to hold hands behind neck when coughing, sitting, turning or getting up/back to bed to reduce postoperative pain and neck muscle strain

   3) Instruct client on self-administration of prescribed anti-thyroid drugs to decrease the vascularity and size of thyroid to minimize risk of hemorrhage

   c. Postoperative care following thyroidectomy

   1) Provide comfort: analgesics, position client in semi-Fowler's position with neck and head supported by pillows to prevent muscle strain, ice collar to wound area for comfort and to prevent edema

   2) Monitor for hemorrhage: tightness of dressing; sanguineous exudate on anterior or posterior neck dressing or on skin of neck, upper chest and upper back, shoulders, and back of neck; auscultate trachea for stridor (indicating edema and narrowed airway); first 24 hours postoperative is time of greatest risk

   3) Promote patent airway: keep head of bed elevated 30 degrees; assess for respiratory distress; keep oral and sterile suction supplies and emergency tracheostomy tray (with tracheostomy kit and IV calcium gluconate or

calcium chloride) within immediate access; maintain humidification of inspired air if ordered; encourage deep breathing exercises hourly; cough only if needed to clear secretions

4) Prevent tetany by early identification of **hypocalcemia** (low serum calcium) evidenced by numbness or tingling of toes, extremities and lips, muscle twitches, positive Chvostek's and Trousseau signs

5) Maintain patent IV site

6) Assess for laryngeal nerve damage noting ability to speak loudly, quality and tone of voice

7. Medication therapy: ethionamide drugs for life to reduce secretion of thyroid hormone, or ablative radioactive I-131 to reduce vascularity and size of thyroid gland and thus reduce thyroid hormone secretion; analgesics to control pain of surgical treatment is done

8. Client education

   a. Instruct client about correct self-administration of medications and that medication use is lifelong

   b. Instruct client about hyperthyroidism, hypothyroidism, and symptoms to report

   c. Instruct client about conditions to report, including signs of hemorrhage, hypocalcemia, incisional infection, respiratory difficulty and discomfort

   d. For exophthalmos, instruct client on methods to protect eyes and adapt to altered visual field

      1) Instruct client to have regular eye exams

      2) Instruct client to call practitioner immediately for any change in vision or appearance of eye; closure of eyelids; eye pain; eye exudate, or **photophobia** (sensitivity to light)

      3) Protect eyes with tinted glasses or eye shields since lids do not cover eyes completely and there may be delayed corneal/blink reflex

      4) Moisten eyes frequently with artificial tears to prevent dry irritation and corneal infection; use caution not to contaminate eyedropper

      5) Soothe dry eye irritation with cool moist compresses

      6) Sleep with head of bed elevated to minimize pressure on optic nerve and wear eye patches to protect eyes during sleep if lids do not close

   e. Surgical client

      1) Ensure that client understands surgical procedure and expected outcomes

      2) Instruct client to support neck with hands; position neck and head with pillows and maintain semi-Fowler's position; avoid hyperextension and sudden quick movements of head and neck

      3) Instruct on wound care

      4) Instruct client to avoid/minimize talking and coughing until wound is healed to prevent strain on laryngeal nerve and vocal cords

   f. Assist client to cope with lifestyle and self-image changes

9. Evaluation: client verbalizes understanding of self-medication administration, eye care, wound care, and symptoms to report; demonstrates support of neck and head; resumes usual social interaction; expresses acceptance of changes and appearance

B. Hypothyroidism

1. Description: occurs when there is an insufficient amount of thyroid hormone (TH) being secreted by the thyroid gland, causing decreased metabolic rate, decreased heat production, and various effects on body systems

2. Etiology and pathophysiology

   a. Primary hypothyroidism accounts for 99 percent of all cases, has a prevalence of 0.8 percent, is 5 to 7 times more common in women, and 50 percent of cases are caused by cell-mediated and antibody-mediated destruction of the thyroid gland

   b. Other causes are thyroiditis, subacute postpartum, external irradiation of the gland, iatrogenic (30 to 40 percent), infections, iodine deficiency, congenital or idiopathic

   c. Secondary hypothyroidism, also called central hypothyroidism, is caused by insufficient secretion of TSH from the pituitary gland or TRH deficiency related to disease of the hypothalamus

3. Assessment

   a. Hypothyroidism is manifested with varying degrees of symptoms, depending on the severity of the condition; general assessments include health history, LOC, vital signs, respiratory effort, activity tolerance and comfort

   b. Clinical manifestations

      1) Depend on the length of time and severity of the lack of thyroid hormone

      2) The thyroid gland gradually enlarges forming a goiter (thickening of the gland) in an attempt to secrete more thyroid hormone

      3) Clients with hypothyroidism may have a large number of symptoms, including lethargy, diminished reflexes, periorbital edema, bradycardia, dysrhythmias, hypotension, reproductive problems (menorrhagia and infertility in females and decreased libido in males), coarse dry hair that is easily lost, coarse dry skin, signs of slowed metabolism (hypothermia, fatigue, weight gain, anorexia), anemia, elevated serum lipids

   c. Assess for myxedema, a life-threatening crisis state of hypothyroidism, characterized by non-pitting edema in connective tissues throughout the body, puffy face and tongue, severe metabolic disorders, hypothermia, cardiovascular collapse, and coma

   d. Diagnostic and laboratory test findings: decreased T_4 and free T_4, normal T_3, and increased TSH levels

4. Therapeutic management: medication to replace T_4

5. Priority nursing diagnosis: Decreased cardiac output; Constipation; Risk for impaired skin integrity; Risk for activity intolerance; Risk for sexual dysfunction; Disturbed body image; Hypothermia; and Deficient knowledge

6. Planning and implementation

   a. Give medication in the morning 1 hour before food intake or 2 hours after food intake to facilitate absorption

   b. Adjust environment with blankets as needed for temperature of comfort; chilling increases metabolic rate, cardiac workload, and oxygen demand

   c. Pace activities with rest periods; instruct client to report shortness of breath, fatigue, dizziness, or any discomfort

   d. Encourage intake of 2,000 mL water daily and a high-fiber diet to promote regular bowel movements

7. Medication therapy: thyroid hormone replacement, such as dessicated thyroid, thyroxine (Synthroid), or triiodothyronine (Cytomel)

8. Client education

   a. Instruct client about hypothyroidism, the importance of wearing a Medic-Alert bracelet, and medication self-administration

   b. Medication is needed for life and should be taken at the same time every morning 1 hr before a meal or 2 hrs after a meal

   c. Instruct the client to take the same brand of medication as brands vary in chemical properties and bioavailability

   d. Instruct client to report weight gain or loss of 5 pounds, activity intolerance, chest pain, heat or cold intolerance, and sleep pattern disturbance

   e. Instruct client to report symptoms of hypothyroidism and hyperthyroidism

9. Evaluation: client verbalizes appropriate medication self-administration; has stabilized weight; is able to do activities of daily living without fatigue, discomfort, or shortness of breath; has normal sleep and elimination pattern; vital signs are within normal range; skin is intact and elastic; client is wearing appropriate Medic-Alert bracelet

V. Disorders of the Parathyroid Gland

A. Hyperparathyroidism

1. Description: increased parathyroid hormone secretion from the parathyroid gland located in the neck; occurs in older adults; is two times more common in women

   a. Primary hyperparathyroidism: hyperplasia or tumor of one of the parathyroid glands, increasing the absorption of calcium in the GI tract

   b. Secondary hyperparathyroidism: gland enlargement due to chronic hypocalcemia in the presence of elevated PTH

   c. Tertiary hyperparathyroidism: parathyroid glands are enlarged and do not respond to changes in serum calcium levels, usually associated with chronic renal failure

2. Etiology and pathophysiology

   a. Increased resorption of calcium and increased excretion of phosphate leads to hypercalcemia and hypophosphatemia

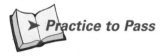

Practice to Pass

Explain why clients with hypothyroidism have increased risk for cardiovascular disease and constipation.

b. Kidneys increase bicarbonate excretion and decrease acid excretion, leading to metabolic acidosis and hypokalemia

c. Bones increase rate of calcium and phosphorus release leading to bone decalcification

d. Hypercalcemia causes calcium deposits in soft tissues, renal calculi, altered neurological function with muscle weakness and atrophy, altered GI function with constipation, abdominal pain, anorexia, and altered cardiovascular system

3. Assessment

    a. General assessments include health history, vital signs, ECG, elimination pattern, nutritional status, activity-exercise tolerance, cognitive-perceptual and sensory function, and neuromuscular function

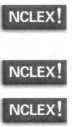

    b. Clinical manifestations: polyuria (early sign) and renal calculi, anorexia, constipation, nausea, vomiting, abdominal pain (from peptic ulcer disease), generalized bone pain, pathologic fractures, muscle weakness and atrophy, CNS signs (depressed deep tendon reflexes, paresthesias, depression, psychosis)

    c. Diagnostic and laboratory test findings: elevated serum levels of total calcium; increased PTH; decreased phosphate; possible bone changes on skeletal x-rays and CT scan

4. Therapeutic management: decrease serum level of calcium with IV normal saline (NS) infusions, diuretics and phosphate replacement; surgery to remove involved parathyroid glands

5. Priority nursing diagnoses: Risk for injury; Pain; Impaired physical mobility; Risk for altered urinary elimination; Risk for constipation; Knowledge deficit

6. Planning and implementation

    a. Promote comfort and safety; client may need to walk with walker to prevent falls

    b. Strain all urine to detect calcium-based urinary stones

    c. Provide 2,000 to 3,000 ml of fluids daily as tolerated and a high-fiber diet

    d. Encourage progressive activity as tolerated, pacing activity with rest periods

    e. Promote nutrition and fluid and electrolyte balance; weigh daily

    f. Provide pre- and postoperative care as described in section IV, A, 6

    g. Prevent tetany caused by surgery or aggressive excretion of calcium through early detection of low serum calcium level; watch for numbness and tingling around mouth and fingertips, muscle twitching of extremities, change in voice, and positive Chvostek and Trousseau signs

7. Medication therapy: analgesics to control pain; diuretics and NS by IV infusion to excrete excess calcium; phosphate and calcitonin (Miacalcin) may be used to inhibit bone reabsorption

8. Client education

    a. Instruct client on appropriate self-administration of medications and about hyperparathyroidism

    b. Instruct client about symptoms to report, including those for hypocalcemia, activity intolerance, and infection

9. Evaluation: client verbalizes pain control, understanding of medications, symptoms to report, postoperative care; and demonstrates appropriate wound care

B. Hypoparathyroidism

1. Description: low PTH levels causing hypocalcemia, usually caused by surgical removal of all or part of the gland

2. Etiology and pathophysiology: hypocalcemia raises the threshold for excitability in nerve and muscle fibers causing the fibers to be easily stimulated; could lead to life-threatening tetany

3. Assessment

    a. General assessments include health history, vital signs, ECG, elimination pattern, nutritional status, activity-exercise tolerance, cognitive-perceptual and sensory function, neuromuscular function

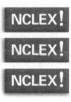

    b. Clinical manifestations: GI symptoms (abdominal pain, nausea, vomiting, diarrhea, anorexia), signs of hypocalcemia (anxiety, headaches, paresthesias, neuromuscular irritability with tremors and muscle spasms), possible difficulty swallowing, possible hoarse voice, sensation of tightness in throat, dry thin hair, patchy hair loss, ridged finger nails

    c. Diagnostic and laboratory test findings: decreased serum PTH, total calcium, free calcium; increased serum phosphate

4. Therapeutic management: supplemental calcium and vitamin D

5. Priority nursing diagnoses: Risk for injury; Anxiety; Knowledge deficit

6. Planning and implementation

    a. Promote comfort and safety; client may need to walk with walker to prevent falls

    b. Encourage progressive activity as tolerated, pacing activity with rest periods

    c. Promote nutrition and fluid and electrolyte balance

7. Medication therapy: calcium supplement orally or by IV infusion; vitamin D orally to promote intestinal absorption of calcium

8. Client education

    a. Instruct client about hypoparathyroidism, to wear Medic-Alert bracelet listing disease and medications, and about self-administration of medication

    b. Instruct client about symptoms to report (as noted above)

    c. Instruct client about diet high in calcium and vitamin D, identifying minimum daily intake; foods high in calcium are cheese, milk, turnip greens, almonds, collard greens, beans, peanuts, frankfurters, and bologna

9. Evaluation: client verbalizes understanding of disease, medications, diet, and the importance of wearing a medical alert bracelet; demonstrates appropriate meal planning

VI. Disorders of the Adrenal Cortex

A. Cushing's syndrome

1. Description: hyperfunction of adrenal gland cortex causing elevated serum cortisol or ACTH levels

2. Etiology and pathophysiology

   a. Elevated serum cortisol causes life-threatening changes in physiological, psychological, and metabolic functioning

   b. Incidence is greater in women; usual age of onset is 30 to 40 years old

   c. Primary Cushing's syndrome is caused by a tumor of the adrenal cortex

   d. Secondary Cushing's syndrome

      1) Disorder of the pituitary or hypothalamus gland causing increased ACTH and hyperplasia of the adrenal cortex; also called Cushing's disease

      2) An ectopic tissue such as an ACTH-producing cancer of the lung, bronchus, or pancreas causes hyperplasia of the adrenal cortex

   e. Iatrogenic: long-term use of glucocorticoid medication such as steroids

3. Assessment

   a. General assessments include health history, vital signs, activity tolerance, skin condition, elimination pattern, nutrition pattern, fluid and electrolyte balance, self-concept, and frequency of blood glucose monitoring

   NCLEX!

   b. Clinical manifestations: generalized weakness with muscle wasting, thin skin that bruises easily, emotional lability (mood swings), skin infections or poor wound healing, striae, hirsutism, hypertension, fluid overload, weight gain, osteoporosis, abnormal fat deposits (truncal obesity, moon facies, fat pad on back of neck), possible amenorrhea, impotence, or decreased libido

   c. Diagnostic and laboratory test findings: elevated serum cortisol, sodium, glucose, calcium, and potassium; serum ACTH can be elevated or decreased; elevated urine 17 KS; positive ACTH suppression test; normal BUN

   NCLEX!

4. Therapeutic management: may include medications to suppress ACTH by the pituitary gland; medications to suppress cortisol secretion by the adrenal cortex; cortisol replacement postoperatively; radiation therapy to the pituitary gland; and single or bilateral adrenalectomy or **hypophysectomy** (removal of the pituitary gland)

   NCLEX!

5. Priority nursing diagnoses: Excess fluid volume; Risk for injury; Risk for infection; Disturbed body image; and Knowledge deficit

   NCLEX!

6. Planning and implementation

   a. Assist client to achieve fluid, electrolyte, glucose, and calcium balance

   b. Analyze daily weights and intake and output

   c. Promote safety: uncluttered walking area, adequate lighting, assistive walking devices to prevent falls as needed, and use of stable, non-skid shoes/slippers

   d. Assist client to pace activities and rest to prevent fatigue

   e. Prevent infection before and after surgery: use standard precautions, provide aseptic wound care, and promote optimal nutrition

   f. Assist client to use effective coping strategies and encourage client to discuss feelings about change in physical appearance

   g. Preoperative care: ensure that client understands the planned surgical procedure, postoperative routines, and expected outcomes

NCLEX!

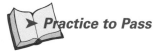

► *Practice to Pass*

Why should the client taking glucocorticosteroids as replacement therapy or to treat an existing disease never miss a dose or suddenly stop taking the medication?

NCLEX!

NCLEX!

NCLEX!

h. Postoperative care

1) Promote effective breathing pattern by encouraging hourly client coughing and deep breathing exercises (clients with transphenoidal surgery should avoid coughing)

2) Explain that mouth-breathing is necessary because of postoperative nasal packing after transphenoidal surgery

3) Assist with turning and repositioning every 2 hours, and encourage ankle dorsiflexion exercises hourly

4) Promote wound healing by minimizing stress on incision line

   a) The adrenalectomy client should log roll to the side to sit up at the bedside and should do the reverse to recline

   b) The client with a transphenoidal incision should avoid blowing nose, sneezing or coughing unless necessary

5) Keep HOB elevated 30 degrees, and use aseptic technique for wound care

6) Examine pituitary surgical wound for cerebrospinal fluid leak

i. Prevent Addisonian crisis: give IV normal saline infusion bolus and cortisol per practitioner's order for the following symptoms: dry, tenting skin, decreased blood pressure, increased pulse, decreased level of consciousness, anorexia, and weakness

7. Medication therapy: may include meturapone (directly inhibits cortisol production and secretion by the adrenal cortex), octreotide (Sandostatin) a somatostatin analog that suppresses ACTH secretion, and mitotane, which suppresses the function of the adrenal cortex and decreases the metabolism of corticosteroids, thus decreasing serum cortisol

8. Client education

   a. Instruct client about Cushing's syndrome, to wear Medic-Alert bracelet listing disease and medications, and self-administration of medication

   b. Instruct client on symptoms to report

   c. Instruct client to eat a diet high in protein and vitamins B and C to support immune system, and also to take supplemental potassium and calcium

   d. Instruct client about wound care and postoperative cortisol replacement

9. Evaluation

   a. Client verbalizes understanding of disease, medication, surgical procedure, planned outcomes, and demonstrates appropriate wound care

   b. Client attains and maintains normal cortisol level, glucose level, vital signs, and is free of infection

   c. Client implements safe behaviors to prevent falls, infection, and other injury

B. Adrenal insufficiency/primary Addison's disease

1. Description: insufficient level of cortisol because of destruction of the adrenal cortex, caused by autoimmune disorder, tuberculosis, septicemia, acquired immunodeficiency syndrome (AIDS), bilateral adrenalectomy, infiltrative diseases, and sudden cessation of long-term high dose steroid medication

2. Etiology and pathophysiology

    a. More common in women age <60 years old

    b. Decreased aldosterone and cortisol levels lead to hyponatremia, **hyperkalemia** (high serum potassium), decreased extracellular fluid, decreased intravascular volume, decreased gluconeogenesis, hypoglycemia, and stress intolerance

    c. High ACTH level leads to hyperpigmentation

3. Assessment

    a. General assessments include: health history, vital signs, LOC, mentation, skin, energy level, activity tolerance, orthostatic BP, ECG (electrocardiogram), nutrition pattern, and elimination pattern

    b. Clinical manifestations

        1) Include hyperpigmentation of skin (eternal tan), delayed wound healing, cardiovascular changes (tachycardia, dysrhythmias, postural hypotension), dehydration and hypovolemia, weight loss, anorexia, nausea, vomiting, diarrhea, depression, lethargy, emotional lability, confusion, muscle weakness and tremors, and muscle and joint pain

        2) Addisonian crisis: a life-threatening response to sudden withdrawal of steroids or exposure to any form of stress, manifested by severe hypotension, circulatory collapse, shock, and coma

    c. Diagnostic and laboratory test findings: decreased serum cortisol, glucose, and sodium; increased serum potassium, BUN and ACTH levels; decreased urine 17 KS; no increase in cortisol with ACTH stimulation test; CT scan can be positive

4. Therapeutic management: replacement of corticosteroids and mineralocorticoids

5. Priority nursing diagnoses: Deficient fluid volume; Risk for ineffective therapeutic regimen management; Deficient knowledge; Risk for electrolyte imbalance (collaborative problem)

6. Planning and implementation

    a. Maintain fluid and electrolyte balance: analyze lab values, intake and output, and daily weight; encourage 3,000 ml of daily oral fluid intake and added sodium in the diet

    b. Promote safety: appropriate walking assistive devices, adequate lighting, clear area for walking, and appropriate slippers or shoes

7. Medication therapy: hydrocortisone (Cortef) to replace cortisol; fludrocortisone (Florinef) to replace mineralocorticoids as needed

8. Client education

    a. Instruct client on Addison's disease, symptoms to report (weight gain, easy bruising or bleeding, weakness, dizziness, lethargy, epigastric discomfort, and change in BP or pulse), need for lifelong medication and disease management, need to consult practitioner before taking any OTC medications, self-administration of medication, and plan for medication adjustment targeting stress response

b. Instruct client to wear Medic-Alert bracelet listing Addison's disease, medications, and contact numbers

c. Instruct client about diet to promote immune system function and foods to increase sodium intake and decrease potassium intake

9. Evaluation

a. Client demonstrates normal cognitive and mentation function, fluid and electrolyte balance, elimination function, and usual level of activity tolerance

b. Client verbalizes understanding of medication, disease, medication administration, stress management, symptoms to report, and wears Medic-Alert bracelet

c. Client demonstrates understanding of diet plan; has stable vital signs; is able to perform activities of daily living; has warm, dry and elastic skin

VII. Disorders of the Pancreas

A. Diabetes mellitus (DM)

1. Description: disorder of the pancreas characterized by insufficient or absolute lack of insulin production causing **hyperglycemia** (elevated blood glucose), requiring life-long lifestyle adjustments, and resulting in multisystem changes in health status (clients with DM have 2 to 4 percent greater incidence of heart disease, 2 to 6 percent greater incidence of stroke/CVA, significant incidence of blindness, nontraumatic amputation, and renal failure)

2. Etiology and pathophysiology

a. The disease effects 4 to 6 percent of the population and is the fourth leading cause of death in the U.S.

b. May be classified as type 1 or type 2

c. Type 1: results from the autoimmune destruction of the beta cells; has a genetic predisposition; is more common in men; can occur at any age but usually occurs in children and adolescents; is also characterized by hyperglycemia and **ketosis** (ketones in the blood resulting from gluconeogenesis of fats)

d. Type 2: exact cause remains unknown although several theories are presented, including compromised ability of beta cells to respond to hyperglycemia, abnormal insulin receptors on the cells, and peripheral insulin resistance; it has a genetic predisposition, can occur at any age, and is more common in obesity, older adults, African-Americans, Hispanic-Americans, and Native Americans

3. Assessment

a. General assessments include: health history, cognitive and mentation function, pattern of weight loss or gain, nutrition pattern, elimination pattern, vital signs, skin/wound healing, eyes/vision, sensory perception, energy level, and activity tolerance

b. Clinical manifestations

1) Type 1: polyuria, polydipsia (excess fluid intake), **polyphagia** (increased food intake), weight loss, malaise, and fatigue

2) Type 2: polyuria, polydipsia, blurred vision, fatigue, **paresthesias** (numbness, tingling, sensitivity), and skin infections

c. See Figure 13-3 for an overview of early and late manifestations of DM

d. Diagnostic and laboratory test findings: elevated random and/or fasting blood glucose, possible positive serum ketones, elevated glycosylated hemoglobin, abnormal oral GTT, urine positive for glucose, and possible positive ketones or acetone

4. Therapeutic management: consists of frequent monitoring of blood and capillary glucose, individualized diet plan, oral antidiabetic medication and/or insulin injections, and exercise plan

a. Diet

1) Follows the diet recommended in the Food Guide Pyramid or the exchange system diet from the American Diabetes Association

2) Caloric intake is based on individual needs, including possible weight loss needs

3) Diet should consist of complex carbohydrate (CHO) in amounts tailored to individual need, avoiding simple sugars; protein at 10 to 20 percent of caloric intake; saturated fat less than 10 percent of calories with cholesterol intake equal to or less than 300 mg/day; sodium intake 2,400 to 3,000 mg/day (same as for general population); dietary fiber 20 to 35 gm/day

4) Diet needs to be tailored to individual and cultural preferences whenever possible to increase adherence

b. Oral antidiabetic medications

1) Are used in type 2 DM only, and are indicated when diet and exercise alone fail to control blood glucose levels

2) Consist of oral sulfonylureas, alpha-glucosidase inhibitor, biguanide, and a miscellaneous agent

3) Instruct clients taking oral sulfonylureas that concurrent use of alcohol can cause a disulfiram-type reaction (hypoglycemia, flushing, headache, nausea, and abdominal cramps)

4) Instruct client about risk of metabolic acidosis and to discuss with primary care provider about need to discontinue medicine if severe diarrhea, infection, or dehydration occur

5) Instruct all clients about manifestations of both hyperglycemia and hypoglycemia, and appropriate corrective actions

c. Insulin therapy

1) Is used in type 1 DM or when diet, exercise, and oral agents are insufficient to control type 2 diabetes

2) Different preparations of insulin are available to maintain near normal blood glucose levels in relation to metabolic demands; insulin is classified according to its source, onset, peak, and duration of action

3) Source: human insulin has a faster onset of action, a shorter peak, and a shorter duration than animal derived insulin; it is preferred to pork or

Figure 13-3

Multi system effects of diabetes mellitus.

Early Manifestations
- Type 1 DM
  – Polyuria
  – Polydipsia
  – Polyphagia
  – Weight loss
  – Glycosuria
  – Fatigue
- Type 2 DM
  – Polyuria
  – Polydipsia
  – Blurred vision

Progressive Complications
- Hyperglycemia
  – Diabetic ketoacidosis
  – Hyperglycemic hyperosmolar nonketotic coma
- Hypoglycemia

Late Complications
Neurologic
- Somatic neuropathies
  – Paresthesias
  – Pain
  – Loss of cutaneous sensation
  – Loss of fine motor control
- Visceral neuropathies
  – Sweating dysfunction
  – Pupillary constriction
  – Fixed heart rate
  – Constipation
  – Diarrhea
  – Incomplete bladder emptying
  – Sexual dysfunction

Sensory
- Diabetic retinopathy
- Cataracts
- Glaucoma

Cardiovascular
- Orthostatic hypotension
- Accelerated atherosclerosis
- Cerebrovascular disease (stroke)
- Coronary artery disease (MI)
- Peripheral vascular disease
- Blood viscosity and platelet disorders

Renal
- Hypertension
- Albuminuria
- Edema
- Chronic renal failure

Musculoskeletal
- Joint contractures

Integumentary
- Foot ulcers
- Gangrene of the feet
- Atrophic changes

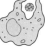

Immune System
- Impaired healing
- Chronic skin infections
- Periodontal disease
- Urinary tract infections
- Lung infections
- Vaginitis

beef insulin (used to be commonly used but had higher incidence of allergic reaction); human insulin is produced through DNA biotechnology by genetically altering strains of *E. coli* and closely resembles insulin produced by the beta cells of the human pancreas

4) Preparations: include rapid-acting (e.g., Insulin lispro, Humalog, regular, Humulin R), intermediate-acting (e.g., NPH, Humulin N), long-acting (e.g., Humulin U), and buffered insulin (e.g., Humulin BR); buffered preparations are used for external insulin pumps

5) Combinations of insulin preparations are usually administered to mimic the pancreatic activity of the pancreas in response to variations in blood glucose levels; for example, rapid and short acting preparations are usually given to cover meal times and intermediate and long acting preparations are used to maintain the basal insulin requirements in between meals

6) Insulin regimens combine short-acting, intermediate-acting, and long-acting preparations to maintain target glucose levels

NCLEX!

7) Only regular insulin may be given intravenously; insulin preparations are usually given via the subcutaneous (SC) route; continuous SC insulin infusion (CSII), also called insulin pump, is also available to deliver a basal rate of insulin and allow for additional bolus doses of insulin based on requirements (e.g., before a meal); insulin patch, nasal spray, and inhaled aerosolized preparations have been developed but are not yet widely used

NCLEX!

8) The nurse should include the following instructions to clients receiving insulin

a) Storage: insulin in use should be stored at room temperature, away from direct sunlight, and should be replaced after 4 weeks; administration of cold insulin causes subcutaneous atrophy (lipoatrophy) or hypertrophy (lipodystrophy), which alters insulin absorption; extra vials of insulin not in use should be stored in the refrigerator

b) Preparation: note date of expiration; discard vial and use a new one if regular insulin appears cloudy; do not shake to avoid inactivation and/or formation of bubbles that lead to dosage errors; roll non-regular insulin gently between the hands to evenly disperse suspended particles; draw regular (clear) insulin first when mixing it with other types of insulin; only mix insulins of the same concentration (e.g., U100 regular and U100 NPH) and from the same source

c) Injection: rotate injection sites with beef or pork insulin to prevent lipoatrophy and lipodystrophy; do not inject insulin in an area that will be involved in exercise, as it will increase the rate of absorption, onset and peak action

d) Monitor for signs of hypoglycemia; have candy or foods with simple carbohydrates available

e) Avoid alcohol while taking insulin because it lowers blood glucose levels and can cause hypoglycemia

5. Priority nursing diagnoses: Ineffective individual coping; Ineffective health maintenance; Risk for infection; Risk for impaired skin integrity; Risk for injury; Risk for disturbed body image; and Knowledge deficit

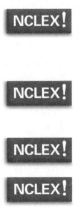

6. Planning and implementation

   a. Promote safety: use appropriate lighting; have client wear protective slippers, socks, and shoes that do not rub or impinge on the skin; analyze symptoms, activity tolerance, and coping effectiveness; monitor blood glucose levels; give medication and appropriate food and fluids

   b. Prevent infection: through appropriate foot care, aseptic injection technique, and fingerstick glucose monitoring technique

   c. Identify the appropriate glucose monitoring protocol and medication administration process depending on client's vision, finances, finger dexterity, living environment, resources, literacy, lifestyle, personal values, work/school environment, and coping status

   d. Coordinate continuing care as appropriate for client's school, work, and other schedules, such as health club

   e. Promote acceptance and effective coping while living with DM

   f. Promote safety: early identification of hypoglycemia; check blood glucose as scheduled; treat hypoglycemia with 15 g CHO snack, such as 8 oz skim milk, 5 Lifesaver candies, 3 large marshmallows, 6 oz juice; and need to check blood glucose

   g. Maintain hydration and avoid hyperglycemia; develop sick day protocol and exercise protocol with client

7. Medication therapy: oral antidiabetic medications and insulin by subcutaneous injection as previously discussed

8. Client education

   a. Instruct client about type of DM, symptoms to report, self-administration of medication, fingerstick glucose monitoring, plan for regular exam by practitioner, need to wear Medic-Alert bracelet indicating DM and medication prescription, need for lifelong medication management and lifestyle adjustments

   b. Instruct client about foot care: keep feet clean and dry; inspect feet daily using mirror to see soles; protect feet by wearing shoes (allow 1/2- to 3/4-inch toe room) or slippers at all times; avoid snug fitting socks or stockings; use cotton socks because they wick perspiration away from skin

   c. Develop with client a plan for sick day management of DM: maintain food and fluid intake, continue to take insulin; increase frequency of blood glucose monitoring, and monitor urine for ketones

   d. Develop with client a diet plan, including considerations for traveling, attendance at parties, sports, and other reasons for altered daily routine

   e. Instruct client on symptoms of hypoglycemia (restlessness, irritability, weakness, hunger, nausea, pale diaphoretic skin, shakiness or trembling, headache, confusion, inability to concentrate, deteriorating LOC to coma, seizures), actions to take, causes of hypoglycemia, and methods to prevent

   f. Discuss with client prevention and management of the acute complications of DM (hyperglycemia, hypoglycemia, diabetic ketoacidosis, and hyperglycemic hyperosmolar non-ketotic coma [HHNK]; and the chronic complications of DM (diabetic retinopathy, nephropathy, and neuropathy)

g. Develop with client a plan for wellness, including exercise

1) Daily cardiovascular exercise decreases the risk for insulin resistance, reduces risk for complications, and improves glucose management

2) Check blood glucose before exercise; check for urine ketones if fasting blood glucose is 250 mg/dl; call practitioner if ketones are present and avoid exercise

3) Monitor for signs of hypoglycemia for up to 24 hours after extensive exercise

9. Evaluation

a. Client verbalizes understanding of DM, medication prescription, need for regular exams, fingerstick glucose monitoring, lifestyle changes, foot care, sick day plan, diet plan, symptoms to report, symptom management, and wellness plan

b. Client demonstrates effective coping through type of questions, normal glycosylated hemoglobin level, emotional response, and behavior

c. Client wears appropriate medical alert bracelet, shoes, and clothing

d. Client demonstrates appropriate meal planning for various situations, foot care, glucose monitoring process, and medication administration

e. Client carries appropriate protein and carbohydrate supplements to treat hypoglycemia

f. Client keeps record of blood glucose levels as instructed

g. Client keeps regular appointments with practitioner

B. Diabetic ketoacidosis (DKA)

1. Description: life-threatening metabolic acidosis resulting from persistent hyperglycemia and breakdown of fats into glucose, leading to presence of ketones in blood; can be triggered by emotional stress, uncompensated exercise, infection, trauma, or insufficient or delayed insulin administration

2. Etiology and pathophysiology: hyperglycemia causes uncompensated polyuria, hemoconcentration, dehydration, hyperosmolarity, and electrolyte imbalance; a significant accumulation of serum ketones leads to acidosis

3. Assessment

a. General assessment includes health history, vital signs, cognitive function and mental status, glucose monitoring log and medication administration, oral intake for past 48 hours, elimination pattern, skin, oxygenation, breath sounds, respiratory effort and pattern, weight, and hourly intake and output

b. Clinical manifestations: thirst, nausea, vomiting, malaise, lethargy, polyuria, warm dry skin, flushed face, acetone (fruity) odor to breath, Kussmaul respirations (deep, nonlabored, rapid respirations)

c. Diagnostic and laboratory test findings: serum glucose >250 mg/dL; plasma pH < 7.35; plasma bicarbonate < 15 mEq/L; serum ketones present; urine positive for glucose and ketones; may have abnormal serum sodium and chloride levels and hyperkalemia

---

NCLEX!

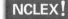

Practice to Pass

How does exercise affect glucose and insulin needs of a person with diabetes mellitus (DM)? If the client with DM is planning an intense exercise activity, when should he check his glucose?

NCLEX!

NCLEX!

4. Therapeutic management: intravenous administration of fluids, electrolytes, and regular insulin to correct hyperglycemia and acidosis; supportive care as indicated such as NPO status, vasopressors, and possible ventilator to respiratory support

a. Insulin

1) A bolus of IV regular insulin is given followed by a continuous IV drip (0.1 unit/kg body weight) until the blood glucose level drops to 250 mg/100 ml or the pH = 7.30

2) Once this blood level is reached, regular insulin is given on a sliding scale according to blood glucose

3) As an alternative to intravenous infusion, intramuscular administration of insulin may be given hourly

4) Bedside blood glucose monitoring is done every 1 to 2 hours to monitor the effectiveness of this therapy

b. Fluid therapy is instituted to diminish the hyperglycemia and to treat the large fluid deficit (dehydration) that accompanies DKA

1) Normal saline solution is usually given at a rate of 1 to 2 L for the first hour, then is decreased to 500 ml/hr as tolerated by cardiac and respiratory systems

2) When the blood glucose level reaches 250 to 300, a 5 percent glucose solution (D$_5$ 1/2NS) is added to prevent hypoglycemia and to prevent cerebral edema

3) Central venous pressure or hemodynamic monitoring may be necessary to evaluate the effectiveness of the therapy

c. Potassium replacement is always necessary in DKA

1) The initial serum potassium (K+) level is usually elevated

2) With the reversal of the acidosis and the administration of insulin, the K+ shifts into the intracellular compartment and the serum level can drop rapidly

3) Replacement therapy is instituted based on the serum K+ level and urinary output

4) Electrocardiographic monitoring is instituted to monitor for cardiac changes due to hyper- and hypokalemia and to monitor the effects of therapy on the serum K+ level

5) Other electrolytes such as phosphate will also be replaced based on the result of laboratory profiles; bicarbonate is not given routinely in DKA because rapid correction of acidosis can cause severe hypokalemia

5. Priority nursing diagnoses: Deficient fluid volume; Risk for injury; Risk for impaired skin integrity; Ineffective breathing pattern; Disturbed sensory perception; Knowledge deficit; Anxiety

6. Planning and implementation

a. Restore fluid, electrolyte and glucose balance with IV infusions, and medications; analyze intake and output, blood glucose, urine ketones, vital signs, oxygenation, and breathing pattern

    b. Maintain skin integrity; promote healing of impaired skin; prevent infection by turning and positioning client every 2 hours; provide pressure relief as indicated; manage incontinence and perspiration with skin protective barriers and cleansing; provide appropriate nutrition and oxygen support

    c. Promote safety by analyzing vital signs, client communication, LOC and emotional response, and activity tolerance; implement falls prevention measures

    d. Assist client to verbalize concerns and cope effectively with illness and fears

    e. Assist client to update Medic-Alert bracelet information as appropriate

7. Medication therapy: IV infusion of NS, regular insulin and electrolyte replacement, including potassium replacement as previously described

NCLEX!

8. Client education: instruct client about the nature and causes of DKA (such as excess glucose intake, insufficient medications, or physiological and/or psychological stressors) and any new medications

9. Evaluation

    a. Fasting blood glucose is within normal range; serum pH is 7.35 to 7.45; urine is negative for ketones

    b. Client's LOC and perceptual function returns to normal; elimination is normal; skin is intact; breathing pattern is normal; and fluid and electrolytes are balanced

    c. Client verbalizes understanding of diabetic ketoacidosis, its causes, methods of prevention, and new medications

C. Hyperglycemic hyperosmolar nonketotic coma (HHNK)

1. Description: life-threatening metabolic disorder of hyperglycemia usually occurring with DM type 2 and triggered by a variety of situations: medications, infection, acute illness, invasive procedure, or a chronic illness

2. Etiology and pathophysiology: increased insulin resistance (caused by one or more of the triggering situations) along with increased carbohydrate intake lead to hyperglycemia, followed by polyuria, decreased plasma volume, decreased glomerular filtration rate (GFR) leading to glucose retention and sodium and water excretion; hyperosmolarity causes dehydration and reduced intracellular water (cell shrinkage)

3. Assessment

    a. General assessments include health history, vital signs, LOC, cognitive and perceptual function, elimination pattern, skin, breathing pattern, breath sounds, reflexes, sensory and motor function, intake and output, weight, electrocardiogram, communication, glucose monitoring log, nutrition pattern, and medications taken within 7 days

NCLEX!

    b. Clinical manifestations: symptoms gradually occur over 24 hours to 2 weeks and include: decreased LOC, dry mucous membranes, polydipsia, hyperthermia, impaired sensory and motor function, positive Babinski sign, and seizures

c. Diagnostic and laboratory test findings: elevated serum sodium, serum osmolality > 340 mOsm/L, serum glucose > 600mg/dL, abnormal serum potassium and chloride, no serum ketones, and normal serum pH

4. Therapeutic management: determine and treat the triggering situation; treat co-existing health deviations; provide fluid and electrolyte replacement; provide regular insulin IV to normalize serum glucose

5. Priority nursing diagnoses: Decreased cardiac output; Deficient fluid volume; Hyperthermia; Disturbed sensory perception; Risk for impaired skin integrity; Risk for aspiration; Deficient knowledge

6. Planning and implementation

   a. Promote normalized cardiac output, sensory perceptual function, fluid and electrolyte balance, normal body temperature by administering fluids, medications, and analyzing intake and output, weight, vital signs, lab values, sensory function, and cognitive function

   b. Maintain intact skin by turning every 2 hours, use of pressure relief aids, nutritional support, use of skin moisturizers and barriers, and management of incontinence

   c. Prevent aspiration by using appropriate feeding precautions, elevate head of bed 15 to 30 degrees during and after feeding for 1 hour; if BP too unstable to elevate head of bed with feeding, then withhold oral feedings

7. Medication therapy: IV infusion of NS to replace fluids and sodium, regular insulin IV to manage the hyperglycemia, and potassium to replace losses and shifts

8. Client education: instruct client on HHNK, symptoms to report, and administration of new medications

9. Evaluation

   a. Client returns to normal LOC and perceptual function, elimination function, and breathing pattern; FBG is within normal range, and skin is intact

   b. Fluid and electrolyte levels are balanced

   c. Client verbalizes understanding of HHNK, symptoms to report, and administration of new medications

Case Study

You have just finished discharging two clients to home when the charge nurse informs you that you will be receiving a client from surgery following a partial thyroidectomy. You will admit the client from the postanesthesia care unit and will be assigned as the primary nurse. Since you have 2 more workdays scheduled, you will be assigned to this client for a total of 3 days.

❶ What supplies should you ask the nurse assistant to place in the room?

❷ Why should vital signs be assessed every 15 minutes for 2 hours, then hourly for 4 hours then every 2 to 4 hours for 24 hours?

❸ What instructions about positioning and transferring the client to the bedside chair should you give to the nurse assistant?

❹ What symptoms and signs should you assess?

❺ What should the client understand about daily thyroid medication?

For suggested responses, see page 739.

Posttest

1 The client is 8 hours post partial thyroidectomy for Graves' disease. What is the best documentation by the nurse of evaluation outcome criteria for the nursing diagnosis risk for Ineffective airway clearance?

(1) Dressing is clean dry and intact, pain minimal and controlled, alert and oriented.
(2) Vital signs stable; client supports neck with hand during change of position.
(3) No tracheal stridor, speaks clearly, and denies numbness or tingling.
(4) Balanced intake and output, vital signs stable, and alert and oriented.

2 Which of the following evaluation data would best lead to nurse to conclude that the client with hyperglycemic hyperosmolar nonketotic coma (HHNK) has demonstrated improvement during the first 24 hours?

(1) Alert and oriented, balanced intake and output, moist mucous membranes
(2) Intake equals output, denies pain and shortness of breath
(3) Alert and oriented, blood and urine without ketones, no orthostatic BP
(4) Respirations easy and even, eats 50 to 75 percent of meals, vital signs stable

3 The nurse is caring for a client with type 1 diabetes mellitus. In developing a teaching plan, which of the following signs and symptoms of hypoglycemia should be included?

(1) Shakiness
(2) Increased thirst
(3) Fever
(4) Fruity breath

4 A client with diabetes is being tested for glycosylated hemoglobin. In explaining the purpose of the laboratory test the nurse explains that glycosylated hemoglobin is used for which of the following purposes?

(1) To check for anemia
(2) To determine the average blood glucose level for up to the previous 4 months
(3) To compare hemoglobin to glucose levels
(4) To calculate the amount of glucose in hemoglobin for the past 6 months

5 A post-surgical client is brought back to the nursing unit following a thyroidectomy. Which of the following methods should the nurse use to assess for bleeding?

(1) Inspect the dressing for signs of hemorrhage.
(2) Change the dressing applied in the operating room.
(3) Check the latest hemoglobin to determine if there has been a drop in value.
(4) Palpate the back of the neck and shoulders for evidence of bleeding.

6 A diabetic client with the flu asks why he should drink juices, check his finger stick glucose every 4 hours and take insulin when he is not eating and is vomiting. Which of the following would be the best explanation by the nurse?

(1) He needs to prevent dehydration, excessive breakdown of fats for glucose, and monitor for hyperglycemia.
(2) He needs to check his blood glucose because vomiting could cause hypoglycemia and drinking fluids will prevent dehydration.
(3) His body uses protein for energy when he is sick, causing increased ketones and hypoglycemia.
(4) If he could substitute water for the juices to prevent dehydration, then he would not need to check his blood glucose levels so often.

7 The client with diabetic ketoacidosis (DKA) is given intravenous normal saline infusion and regular insulin. In addition to hourly blood glucose monitoring, what assessment data are early signs of clinical improvement?

(1) Respiratory rate of 12 to 15 and normal BP in the standing position
(2) Temperature and pulse in normal range
(3) Improved level of consciousness and decreasing urine output
(4) Client eats a full meal and respiratory rate is normal

8 The nurse is preparing to discharge a client newly diagnosed with diabetes mellitus. The client states, "I should eat a candy bar or cup of ice cream every time I feel shaky, hungry, or nauseated." Which of the following is the best response by the nurse?

(1) "Yes, a candy bar or cup of ice cream is needed to treat the hypoglycemia."
(2) "Yes, you should eat the snack, then have a meal as soon as possible."
(3) "No, you should quickly eat a meal; the candy will cause hyperglycemia."
(4) "No, these have too much sugar and fat, 5 Lifesavers candy or skim milk are better."

9 The client had a bilateral adrenalectomy for Cushing's syndrome. He is being sent home with a new prescription for hydrocortisone. The best statement indicating understanding of the drug and associated risk is:

(1) "I am taking this drug to replace the hormones usually secreted by the adrenal medulla."
(2) "I should take this pill every morning before breakfast."
(3) "This pill may cause weight gain, so I should exercise more and eat less."
(4) "I should call the doctor if I think I am starting a cold, and I should not take aspirin."

10 An obese, elderly client is being given a high-dose steroid protocol as emergency treatment of a spinal cord injury. The client's family has requested frequent refills for his cup of chipped ice and his urine output is 600 mL for the first 4 hours and 900 mL in the second 4 hours. The family states that the client was often thirsty at home, even prior to the injury. The nurse should take which of the following most appropriate actions?

(1) Obtain finger stick blood glucose and tabulate the client's 24 hour intake and output.
(2) Restrict the client's intake to prevent fluid volume excess and electrolyte imbalance.
(3) Obtain and monitor CBC, hemoglobin and hematocrit, and vital signs for hypervolemia.
(4) Evaluate the client's breathing pattern and understanding of current treatment plan.

See pages 519–520 for Answers and Rationales.

Answers and Rationales

Pretest

1 Answer: 2 *Rationale:* Clients receiving doses of I-131 that are greater than 30 mCi may not have visitors for 24 or more hours based on radiation dose. For dose of 30 mCi or less, visitors must remain several feet away from client and client may not hold/cuddle children or sleep in same room as another person for 8 days (to protect them from radiation exposure). Clients who are allergic to shellfish are also allergic to iodine but egg allergy is irrelevant (option 1). Options 3 and 4 are unrelated to this medication.
Cognitive Level: Application
Nursing Process: Implementation; *Test Plan:* HPM

2 Answer: 3 *Rationale:* The parathyroid glands, located near the thyroid gland, may have been injured or accidentally removed, resulting in hypocalcemia. Hypocalcemia is life-threatening; thus it is important to identify early signs. Numbness and/or tingling of the mouth, face, or extremities are early symptoms of low serum calcium. Reduced thyroid hormone levels are expected results of surgery (option 1). Option 2 should refer to the pituitary gland. Option 4 is possible, but could be detected by hoarseness or weak voice.
Cognitive Level: Application
Nursing Process: Assessment; *Test Plan:* PHYS

3 Answer: 2 *Rationale:* Iodine intake is needed for the thyroid gland to produce thyroid hormone. Insufficient iodine intake leads to low thyroid hormone production and symptoms of hypothyroidism, which includes constipation, weight gain, and muscle stiffness, among others. The other options are incorrect.
Cognitive Level: Application
Nursing Process: Implementation; *Test Plan:* HPM

4 Answer: 2 *Rationale:* Clients with Addison disease should be assessed for signs of Addisonian crisis following a stressful event such as surgery. Signs of Addisonian crisis include decreased urine output, decreased blood pressure, dry skin, and altered level of consciousness. Options 1, 3, and 4 do not apply to the necessary priority assessments related to Addisonian crisis, although they are good general postoperative assessments.
Cognitive Level: Analysis
Nursing Process: Planning; *Test Plan:* PHYS

5 Answer: 1 *Rationale:* Research by the National Institute of Health and the American Diabetes Association demonstrates a strong correlation between chronic hyperglycemia and complications of retinopathy, nephropathy, and neuropathy. Thus, there is damage to the eyes, kidneys, and peripheral nerves, respectively. Lactic acidosis occurs with diabetic ketoacidosis (option 2). Option 3 is a false rationale for the client in the question. Insulin is needed to carry glucose across the cell membrane into the cell, not to be transported in the blood (option 4).
Cognitive Level: Analysis
Nursing Process: Implementation; *Test Plan:* PHYS

6 Answer: 4 *Rationale:* In SIADH there is excess secretion of ADH that causes fluid retention, dilutes the plasma causing suppression of aldosterone, and increases renal excretion of sodium. Water then moves into the cells from the plasma and interstitial spaces causing cellular edema. The treatment is fluid restriction and hypertonic saline infusion. Options 1 and 3 are the opposite of standard treatment and are therefore incorrect. Option 2 is unrelated to this client.
Cognitive Level: Application
Nursing Process: Evaluation; *Test Plan:* PHYS

7 Answer: 3 *Rationale:* Diabetes insipidus (DI) can develop with head injury, tumors, and other conditions that cause increased intracranial pressure. Excessive urine output of 350 cc/hr or more is a classic early symptom of DI. The specific gravity provides valuable information about renal function and response to ADH. Using critical inquiry to analyze the urine output, specific gravity and other characteristics of the urine, the nurse assesses for classic signs of DI that can occur following a head injury. Options 1 and 4 are false. Option 2 would be insufficient fluid replacement.
Cognitive Level: Analysis
Nursing Process: Assessment; *Test Plan:* PHYS

8 Answer: 4 *Rationale:* Option 4 addresses the lifelong hormone replacement of thyroid, glucocorticoids, and gonadotropin needed when the entire pituitary gland is removed. Options 1 and 3 are incorrect. Option 2 relates to the immediate postoperative time while the client's comments relate to long-term outcome.
Cognitive Level: Application
Nursing Process: Evaluation; *Test Plan:* PHYS

9 Answer: 2 *Rationale:* DKA is associated with excessive urine output, dehydration, and hypokalemia, placing the client at risk for decreased cardiac output

and cardiac dysrhythmias. Option 1 is false regarding output and does not address the metabolic problem. Options 3 and 4 may apply to the client but are not the priority needs; in addition, option 3 will resolve as the DKA is treated.
Cognitive Level: Analysis
Nursing Process: Analysis; *Test Plan:* PHYS

10   Answer: 4   *Rationale:* Daily total baths remove the protective sebum from the skin, placing the client at risk for altered skin integrity. Since the client's level of participation in the bath or other self-care activity is not presented, the other 3 options are inappropriate. In addition, options 2 and 3 are not specific and measurable enough to meet criteria for an outcome statement.
Cognitive Level: Application
Nursing Process: Planning; *Test Plan:* HPM

Posttest

1   Answer: 3   *Rationale:* Early signs of edema of the larynx leading to airway obstruction are tight-fitting dressing, stridor, stertor, and/or weak or harsh voice. Numbness or tingling of the extremities, lips or mouth are signs of hypocalcemia that can lead to respiratory distress due to tetany. The data in the other options are important routine postoperative assessments, but they do not relate to the client's airway.
Cognitive Level: Application
Nursing Process: Evaluation; *Test Plan:* PHYS

2   Answer: 1   *Rationale:* HHNK results from hyperglycemia, causing excessive loss of water and retention of glucose that leads to dehydration, hypernatremia and hypokalemia. Symptoms are dry, tenting skin, dry mucous membranes, altered level of consciousness and hyperthermia. Ketones are not present in HHNK; thus, monitoring for ketones is inappropriate (option 3). Options 2 and 4 do not address the primary problems that occur with HHNK.
Cognitive Level: Application
Nursing Process: Evaluation; *Test Plan:* PHYS

3   Answer: 1   *Rationale:* The signs of hypoglycemia include hunger, shakiness, sweating, pale cool skin, and irritability. These signs may be manifestations of impaired cerebral function from the hypoglycemia. The other options are all signs of hyperglycemia.
Cognitive Level: Application
Nursing Process: Planning; *Test Plan:* PHYS

4   Answer: 2   *Rationale:* Glycosylated hemoglobin reflects the average blood glucose over the life of the RBC, usually 4 months. This test is not a ratio of he-

moglobin to glucose content (option 3) nor is it helpful in diagnosing anemia (option 1). The time frame in option 4 is too long.
Cognitive Level: Application
Nursing Process: Implementation; *Test Plan:* PHYS

5   Answer: 4   *Rationale:* The danger of hemorrhage is greatest during the first 24 hours following thyroid surgery. The tendency is for blood to flow down at the sides and posteriorly if hemorrhage occurs in the area of the neck. Inspecting the dressings for signs of hemorrhage may not reveal bleeding (option 1). Changing dressings immediately after surgery is not appropriate (option 2). A drop in hemoglobin may be a clue to bleeding but is not the best initial assessment action (option 3).
Cognitive Level: Application
Nursing Process: Assessment; *Test Plan:* SECE

6   Answer: 1   *Rationale:* Starvation-induced ketosis can be prevented by drinking juices that equal the prescribed carbohydrate meal pattern. Fluids are needed to prevent dehydration and hyperosmolality, which could result from large fluid losses from persistent vomiting. The liver breaks down fats to form glucose for energy and ketones, leading to DKA. The other options do not address the key issues of dehydration and hyperglycemia.
Cognitive Level: Application
Nursing Process: Planning; *Test Plan:* PHYS

7   Answer: 3   *Rationale:* Level of consciousness responds quickly to early changes in pH and restoration of fluid and electrolyte balance. Urine output decreases as hyperglycemia is resolved. The respiratory buffer system takes a few hours to respond to change in pH. Dehydration is usually so severe that several hours of rehydration are needed to reduce pulse (option 2) and resolve orthostatic BP (option 1). Option 4 is inappropriate because eating a full meal is not an early sign of improvement.
Cognitive Level: Analysis
Nursing Process: Evaluation; *Test Plan:* PHYS

8   Answer: 4   *Rationale:* The candy bar and ice cream may have too much glucose and fat, potentially leading to hyperglycemia. In addition the fat may delay glucose absorption. Immediate absorption of glucose is needed in hypoglycemia. The client should also check the blood glucose within 15 minutes of taking glucose because of signs of hypoglycemia.
Cognitive Level: Application
Nursing Process: Implementation; *Test Plan:* HPM

9 **Answer: 4** *Rationale:* Usually the cortex of the adrenal gland (not the medulla as in option 1) increases secretion of cortisol to stimulate the immune system in response to an infection. Thus the replacement dose during illness may need to be adjusted once a client's adrenal glands are removed. Hydrocortisone can irritate gastric mucosa and so clients should not take gastric irritants such as aspirin or nonsteroidal anti-inflammatory drugs (NSAIDs). Dosage may be adjusted during illness. Options 2 and 3 do not address the risk of the drug, which is the issue of the question.
Cognitive Level: Analysis
Nursing Process: Evaluation; *Test Plan:* HPM

10 **Answer: 1** *Rationale:* The client is at risk for type 2 diabetes mellitus (DM). Polydipsia and polyuria are signs of hyperglycemia, a symptom of DM. Steroids may also increase carbohydrate metabolism, leading to hyperglycemia in clients with insufficient insulin. Thus the nurse should assess the client's blood glucose. Since hyperglycemia places the client at risk for fluid volume deficit the nurse should calculate the client's fluid balance. The nurse also needs to record the assessment data and report it to the physician. The client is not at risk for hypervolemia (options 2 and 3). Option 4 is not a priority.
Cognitive Level: Application
Nursing Process: Planning; *Test Plan:* PHYS

References

Corbett, J. V. (2000). *Laboratory tests and diagnostic procedures with nursing diagnoses* (5th ed.). Upper Saddle River, NJ: Prentice Hall, pp. 69–72, 111–119, 138–142, 167–169, 176–211, 385–398, 400–419, 527, 538, 559–568, 577, 592–593, 731–738.

Doenges, M. E. & Moorhouse, M. F. (2000). *Nurse's pocket guide: Diagnoses, interventions, and rationales* (7th ed.). Philadelphia: F. A. Davis, pp. 54–58, 214–226, 555–556.

Elliot, B. (2000). Case report: Diagnosing and treating hypothyroidism. *The Nurse Practitioner: 25* (3): 92–105.

Gulanick, M., Klopp, K., Galanes, S., Gradishar, D., & Puzas, M.K. (1998). *Nursing care plans: Nursing diagnosis and intervention* (4th ed.). St. Louis, MO: Mosby.

Ignatavicius, D. D., Workman, L. M., & Mishler, M. A., (1999). *Medical-surgical nursing across the health care continuum* (3rd ed.). Philadelphia: Saunders, pp. 293–303, 1594–1599, 1690.

Kozier, B., Erb, G. Berman, A. J., & Burke, K. (2000). *Fundamentals of nursing: Concepts, process and practice* (6th ed). Upper Saddle River, NJ: Prentice Hall, pp. 496–619, 700–701, 888–905, 1000–1060, 1115–1363.

Lemone, P. & Burke, K. (2000). *Medical-surgical nursing: Critical thinking in client care* (2nd ed.). Upper Saddle River, NJ: Prentice Hall, Inc., pp. 106–132, 149–160, 364, 683–764.

Martini, F. H. & Bartholomew, E. F. (2000). *Essentials of anatomy & physiology* (2nd ed.). Upper Saddle River, NJ: Prentice-Hall, Inc., pp. 306–323.

Porth, C. M. (1998). *Pathophysiology: Concepts of altered health states* (5th ed.). Philadelphia: Lippincott, pp. 604–605, 778–782.

Rakel, R. (Ed.) (1999). *Conn's current therapy.* Philadelphia: Saunders, pp. 622–630, 638–639, 652–663, 672–673, 1263.

Terpstra, T. L. & Terpstra, T. L. (2000). Syndrome of inappropriate antidiuretic hormone secretion: Recognition and management, *Medsurg Nursing 9* (2): 61–70.

Wilkinson, J. M. (2000). *Nursing diagnosis handbook with NIC interventions and NOC outcomes* (7th ed). Upper Saddle River, NJ: Prentice Hall, Inc., pp. 159–163.

Wilson, B. A., Shannon, M. T., & Stang, C. L. (2003). *Nurses drug guide 2003.* Upper Saddle River, NJ: Prentice Hall.

CHAPTER **14**

Hematologic Disorders

Tomas M. Madayag, ARNP, MEd, MSN, EdD

CHAPTER OUTLINE

OBJECTIVES

▌ Identify basic structures and functions of the hematologic system.

▌ Describe the pathophysiology and etiology of common hematologic disorders.

▌ Discuss expected assessment data and diagnostic test findings for selected hematologic disorders.

▌ Identify priority nursing diagnoses for selected hematologic disorders.

▌ Discuss therapeutic management of selected hematologic disorders.

▌ Discuss nursing management of a client experiencing a hematologic disorder.

▌ Identify expected outcomes for the client experiencing a hematologic disorder.

[Media Link]

Use the CD-ROM enclosed with this text, or log onto the address given to access the free, interactive Companion Website created for this series. The CD-ROM and Companion Website accompanying this book offer additional practice opportunities and information—NCLEX Review, Case Studies, Glossary, In Depth with NCLEX, and more.

www.prenhall.com/hogan

REVIEW AT A GLANCE

anergy *a decreased reaction to skin sensitivity tests*

bands *granulocytes that are less mature than a fully developed neutrophil*

cheilosis *cracks in the corners of the mouth*

consumption coagulopathy *another term for disseminated intravascular coagulopathy, a syndrome characterized by abnormal initiation and acceleration of clotting and simultaneous hemorrhage*

culling *the destruction of red blood cells*

erythropoiesis *the production of red blood cells*

erythromyalgia *burning sensation of the fingers and toes*

ferritin *measures the iron in plasma, which is also a direct reflection of total iron stores*

fibrinolysis *the process whereby a clot is dissolved after tissue repair is completed*

glossitis *smooth, sore, beefy red tongue*

hemarthrosis *joint bleeding, swelling and damage*

hemostasis *the series of reactions that lead to the formation of a platelet and clot where there is damage or injury to an area*

hypochromic *having less pigmentation, refers to erythrocytes*

leukocytosis *abnormal elevation of the white blood cell count*

leukopenia *a decrease in the number of white blood cells*

microcytic *small in size; refers to erythrocytes*

plethora *a ruddy (dark, flushed) color of the face, hands, feet, ears, and mucous membranes resulting from the engorgement or distention of blood vessels*

priapism *abnormal, painful, continuous erection of the penis*

shift to the left *describes the increase in immature neutrophils resulting from activation of the bone marrow to produce white blood cells in response to infectious processes*

thrombocytopenia *decrease in the number of platelets*

Pretest

1 A client asks the nurse why vitamin B_{12} is important for red blood cell formation. The nurse responds with the knowledge that Vitamin B_{12} deficiency causes which of the following changes in the red blood cell?

(1) Decreased mean corpuscular volume (MCV)
(2) Increased hemoglobin in the red blood cell
(3) Makes the cell irregular and oval-shaped
(4) Makes the cell smaller in shape and deficient in hemoglobin

2 A nurse is discussing the role of hypoxia in red blood cell (RBC) production. Which of the following statements is accurate?

(1) Hypoxia stimulates the hemoglobin content of the RBC to increase.
(2) Hypoxia stimulates the release of erythropoietin in the kidneys.
(3) Reticulocytes become erythrocytes faster with hypoxia.
(4) RBC destruction is increased with hypoxia therefore stimulating RBC production.

3 The destruction of old red blood cells occurs as senescent cells decrease their ATP content. Which statement accurately describes what happens to the heme molecule during this phase?

(1) It is converted to bilirubin that is conjugated and excreted as bile.
(2) It binds with a plasma protein to form haptoglobin.
(3) The kidneys excrete the heme molecule.
(4) The heme molecule is conjugated with glucorinide in the spleen.

4 A client with a hemolytic blood disorder presents to the primary care center with jaundice. The nurse explains to the client that the jaundice is most likely caused by which of the following?

(1) Increased bilirubin in plasma
(2) Increased haptoglobin in plasma
(3) Hepatitis infection
(4) Loss of plasma proteins

5 A nurse is evaluating the response of a patient with anemia to therapy. Which of the following laboratory tests would the nurse look to that best reflects bone marrow production of red blood cells?

(1) Hematocrit
(2) Hemoglobin
(3) Serum ferritin
(4) Reticulocyte count

6 The nurse who is assessing a client with iron-deficiency anemia notes that the tongue is inflamed. The nurse documents this observation as:

(1) Cheilitis.
(2) Achlorhydria.
(3) Glossitis.
(4) Cheilosis.

7 The nurse is teaching a client about measures to increase the absorption of the prescribed oral iron preparation. Which of the following instructions would the nurse give to the client?

(1) Take the medicine with milk.
(2) Take the pill with a drink that contains vitamin C.
(3) Take the iron with meals.
(4) Take the iron after meals.

8 Which of the following statements made by a client with iron-deficiency anemia indicates the need for further teaching?

(1) "I should stop taking the medicine if my stools turn black."
(2) "I should dilute the liquid iron preparation and use a straw when taking it."
(3) "I can prevent the constipation by increasing the intake of fluids and fiber."
(4) "I should return to the clinic if my stomach upset worsens with this medication."

9 Which of the following food choices made by a client with anemia best indicates that the teaching regarding selection of foods high in iron has been successful?

(1) Citrus fruits
(2) Green leafy vegetables
(3) Eggs, milk, and milk products
(4) Liver and muscle meats

10 A nurse is preparing to administer an intramuscular (IM) dose of iron to a client with anemia. Which of the following precautions should the nurse take?

(1) Administer the drug utilizing a Z tract technique.
(2) Use a 1-inch, 19-gauge needle.
(3) Administer the drug deep in the deltoid muscle.
(4) Massage the area vigorously after administering the iron.

See pages 560–561 for Answers and Rationales.

I. Overview of Anatomy and Physiology

A. Blood components

1. Plasma: a straw-colored liquid portion of the blood in which the cells and platelets are suspended; makes up approximately 50 to 55 percent of a blood sample; consists of water (approximately 92 percent), amino acids, proteins, carbohydrates, lipids, vitamins, hormones, electrolytes, and cellular wastes

2. Serum is essentially the same as plasma only without the fibrinogen and clotting factors; if whole blood is allowed to clot and the clot is removed, the remaining fluid is known as serum

3. Blood cells along with platelets comprise the remaining blood sample

4. The volume of blood is approximately 8 percent of total body weight

B. Red blood cells

NCLEX!

1. Non-nucleated, biconcave, disc-shaped cells also known as erythrocytes; they are the most abundant type of blood cell making up 99 percent of blood cells; the shape serves to increase the surface area for diffusion of oxygen

Figure 14-1

Erythropoiesis. RBCs being formed within the bone marrow as erythroblasts. These mature into normoblasts, which eventually eject their nucleus and organelles to form reticulocytes. The reticulocytes mature within the blood or spleen and become erythrocytes.

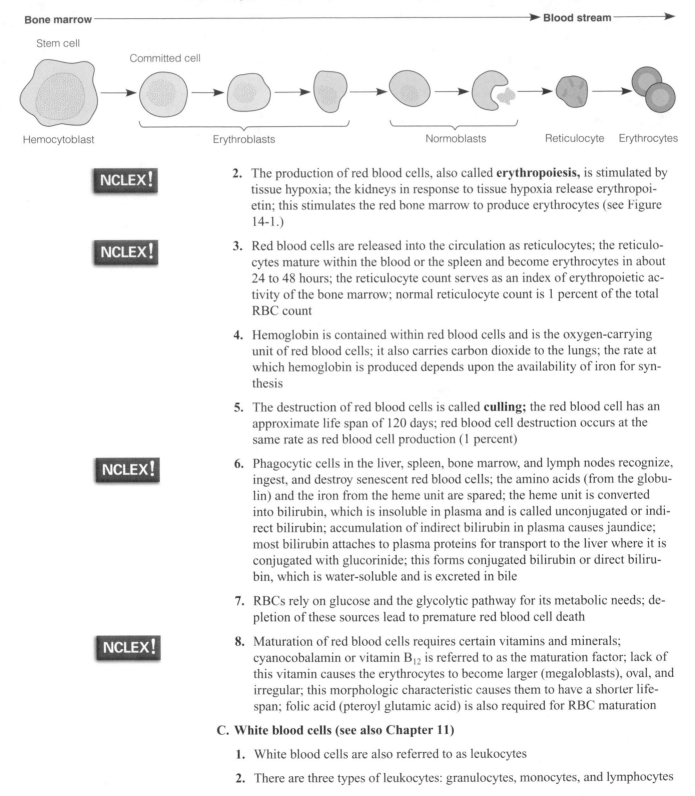

Bone marrow ——————————————————————————→ Blood stream ——→

Stem cell

Committed cell

Hemocytoblast   Erythroblasts   Normoblasts   Reticulocyte   Erythrocytes

NCLEX!

2. The production of red blood cells, also called **erythropoiesis,** is stimulated by tissue hypoxia; the kidneys in response to tissue hypoxia release erythropoietin; this stimulates the red bone marrow to produce erythrocytes (see Figure 14-1.)

NCLEX!

3. Red blood cells are released into the circulation as reticulocytes; the reticulocytes mature within the blood or the spleen and become erythrocytes in about 24 to 48 hours; the reticulocyte count serves as an index of erythropoietic activity of the bone marrow; normal reticulocyte count is 1 percent of the total RBC count

4. Hemoglobin is contained within red blood cells and is the oxygen-carrying unit of red blood cells; it also carries carbon dioxide to the lungs; the rate at which hemoglobin is produced depends upon the availability of iron for synthesis

5. The destruction of red blood cells is called **culling;** the red blood cell has an approximate life span of 120 days; red blood cell destruction occurs at the same rate as red blood cell production (1 percent)

NCLEX!

6. Phagocytic cells in the liver, spleen, bone marrow, and lymph nodes recognize, ingest, and destroy senescent red blood cells; the amino acids (from the globulin) and the iron from the heme unit are spared; the heme unit is converted into bilirubin, which is insoluble in plasma and is called unconjugated or indirect bilirubin; accumulation of indirect bilirubin in plasma causes jaundice; most bilirubin attaches to plasma proteins for transport to the liver where it is conjugated with glucorinide; this forms conjugated bilirubin or direct bilirubin, which is water-soluble and is excreted in bile

7. RBCs rely on glucose and the glycolytic pathway for its metabolic needs; depletion of these sources lead to premature red blood cell death

NCLEX!

8. Maturation of red blood cells requires certain vitamins and minerals; cyanocobalamin or vitamin B_{12} is referred to as the maturation factor; lack of this vitamin causes the erythrocytes to become larger (megaloblasts), oval, and irregular; this morphologic characteristic causes them to have a shorter lifespan; folic acid (pteroyl glutamic acid) is also required for RBC maturation

C. White blood cells (see also Chapter 11)

1. White blood cells are also referred to as leukocytes

2. There are three types of leukocytes: granulocytes, monocytes, and lymphocytes

3. Granulocytes contain granules in their cytoplasm and act as phagocytes; three types of granulocytes are: neutrophils, eosinophils, and basophils, which are referred to as the polymorphonuclear leukocytes (PMNs)

   NCLEX!

   a. Neutrophils: act as phagocytes; develop from metamyelocytes and become bands; **bands** are granulocytes that are less mature than a fully developed neutrophil; a **shift to the left** describes the increase in immature neutrophils resulting from activation of the bone marrow to produce white blood cells in response to infectious processes; as the bands mature, the nucleus becomes segmented and develop into neutrophils, which is why neutrophils are often referred to as "segs"

   b. Eosinophils are also phagocytes but not as efficient in this role compared to the neutrophils; they have the ability to engulf antigen-antibody complexes from allergic responses; they also have the ability to protect the individual from parasitic infections

   c. Basophils contain histamine, heparin, and serotonin; these are similar to the mast cell activity seen in allergic and inflammatory reactions; basophils have limited phagocytic activity

4. Monocytes

   a. Large phagocytic cells produced in the bone marrow; once they leave the circulation, they reside in tissues to become macrophages

   b. Macrophages are responsible for removing dead and senescent cells as well as having the ability to engulf microorganisms

5. Lymphocytes

   a. Originate primarily from the lymph nodes and also from the bone marrow

   b. There are two types of lymphocytes: T lymphocytes and B lymphocytes

   c. T lymphocytes originate from the thymus; they are involved in cell-mediated immunity

   d. B lymphocytes are involved in humoral immunity

D. Platelets (thrombocytes)

1. Majority of platelets are present in circulation; the spleen contains the remainder of platelets; approximately 20,000 to 40,000 new platelets per cubic millimeter of blood are produced each day; life span of platelets is approximately 10 days

2. The major function of platelets is to maintain hemostasis and coagulation; they have the ability to plug breaks in blood vessels and therefore are able to maintain the integrity of these vessels

3. Platelets also release thromboplastin (factor III) necessary for the conversion of prothrombin to thrombin, which is the first step of the coagulation mechanism

E. Normal clotting mechanisms

1. **Hemostasis** and coagulation refer to the series of reactions that lead to the formation of a platelet and clot where there is damage or injury to an area; it involves three mechanisms: vascular spasm, the formation of a platelet plug, and

Figure 14-2

Flow diagram of factor activation leading to clot formation. Clotting may be mediated by chemical factors in either of two independent pathways: the longer intrinsic pathway and the "short-cut" extrinsic pathway. Both pathways eventually activate factor X, which begins the series of events leading to clot formation. Once factor X is activated, four sequential steps occur: (1) Factor X combines with other factors to form prothrombin activator; (2) prothrombin activator transforms fibrinogen into long fibrin strands; and (3) thrombin also activates factor XIII, which (4) draws the fibrin strands together into a dense meshwork. The complete process of clot formation occurs within 3 to 6 minutes after blood vessel damage.

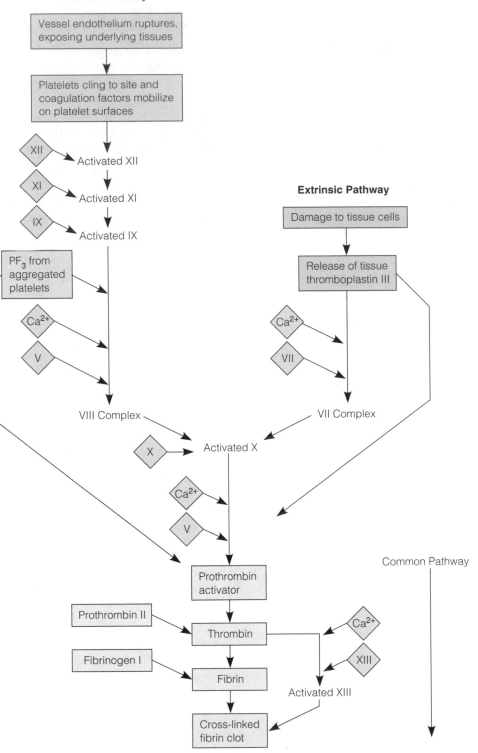

the activation of clotting factors; the fibrin clot is produced through either the intrinsic or extrinsic pathways; either pathway ends in a common pathway, a process known as coagulation cascade (see Figure 14-2)

  a. Intrinsic pathway: stimulated by contact with foreign surfaces in the absence of tissue damage; is a secondary clotting mechanism initiated by activation of the Hageman factor; in the presence of calcium ions, the activated factor triggers a series of changes leading to the formation of prothrombin activator

  b. Extrinsic pathway: is triggered by the release of tissue thromboplastin from damaged tissues

2. After a clot is formed, clot retraction and dissolution occurs; **fibrinolysis** is the process whereby a clot is dissolved after tissue repair is completed; plasminogen, which is present in the blood clot, is transformed into plasmin; plasmin dissolves the fibrin strands of the clot; fibrinolysis continues until the blood clot is dissolved

II. Diagnostic Tests and Assessments

A. Red blood cell count (see Table 14-1)

B. Hemoglobin and hematocrit

1. Hemoglobin measures the hemoglobin available in circulation, which is the gas-carrying capacity of an erythrocyte

2. Hematocrit is the ratio of the RBC volume to the volume of whole blood

C. RBC indexes

1. MCV (mean corpuscular volume): estimates size of the RBC

2. MCH (mean corpuscular hemoglobin): measures the content of Hgb in RBCs from a single cell

Table 14-1

Normal Laboratory Values for Red Blood Cells and Platelets

Laboratory Test	Normal Value
Red blood cell count	
Men	4.2–5.4 million/mm³
Women	3.6–5.0 million/mm³
Reticulocytes	1.0–1.5% of total RBC
Hemoglobin (Hgb)	
Men	14–16.5 g/dL
Women	12–15 g/dL
Hematocrit (Hct)	
Men	40–50%
Women	37–47%
Mean Corpuscular Volume (MCV)	85–100 fL/cell
Mean corpuscular hemoglobin concentration (MCHC)	31–35 g/dL
Mean corpuscular hemoglobin (MCH)	27–34 pg/cell
Platelet count	150,000–400,000/mm³

Source: Lemone, P. & Burke, K. (2000). *Medical-surgical nursing* (2nd ed.). Upper Saddle River, NJ: Prentice Hall, p. 1302.

3. MCHC (mean corpuscular hemoglobin concentration): a more accurate measurement of the Hgb content of RBC as it measures the entire volume of RBCs

D. Serum ferritin, transferrin, and total iron-binding capacity (TIBC): these tests are used to evaluate iron levels; **ferritin** measures the iron in plasma, which is also a direct reflection of total iron stores; transferrin is the major iron-transport protein

E. White blood cell count (see Table 14-2)

1. Abnormal elevation of the WBC is referred to as **leukocytosis**

2. **Leukopenia** is a decrease in the number of white blood cells

3. Differential count refers to the breakdown of the different types of cells

F. Coagulation studies

1. *Bleeding time:* normal range is 1 to 4 minutes; it is used in evaluation of platelet function; extended bleeding times are seen with thrombocytopenia and aspirin therapy

2. *Prothrombin Time (PT):* is the rapidity of blood clotting; normal range is 11 to 16 seconds; PT evaluates extrinsic coagulation pathway which include factors I, II, V, VII, X; INR is often currently used instead of PT because it is a standardized value (therapeutic range often varies from 2 to 3 depending on condition)

3. *Partial thromboplastin time (PTT):* normal range is 60 to 70 seconds, which evaluates the intrinsic coagulation pathway or fibrin clot formation

4. *Activated partial thromboplastin time (APTT):* normal range is 30 to 45 seconds; is a modified PTT, preferred because it is quicker to perform; APTT is used in heparin therapy and in the evaluation of hemophilia; APTT is increased in anticoagulation therapy, liver disease, vitamin K deficiency, and disseminated intravascular coagulation (DIC)

5. *Fibrinogen:* normal range is 150 to 400 mg/dL; it is a soluble plasma protein that is decreased in DIC and fibrinogen disorders and increased in acute infections, hepatitis, and oral contraceptive use

6. *Fibrin degradation products (FDP):* normal value is < 10 μg/mL; FDP is increased in fibrinolysis, thrombolytic therapy, and DIC

	Laboratory Test	**Value**
Table 14-2		
Normal Laboratory Values: White Blood Cells	WBC count	5,000–10,000/mm^3
	Differential	
	Neutrophils	60–70% or 3,000–7,000/mm^3
	Eosinophils	1–3% or 50–400/mm^3
	Basophils	0.3–0.5% or 25–200/mm^3
	Lymphocytes	20–30% or 1,000–4,000/mm^3
	Monocytes	3–8% or 100–600/mm^3

Source: Lemone, P. & Burke, K. (2000). *Medical surgical nursing* (2nd ed.). Upper Saddle River, NJ: Prentice Hall, p. 1277.

7. *Fibrin D-dimer:* normal is 0 to 0.5 µg/mL; D-dimer is the most sensitive indicator to differentiate DIC from primary fibrinolysis; it is elevated in DIC

G. Bone marrow examination

1. Specimens obtained during a bone marrow examination may include those obtained by aspiration or biopsy

2. Sites for bone marrow aspiration may include: sternum, iliac crest (most common), and tibia; the most common site for bone marrow biopsy is the posterosuperior iliac spine; the sternum also is used

3. Aspiration is the most common procedure for obtaining a marrow sample

4. The client is positioned based on the site selected by the physician; the skin and periosteum are anesthetized to decrease pain with anesthetic such as procaine; the marrow aspiration needle is then inserted; after the marrow cavity is entered, the marrow stylet is removed from the needle and a sterile syringe is attached; the syringe plunger is drawn back until marrow appears in the syringe

5. During the withdrawal of aspirate, the client will experience sharp pain often described as a burning pain

6. After the needle is removed, a pressure dressing is applied over the puncture site, where only minimal bleeding should occur; if the patient has thrombocytopenia, pressure is applied for 3 to 5 minutes

7. The nurse should check on the facility's procedure manual as to the disposition of specimens

8. Most clients experience little, if any, pain or discomfort after the procedure; some persons will complain of tenderness and ache at the aspiration site for a few days

9. The procedure for a bone marrow biopsy is essentially the same as for aspiration; the biopsy needle most commonly used is a Jamshidi needle, which allows a second needle, called a stylet to be inserted within in the initial biopsy needle and a core of marrow to be collected and withdrawn through the sleeve of the needle; after the procedure, clients are assessed for bleeding from the puncture site

H. Lymphangiography

1. Is visualization of the lymph system radiographically after injection of a dye

2. It is used primarily in staging of Hodgkin's and non-Hodgkin's lymphoma

I. Lymph node biopsy

1. Can either be done utilizing a closed needle biopsy done at the bedside or an open biopsy performed in the operating room

2. The purpose is to obtain lymph tissue for histologic analysis

III. Common Nursing Procedures of the Hematologic System

A. Administration of blood and blood products

1. Check the agency's policy and procedure pertaining to blood transfusion and transfusion of blood products

NCLEX!

> **Practice to Pass**

A client undergoes a bone marrow biopsy. What nursing interventions should you implement?

NCLEX!

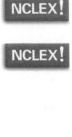

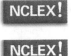

2. Verify the physician's order for the transfusion noting the blood product ordered, the time specified for transfusion (if any), and any medications to be given before transfusion

3. Check that the client has given consent for receiving blood transfusion

4. Check that a typing and crossmatch has been performed

5. Obtain blood from the blood bank when an intravenous access line is available; the IV line should be maintained with normal saline while waiting for the blood or blood product to be delivered to the nursing unit; return blood to the blood bank immediately if transfusion is not possible; blood may not be returned to the blood bank after 20 minutes; do not keep blood or blood products in the nursing unit refrigerator; blood is refrigerated under strict and controlled conditions only in the blood bank

6. Validate data on the blood or blood product with another nurse; the client's ID bracelet should match the blood bank number on the unit of blood

7. Validate with another nurse that the client's name, ID number, blood type, and Rh match the unit of blood to be transfused

8. Note the expiration date indicated on the blood product

9. Observe the unit of blood for bubbles or discoloration; return unit of blood to the blood bank if break in the bag is noted or if signs of contamination are evident

10. Obtain pre-transfusion vital signs, and the vital signs 15 minutes after the transfusion is initiated and immediately after the completion of the transfusion; a pre-transfusion temperature of 100°F or higher should be reported to the physician before initiating the transfusion; any increase in 2°F in the client's temperature may indicate a transfusion reaction and should be reported to the physician

11. Start blood transfusion slowly, administering 25 to 50 mL during the first 15 minutes; most untoward reactions occur during the first 15 minutes; stay with the client during this period of time

12. Do not administer any medications through the blood transfusion tubing; use tubing specific for the blood product being transfused; a blood filter is used to prevent clots and other particles from entering the venous system

13. Use only agency-approved blood-warming devices; do not warm blood in hot water or microwave ovens

14. Blood products should not be infused longer than 4 hours; the longer a blood product is in room temperature, the greater the chances of bacterial contamination

15. Discard tubings and bags used in the transfusion in a biohazard receptacle

16. Follow the agency's protocol for any suspected transfusion reactions

B. Protocol for suspected blood transfusion reaction

1. Check the specific policy and protocol of the agency

2. If blood transfusion reaction is noted or suspected, stop the infusion immediately; change IV tubing and keep vein open with normal saline; the IV access might be needed for the administration of emergency drugs

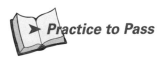

Practice to Pass

Your client is to receive a unit of packed red blood cells. When the unit of blood is delivered to the nursing unit, you are unable to initiate an IV access. What actions should you take?

Box 14-1

**Signs and Symptoms
of Blood Transfusion
Reaction**

Hemolytic: Chills, fever, urticaria, tachycardia, chest pain or complaints of chest tightness, shortness of breath, dyspnea, lumbar pain, nausea, vomiting, rales, hematuria, hypotension, wheezing
Bacterial (pyrogenic): Hypotension, fever, chills, flushed skin, abdominal pain, pain in extremities, vomiting, diarrhea
Allergic reaction: Urticaria, pruritus, swelling of the tongue, swelling of the face, difficulty of
breathing, pulmonary edema, shock
Circulatory overload: Chest pain, tightness of the chest, cough, rales, pulmonary edema, tachycardia, elevated blood pressure

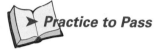

Practice to Pass

Your client is receiving
a unit of packed red
blood cells. Twenty
minutes after the start
of transfusion, the client
complains of chills.
Describe the actions
you would take.

3. Assess the client for other signs and symptoms of transfusion reaction (see
   Box 14-1)

4. Notify the physician and the blood bank

5. Send the unit of blood and tubing used to the blood bank; this will help determine the cause of the reaction

6. Urine and blood samples will be required; follow the agency's protocol

7. Administer drugs that are prescribed and continue to monitor the client

8. Document the reaction and interventions

IV. Common Disorders of the Hematologic System

A. Iron-deficiency anemia (IDA)

1. Description: anemia that results when the supply of iron is inadequate for optimal formation of RBCs related to excessive iron loss caused by bleeding, decreased dietary intake, or malabsorption

2. Etiology and pathophysiology

   a. Iron deficiency accounts for 60 percent of anemias in clients over age 65;
      the most common cause of IDA is blood loss from gastrointestinal or geni-
      tourinary system

   b. Normal iron excretion is less than 1 mg/day through the urine, sweat, bile,
      feces, and from desquamated cells of the skin; the average woman loses 0.5
      mg of iron daily or 15 mg monthly during menstruation; menstruation is
      the most common cause of iron deficiency in women, while gastrointestinal
      bleeding is the most common cause in men

   c. Anemia reduces the oxygen-carrying capacity of the blood, producing tis-
      sue hypoxia

NCLEX!

   d. Iron is stored in the body as ferritin, an iron-phosphorus-protein complex
      that contains about 23 percent iron; it is formed in the intestinal mucosa,
      when ferritin iron joins with the protein apoferritin; ferritin is stored in the
      tissues, primarily in the reticuloendothelial cells of the liver, spleen, and
      bone marrow

   e. Develops slowly through three phases: body's stores of iron used for ery-
      thropoiesis are depleted, insufficient iron is transported to the bone marrow
      and iron deficient erythopoiesis begins, allowing small hemoglobin defi-
      cient cells to enter the peripheral circulation in large numbers; iron is
      needed on the hemoglobin so the oxygen molecule will attach

f. Adequate iron in the RBC is essential since the oxygen molecule attaches to it

g. An average diet supplies the body with 12 to 15 mg/day of iron, of which only 5 to 10 percent is absorbed

3. Assessment

   a. Clinical manifestations (usually develop gradually with the client not seeking attention until the hemoglobin drops to 7 to 8 g/dL)

      1) Fatigue

      2) Weakness

      3) Shortness of breath

      4) Pallor (ear lobes, palms, and conjunctiva)

      5) Brittle spoon-like nails

      6) **Cheilosis** (cracks in the corners of the mouth)

      7) Smooth, sore tongue

      8) Dizziness

      9) Pica (craving to eat unusual substances such as clay or starch)

   b. Diagnostic and laboratory tests

      1) Is considered a **microcytic** and **hypochromic** anemia (small RBC diameter <6 with decreased pigmentation) with an increase in the red cell size distribution width (RDW)

      2) Erythrocytes are small (microcytic) and pale (hypochromic); mean corpuscular volume (MCV; measures size) is decreased and mean corpuscular hemoglobin (MCH) or mean corpuscular hemoglobin concentration or MCHC (calculated value of the hemoglobin present in the RBC compared to its size) will be decreased; the MCV, MCH, and MCHC should be analyzed only when the hemoglobin is low

      3) Low serum iron level and elevated serum iron-binding capacity or low serum ferritin levels

4. Therapeutic management

   a. The cause for the anemia is usually explored; stools are examined for occult blood; endoscopic examination and other diagnostic procedures may be performed to rule out possible sources of bleeding, which is a common cause of iron deficiency

   b. Increase intake of iron-rich foods (see Box 14-2)

   c. Vitamin supplementation; administration of oral iron preparation in the form of ferrous sulfate

   d. Parenteral administration of iron

5. Priority nursing diagnoses: Activity intolerance; Risk for decreased cardiac output; Risk for injury; Ineffective health maintenance

Box 14-2	Organ meat	Beans
Sources of Dietary Iron	Meat	Molasses
	Green leafy vegetables	Raisins

6. Planning and implementation

NCLEX!

 a. Administer oral iron preparation with orange juice or vitamin C to increase absorption; antacids interfere with the absorption of iron

NCLEX!

 b. Administer parenteral iron deep intramuscularly via the Z-track method

 c. Identify/implement energy-saving techniques, e.g., shower chair, sitting to perform tasks

 d. Promote quiet environment to facilitate sleep/rest

 e. Monitor for dizziness, suggest position changes be made slowly

 f. Provide/recommend assistance with activities/ambulation as needed, allowing patient independence as much as needed

 g. Monitor laboratory studies, e.g., Hgb/Hct, RBC count

 h. Administer medications, blood or blood products as indicated; monitor closely for transfusion reactions

 i. Encourage/assist with good oral hygiene before and after meals, using soft bristled toothbrush for gentle brushing of fragile gums

 j. Determine stool color, consistency, frequency, and amount

 k. Encourage fluid intake of 2,500 to 3,000 mL day

 l. Discuss use of stool softeners, bulk-forming laxatives, mild stimulants, or enemas if indicated; monitor effectiveness

NCLEX!

 m. Oral liquid form of iron can stain the teeth; clients should use a straw or place spoon at the back of the mouth to take the supplement and rinse mouth thoroughly afterward

 n. Caution client that bowel movement may appear greenish black/tarry

 o. Deep IM, Z-track administration of medication; use separate needles for withdrawing and injecting the medication

 p. Caution regarding possible systemic (allergic) reactions to the medication, e.g., (flushing, nausea/vomiting, myalgias) and the importance of reporting symptoms

 q. Refer to appropriate community resources when indicated, e.g., social services for food stamps, meals on wheels

7. Medication therapy

 a. Usual therapy is oral ferrous sulfate ($FeSO_4$) 300 to 325 mg t.i.d., given 1 hr before meals for 6 months; other oral forms may include ferrous gluconate (Fergon) and ferrous fumarate (Ircon, Femiron)

      b. If the client is unable to tolerate oral therapy, iron dextran (INFeD) may be given by deep IM (Z-track) route or as IV therapy; there is risk of anaphylaxis with parenteral administration; therefore, before a full dose is given a small test dose is administered

      c. Transfusion of packed RBCs may be necessary if anemia is severe

  8. Client education

      a. Teach clients to maintain good nutrition; the elderly and those with limited economic means may have dietary deficiencies requiring referrals to appropriate agencies (e.g., Meals on Wheels)

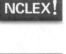

      b. Teach client to take iron on an empty stomach; absorption of iron is decreased with food; absorption may be enhanced when taken with an acidic beverage (such as one with vitamin C); but avoid grapefruit juice

      c. Inform clients that their stools will appear black with the oral intake of iron

      d. Teach the client to report to the healthcare provider persistent GI symptoms secondary to iron intake

      e. Clients should be informed that iron preparations cause constipation; the addition of a stool softener may be necessary; other measures such as increasing oral intake of fluids and fiber will prevent constipation

      f. Review required diet alterations to meet specific dietary needs; foods high in iron include organ meats (beef or calf's liver, chicken liver), other meats, beans (black, pinto, and garbanzo), leafy green vegetables, raisins, and molasses

  9. Evaluation

      a. Client verbalizes dietary sources of iron

      b. Client demonstrates increasing activity tolerance

      c. Client reports decrease in or resolution of symptoms

B. Megaloblastic anemia

  1. Vitamin B_{12} deficiency anemia

      a. Description: a type of anemia characterized by macrocytic red blood cells

      b. Etiology and pathophysiology

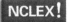

         1) Inevitably develops after total gastrectomy, with 15 percent of clients developing pernicious anemia after partial gastrectomy or gastrojejunostomy

         2) Lack of vitamin B_{12} alters the structure and disrupts the function of the peripheral nerves, spinal cord, and brain

         3) Lack of vitamin B_{12} impairs cellular division and maturation especially in rapidly proliferating RBCs

         4) Pernicious anemia is the body's inability to absorb vitamin B_{12} because of a lack of intrinsic factor, a substance secreted by the parietal cells of the gastric mucosa

c. Assessment

   1) Clinical manifestations: signs and symptoms include pallor or slight jaundice with a complaint of weakness; smooth, sore, beefy red tongue (**glossitis**), with diarrhea; paresthesias (altered sensations such as numbness or tingling in the extremities), impaired proprioception (difficulty identifying one's position in space, which may progress to difficulty with balance); clients with this anemia tend to be fair-haired or prematurely gray

   2) Diagnostic and laboratory tests

     a) Macrocytic (megaloblastic) anemia (RBC diameter > 8)

     b) Laboratory examination shows an increase in the MCV and MCHC

     c) Gastric secretion analysis reveals achlorhydria: the absence of free hydrochloric acid in a pH maintained at 3.5

     d) 24 hour urine for Schilling test (a vitamin B_{12} absorption test that indicates if a client lacks intrinsic factor by measuring the excretion of orally administered radionuclide labeled B_{12}) confirms the diagnosis of pernicious anemia

d. Therapeutic management

   1) Review required diet alterations to meet specific dietary needs; if the deficiency is caused by a vegetarian diet, fortified soy milk may be added to the diet, or oral supplements of B_{12} may be added

   2) If the deficiency is caused by gastric malabsorption such as deficiency of intrinsic factor, lifelong replacement therapy is required; an intramuscular injection of B_{12} is required and in some situations megadoses or oral vitamins may be given

e. Priority nursing diagnoses: Risk for injury; Activity intolerance; Altered oral mucous membrane

f. Planning and implementation: the major nursing consideration in the care of the client with this type of anemia is client education pertaining to nutrition and medications (see section h below); the client should be assessed carefully for neurologic deficits and incorporate in the plan of care interventions relating to prevention of injury

g. Medication therapy: parenteral vitamin B_{12}, 100 to 1000 micrograms subcutaneously daily for 7 days, then once a week for 1 month, then monthly for the remainder of life is usually prescribed to clients with this type of anemia

h. Client education

   1) Inform client that the burning sensation felt after a parenteral dose of vitamin B_{12} is temporary

   2) Discuss dietary sources of vitamin B_{12} like dairy products, animal proteins, and eggs

   3) For clients who have pernicious anemia, discuss the regular schedule of parenterally administered vitamin B_{12} and the importance and necessity for continued treatment

     i. Evaluation

       1) Client reports resolution of paresthesia

       2) No injuries are sustained secondary from loss of balance

       3) Self-reports of increased tolerance to activity

  2. Folic acid deficiency anemia

     a. Description: anemia caused by a deficiency of folic acid resulting in the interruption of DNA synthesis and normal maturation of red blood cells

     b. Etiology and pathophysiology

       1) Causative etiology: poor nutrition, malabsorption syndrome, medications that impede the absorption (oral contraceptives, anticonvulsants, methotrexate [MTX]), alcohol abuse, and anorexia

       2) Alcoholics and those receiving total parenteral nutrition are at risk

       3) Pregnant women, infants, and teenagers are also at risk for the development of folic acid deficiency

       4) Clients on hemodialysis are also at risk for the development of folic acid deficiency

       5) Lack of folic acid causes the formation of megaloblastic cells; these cells are fragile

     c. Assessment

       1) Clinical manifestations: pallor, progressive weakness, fatigue, shortness of breath, cardiac palpitations; GI symptoms are similar to B_{12} deficiency, but usually more severe (glossitis, cheilosis, and diarrhea); neurological symptoms seen in B_{12} deficiency are not seen in folic acid deficiency and therefore assist in the differentiation of these two types of anemia

       2) Diagnostic and laboratory tests

         a) Macrocytic (megaloblastic) anemia (RBC diameter > 8)

         b) MCV high with low hemoglobin

         c) Low serum folate level

     d. Therapeutic management: includes dietary counseling and the administration of folic acid

     e. Priority nursing diagnoses: Activity intolerance; Constipation; Diarrhea; Risk for infection

     f. Planning and implementation

       1) Identify/implement energy-saving techniques, e.g., shower chair, sitting to perform tasks

       2) Monitor for dizziness, suggest position changes be made slowly

       3) Provide/recommend assistance with activities/ambulation as needed, allowing client independence as much as needed

       4) Monitor laboratory studies, e.g., Hgb/Hct, RBC count

5) Encourage/assist with good oral hygiene before and after meals, using soft bristled toothbrush for gentle brushing of fragile gums

6) Refer to appropriate community resources when indicated, e.g., social services for food stamps, Meals on Wheels, Alcoholics Anonymous

g. Medication therapy: oral folate, 1 to 5 mg/day for 3 to 4 months; folate should be given along with vitamin B_{12} when both are deficient

h. Client education

1) Discuss with client the dietary sources of folic acid such as green leafy vegetables, fish, citrus fruits, yeast, dried beans, grains, nuts, and liver

2) Teach clients who are at risk for the development of folic acid deficiency (alcoholism, clients on hemodialysis and certain drugs) to increase their dietary intake through diet selection and supplementation

3) Discuss with client strategies to decrease pain associated with glossitis such as eating bland and soft foods

i. Evaluation

1) The client verbalizes decrease in or resolution of symptoms

2) The client selects foods that are high in folic acid

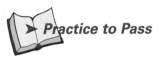

Practice to Pass

A client with folic acid deficiency anemia asks you why he developed this type of anemia. What would your response be?

C. Aplastic anemia

1. Description: aplastic anemia is a form of anemia resulting in decreased production of bone marrow elements, namely erythrocytes, leukocytes, and platelets

2. Etiology and pathophysiology

a. Affects all age groups and both genders

b. Two classifications of aplastic anemia include congenital or acquired; congenital aplastic anemia is caused by a chromosomal alteration; acquired form of the disease may be caused by radiation, chemical agents and toxins, drugs, viral and bacterial infections, pregnancy, and idiopathic; in about 50 percent of cases, the cause is unknown

c. There is a decrease or cessation of production of RBCs (anemia), WBCs (leukopenia), and platelets (**thrombocytopenia**); the decrease may result from damage to bone marrow stem cells, the bone marrow itself, and the replacement of bone marrow with fat; depending on the causative factor, the condition may be acute or chronic

3. Assessment

a. Clinical manifestations

1) Pallor

2) Fatigue

3) Palpitations

4) Exertional dyspnea

5) Infections of the skin and mucous membranes

6) Bleeding from gums, nose, vagina, or rectum

7) Purpura (bruising)

8) Retinal hemorrhage

b. Diagnostic and laboratory tests

1) Blood counts reveal pancytopenia (decreased RBC, WBC, and platelets)

2) Decreased reticulocyte count

3) Bone marrow examination reveals decrease in activity of the bone marrow or no cell activity

4. Therapeutic management

a. Identification of the cause of bone marrow suppression

b. Bone marrow transplantation

c. Immunosuppression

d. Transfusion of leukocyte-poor RBCs

e. Splenectomy

5. Priority nursing diagnoses: Risk for infection; Risk for bleeding; and Activity intolerance

6. Planning and implementation

a. Institute reverse isolation

b. Limit visitors and potential sources of infection

c. Monitor for evidence of bleeding

d. Avoid invasive procedures including rectal temperatures

e. Provide frequent rest periods

f. Monitor tolerance to activities

7. Medication therapy

a. Agents that suppress lymphocyte activity such as antilymphocyte globulin (ALG), antithymocyte globulin (ATG), and cyclosporine (Sandimmune)

b. Immunosuppresive agents such as prednisone and cyclophosphamide (Cytoxan)

8. Client education

a. Teach client ways to prevent infection such as avoiding crowds, maintaining good hygiene, handwashing, and elimination of uncooked foods from the diet

b. Discuss ways to prevent hemorrhage such as using a soft toothbrush, avoiding contact sports, and use of an electric razor

c. Emphasize the avoidance of drugs that increase bleeding tendency such as aspirin

d. Teach client to balance activity with adequate rest periods to avoid fatigue

e. Teach client about symptoms to report to the healthcare provider including signs of infection, bleeding, and increasing intolerance to activity

9. Evaluation

    a. Client verbalizes ways to prevent infection, bleeding, and fatigue

    b. Client does not develop infection

    c. Client does not develop hemorrhage

D. Sickle cell disease

  1. Definition: a hereditary, chronic form of hemolytic anemia

  2. Etiology and pathophysiology

    a. Eight percent of African-Americans are heterozygous (carriers) for sickle cell anemia thereby inheriting one affected gene or the sickle cell trait

    b. One percent of African-Americans are homozygous (identical genes) for the disorder, thereby inheriting a defective gene from both parents or sickle cell anemia and are likely to experience sickle cell crisis

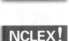

    c. Sickle cell trait (heterozygous state) is a generally mild condition that produces few, if any, manifestations

    d. Sickle cell anemia is caused by an autosomal genetic defect (one gene affected) that results in the synthesis of hemoglobin S

    e. Produced by a mutation in the beta chain of the hemoglobin molecule through a substitution of the amino acid valine for glutamine in both beta chains

    f. During decreased oxygen tension in the plasma, the hemoglobin S causes the RBCs to elongate, become rigid, and assume a crescent, sickled shape causing the cells to clump together, obstruct capillary blood flow causing ischemia and possible tissue infarction

    g. Conditions likely to trigger a sickle cell crisis include: hypoxia, low environmental and/or body temperature, excessive exercise, high altitudes, or inadequate oxygen during anesthesia

    h. Other causes of sickle cell crisis include: elevated blood viscosity/decreased plasma volume, infection, dehydration, and/or increased hydrogen ion concentration (acidosis)

    i. With normal oxygenation, the sickled RBCs resume their normal shape; repeated episodes of sickling and unsickling weaken the cell membrane, causing them to hemolyze and be removed

    j. Crisis is extremely painful and can last from 4 to 6 days

  3. Assessment

    a. Clinical manifestations

      1) Pallor

      2) Jaundice

      3) Fatigue

      4) Irritability

      5) Large joints and surrounding tissue may become swollen during crisis

      6) **Priapism** (abnormal, painful, continuous erection of the penis) may occur if penile veins are obstructed

      7) Pain

   b. Diagnostic and laboratory tests

      1) Anemia with sickled cells noted on a peripheral smear

      2) Hemoglobin electrophoresis: a blood test that causes the hemoglobin molecule to migrate in solution in response to electric currents to determine the presence and percentage of hemoglobin S; used for a definitive diagnosis

      3) Elevated serum bilrubin levels

      4) Elevated reticulocyte count

4. Therapeutic management

   a. Bone marrow transplantation

   b. Blood transfusions

   c. Management of pain

   d. Use of chemotherapy drug hydroxyurea (Droxia) to increase hemoglobin F and decrease sickling

5. Priority nursing diagnoses: Pain; Ineffective tissue perfusion; Impaired gas exchange; Risk for infection; and Knowledge deficit

6. Planning and implementation

   a. Teach clients ways to prevent development of sickle cell crisis (see client education)

   b. Refer to appropriate agency for genetic counseling and family planning

   c. Clients who are in crisis should have the following included

      1) Management of pain

      2) Administration of oxygen

      3) Promoting hydration to decrease blood viscocity; the client in crisis should have an oral intake of at least 6 to 8 quarts/day or IV fluids of 3 liters/day

      4) Monitor for complications such as vaso-occlusive disease (thrombosis), hypoxia, CVA, renal dysfunction, priapism leading to impotence, acute chest syndrome (fever, chest pain, cough, pulmonary infiltrates, and dyspnea), and substance abuse

      5) Management of infection

   d. Administer care with attention to culture; avoid racial bias or cultural insensitivity

7. Medication therapy

   a. Nifedipine (Procardia) may be used for priapism

   b. Hydroxyurea (Droxia) to increase hemoglobin F and decrease sickling

NCLEX!

    c. Narcotic (opioid) analgesics during the acute phase of sickle cell crisis, often at large doses

    d. Broad-spectrum antibiotics to manage acute chest syndrome

    e. Folic acid supplements

8. Client education

NCLEX!

    a. Teach client ways to prevent sickle cell crisis; these instructions should include:

        1) Maintain adequate fluid intake; clients with sickle cell disease should maintain an oral intake of at least 4 to 6 quarts/day; avoid conditions that might predispose them to dehydration

        2) Avoid high altitudes

        3) Prevent and promptly treat infections

        4) Stress-reduction strategies

        5) Avoid exposure to cold

        6) Avoid overexertion

    b. Discuss the importance of adhering to vaccination schedules for pneumococcal pneumonia, haemophilus influenza type B, and hepatitis B

    c. Importance of regular medical follow-up

9. Evaluation

    a. Client verbalizes pain relief

    b. Client does not develop an infection

    c. Client adheres to vaccination schedule

    d. Client identifies precipitating factor/s leading to crisis state

E. Polycythemia

1. Description: an increase in the number of circulating erythrocytes and the concentration of hemoglobin in the blood; also known as polycythemia vera, PV, or myeloproliferative red cell disorder; polycythemia can be primary or secondary

2. Etiology and pathophysiology

    a. Primary

        1) Common in men of European Jewish descent

        2) Neoplastic stem cell disorder characterized by increased production of RBCs, granulocytes, and platelets

        3) With the overproduction of erythrocytes, increased blood viscocity results in congestion of blood in tissues, the liver, and spleen

        4) Thrombi form, acidosis develops, and tissue infarction occurs as a result of the diminished circulatory flow of blood caused by the increased viscosity

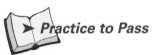

Practice to Pass

A client with sickle cell trait asks you the implications if she gets married to someone with sickle trait. How should you respond?

    b. Secondary

       1) Most common form of polycythemia vera

       2) The disturbance is not in the development of red blood cells but in the abnormal increase of erythropoietin, causing excessive erythropoiesis

       3) The increase in red blood cell production caused by increased erythropoietin release is a physiologic response to hypoxia; hypoxia stimulates the release of erythropoietin in the kidney

       4) Chronic hypoxic states may be produced by prolonged exposure to high altitudes, pulmonary diseases, hypoventilation, and smoking

       5) The results of an increased RBC production include the increased viscosity of blood, which alters circulatory flow

3. Assessment

    a. Clinical manifestations

       1) **Plethora:** a ruddy (dark, flushed) color of the face, hands, feet, ears, and mucous membranes resulting from the engorgement or distention of blood vessels

       2) Symptoms associated with increased blood volume including headaches, vertigo, blurred vision, and tinnitus

       3) Distended superficial veins

       4) Itching unrelieved by antihistamines

       5) Symptoms associated with impaired tissue oxygenation including angina, claudication, or dyspnea

       6) **Erythromyalgia,** or burning sensation of the fingers and toes

       7) Splenomegaly in majority of those with primary polycythemia vera

       8) Epistaxis, GI bleeding

    b. Diagnostic and laboratory tests

       1) Elevated hemoglobin and erythrocyte count

       2) Decreased MCHC

       3) Increased WBC and basophilia

       4) Increased platelets

       5) Elevated leukocyte alkaline phosphatase

       6) Elevated uric acid

       7) Elevated cobalamin levels

       8) Increased histamine levels

       9) Bone marrow examination shows hypercellularity

4. Therapeutic management

    a. Management of the underlying condition (such as COPD) causing the chronic hypoxia

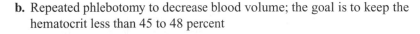

    b. Repeated phlebotomy to decrease blood volume; the goal is to keep the hematocrit less than 45 to 48 percent

    c. Hydration to decrease blood viscosity

5. Priority nursing diagnoses: Impaired gas exchange; Pain; Risk for infection

6. Planning and implementation

    a. Assist in phlebotomy

    b. Measures to relieve pruritus including cool and tepid baths

    c. Accurate monitoring of fluid intake and output

    d. Nursing measures to prevent thrombotic events including early ambulation, passive leg exercises when on bed rest, avoid crossing legs, and maintaining adequate hydration

    e. Administration of medications for the prevention of complications including anticoagulants

7. Medication therapy

    a. Myelosuppressive agents to inhibit bone marrow activity including hydroxyurea (Hydrea), melphalan (Alkeran), and radioactive phosphorus

    b. Allopurinol to manage gout

    c. Antiplatelet agents to prevent thrombotic complications

8. Client education

    a. Teach client about the importance of maintaining good hydration; the client should drink at least 3 liters of fluid per day

    b. Teach client about the disease and ways in which it can be controlled, such as smoking cessation

    c. Discuss signs and symptoms of complications associated with the disorder including signs of vaso-occlusive states (MI, CVA) and bleeding that require immediate medical attention

    d. Teach client to prevent bleeding states such as using a razor, using soft-bristled toothbrush, not flossing, and avoiding the use of aspirin and aspirin-containing products

    e. Emphasize the importance of a regular medical check-up

    f. Teach client to avoid products that contain iron

    g. Discuss ways of preventing thrombosis

9. Evaluation

    a. The hematocrit is within normal range

    b. The client does not develop complications associated with thrombus formation

    c. The client maintains adequate hydration

F. Thrombocytopenia

1. Definition: a decrease in the number of circulating platelets or a platelet count of less than 100,000 platelets per milliliter of blood resulting in problems of hemostasis

2. Etiology and pathophysiology

   a. The decrease in the number of circulating platelets may be a result of three mechanisms: decreased production, increased destruction, or increased consumption

   b. The cause of decreased production of platelets may be inherited or acquired

   c. Increased destruction of platelets may be caused by an immune system defect; the platelets become coated with an antibody; when these antibody coated platelets reach the spleen, they are recognized as foreign and are destroyed; platelets normally have a circulating life of 8 to 10 days but this immune response shortens their life cycle; this condition is referred to as immune thrombocytopenic purpura (ITP); the acute form of this disorder is more common in children whereas the chronic form is more common in women between the ages of 20 to 50

   d. Other causes of increased destruction of platelets include non–immune-related factors such as infection or drug-induced effects

   e. A decrease in the number of functional platelets leads to bleeding disorders; cerebral and pulmonary hemorrhage can occur when platelet counts drop below 10,000/mm^3

3. Assessment

   a. Clinical manifestations

      1) Petechiae and purpura most commonly found in the anterior thorax, arms, and neck

      2) Epistaxis, gingival bleeding, menorrhagia, hematuria, and gastrointestinal bleeding

      3) Signs of internal hemorrhage

   b. Diagnostic and laboratory tests

      1) Decreased hemoglobin and hematocrit if bleeding is present

      2) Decreased platelet count

      3) Prolonged bleeding time

      4) Bone marrow examination to determine the etiology; may reveal decreased platelet activity or increased megakaryocytes

4. Therapeutic management

   a. Treatment of the underlying cause or removal of the causative agent

   b. Use of immunosuppressive and chemotherapeutic agents in cases of ITP

   c. Platelet transfusions if there is active bleeding; little benefit in ITP

   d. Splenectomy in ITP

5. Priority nursing diagnoses: Risk for Injury: bleeding; Fatigue; Altered oral mucous membrane

6. Planning and implementation

   a. Institute bleeding (thrombocytopenic) precautions

     1) Avoid intramuscular or subcutaneous injections

     2) Avoid indwelling catheters

     3) If absolutely necessary use smallest-gauge needles for injections or venipunctures; apply pressure on injection sites for 5 minutes or until bleeding stops

     4) Discourage straining at stool, vigorous coughing, and nose blowing

     5) Avoid rectal manipulation such as rectal temperatures, suppositories, or enemas

     6) Discourage the use of razors; use only electric shavers

     7) Use soft-bristled toothbrush or toothettes and avoid flossing

     8) Pad side rails if necessary and avoid tissue trauma

     9) Avoid the use of aspirin and drugs that interfere with blood coagulation

   b. Monitor for signs of bleeding; test stools for occult blood

   c. Monitor CBC and platelet counts

   d. Administer platelets as ordered

   e. Monitor response to therapy

7. Medication therapy

   a. Steroids and immunoglobulins may be used to suppress the immune response in ITP

   b. Immunosuppressive agents may be used such as vincristine (Oncovin) and cyclophosphamide (Cytoxan)

   c. Platelet growth factor such as oprelvekin (Neumega)

8. Client education

   a. Teach the client and family to monitor for signs of bleeding and when to contact the primary care provider

   b. Include instructions on bleeding precautions such as the use of soft-bristled toothbrush, avoidance of flossing, prevention of tissue trauma and injury including vigorous sexual intercourse, and using an electric razor for shaving

   c. Teach client to avoid drugs that contain aspirin and others that interfere with coagulation

   d. Discuss medication dosing, schedule, and side effects

   e. Teach the importance of regular medical follow-up and platelet monitoring

9. Evaluation

   a. There is no evidence of bleeding

   b. Client has increased platelet count

      c. Client verbalizes knowledge of medication actions and precautions

      d. Client identifies methods to monitor for signs of occult bleeding

G. Hemophilia

    1. Description: a group of hereditary clotting factor disorders characterized by prolonged coagulation time that results in prolonged and sometimes excessive bleeding

    2. Etiology and pathophysiology

      a. Hemophilia A and B are X-linked recessive disorders transmitted by female carriers, displayed almost exclusively in males

      b. *Hemophilia A* (classic hemophilia) is a deficiency in Factor VIII (an alpha globulin that stabilizes fibrin clots; it is the most common form of hemophilia

      c. *Hemophilia B* (Christmas disease) is a deficiency in Factor IX; (a vitamin-dependent beta globulin essential in stage 1 of the intrinsic coagulation system as an influence on the amount of thromboplastin available)

      d. Despite the difference in factor deficiency, hemophilia A and B are clinically identical

      e. In clients with hemophilia A and B, platelet plugs are formed at the site of bleeding, but the clotting factor impairs the coagulation response and the capacity to form a stable clot

      f. *Von Willebrand's disease* is a related disorder caused by a deficiency of the von Willebrand's factor (vWF), which is necessary for factor VIII activity and platelet adhesion; this disorder affects men and women equally

    3. Assessment

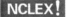

      a. Clinical manifestations

        1) Persistent and prolonged bleeding from small cuts and injuries

        2) Delay of onset of bleeding after an injury

        3) Subcutaneous ecchymosis and subcutaneous hematomas

        4) Gingival bleeding

        5) Gastrointestinal bleeding, which may be manifested by hematemesis (vomiting blood), occult blood in the stools, gastric pain, or abdominal pain

        6) Urinary tract bleeding (hematuria)

        7) Pain, paresthesias, or paralysis resulting from nerve compression of the hematomas

        8) **Hemarthrosis** (joint bleeding, swelling and damage)

      b. Diagnostic and laboratory tests

        1) Specific factor assays are used to determine the type of hemophilia present

        2) APTT is increased in all types of hemophilia

   3) Bleeding time is prolonged in von Willebrand's disease

   4) Decreased factor VIII in hemophilia A, vWF in von Willebrand's disease, and factor IX in hemophilia B

4. Therapeutic management

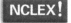

   a. Treatment is the replacement of the deficient coagulation factor(s)

   b. Hemophilia A: cryoprecipitate containing 8 to 100 units of factor VIII per bag at 12-hour intervals until bleeding ceases; freeze-dried concentrate of factor VIII may also be given

   c. Hemophilia B: plasma or factor IX concentrate given q 24 hours or until bleeding ceases

   d. Von Willebrand's disease: cryoprecipitate containing 8 to 100 units of factor VIII per bag at 12-hour intervals until bleeding ceases; desmopressin (DDAVP) given intravenously may also be used

   e. Supportive treatment for hemarthrosis including arthrocentesis and physiotherapy

   f. Control of topical bleeding with hemostatic agents, pressure, and application of ice

   g. Management of complications associated with hemorrhage

5. Priority nursing diagnoses: Risk for injury, bleeding; Decreased cardiac output; Deficient fluid volume; and Risk for ineffective therapeutic regimen management

6. Planning and implementation

   a. Teach the client and family about the disease and therapeutic regimen

   b. Refer for genetic counseling and family planning

   c. Refer to the National Hemophilia Foundation for support and counseling

   d. Monitor for signs of complications including hemarthrosis and intracranial bleeding

   e. Assist in the management of pain associated with hemarthrosis; measures include joint immobilization, application of ice, and administration of analgesics; aspirin and drugs affecting coagulation are avoided

   f. Control bleeding and maintain hemostasis through direct pressure, application of topical hemostatic agents, and application of ice

   g. Administer medications as prescribed

7. Medication therapy: see therapeutic management

8. Client education

   a. Discuss with client and family signs and symptoms requiring immediate medical attention, which includes severe joint pain, trauma or injury, and signs of uncontrolled internal bleeding

   b. Teach the client and family precautions to prevent bleeding including the use of soft bristled toothbrush, avoid flossing, use of electric razor, avoiding contact sports or activities most likely to cause injury, and avoidance of aspirin and other drugs that interfere with coagulation

   c. Teach the client about the importance of wearing a Medic-Alert bracelet indicating the hemophilia

   d. Emphasize the need to maintain good dental hygiene to decrease the necessity of invasive dental procedures

   e. Emphasize the importance of adhering to scheduled visits and follow-up care with the primary health provider

9. Evaluation

   a. The client identifies strategies to prevent injury and bleeding precautions

   b. There is no evidence of internal bleeding including hemarthrosis

   c. The client and family seek support from the local chapter of the National Hemophilia Society

H. Disseminated intravascular coagulopathy (or coagulation)

1. Description: disseminated intravascular coagulopathy or **consumption coagulopathy** is a syndrome characterized by abnormal initiation and acceleration of clotting and simultaneous hemorrhage; the paradoxical bleeding that occurs is a result of the consumption of clotting factors and platelets; the syndrome is usually precipitated by an underlying pathologic condition

2. Etiology and pathophysiology

   a. Mortality rate associated with DIC is as high as 80 percent with the most frequent sequela being hemorrhage

   b. The syndrome is precipitated by conditions such as widespread tissue damage, hemolysis, hypotension, hypoxia, and metabolic acidosis (see Box 14-3)

   NCLEX!

   c. The underlying condition causes initiation and widespread formation of clots in the vascular system either through the activation of factor XII, factors II and X, or the release of tissue thromboplastin; substances necessary for clotting are used at a more rapid rate than they can be replaced

   d. As the clotting continues, the fibrinolytic pathway is activated to dissolve the clots formed; clotting factors become depleted while fibrinolysis continues; platelets decrease, clotting factors II, V, VIII, and fibrinogen are depleted

   e. Fibrin degradation products (FDP) are released as a result of fibrinolysis; fibrin degradation products (FDP), which are potent anticoagulants used to lyse the clots further, increase the bleeding state

Box 14-3		
Risk Factors for DIC	Venomous snakebite	Tissue necrosis
	Sepsis	Drug reactions
	Trauma	Liver disease
	Obstetric complications	Acute hemolysis
	Neoplasms	Extensive burns
	Vascular disorders	Prosthetic devices
	Hypoxia	

    f. With the depletion of clotting factors and the increase in fibrin degradation products, stable blood clots no longer form and hemorrhage occurs

3. Assessment

    a. Clinical manifestations (see Box 14-4)

    b. Diagnostic and laboratory tests

        1) Prothrombin time: prolonged

        2) Partial thromboplastin time: prolonged

        3) Thrombin time: prolonged

        4) Fibrinogen: decreased

        5) Platelets: decreased

        6) Fibrin split (degradation) products: elevated

        7) Factor assays (factors V, VII, VIII, X, XIII): reduced

        8) D-dimers: elevated

NCLEX!

4. Therapeutic management

    a. The priority of therapeutic management is to initiate treatment of the underlying medical condition that precipitated DIC

    b. Supportive treatment for the manifestations of DIC such as the control of bleeding; life-threatening hemorrhage may be treated by administering specific blood components based on the identified deficiency: platelets for

---

Box 14-4

Clinical Manifestations of DIC

Integumentary
Decreased skin temperature
Pallor
Purpura
Ecchymoses
Hematomas
Acral cyanosis
Altered sensation
Superficial gangrene
Gingival bleeding
Bleeding from puncture sites

Gastrointestinal
Hemoptysis
Melena
Occult blood in stool or vomitus
Abdominal distention
Abdominal pain

Respiratory
Dyspnea
Tachypnea
Orthopnea
Decreased breath sounds
Chest pain

Cardiovascular
Decreased pulses
Decreased capillary filling time
Tachycardia
Venous distention

Genitourinary
Hematuria
Oliguria

Nervous System
Vision changes
Dizziness
Headache
Irritability
Anxiety
Confusion
Seizures

Musculoskeletal
Joint pain
Bone pain
Weakness

thrombocytopenia; cryoprecipitate to replace fibrinogen, and factors V and VII; and fresh frozen plasma to replace all clotting factors except platelets

    c. Use of heparin or antithrombin III (AT-III) to control intravascular clotting; their use is controversial

5. Priority nursing diagnoses: Impaired gas exchange; Ineffective tissue perfusion; Risk for deficient fluid volume; Pain; and Decreased cardiac output

6. Planning and implementation

    a. Assess client carefully for evidence of bleeding and altered tissue oxygenation

    b. Institute thrombocytopenic precautions (refer to previous discussion on thrombocytopenia)

    c. Monitor intake and output hourly

    d. Administer blood products as indicated by the healthcare provider

    e. Monitor for signs of complications such as renal failure, pulmonary embolism, cerebrovascular accident, and acute respiratory distress syndrome

    f. Monitor effectiveness of therapy and pharmacologic interventions

    g. Provide emotional support to client and family

7. Medication therapy

    a. Heparin and antithrombin III, although their use is controversial; these drugs are usually indicated to manage thrombosis

    b. Epsilon aminocaproic acid (Amicar) to inhibit fibrinolysis

    c. Blood products (FFP, platelets, and cryoprecipitate)

8. Client education

    a. Teach the client and family regarding the syndrome and explain treatments and interventions

    b. Teach the client to report symptoms of complications including abdominal pain, headache, visual disturbances, and pain

    c. Discuss with the client and family thrombocytopenic precautions (see client education in the discussion of thrombocytopenia)

9. Evaluation

    a. The client's hemodynamic status is maintained

    b. Peripheral pulses remain intact

    c. Skin remains intact

I. Neutropenia

1. Description: refers to a decrease (less than 2,000/mm^3) in the neutrophil count either as a result of decreased production or increased destruction; the neutrophil plays a major role in phagocytosis of disease-producing microorganisms; consequently, a decrease in their numbers increases the individual's risk for infection

2. Etiology and pathophysiology

   a. Neutropenia is not a disease but a syndrome

   b. Neutropenia may occur as a primary hematologic disorder but may also be caused by drugs, autoimmune disorders, infections, and other medical conditions such as severe sepsis and nutritional deficiencies

   c. If the leukocyte count is decreased, or if immature white blood cells predominate in the circulation, the normal phagocytic function of these cells is impaired; when phagocytic activity is decreased, the client with neutropenia is susceptible to both exogenous and endogenous sources of infection; minor infections may progress to the more serious sepsis

   d. Neutrophils constitute about 70 percent of the total circulating white blood cells. Normally, the neutrophil count is above 2,000/mm^3; the absolute neutrophil count (ANC) is determined by the following formula:

   $$\frac{\%\ \text{neutrophils} + \%\ \text{bands}}{100} \times \text{total WBC count} = \text{ANC}$$

3. Assessment

   a. Clinical manifestations: there are no real symptoms associated with neutropenia

   b. Diagnostic and laboratory tests

      1) Neutrophil count less than 1,000 to 1,500

      2) Bone marrow examination to examine cell morphology helps distinguish the etiologic factor causing the neutropenia

4. Therapeutic management

   a. If the etiology of neutropenia is drug-induced, discontinuation of the medication is indicated

   b. Corticosteroids are used if the etiology is immunologic

   c. If the etiology is decreased production, growth factors (granulocyte/macrophage colony stimulating factor or GM-CSF) may be used

   d. If client develops a fever, identification and treatment of the infection is instituted

5. Priority nursing diagnoses: Risk for infection; Knowledge deficit; and Anxiety

6. Planning and implementation

   a. Monitor for signs of infection; monitor temperature elevations

   b. Obtain cultures suspected as sites of infection

   c. Administer antibiotics as prescribed and evaluate their effectiveness

   d. Administer medications that stimulate the production of neutrophils

   e. Enforce strict hand-washing by all individuals in contact with the client

   f. Institute reverse isolation; use private room with HEPA filtration if possible

   g. Avoid invasive procedures

   h. Fresh flowers and fruits should not be permitted in the client's room

7. Medication therapy: Growth factors such as G-SF (Neupogen) or granulocyte/macrophage-colony-stimulating factor (Leukine) is given to increase the neutrophil count

NCLEX!

8. Client education

   a. Teach client and family to report signs of fever

   b. Teach the client and individuals who come in contact with the client about strict hand-washing and reverse isolation procedure

   c. Teach client methods to maintain good personal hygiene

   d. Explain to the client and family about the condition and the rationale of therapeutic interventions

9. Evaluation

   a. The absolute neutrophil count normalizes

   b. The client is free of infection

   c. The client and family verbalize methods of limiting exposure to pathogens

J. Leukemia

1. Definition: a malignant disorder of the blood-forming tissues of the bone marrow, spleen, and lymph system characterized by unregulated proliferation of WBCs and their precursors

2. Etiology and pathophysiology

NCLEX!

   a. The type of WBC affected (granulocyte, lymphocyte, monocyte) and the duration of the disease (acute or chronic) is the basis of the classification of the different types of leukemia; if the majority of the leukemia cells are primitive, the leukemia is classified as acute; if the leukemic cells are mostly mature (well-differentiated), the leukemia is classified as chronic

      1) Acute lymphocytic/lymphoblastic leukemia (ALL)

         a) Peak incidence at 2 to 4 years of age

         b) Immature granulocytes proliferate and accumulate in the marrow

      2) Chronic lymphocytic leukemia (CLL)

         a) More common in men and mainly between the ages of 50 and 70

         b) Abnormal and incompetent lymphocytes proliferate and accumulate in the lymph nodes and spreads to other lymphatic tissues and the spleen; most of the circulating cells are mature lymphocytes

      3) Acute myelogenous/myelocytic leukemia (AML)

         a) All age groups are affected with a peak incidence at age 60

         b) There is uncontrolled proliferation of myeloblasts, which are the precursors of granulocytes; they accumulate in the bone marrow

      4) Chronic myelogenous leukemia (CML)

         a) Uncommon in people under 20 years of age; the incidence rises with age

b) There is uncontrolled proliferation of granulocytes resulting in increased circulating blast (immature) cells; the marrow expands into long bones because of this proliferation and also extends into the liver and spleen

NCLEX!

c) In most cases the Philadelphia chromosome, a characteristic chromosomal abnormality, is present

b. Abnormal or immature WBCs do not function properly because of the massive proliferation of these abnormal immature cells; abnormal cells can continue to multiply, infiltrate, and damage the bone marrow, spleen, lymph nodes, liver, kidneys, lungs, gonads, skin, and central nervous system (CNS)

c. Normal bone marrow becomes diffusely replaced with abnormal or immature WBCs, interfering with the bone marrow's ability to produce other types of cells such as erythrocytes and thrombocytes; the bone marrow becomes functionally incompetent with resulting bone marrow suppression

d. Acute leukemia has a rapid onset, progresses rapidly, with a short clinical course; left untreated, death will result in days or months; the symptoms of acute leukemia relate to a depressed bone marrow, infiltration of leukemic cells into other organ systems, and hypermetabolism of leukemia cells

NCLEX!

e. Chronic leukemia has a more insidious onset with a more prolonged clinical course; clients with the chronic form of leukemia are usually asymptomatic early in the disease; the life expectancy may be more than 5 years; symptoms of chronic leukemia relate to hypermetabolism of leukemia cells infiltrating other organ systems; the cells in this type of leukemia are more mature and function more effectively

3. Assessment

NCLEX!

a. Clinical manifestations

1) Fever

2) Night sweats

3) Bleeding

4) Ecchymoses

5) Lymphadenopathy

6) Weakness

7) Fatigue

8) Pruritic vesicular lesions

9) Anorexia

10) Weight loss

11) Shortness of breath

12) Decreased activity tolerance

13) Bone or joint pain

14) Visual disturbances

15) Gingival bleeding

16) Epistaxis

17) Pallor

18) Splenomegaly

19) Hepatomegaly

    b. Diagnostic and laboratory tests

1) Increased WBC (in CLL and CML)

2) A normal, decreased or increased WBC (in ALL and AML)

3) Decreased reaction to skin sensitivity tests (**anergy**)

4) Bone marrow tests reveal excessive blast cells in AML

5) Philadelphia chromosome found in 90 to 95 percent in clients with CML; BCR/ABL gene is present in virtually all clients with CML

6) Bone marrow biopsy and aspirate is the definitive diagnostic test

4. Therapeutic management

    a. Induction of remission with chemotherapy and radiation therapy

    b. Bone marrow and stem cell transplantation

5. Priority nursing diagnoses; Risk for infection; Risk for bleeding; Imbalanced nutrition: less than body requirements; Fatigue; Activity intolerance; Pain; Anticipatory grieving

6. Planning and implementation

    a. Review and institute the care of a client receiving chemotherapy (see Chapter 12)

    b. Review and implement the nursing care of a client undergoing radiation therapy (see oncology chapter)

    c. Assist in bone marrow biopsy; apply pressure on the site for 5 minutes or until bleeding stops; frequently assess the site for signs of bleeding up to 4 hours after the procedure

    d. Institute neutropenic and bleeding precautions (see previous discussion)

    e. Plan activities to prevent fatigue; provide measures for uninterrupted rest and sleep

    f. Provide for diversionary activities

    g. Maintain good nutrition; enlist the assistance of a dietician in maximizing and meeting the nutritional needs of the client

    h. Assist the client in maintaining good personal hygiene; measures to promote oral hygiene should be instituted

    i. Refer client and family to appropriate agencies such as Meals on Wheels, American Cancer Society, and the Leukemia Society

    j. Provide emotional support to the client and family; refer to appropriate agency, organization, or professional for counseling and support

    k. Administer drugs that are prescribed and monitor for side effects

    l. Monitor laboratory results to evaluate effectiveness of interventions and therapy

    m. Prepare the client for bone marrow transplantation if this is included in the treatment plan

7. Medication therapy: chemotherapeutic drugs include alkylating agents (Busulfan [Myleran]), anthracyclines (Doxorubicin [Adriamycin]), antimetabolites (Fludarabine [Fludara]), corticosteroid (Prednisone), plant alkaloids (Vincristine [Oncovin]) and others

8. Client education

    a. Teach client and family about precautions to prevent bleeding (see previous discussion)

    b. Teach client and family about neutropenic precautions as previously discussed

    c. Teach client to maintain good oral hygiene including measures to keep the oral cavity moist; these measures can include rinsing mouth with saline, lubricating the lips and oral mucosa with water-soluble lubricants every 2 hours; alcohol-based mouthwash solutions should be avoided; sponge-tipped applicators should be used for oral hygiene if the neutrophil and platelet counts are low

    d. Teach client measures to prevent peri-rectal complications; the area should be washed and cleansed thoroughly after each bowel movement

    e. Discuss with client and family therapeutic plans and interventions

9. Evaluation

    a. The client has no infection

    b. The client has no bleeding episodes

    c. Client reports adequate pain control

    d. Client tolerates activities of daily living

K. Malignant lymphomas

1. Definition: lymphoma is a group of malignant neoplasms that affects the lymphatic system resulting in the proliferation of lymphocytes; lymphomas can be classified as Hodgkin's disease and non-Hodgkin's lymphoma

2. Etiology and pathophysiology

    a. Hodgkin's disease

        1) More common in men and has two peaks; 15 to 35 years of age and 55 to 75 years of age; incidence is higher in whites than in African-Americans

        2) The cause of the disease is unknown although several factors have been identified to contribute to the development of the disease; these factors include infection with the Epstein-Barr virus (EBV), familial pattern, and exposure to toxins

NCLEX!

3) Hodgkin's disease is characterized by the presence of Reed-Sternberg cell, a multinucleated and gigantic tumor cell thought to be of lymphoid origin

4) The tumor originates in a lymph node (in majority of cases from the cervical nodes) and infiltrates the spleen, lungs, and liver

  b. Non-Hodgkin's lymphoma

1) Most common form of lymphoma; affects usually adults from 50 to 70 years old; it is more common in men than women and in whites

2) There is no known cause but the incidence of non-Hodgkin's lymphoma is linked to viral infections, immune disorders, genetic abnormalities, exposure to chemicals, and infection with *Helicobacter pylori*

3) Non-Hodgkin's lymphoma has a similar pathophysiology to Hodgkin's disease, although Reed-Sternberg cells are absent and the method of lymph node infiltration is different

4) In majority of cases, the disease involves malignant B cells; the lymphoma usually originates outside the lymph nodes; the lymphoid tissues involved become infiltrated with malignant cells; the cells that make up the lymphoid tissue become abnormal and crowd out normal cells

3. Assessment

  a. Clinical manifestations

1) Hodgkin's disease

NCLEX!

NCLEX!

NCLEX!

  a) Usually begins with a firm and painless enlargement of one or more lymph nodes on one side of the neck

  b) Fatigue

  c) Weakness

  d) Anorexia

  e) Dysphagia

  f) Dyspnea

  g) Pruritus

  h) Development of severe but brief pain at the site of Hodgkin's after ingestion of alcohol

  i) Cough

  j) Jaundice

  k) Abdominal pain

  l) Bone pain

NCLEX!

NCLEX!

  m) B symptoms: fever without chills; night sweats, and unintentional 10 percent weight loss

  n) Enlarged lymph nodes, liver, and spleen

2) Non-Hodgkin's lymphoma

a) Painless lymph node enlargement

b) B symptoms (see above)

c) Abdominal pain, nausea, vomiting

d) Hematuria

e) Peripheral neuropathy, cranial nerve palsies, headaches, visual disturbances, changes in mental status, and seizures

f) Shortness of breath, cough, and chest pain

b. Diagnostic and laboratory tests

1) Hodgkin's disease

a) Normocytic, normochromic anemia

b) Neutrophilia, monocytophilia, and lymphopenia

c) Presence of Reed-Sternberg cells in excisional bone biopsy

d) Mediastinal lymphadenopathy revealed by chest x-ray, CT scan, and radioisotope studies

e) Mediastinal mass and pulmonary infiltrates may be seen on chest x-ray

f) Absent or decreased response to skin sensitivity testing known as anergy

2) Non-Hodgkin's lymphoma

a) Lymphocytopenia

b) X-ray may reveal pulmonary infiltrates

c) Lymph node biopsy helps to identify the cell type and pattern

4. Therapeutic management

a. Hodgkin's disease

1) Lymphangiography is used to evaluate abdominal nodes

2) Staging laparotomy is performed to obtain specimen of retroperitoneal lymph nodes and to remove the spleen

3) Staging of the disease to determine the extent of the disease and appropriate therapy is instituted; stage I indicates involvement of a single lymph node region; stage IV (for Hodgkin's disease only) indicates diffuse or disseminated involvement of 1+ extralymphatic organs, with or without lymph node involvement (liver, lung, marrow, skin)

4) Radiation therapy for stages IA, IB, IIA, and IIB

5) Combination chemotherapy for stages III, IV, and all B stages

6) Combination radiation and chemotherapy for stages IA and IB

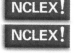

  b. Non-Hodgkin's lymphoma

    1) Staging of the disease is undertaken; this is based on data obtained from CT scans and bone marrow biopsies

    2) Combination chemotherapy

    3) Radiation alone or in combination with chemotherapy for stage I and II

    4) Biologic therapy with alpha interferon, interleukin-2, and tumor necrosis factor

    5) Administration of rituximab (Rituxan), a monoclonal antibody against the CD20 of malignant B lymphocytes, which causes cell lysis and death

5. Priority nursing diagnoses: Risk for infection; Activity intolerance; Ineffective protection; Fatigue; Imbalanced nutrition: less than body requirements; Disturbed body image; Hoplessness

6. Planning and implementation

  a. Institue nursing interventions for clients on chemotherapy or radiation therapy

  b. Assist in balancing activity with periods of rest

  c. Provide and assist in maintaining good nutritional state

  d. Provide measures to diminish the discomfort associated with pruritus

  e. Provide interventions to enable client to deal with body image changes such as alopecia, weight loss, and sterility

  f. Refer client and family to appropriate agencies for support such as the American Cancer Society

  g. Plan interventions for the prevention of infection

7. Medication therapy

  a. Chemotherapeutic agents

  b. Biologic therapy agents

8. Client education

  a. Discuss with client and family the nature of the disease, the course of therapy, and associated interventions

  b. Teach the client and family about the medications prescribed, precautions, and side effects

  c. Teach the client and family symptoms necessitating immediate medical intervention such as the occurrence of bleeding, infection, or fever

9. Evaluation

  a. The client does not develop complications of bleeding or infection

  b. The client regains normal weight

  c. The client verbalizes absence of pain

  d. The client and family verbalize understanding of reasons of ongoing treatment and interventions

Case Study

You are the nurse assigned to a client who was admitted 3 days ago with a diagnosis of septic shock. During your initial assessment, you note that the client's capillary refill on the left lower extremity is delayed. The dorsalis pedis and posterior tibial pulses on the left are significantly less (1+) than the right (2+). The extremity is cold, and the client claims to have pain on that side. On further examination, you notice that the client is oozing blood from previous IV and injection sites. His Foley catheter is draining pink-tinged urine. You suspect disseminated intravascular coagulopathy (DIC).

❶ What factor/s may have contributed to the development of DIC?

❷ What immediate nursing interventions will you take?

❸ What laboratory tests do you anticipate the physician will recommend and why?

❹ If your hunch was correct that the client is in DIC, what would you expect the laboratory results to be ?

❺ Identify three priority nursing diagnoses for this client.

For suggested responses, see page 739.

Posttest

1 The nurse would assess a client who has undergone a small bowel resection of the ileum for development of which type of anemia?

(1) Iron-deficiency anemia
(2) Vitamin B_{12} deficiency anemia
(3) Anemia of chronic disease
(4) Aplastic anemia

2 A client has an order for a test to determine if pernicious anemia is present. For which of the following tests should the nurse schedule the client?

(1) Serum folate level
(2) Schilling test
(3) Serum iron and total iron-binding capacity (TIBC)
(4) Bone marrow aspiration

3 The nurse is assessing a group of clients and identifies which of the following as being at high risk for the development of folic acid deficiency anemia?

(1) Obese individuals
(2) Alcoholics
(3) Young adults
(4) Athletes

4 Which of the following questions during the data-gathering phase is important for the nurse to ask a client suspected of having a nutritional anemia?

(1) "Do you have a sore tongue?"
(2) "How has the consistency of your stools been?"
(3) "Do you experience any tingling or numbness?"
(4) "Have you had blood transfusions in the past?"

5 A couple seeks genetic counseling for sickle cell. Both have sickle cell traits. The nurse understands that the chances of the couple's offspring developing sickle cell disease with each pregnancy is described best by which of the following?

(1) None of the offspring will develop sickle cell disease.
(2) There is a twenty-five percent chance that their offspring will develop sickle cell disease.
(3) There is a fifty percent chance that their offspring will develop sickle cell disease.
(4) All their children will have sickle cell traits, but none will have the disease.

6 The nurse is preparing a teaching plan for a client with sickle cell disease about ways to prevent crisis episodes. Which of the following should be emphasized to prevent sickle cell crisis?

(1) Eat nutritious foods that are high in iron.
(2) Seek treatment for infections as soon as possible.
(3) Take adequate amounts of supplemental vitamins and minerals.
(4) Avoid any type of physical activity.

7 Which of the following nursing diagnoses should receive the highest priority in a client with sickle cell crisis?

(1) Pain
(2) Self-care deficit
(3) Activity intolerance
(4) Altered health maintenance

8 The nurse is reviewing laboratory results of a client. Which of the following laboratory results indicate that a client has sickle cell disease?

(1) 30 percent HbS
(2) 90 percent HbS
(3) Hematocrit of 40 percent
(4) Hematocrit of 50 percent

9 Which of the following statements made by a client with sickle cell trait indicates the need for further teaching?

(1) "I don't have to worry about developing sickle cell crisis since I only have the trait."
(2) "I will need to seek genetic counseling before I get married and plan children."
(3) "I will need to plan my activities avoiding those that decrease my oxygen levels."
(4) "I need to avoid the use of recreational drugs and alcohol."

10 Which of the following nursing observations indicate that a positive outcome for a client with sickle cell crisis has been met?

(1) The client has an intake of 3,000 mL per day.
(2) The urinary output is 20 cc per hour.
(3) Client complains of persistent joint pain.
(4) The client has a temperature of 100° F.

See pages 561–562 for Answers and Rationales.

Answers and Rationales

Pretest

1 Answer: 3 Rationale: Vitamin B_{12} deficiency anemia causes the production of abnormally large red blood cells. This deficiency causes the red blood cell to be irregular and oval, rather than the biconcave shape of a normal red blood cell. This shape predisposes the cells to a shorter lifespan. In this type of anemia, there is an increase in the MCV (option 1) and a decrease in the hemoglobin (option 2). Option 4 is characteristic of iron deficiency anemia.
Cognitive Level: Application
Nursing Process: Implementation; *Test Plan:* PHYS

2 Answer: 2 Rationale: Hypoxia stimulates the release of the hormone erythropoietin from the kidney and increases bone marrow production of RBCs. The hemoglobin does not increase in size with hypoxia. Reticulocytes mature in 24 to 48 hours, and their maturation is not influenced by hypoxia.
Cognitive Level: Comprehension
Nursing Process: Analysis; *Test Plan:* PHYS

3 Answer: 1 Rationale: After the destruction of red blood cells, the iron is recycled by transferrin. The heme unit is converted to bilirubin, which is conjugated with glucorinide in the liver and eventually excreted in bile. Hemoglobin binds with haptoglobin to prevent renal excretion during the destruction of the RBC membrane.
Cognitive Level: Comprehension
Nursing Process: Analysis; *Test Plan:* PHYS

4 Answer: 1 Rationale: Lysis of red blood cells causes retention of iron and other substances including bilirubin to accumulate in plasma. The accumulation of bilirubin causes jaundice. Although hepatitis infection may also be the reason for jaundice, the hemolytic anemia present most likely caused the jaundice to occur.
Cognitive Level: Application
Nursing Process: Analysis; *Test Plan:* PHYS

5 Answer: 4 Rationale: The reticulocyte (immature RBC) count is an indicator that new red blood cells

are being produced by the bone marrow. An increase in the reticulocyte count in an anemic client indicates that the bone marrow is responding to the decrease in RBCs. The hematocrit count measures the percent of RBCs in the total blood volume. Hemoglobin is not directly linked to bone marrow activity. Serum ferritin levels reflect available iron stores.
Cognitive Level: Application
Nursing Process: Assessment; *Test Plan:* PHYS

6 **Answer: 3** *Rationale:* Iron-deficiency anemia is manifested clinically by glossitis or inflammation of the tongue. After pallor, this is the second most frequent manifestation of this type of anemia. Cheilitis or inflammation of the lips is another finding in this type of anemia. Achlorhydria, or the absence of free hydrochloric acid is a manifestation of a depressed parietal cell function and is associated with vitamin B_{12} deficiency anemia. Cheilosis is cracking of lips at the angles of the mouth.
Cognitive Level: Application
Nursing Process: Assessment; *Test Plan:* PHYS

7 **Answer: 2** *Rationale:* An acidic environment (such as in the presence of vitamin C) enhances the absorption of iron. Administering the medication with meals binds the iron with food and interferes with its absorption.
Cognitive Level: Application
Nursing Process: Implementation; *Test Plan:* PHYS

8 **Answer: 1** *Rationale:* The client on an oral iron preparation should be taught to expect the stools to turn black because of the excessive iron that is eliminated. All the other choices should be included in the teaching plan. The health care practitioner may change the iron preparation prescribed to the client if gastrointestinal symptoms become intolerable.
Cognitive Level: Analysis
Nursing Process: Evaluation; *Test Plan:* SECE

9 **Answer: 4** *Rationale:* Liver and muscle meats are excellent sources of iron. The other foods are also beneficial for the dietary management of anemia, but option 4 is specifically an excellent source of iron.
Cognitive Level: Analysis
Nursing Process: Evaluation; *Test Plan:* HPM

10 **Answer: 1** *Rationale:* When administering an iron preparation intramuscularly, it should be given deep in the muscle. The site should be in the upper outer quadrant of the buttocks utilizing the Z tract technique. No more than 2 mL of the solution should be administered and the length of the needle should be 2 to 3 inches. The area should not be massaged after the injection.
Cognitive Level: Application
Nursing Process: Implementation; *Test Plan:* PHYS

Posttest

1 **Answer: 2** *Rationale:* Resection of the distal ileum results in the impaired absorption of vitamin B_{12}. The other cause of vitamin B_{12} deficiency is the loss of intrinsic factor-secreting surfaces that are normally secreted by parietal cells.
Cognitive Level: Application
Nursing Process: Implementation; *Test Plan:* SECE

2 **Answer: 2** *Rationale:* Schilling test involves the administration of radioactive vitamin B_{12}. Increased absorption of vitamin B_{12} when intrinsic factor is given parenterally is indicative of pernicious anemia.
Cognitive Level: Application
Nursing Process: Planning; *Test Plan:* PHYS

3 **Answer: 2** *Rationale:* Individuals who are chronically undernourished including the elderly, alcoholics, substance abusers; those with high metabolic requirements and on total parenteral nutrition are also at risk for folic acid deficiency anemia. Alcoholics are particularly at risk because alcohol interferes with folate metabolism.
Cognitive Level: Application
Nursing Process: Analysis; *Test Plan:* PHYS

4 **Answer: 3** *Rationale:* The differentiating symptom of vitamin B_{12} and folic acid deficiency anemia is the absence of neurologic symptoms such as numbness and altered proprioception in folic acid deficiency anemia. The gastrointestinal symptoms of cheilosis, glossitis, and diarrhea are present in both forms of nutritional anemia although usually more severe in folic acid deficiency anemia.
Cognitive Level: Application
Nursing Process: Assessment; *Test Plan:* PHYS

5 **Answer: 2** *Rationale:* Sickle cell disease is an autosomal recessive genetic disorder where the individual is homozygous for the abnormal hemoglobin. If both parents have sickle cell traits, there is a 25 percent chance that each pregnancy will produce a child with the disease.
Cognitive Level: Analysis
Nursing Process: Analysis; *Test Plan:* HPM

6 **Answer: 2** *Rationale:* Clients with sickle cell disease have scarred spleen resulting in decreased ability to fight off infection. The individual with sickle cell disease must seek early treatment of infections.

Pneumonia is one of the most common infections affecting individuals with sickle cell disease. Option 4 is inaccurate in that vigorous physical activity should be avoided.
Cognitive Level: Application
Nursing Process: Planning; *Test Plan:* HPM

7   **Answer: 1** *Rationale:* The client in sickle cell crisis will have pain related to ischemic tissue injury resulting from obstruction of blood flow. The other diagnoses although important are of lesser priority than the nursing diagnosis of pain.
Cognitive Level: Analysis
Nursing Process: Analysis; *Test Plan:* PHYS

8   **Answer: 2** *Rationale:* Clients with sickle cell disease express 80 to 90 percent of HbS. Clients with sickle cell trait usually express less than 40 percent of HbS. The hematocrit of clients with sickle cell disease is usually decreased between 20 to 30 percent.
Cognitive Level: Application
Nursing Process: Analysis; *Test Plan:* PHYS

9   **Answer: 1** *Rationale:* Clients with sickle cell trait may also develop sickle cell crisis although their symptoms are often milder since only about 30 percent of their hemoglobin is abnormal. The other options are rational lifestyle adjustments the client makes in order to deal with the disease.
Cognitive Level: Application
Nursing Process: Evaluation; *Test Plan:* HPM

10   **Answer: 1** *Rationale:* An observation for the client in sickle cell crisis that indicates a positive outcome includes stable vital signs, an oral intake of 3,000 mL/day, and verbalization of pain control. Maintaining an adequate intake is essential to maintain blood flow, decrease pain, and prevent renal damage.
Cognitive Level: Analysis
Nursing Process: Evaluation; *Test Plan:* SECE

References

Bullock, B. L., & Henze, R. L. (2000). *Focus on pathophysiology.* Philadelphia: Lippincott.

Crowley, L. V. (2001). *An introduction to human disease: Pathology and pathophysiology correlations* (5th ed.). Boston: Jones and Barlett.

Huether, S. E., & McCance, K. L. (2000). *Understanding pathophysiology.* St. Louis, MO: Mosby.

Ignatavicius, D., & Workman, M. L., (2002). *Medical-surgical nursing across the health care continuum* (4th ed.). Philadelphia: Saunders.

Lemone, P. & Burke, K. (2003). *Medical surgical nursing: Critical thinking in client care* (3rd ed.). Upper Saddle River, NJ: Prentice Hall.

Lewis, S., Heitkemper, M., & Dirksen, S. (2000). *Medical-surgical nursing: Assessment and management of clinical problems* (5th ed.). St. Louis, MO: Mosby.

Phipps, W., Monahan, F., Sands, J., Marek, J. & Neighbors, M. (2003). *Medical surgical nursing: Health and illness perspectives* (7th ed.). St. Louis, MO: Mosby-Year Book, Inc.

Smeltzer, S. C., & Bare, B. G. (2000). *Brunner and Suddarth's textbook of medical-surgical nursing* (9th ed.). Philadelphia: Lippincott Williams & Wilkins.

Smith, S., Duell, D., & Martin, B. (2000). *Clinical nursing skills* (5th ed.). Upple Saddle River, NJ: Prentice Hall, Inc.

CHAPTER 15

Reproductive and Sexual Disorders

Sammie L. Justesen, RN

CHAPTER OUTLINE

OBJECTIVES

▌ Identify basic structures and functions of the reproductive system.

▌ Describe the pathophysiology and etiology of common reproductive and sexual disorders.

▌ Discuss expected assessment data and diagnostic test findings for selected reproductive and sexual disorders.

▌ Identify priority nursing diagnoses for selected reproductive and sexual disorders.

▌ Discuss therapeutic management of a client experiencing reproductive and sexual disorders.

▌ Discuss nursing management of a client experiencing reproductive and sexual disorders.

▌ Identify expected outcomes for the client experiencing reproductive and sexual disorders.

[*Media Link*]

Use the CD-ROM enclosed with this text, or log onto the address given to access the free, interactive Companion Website created for this series. The CD-ROM and Companion Website accompanying this book offer additional practice opportunities and information—NCLEX Review, Case Studies, Glossary, In Depth with NCLEX, and more.

www.prenhall.com/hogan

REVIEW AT A GLANCE

amenorrhea *absence of menstruation*

colposcopy *procedure for visualization of the cervix*

cystocele *herniation of the bladder into the vagina*

dysmenorrhea *pain associated with menstruation*

hydrocele *abnormal fluid collection within layers of the tunica vaginalis, surrounding the testes*

infertility *inability to conceive after 1 year of regular intercourse with no contraceptive measures, or inability to deliver a live fetus after 3 consecutive conceptions*

laparoscopy *procedure to visualize internal pelvic organs, using scope inserted through incision in abdominal wall*

menorrhagia *excessive or prolonged menstruation*

metrorrhagia *bleeding between menstrual periods*

oligomenorrhea *scant menses, usually related to hormonal imbalance*

orchitis *infection or inflammation of the testicles*

phimosis *constriction of the foreskin so it can't be retracted over the glans penis*

priapism *sustained, painful erection not associated with sexual arousal*

rectocele *herniation of the rectum into the vagina*

testicular torsion *twisting of the testes and spermatic cord*

uterine prolapse *downward displacement of the uterus into the vaginal canal*

varicocele *cluster of dilated veins in spermatic cord*

vulvitis *inflammation or infection of the vulva*

Pretest

1 The nurse caring for a client with benign prostatic hyperplasia (BPH) explains that currently the cause of this disorder is:

(1) Linked to sexual activity.
(2) Linked to diet.
(3) Unknown.
(4) Related to racial origins.

2 A male client presents to the emergency room with priapism, or sustained erection. The nurse understands that this client needs which of the following?

(1) Immediate medical attention
(2) A relaxing environment so his erection will recede
(3) Warm soaks to the penis
(4) An evaluation for sexual dysfunction

3 The nurse is evaluating a client with erectile dysfunction. Which of the following medications currently used by the client could be an underlying cause?

(1) Propranolol (Inderal)
(2) Acetylsalicylic acid (aspirin)
(3) Penicillin
(4) Furosemide (Lasix)

4 A 68-year-old female client presents to the gynecology clinic with complaints of painless vaginal bleeding. The nurse should be certain the client is tested for which of the following health problems?

(1) Ovarian cyst
(2) Cervical or uterine cancer
(3) Hormonal imbalances
(4) Endometriosis

5 The nurse concludes that a client who undergoes nocturnal penile tumescence and rigidity (NPTR) monitoring is most likely being evaluated for which of the following disorders?

(1) Prostate cancer
(2) Infertility
(3) Erectile dysfunction
(4) Phimosis

6 When examining a female client, the nurse observes tissue protruding from the vagina. The nurse checks the medical record for a documented history of which of the following disorders?

(1) Rectocele
(2) Cystocele
(3) Vaginal infection
(4) Uterine prolapse

7 A client has just had a Papanicolaou (Pap) test. The nurse would write which of the following indications for the test on the laboratory requisition?

(1) Infertility
(2) Sterility
(3) Human papilloma virus (HPV) infection
(4) Acquired immunodeficiency syndrome (AIDS)

8 When evaluating a client for breast cancer, the nurse recognizes that which of the following client-related factors is a risk for developing this disease?

(1) Use of foam contraceptives
(2) Early menopause, before age 45
(3) First birth before age 20
(4) Early menarche, before age 12

9 When teaching a female client to perform breast self-examination (BSE), the nurse should instruct her to perform the exam:

(1) During menstrual flow.
(2) At the same time each month.
(3) At a random time each month.
(4) Every 2 months.

10 When caring for a client with syphilis, the nurse instructs the client that syphilis may be transmitted by which of the following methods?

(1) Kissing
(2) Open lesions during any sexual contact
(3) Sharing eating utensils
(4) Shaking hands

See pages 624–625 for Answers and Rationales.

I. Overview of Anatomy and Physiology

A. External male reproductive structures (see Figure 15-1)

1. Scrotum: skin-covered sac suspended from the perineal region in front of the anus; covers, protects, and regulates temperature of the testes

2. Testes: male reproductive glands; paired organs suspended in the scrotum by the spermatic cord

   a. Develop in abdominal cavity of fetus and descend into scrotum

   b. Produce sperm and the male hormone testosterone

3. Epididymis: a long, coiled tube attached to the side and top of each testis; final area for storage and maturation of sperm; contracts to propel sperm through the vas deferens, to the ampulla where they are stored until ejaculation

4. Ductus deferens (vas deferens): located between the epididymis and the ejaculatory duct; stores and transports sperm

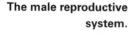

Figure 15-1

The male reproductive system.

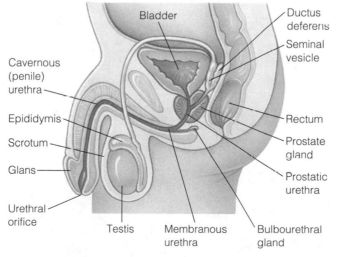

Bladder

Ductus deferens

Seminal vesicle

Cavernous (penile) urethra

Epididymis

Scrotum

Glans

Urethral orifice

Rectum

Prostate gland

Prostatic urethra

Testis

Membranous urethra

Bulbourethral gland

   5. Penis: attached to pubic area in front of scrotum; genital organ that encloses the urethra; comparable to female clitoris

   a. Shaft: main part of penis; contains three columns of erectile tissue; two lateral columns are called corpora cavernosa, and central mass is called corpus spongiosum

   b. Glans: tip of penis

   c. Foreskin: double fold of skin covering the glans

B. Internal male genitalia (refer again to Figure 15-1)

   1. Urethra: begins at bladder and passes through prostate and penis; pathway for eliminating urine and semen

   NCLEX!

   2. Prostate: encircles urethra just below the urinary bladder; walnut-sized gland containing muscle tissue

   a. Secretes thin, milky alkaline fluid into excretory ducts that open into the urethra

   b. Alkalinity helps protect sperm from acid present in the male urethra and female vagina, thus increasing sperm mobility

   3. Seminal vesicles: located on posterior bladder wall in front of rectum; secrete alkaline fluid containing large amounts of fructose and prostaglandins to help nourish and activate sperm

   4. Bulbourethral glands (Cowper's glands): two pea-sized structures located on each side of urethra, inferior to the prostate; secrete alkaline fluid into urethra and neutralize traces of acidic urine in the urethra

   5. Semen (seminal fluid): milky, viscous liquid with pH of about 7.5; contains about 120 million sperm per mL, plus glandular secretions

C. Male reproductive physiology

   1. Hypothalamic-pituitary-testicular axis

   a. Gonadotropin-releasing hormone from the hypothalamus stimulates the anterior pituitary to secrete interstitial cell-stimulating hormone

   b. Interstitial cell-stimulating hormone in turn stimulates hyperplasia of the interstitial cells of the testes, leading to production of testosterone

   2. Spermatogenesis: sperm produced at rate of 300 million per day; continues throughout male life cycle, but diminishes with age

   3. Erection: enlargement and hardening of penis in response to physical or psychological stimuli; afferent input from stimuli are transmitted by pudendal nerve to the cerebrum; efferent nerve fibers transmit impulses to sacral portion of parasympathetic nervous system, resulting in dilation of penis

   4. Ejaculation: expulsion of semen from urethra to outside; reflex centered in lumbar section of spinal cord sends impulses to genital organs, carrying peristaltic contractions that propel sperm into the urethra; ejaculation occurs when impulses reach pudendal nerves and stimulate skeletal muscles at base of penis

| Figure 15-2 | The internal organs of the female reproductive system. |

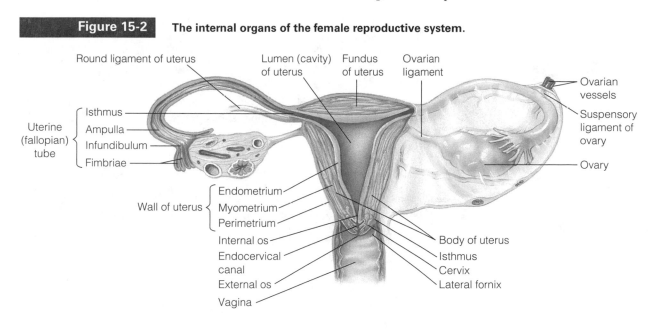

D. Female reproductive structures (see Figure 15-2)

1. Ovaries: flat, almond-shaped structures on each side of the uterus; comparable to the male testes; produce and discharge ova

   a. Attached to uterus by a ligament

   b. Store female germ cells and produce estrogen and progesterone, female hormones

   c. Play essential role in menstrual cycle and pregnancy

2. Uterus: pear-shaped, muscular organ with thick walls; located between bladder and rectum; contains three parts—fundus, body, and cervix

   a. Supported by four ligaments

   b. Receives fertilized ovum and provides site for growth and development of the fetus

   c. Uterine wall has three layers: perimetrium (outer serous layer), myometrium (middle layer), and endometrium (inner lining)

3. Cervix: portion of the uterus that forms pathway between uterus and vagina; softens in response to hormones during pregnancy

   a. Internal os: uterine opening of cervix

   b. External os: vaginal opening of cervix

   c. Endocervical canal: space between the two openings

4. Fallopian tubes: thin, cylindrical structures about 4 inches long, attached to uterus on one end and supported by the broad ligament; propel ovum from the ovaries to the uterus

   a. Lateral ends are open and made of projections called fimbriae that drape over each ovary; fimbriae pick up the ovum (egg) after it is discharged from the ovary

b. Tubes are lined with ciliated cells and muscle tissue that propel ovum toward the uterus

c. Fertilization of ovum usually occurs in the outer portion of one of the fallopian tubes

5. Vagina: fibromuscular tube about 3 to 4 inches long located behind bladder and urethra, in front of rectum; upper end connects with cervix; serves as route for excretion of secretions (menstrual fluid) and is organ of sexual response

6. External genitalia

a. Mons pubis: soft mound of adipose tissue located in front of symphysis pubis; protects and cushions symphysis pubis; enhances sexual sensations

b. Labia majora: two longitudinal folds of tissue that begin at mons pubis and surround each side of vaginal opening; protects other structures and enhances sexual arousal

c. Labia minora: smaller tissue folds enclosed by labia majora; protect clitoris, lubricate vulva, and enhance sexual arousal

d. Vestibule: area enclosed by the labia minora

e. Bartholin's glands: located on each side of vaginal opening; secrete clear mucus during intercourse

f. Skene's glands: open onto the vestibule on each side of urethra; drain urethral glands and produce lubricating mucus

g. Clitoris: small bud of erectile tissue just below the joining of the labia minora; stimulates and elevates sexual arousal

h. Perineum: skin-covered muscular area between vaginal opening and anus; provides support for pelvic organs

7. Breasts: mammary glands located between 3rd and 7th ribs on the anterior chest wall; supply nourishment for an infant

a. Areola: pigmented area containing sebaceous glands and a nipple

b. Cooper's ligaments support the breast and divide each into 15 to 25 lobes; each lobe contains alveolar glands connected by ducts that open to the nipple

E. **Female reproductive physiology**

1. Female sex hormones produced by ovaries

a. Estrogens: steroid hormones that occur in three forms (estradiol and estrone naturally produced by ovaries and estriol, their metabolic product); essential for development and maintenance of secondary sex characteristics and help stimulate female reproductive organs to prepare for growth of fetus; also serve other functions in body

b. Progesterone: affects development of breast glandular tissue and the endometrium

c. Androgens: responsible for normal hair growth patterns at puberty and have metabolic effects

2. Menstruation cycle: periodic hormonal cycle involving hypothalamus, anterior pituitary gland, uterus, and ovaries; prepares body for pregnancy through release of a single mature ovum and prepares uterus for implantation; cycle begins at puberty (often ages 12–15) and ends with menopause (often in 40s or 50s); 28 days is average length of cycle

   a. Menstrual phase: from day 1 to 5; inner-endometrial layer of uterus detaches and is expelled as menstrual fluid

   b. Proliferative phase: days 6 to 14; begins as maturing follicle begins to produce estrogen, which stimulates rapid growth of endometrium

   c. Secretory phase: days 14 to 28; corpus luteum produces progesterone, and rising levels increase vascularity of the endometrium and change the inner layer to secretory mucosa; these changes facilitate passage of sperm into the uterus; if fertilization does not occur, hormone levels fall

   d. Ischemic phase: without fertilization, spasm of the spiral arteries causes hypoxia of endometrial cells, which degenerate and slough off; this leads to the menstrual phase

F. Gestation

1. Fertilization occurs when the ovum is penetrated by one sperm cell in the fallopian tube; each reproductive cell (one gamete) carries 23 chromosomes; after fertilization, the fertilized egg descends to the uterus

2. Embryo: the fertilized ovum during the first 2 months of development

   a. First 8 weeks, when major organs develop, is most vulnerable period

   b. Cells arrange themselves in 3 layers: ectoderm (outer layer), endoderm (inner layer), and mesoderm (middle layer)

3. Fetal membranes: membranes surrounding the fetus; composed of two layers

   a. Amnion: glistening inner membrane; forms during 2nd week of life; encloses the amniotic cavity

   b. Chorion: outer membrane

4. Amniotic fluid: forms within amniotic cavity and surrounds embryo; consists of 500 to 1,000 mL of fluid by end of pregnancy

5. Placenta: organ that provides for exchange of nutrients and waste products between mother and fetus; also acts as endocrine organ

   a. Develops by third month; formed by union of chorionic villi and decidua basalis

   b. Provides oxygen and removes carbon dioxide from fetal system

   c. Maintains fetal fluid and electrolyte and acid–base balance

   d. Exchange takes place through diffusion; nutrients pass through, along with drugs, antibodies to some diseases, and certain viruses

   e. Human chorionic gonadotropin (HCG): placental hormone detected in urine 15 days after implantation; stimulates corpus luteum to maintain endometrium and is the basis of immunological test of pregnancy

   f. Human placental lactogen (HPL): similar effects to growth hormone

   g. Estrogen and progesterone: hormones produced by placenta

6. Umbilical cord: extends from fetus to center of the fetal surface of placenta; contains blood vessels that supply nutrients to the fetus and remove waste products

7. Fetal circulation

   a. Arteries carry venous blood

   b. Veins carry arterial blood

   c. Circulation bypass occurs because of nonfunctioning lungs: ductus arteriosus (between pulmonary artery and aorta) and foramen ovale (between right and left atrium)

   d. Ductus venosus bypass occurs because fetal liver is not used for waste exchange

   e. Bypasses must close after birth to permit blood flow through lungs and liver

G. Lactation

1. Hormonal stimulation during pregnancy causes proliferation of glandular tissue within the breasts

2. Breasts secrete colostrum for 2 to 3 days postpartum, a nutrient-rich fluid that also contains maternal antibodies and is a precursor to breast milk

3. Anterior pituitary: stimulates secretion of prolactin once placental hormones that inhibited the pituitary are absent

4. Breasts become full, distended, tender, and warm within 3 to 4 days, indicating production of milk

5. Milk usually produced with stimulus of sucking infant

6. Posterior pituitary discharges oxytocin, causing alveoli to contract and allow flow of milk in response to sucking—"let-down reflex"

H. Menopause: permanent cessation of menstruation resulting from the loss of ovarian follicular activity

1. Usually occurs between 40 to 50 years of age

2. Perimenopause: period just before, during, and after menopause

3. Physical changes

   a. Ovaries lose ability to respond to pituitary stimulation and normal ovarian function ceases

   b. Monthly flow becomes smaller, irregular, and gradually ceases

   c. Vagina becomes smaller and secretions diminish

   d. Uterus, bladder, rectum, and supporting structures lose tone, leading to uterine prolapse, rectocele, and cystocele

   e. Atherosclerosis and osteoporosis are more likely to develop

   f. Hot flashes, psychological symptoms (such as irritability, mood swings, depression, anxiety), insomnia, weakness, headache, and dizziness are common symptoms of perimenopause

NCLEX!

    g. Hormone replacement therapy (HRT) is used to manage clients undergoing menopause, which includes estrogen and progestin (progesterone); estrogen given alone can lead to gynecological cancers and thromboembolic disorders

II. Diagnostic Tests and Assessments

A. Laboratory tests

1. Androstenedione level: blood tests for androgen (male sex hormone) levels; normal results are lower in postmenopausal women than in men and adult premenopausal women

2. Estradiol, serum: measures hormone levels to identify causes of infertility, menstrual irregularity, or precocious puberty; oral contraceptives lower estradiol levels

3. Estriol: measures fetal viability by measuring urine levels of placental estriol, the predominant estrogen excreted in urine during pregnancy; a steady rise in estriol reflects a properly functioning placenta

4. Estrogen-progesterone receptor assay: estrogen and progesterone receptors are cellular proteins that bind the hormones before they can elicit a cellular response

   a. Tissue samples in a client with breast cancer help predict the client's response to therapy

   b. Clients with tumors positive for estrogen and progesterone receptors respond best to hormonal therapy

5. Estrogen, urine: measures the quantity of estradiol, estrone, and estriol (major estrogen hormones) in urine; clinical indications for the test include tumors of ovarian, adrenocortical, or testicular origin

6. Follicle stimulating hormone (FSH), serum: tests gonadal function by measuring plasma levels of FSH

   a. Aids diagnosis of infertility and disorders of menstruation, such as amenorrhea (lack of menstruation)

   b. Aids diagnosis of precocious puberty or hypogonadism

7. FTA-ABS: fluorescent treponemal antibody absorption test; detects antibodies to the spirochete that causes syphilis; used to confirm primary or secondary syphilis and verify suspected false-positive results to VDRL

8. Gram stain: uses staining technique to identify infectious organisms in body fluid (blood, urine, etc.)

9. Human chorionic gonadotropin (hCG), serum: measures the glycoprotein hormone hCG, which should increase steadily during first trimester of pregnancy; levels then fall to less than 10 percent of peak

   a. Detects early pregnancy

   b. Determines adequacy of hormone production in high-risk pregnancies

   c. Aids diagnosis of certain tumors

   d. Monitors treatment for induction of ovulation and conception

10. Luteinizing hormone, plasma: part of infertility studies for women and men; hormone levels help detect ovulation, assess male or female infertility, evaluate amenorrhea, and monitor ovulation-inducing therapy

11. Pregnanetriol, urine: tiny amounts of pregnanetriol are normally excreted in urine; increased amounts help diagnose adrenogenital syndrome

12. Progesterone, plasma: provides information about corpus luteum function in infertility studies, or placental function in pregnancy; used in conjunction with basal body temperature readings to aid in confirming ovulation

13. Prolactin, serum: measures the hormone needed to begin and maintain lactation; aids diagnosis of pituitary or hypothalamic dysfunction, and evaluates secondary amenorrhea

14. PSA: prostate-specific antigen; helps track course of prostate cancer and evaluate response to treatment; is becoming increasingly used as a screening procedure for prostate cancer in men over 50 years old, but should not be used alone without concurrent physical examination of the prostate by digital rectal exam

15. Prostatic acid phosphatase; measures phosphatase enzymes found mostly in the prostate; above the normal levels suspicious for prostate cancer

16. Semen analysis: collected directly from the client, from the vagina of a sexual partner, or from the vagina or skin of a rape victim; used to evaluate male fertility, substantiate effectiveness of a vasectomy, or to detect semen on the body or clothing of a suspected rape victim

17. Testosterone, serum or plasma: to evaluate male infertility or sexual dysfunction, diagnose male sexual precocity, and evaluate female hirsutisim (excessive body hair) and virilization (male characteristics)

18. VDRL: venereal disease research laboratory test; used to screen for primary and secondary syphilis and monitor response to treatment

B. Radiology studies

1. Soft tissue mammography: low-dose X-ray examination of the breast used to detect breast lesions before they can be felt; also allows comparison of current breast status with that shown by previous films

2. Contrast mammography: magnetic resonance imaging (MRI) technique to investigate the breast for cancer; uses a contrast medium that is picked up by vascular tumors; provides additional information after an abnormal mammogram

3. Ultrasonography: high-frequency sound waves are recorded as they strike tissues of different densities, providing an image of the tissues; used to investigate questionable areas detected by physical exam or mammogram

4. Computed tomography (CT) scan: multiple x-rays are passed through the tissues, providing computer-reconstructed images that offer cross-sectional views

C. Cytology

1. Papanicolaou (Pap) smear: used to screen for cervical cancer, assess client's hormonal status, and identify presence of sexually transmitted diseases, such

as human papilloma virus infection; obtained during a pelvic exam by scraping tissue from the cervical os

2. Nipple discharge examination: nipple discharge is examined under a microscope; usually indicated whenever bloody or red-brown discharge is noted; may reveal the presence of cancer cells

3. Breast biopsy: tissue is removed from a breast lesion for histologic examination to determine whether cancer is present

   a. Aspiration biopsy: also called fine-needle aspiration biopsy; a fine needle is used to remove cells or fluid from the breast lesion; mammography and a computer are used to guide the needle

   b. Incisional biopsy: a larger piece of tissue is surgically removed from the breast

   c. Excisional biopsy: the entire breast lesion is surgically removed, along with surrounding tissue

   d. Tru-cut or core biopsy: a plug of tissue from a breast lesion is removed with a hollow-core needle

   e. Stereotactic needle biopsy: involves computer guided breast tissue removal using mammographic images from nonpalpable breast lesions

D. **Colposcopy:** cervix is visualized and magnified in bright light to identify abnormal areas; a colposcope (low-power microscope) is used for the procedure; used when Pap tests indicate pathologic changes

E. **Laparoscopy:** procedure to visualize internal pelvic organs, using a laparoscope inserted through an incision in the abdominal wall

   a. Diagnostic: allows identification of endometriosis, ectopic pregnancy, pelvic inflammatory disease, and signs of malignancy

   b. Therapeutic: most often used for tubal sterilization; also useful for removal of peritubal lesions and aspiration of ova for in vitro fertilization

F. **Hysteroscopy:** an endoscopic exam to visualize the interior of the uterus and the cervical canal; used to remove intrauterine devices, and complement other diagnostic tests for unexplained bleeding and infertility

G. **Nocturnal penile tumescence tests:** measures penile tumescence or rigidity during sleep to document the presence of sleep-associated erections; based on the assumption that men with psychogenic impotence have normal erections during sleep, whereas men with organic impotence have impaired erections during sleep

H. **Digital rectal examination:** used to palpate the prostate gland; a gloved, lubricated index finger is inserted in the rectum; the normal prostate should be wide, nontender, and should feel smooth and rubbery

III. **Common Nursing Techniques and Procedures**

A. **Self breast-examination (BSE):** client education (see Figure 15-3)

   1. Teach client to observe breasts in front of a mirror in four positions

      a. With arms relaxed and down

      b. With arms lifted overhead

| Figure 16-3 | Teaching breast self-examination.

Teaching Breast Self-Examination (BSE)

Step 1 Teach the client to observe her breasts in front of a mirror and in good lighting. Tell her to observe her breasts in four positions:

With her arms relaxed and at her sides

With her arms lifted over her head

With her hands pressed against her hips

With her hands pressed together at her waist, leaning forward

Instruct her to look at each breast individually, and then to compare them. She should observe for any visible abnormalities, such as lumps, dimpling, deviation, recent nipple retraction, irregular shape, edema, discharge, or asymmetry.

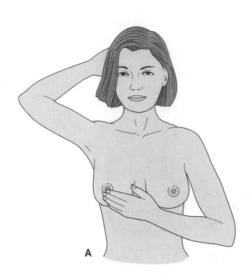

A

Step 2 Teach the client to palpate both breasts while standing or sitting, with one hand behind her head (Figure A). Tell her that many women palpate their breasts in the shower because water and soap make the skin slippery and easier to palpate. Show the woman how to use the pads of her fingers to palpate all areas of her breast, using the concentric circles technique (Figure B). Tell her to press the breast tissue gently against the chest wall, and to be sure to palpate the axillary tail.

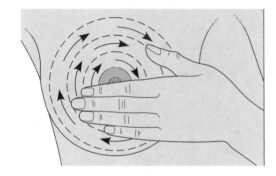

B

Step 3 Instruct the client to palpate her breasts again while lying down, as described in Step 2. Suggest that she place a folded towel under the shoulder and back on the side to be palpated. The arm on the examining side should be over the head, with the hand under the head (Figure C).

Step 4 Teach the client to palpate the areola and nipples next. Show her how to compress the nipple to check for discharge (Figure D).

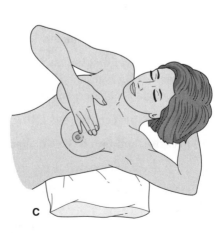

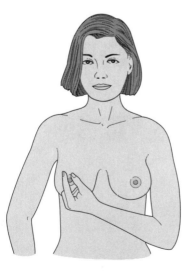

Step 5 Remind the client to use a calendar to keep a record of when she performs BSE. Teach her to perform BSE at the same time each month, usually 5 days after the onset of menses, when there is less hormonal influence on tissues.

C

D

    c. With hands pressed against hips

    d. With hands pressed together at the waist, leaning forward

  2. Teach client to palpate both breasts while standing or sitting, holding one hand behind her head (see Figure 15-3, A); demonstrate using pads of fingers to palpate all areas, using concentric circles (Figure 15-3, B)

  3. Palpate breasts as described in step 2 while lying down (Figure 15-3, C)

  4. Teach client to palpate the areola and nipples, compressing the nipple to check for discharge (Figure 15-3, D)

  5. Remind client to perform BSE once a month at the same time, usually 5 days after menstrual period begins; postmenopausal women should perform BSE on the same day of each month

B. Self-testicular examination: client education

  1. Teach client to examine testicles with soapy hands during a warm shower or bath

  2. Gently roll each testicle between thumb and forefinger of each hand; if lumps are noted or one testicle feels significantly larger than the other, notify physician

  3. Check for any hard lump felt directly on the testicle—this is abnormal

  4. Perform the exam on the same day, at least once each month

IV. Care of the Postoperative Client

A. Nursing management of the client undergoing prostate surgery

  1. Maintain usual postoperative assessment

  2. If dressings are present, monitor for drainage and change as needed

  3. Monitor vital signs closely for 24 hours, observing for signs of hemorrhage (frank blood in urine, large blood clots, decreased hemoglobin and hematocrit, tachycardia, and hypotension)

  4. In clients who have a urinary catheter following surgery, traction may be applied against the prostatic fossa to prevent bleeding; the balloon at the tip of the catheter exerts pressure to prevent hemorrhage; the surgeon positions the external end of the catheter by anchoring it tightly to the client's inner thigh to maintain traction; the catheter should not be repositioned

  5. A client who has a large indwelling catheter may feel the urge to void, which results from stimulation of the micturition center; explain to the client that this is a normal sensation; efforts by the client to void or strain will increase the risk of bleeding and aggravate pain

  6. Continuous bladder irrigation (CBI) may be ordered on a client postoperatively

    a. The purpose of the CBI is to prevent the formation of blood clots

    b. If blood clots do form, the urinary catheter will become plugged and prevent outflow of urine; the obstruction will also cause bladder spasms and pain

    c. A key nursing intervention for the client on CBI is to keep the outflow from the catheter light pink or clear; the rate of administration of the irrigating solution is therefore titrated to keep the color of the outflow this color and prevent blood clots from forming; it is essential to calculate intake and output to determine true urine output

   d. Indications that the rate of the irrigation is inadequate include: decreased outflow from the catheter; bladder spasms; and dark-colored or frankly bloody drainage

7. Monitor the client for signs of hemorrhage; bladder spasms and frank bloody output may indicate bleeding

8. The irrigating solution used during and after surgery may be absorbed causing fluid shifts and dilutional hyponatremia, referred to as the TURP syndrome; monitor the client for signs of hyponatremia and bradycardia, nausea, and vomiting; monitor serum sodium levels, and hemoglobin and hematocrit (lowered with dilutional effect); in addition, other signs of volume excess will also be evident, including hypertension and confusion

9. If manual irrigations are ordered, maintain sterile technique

10. Medicate as needed for pain

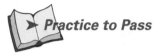

B. Nursing management of the client undergoing a mastectomy

   1. Maintain usual postoperative assessment

   2. Begin emotional support before surgery and continue in postoperative period

   3. Turn, cough, and deep breathe to prevent respiratory complications; restrictive surgical dressing may decrease chest expansion

A client who is receiving continuous bladder irrigation complains of severe bladder spasms. What is your nursing action?

   4. Position client on back or unaffected side

   5. Jackson-Pratt drain or Hemovac may be in place to drain fluids that accumulate when lymph nodes are removed

   6. Note signs of bleeding on dressing and reinforce pressure dressing as needed

   7. Encourage early range of motion exercise to prevent contractures and lymphedema

   8. Use unaffected arm only to provide IV fluids and take blood pressure

   9. Discharge instructions

      a. Use caution when lifting heavy objects with arm on affected side

      b. Avoid injury and infection on affected side; wear rubber gloves when washing dishes and garden gloves when working outside

      c. Don't allow procedures, such as blood pressure or venipuncture, on the affected side

      d. Refer clients to support group for psychosocial support

V. Disorders of the Male Reproductive System

   A. Priapism

      1. Description: sustained, painful erection that lasts at least 4 hours and is not associated with sexual arousal

2. Etiology and pathophysiology

   a. High-flow, or arterial priapism may follow trauma to the perineal area or injection of vasodilating drugs into penis to treat impotence

   b. Veno-occlusive, or ischemic priapism is caused by blood trapped within the penis, possibly caused by clotting or failure of normal autonomic responses that cause detumescence

   c. Conditions such as sickle-cell anemia, leukemia, multiple sclerosis, and metastatic tumors may lead to priapism

   d. May lead to tissue fibrosis and impotence if untreated

3. Assessment

   a. Clinical manifestations

      1) Sustained erection not associated with sexual arousal

      2) Client claims erection is harder than normal

      3) Discoloration of the penis

      4) Penile pain

      5) Urinary retention

      6) Bladder distention

   b. Diagnostic and laboratory tests: none

4. Therapeutic management

   a. Analgesia

   b. Sedation

   c. Hydration

   d. Treatment of the underlying condition

   e. Aspiration and irrigation of corpus cavernosum and injection of dilute vasoconstrictive agents are possible treatments

   f. Surgery may be required if other treatments fail; under local anesthesia, a large needle is passed through glans penis down to distal shaft, and a core of tissue is removed; this is repeated to create fistulas from which blood can drain into the corpus spongiosum

5. Priority nursing diagnoses: Pain; Risk for urinary retention; Risk for sexual dysfunction

6. Planning and implementation

   a. Administer analgesics and sedative promptly, before pain becomes severe and difficult to control

   b. Apply ice packs to penis as ordered for pain relief and edema control

   c. Facilitate voiding by helping the patient to a standing position, offering fluids, and running water in the sink

   d. Report signs of urinary retention: inability to void or voiding in small amounts

7. Medication therapy: analgesics and sedation for pain relief; alpha-adrenergic drugs injected into corpora cavernosa to reverse effects of vasodilating drugs when priapism is caused by intracavernosal injection; and intracavernosal injection of alpha-adrenergic drug (epinephrine or phenylephrine) for decompression and detumescence

8. Client education

   a. Assess client's understanding of treatment and causes of his condition

   b. Instruct client to seek medical attention early if priapism recurs

   c. Reassure client that sexual potency is usually maintained after shunting procedure

   d. Instruct client to report difficulty voiding or painful urination

   e. If surgery is performed, teach client how to care for sutures

9. Evaluation: client reports diminished pain; initiates voiding with output of at least 120 mL; discusses concerns and prognosis with his sexual partner

B. Phimosis

1. Description: constriction of the foreskin so that it cannot be retracted over the glans penis

2. Etiology and pathophysiology

   a. May be congenital or related to chronic infections under foreskin (balanoposthitis), leading to adhesions

   b. Phimosis prevents adequate hygiene, which may lead to malignant changes and stenosis of the meatus

   c. Phimosis interferes with erection; penile edema may cause severe pain

3. Assessment

   a. Clinical manifestations

      1) Non-retractable foreskin

      2) Signs of infection: swelling, redness, purulent discharge, and pain

      3) Painful erections

      4) Decreased urinary flow, painful urination, and straining to void

   b. Diagnostic and laboratory tests: none

4. Therapeutic management

   a. A dorsal slit of the foreskin may be necessary as an emergency measure

   b. Stretching of the foreskin by repeated retraction behind the glans

   c. Circumcision

5. Priority nursing diagnoses: Pain; Risk for urinary retention; Risk for infection

6. Planning and implementation

   a. Administer antibiotics and apply warms soaks

   b. Monitor client's urinary status, including his ability to void

    c. Encourage fluids to increase urinary output

    d. Apply ice packs to area for pain relief and to decrease edema

    e. Be aware that circumcision is usually indicated after obstruction and infection are resolved

  7. Medication therapy: antibiotics to treat infection; analgesics for pain relief

  8. Client education

    a. If circumcision or dorsal slit is performed, teach client how to care for incisions; a dry dressing may cover petrolatum gauze dressing, and may need to be changed with each voiding; sutures will be absorbed

    b. Sexual intercourse is usually permitted 1 week after surgery

    c. Instruct in personal hygiene measures, especially if circumcision is not performed

    d. Instruct client to report purulent drainage, redness, or edema of penis

  9. Evaluation: client reports that pain is decreased or resolved; voids at least 200 mL of urine within 8 hours after treatment or surgery; foul-smelling or purulent drainage is absent; client describes proper hygiene and wound care; client describes signs of infection

C. Erectile dysfunction

  1. Description

    a. Inability to attain and maintain an erection sufficient to perform satisfactory sexual intercourse

    b. The term *impotence* is synonymous with erectile dysfunction; may describe total inability to achieve erection, or inconsistent erections, or ability to sustain only brief erections

  2. Etiology and pathophysiology

    a. Age-related changes involve cellular and tissue changes in penis, decreased sensory activity, decreased testosterone levels, and effects of chronic illness such as diabetes

    b. Veno-occlusive mechanism prevents blood from leaving the penis; problems with this mechanism cause incomplete erections

    c. Damage to arteries, smooth muscles and fibrous tissues by disease is the most common cause of impotence (diabetes, kidney disease, chronic alcoholism, atherosclerosis, and vascular disease cause 70 percent of erectile dysfunctions)

    d. Prostate surgery may damage innervation and blood flow to the penis

NCLEX!

    e. Many medications, such as antihypertensive agents or psychotropic agents (haloperidol [Haldol], chlorpromazine [Thorazine]), can lead to impotence

    f. Psychogenic causes include depression, stress, fatigue, and fear of failure

    g. Substance abuse often causes erectile dysfunction

3. Assessment

   a. Clinical manifestations

      1) Inability to have an erection

      2) Inability to maintain an erection

      3) Inability to penetrate for intercourse because erection is not hard enough

   b. Diagnostic and laboratory tests

      1) Blood profiles

      2) Nocturnal penile tumescence and rigidity (NPTR)

      3) Cavernosometry (used to evaluate arterial inflow and venous outflow of the penis)

      4) Intracavernous injections to differentiate between physical and psychological causes of erectile dysfunction

      5) Psychological evaluation

4. Therapeutic management

   a. External mechanical devices such as vacuum constriction device (VCD)

   b. Counseling and sex therapy

   c. Implantation of prosthetic devices

   d. Vascular reconstructive surgery

5. Priority nursing diagnoses: Sexual dysfunction; Disturbed self-esteem; Ineffective role performance; and Ineffective coping

6. Planning and implementation

   a. Be aware that some clients feel intense shame and have difficulty discussing erectile dysfunction

   b. Vacuum devices may be used, but they are clumsy and reduce spontaneity

7. Medication therapy

   a. Sildenafil (Viagra) may be used to increase smooth muscle relaxation in the corpus cavernosum, increasing the ability to maintain an erection; assess medication history (drug is contraindicated for men taking nitrates because of risk of hypotension); assess risk of priapism (men with sickle-cell disease, leukemia, or physical abnormality of penis)

   b. Self-administered intracavernous injections of papaverine or prostaglandin E may be used

   c. Transdermal nitroglycerin paste may occasionally restore erectile function caused by arteriolar dilation

   d. Alprostadil (Muse), a single use urethral suppository with applicator, leads to erection within approximately 10 minutes, but reduces spontaneity and can cause burning of the urethra

NCLEX!

8. Client education

   a. Provide list of support services for client and his sexual partner

   b. Encourage discussion of alternate sexual practices

   c. Teach the use of mechanical devices, such as vacuum constriction device

   d. As appropriate, discuss causes of client's sexual dysfunction that can be controlled, such as smoking, alcohol use, and drug abuse

   e. Instruct in technique of intracavernous injection and use of topical medications, if ordered

   f. For clients who take sildenafil (Viagra): take drug approximately 1 hour before sexual activity; do not use drug more than once a day; taking drug after a high-fat meal may delay the effect; discontinue drug and notify physician if chest pain or shortness of breath occur with use

9. Evaluation: demonstrates use of mechanical device; verbalizes actions and use of medication; states satisfaction with and acceptance of alternative sexual practices; understands cause of sexual dysfunction and verbalizes appropriate treatment

D. Orchitis

1. Description: infection or inflammation of one or both of the testicles

2. Etiology and pathophysiology

   a. Rarely a primary infection; usually caused by ascending infection from the epididymis, or spread from another part of the body by the lymph nodes

   b. Many different organisms lead to infection, including bacteria, viruses, parasites, and fungi

   c. Trauma or surgery may cause inflammation of the testes

   d. Orchitis related to mumps usually occurs 4 to 6 days after inflammation of the parotid glands

   e. Testicular abscesses, atrophy, fibrosis, and infertility may result from orchitis

3. Assessment

   a. Clinical manifestations

      1) Fever, chills, and sudden pain that involves the testes radiating to groin

      2) Nausea and vomiting may accompany pain

      3) Tenderness, redness, and warmth; scrotal skin may also be red and edematous

      4) Some men experience few symptoms and may complain only of scrotal edema

      5) Presence of other infections, including mumps, urinary tract infection, or epididymitis

   b. Diagnostic and laboratory tests: urine culture to determine presence of infection, and sensitivity test to determine appropriate antibiotic treatment

4. Therapeutic management

   a. Antibiotics

   b. Aspiration of fluid if hydrocele is present

5. Priority nursing diagnoses: Pain (scrotal); Risk for infection; Hyperthermia; and Fear

6. Planning and implementation

   a. Bedrest, scrotal elevation, and cold applications are used to decrease inflammation of the testes

   b. Administer antibiotic therapy based on causative organism

   c. Monitor symptoms, including fever, pain, nausea, and vomiting

7. Medication therapy: antibiotics to treat infection, analgesics for discomfort, antiemetics for nausea, anti-inflammatory agents for inflammation, and corticosteroids to reduce symptoms

8. Client education

   a. Explain medication therapy and the importance of finishing antibiotic regime, even after symptoms resolve

   b. If incision and drainage were done, teach dressing change procedure; observe wound for redness and drainage; cleanse site gently with sterile water or saline

   c. Explain how to apply a scrotal support to provide elevation and secure dressing

   d. Teach client that exposure to mumps can result in sterility

9. Evaluation: client verbalizes purpose and correct use of medications, demonstrates dressing change procedure and use of scrotal support, states that pain is diminished or absent, temperature is reduced or normal, and describes measures to prevent recurrences

E. **Epididymitis**

   1. Description: infection or inflammation of the epididymis, a small structure that rests on the testes

   2. Etiology and pathophysiology

      a. Most common intrascrotal infection, but causes differ among younger and older men

      b. In younger men, most often caused by sexually transmitted urethritis caused by *Chlamydia trachomatis* or *Neiserria gonorrhoeae*

      c. In older men, usually associated with urinary tract infection or prostatitis

      d. Usually unilateral and caused by infection; may be a complication of invasive urinary tract procedures, such as catheterization or cystoscopy

   3. Assessment

      a. Clinical manifestations

         1) Scrotum may be red and swollen

         2) Urethral discharge may be present

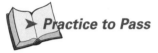

Practice to Pass

How would you explain to an adult male client that mumps could lead to sterility?

3) Severe pain and tenderness in the groin and scrotum on affected side

4) Fever, nausea, and vomiting

5) Burning on urination, frequency, and urgency

6) Client may walk with a "duck waddle" to avoid pressure on the groin and scrotum

b. Diagnostic and laboratory tests

1) White blood cell count may be elevated (between 20,000 and 30,000/mm^3)

2) Urinalysis shows increased WBC and presence of bacteria

3) Urine culture to identify organism

4) Scrotal ultrasound

5) Radionuclide scan

6) Aspiration of fluid from the epididymis

4. Therapeutic management

   a. Antibiotic therapy

   b. Anti-inflammatory drugs

5. Priority nursing diagnoses: Pain, Hyperthermia, and Fear

6. Planning and implementation

   a. Enforce bedrest for 5 to 7 days or until pain-free

   b. Elevate client's scrotum and provide cold packs to control pain and edema

   c. Administer antibiotics as ordered; severe cases require IV antibiotics

   d. Inspect the scrotal area for changes

   e. Monitor temperature and provide antipyretics as prescribed; offer fluids to replace fluid lost through diaphoresis and increased metabolism

7. Medication therapy: antibiotics to treat infection, antipyretics for fever, analgesics for pain relief, antiemetics to treat nausea

8. Client education

   a. Teach client to elevate scrotum with a towel or scrotal support to reduce pain and edema; scrotal support may continue to be worn up to 6 weeks as necessary

   b. Instruct client in applying intermittent cold compresses to the scrotum or taking sitz baths

   c. Instruct in the purpose, use, and potential adverse effects of antibiotics; instruct client to take all of his medication, even if symptoms resolve

   d. Encourage client to ask questions about effects of the infection on his fertility; sterility is usually a complication of bilateral epididymitis and may develop with recurrences of infection; erectile dysfunction is not a concern

   e. Explain cause of epididymitis and reasons for treatment; provide information to prevent recurrence of infection (drink 3,000 mL of fluid daily to prevent UTI) and other measures to decrease risk of reinfection

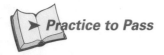

Practice to Pass

What advice would you give a client who contracted epididymitis from a sexual partner?

f. If caused by a sexually transmitted organism, advise client to avoid sexual intercourse until his partner has been examined and treated

9. Evaluation: client states that pain is diminished or absent; temperature is reduced or returned to normal; discusses concerns about sterility and sexual function; states the cause of his infection; correctly describes self-care activities; describes measures to prevent recurrences

F. Hydrocele

1. Description: abnormal fluid collection within the layers of the tunica vaginalis, which surrounds the testis

2. Etiology and pathophysiology

    a. May be unilateral or bilateral

    b. In adults, may be secondary to epididymo-orchitis, scrotal trauma, testicular cancer, or hypoalbuminemia

    c. Caused by increased production of fluid within the scrotum, or decreased reabsorption of the fluid; size of hydrocele depends on the extent of imbalance between fluid production and reabsorption

    d. Large hydrocele can impair physical activity and compromise blood supply to the testis

    e. Fluid characteristics depend on the cause; fluid associated with infection may be cloudy and contain bacteria

3. Assessment

    a. Clinical manifestations

        1) Swelling of the testes

        2) Discrepancies in size of the testes

        3) Pain and tenderness of the testes

    b. Diagnostic and laboratory tests: transillumination with a bright light shows fluid collection in the mass

4. Therapeutic management

    a. No treatment is needed unless the mass increases in size and causes discomfort

    b. Aspiration via a needle and syringe

    c. Hydrocelectomy (removal of fluid-filled sac)

5. Priority nursing diagnoses: Risk for sexual dysfunction, Risk for infection

6. Planning and implementation

    a. Observe and monitor degree of scrotal edema

    b. Treatment may be unnecessary, but provide supportive care for client

    c. Fluid aspiration is most conservative treatment; provide information as needed and allow client to verbalize his concerns and questions

    d. Provide medication for pain control as needed

e. If hydrocelectomy is performed, make standard postoperative assessments, note color and amount of wound drainage; provide scrotal support, cold packs, and pain medication

7. Medication therapy: analgesics for pain control; sclerosing drug, such as 5 percent tetracycline, may be injected into scrotal sac after aspiration of fluid

8. Client education instructions after hydrocelectomy

   NCLEX!

   a. Apply ice packs to scrotum as instructed

   b. Change dressing daily and as needed; cleanse wound with soap and water

   c. Reapply clean scrotal support

   NCLEX!

   d. Keep scrotum elevated until edema resolves

   e. Remind client that scrotal edema will disappear in 2 to 4 weeks

   f. Avoid sexual intercourse and strenuous activity until directed by care provider

   g. Sutures are absorbable

9. Evaluation: client describes procedure for applying cold packs to scrotum; demonstrates changing scrotal wound dressing; verbalizes reason for elevating scrotum; lists symptoms to be reported; reports that symptoms are relieved

G. Varicocele

1. Description: a cluster of dilated veins from the pampiniform venous complex on the spermatic cord that form a soft mass that can cause pain

2. Etiology and pathophysiology

   a. Usually occurs in men between ages 15 and 40, with no known cause

   b. Occasionally caused by defect in valves of the internal spermatic veins

   c. Commonly associated with infertility, for unclear reasons; venous enlargement may increase scrotal temperature, thus impairing sperm production and motility

3. Assessment

   a. Clinical manifestations

   NCLEX!

      1) Dull ache or feeling of heaviness in the scrotum on the affected side

      2) Many men are asymptomatic

      3) Dilated, tortuous veins may be palpated posterior to and above the affected testes when client is standing; mass usually disappears when client lies down

      4) Rush of blood can be felt in scrotum when client performs Valsalva maneuver

   b. Diagnostic and laboratory tests: doppler ultrasonogram or venogram may confirm diagnosis

4. Therapeutic management

   a. Surgical repair of the varicocele (varicocelectomy)

b. Embolization (occluding the internal spermatic vein on the affected side, using a balloon-tipped catheter, coil, or sclerosing agent) may be performed in conjunction with venography

c. Ligation of the spermatic vein

5. Priority nursing diagnoses: Pain, Risk for ineffective health maintenance

6. Planning and implementation

   a. Apply scrotal support to relieve client's discomfort

   b. Prepare client for surgery as indicated; client usually returns home within a few hours of surgery

7. Medication therapy: sclerosing agent injected into internal spermatic vein; analgesic medications for discomfort

8. Client education after varicocelectomy

   a. Remain at home for about 5 days and avoid driving for 1 week

   b. Avoid strenuous physical activity for 3 weeks

   c. Follow healthcare provider's instructions for resuming sexual activity

   d. Instruct client that fertility may not be restored by the procedure, and effects won't be known for several months

   e. Remove soiled dressing and cleanse wound gently with soap and water

   f. Wear scrotal support to decrease edema

9. Evaluation: client describes importance of wearing scrotal support; demonstrates changing wound dressing; verbalizes reason for elevating scrotum; lists symptoms to be reported

H. Testicular torsion

1. Description: twisting of the testes and spermatic cord

2. Etiology and pathophysiology

   a. Is considered a surgical emergency; compromised blood flow may lead to testicular ischemia and necrosis on the affected side

   b. Almost always occurs between birth and age 20

   c. Cause is not well understood; possibly related to elevated hormone levels and abnormal attachment of the testicles to the scrotum

   d. Three types of testicular torsion: intravaginal (twisting of the testicle within its outer coat), extravaginal (strangulation of the spermatic cord at the external inguinal ring), and torsion of the appendix teste (twisting of one of the four testicular appendages)

3. Assessment

   a. Clinical manifestations (see Box 15-1 for clinical signs of testicular torsion)

      1) Acute onset of pain localized to testes that may radiate to the lower abdomen and groin; acute on-and-off pain suggests intermittent torsion

      2) Swollen, reddened and tender testis; the affected side is usually elevated

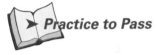

Practice to Pass

At what ages are male clients most likely to develop a varicocele?

NCLEX!

NCLEX!

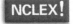

NCLEX!

NCLEX!

Box 15-1

Clinical Signs of Testicular Torsion

Intravaginal Torsion: Caused by twisting of the testicle within its outer coat
- Sudden onset of scrotal pain, sometimes related to trauma
- Nausea and vomiting
- Cremasteric reflex depressed or absent

Extravaginal Torsion: Caused by strangulation of the spermatic cord at the external inguinal ring
- Symptoms similar to those of intravaginal torsion

Torsion of the Appendix Teste: Caused by twisting of one of the four testicular appendages
- Less severe symptoms
- Cremasteric reflex present

    3) Tender epididymis

    4) Negative cremasteric reflex on the same side of torsion (stroke or gently pinch the skin of the upper inner thigh while observing the scrotum; a normal response is contraction of the cremasteric muscles of the scrotum, with elevation of the testis)

    5) Nausea and vomiting

  b. Diagnostic and laboratory tests

    1) Urinalysis usually is normal

    2) Orchiogram or testicular scan shows diminished or obstructed blood flow

    3) Doppler study identifies reduced blood flow

4. Therapeutic management

  a. Detorsion (surgical untwisting of the spermatic cord)

  b. Orchiopexy (surgical fixation of the testis to the scrotal wall)

  c. Orchiectomy (surgical excision of the testicle)

5. Priority nursing diagnoses: Pain, Anxiety, Disturbed body image, Deficient knowledge

6. Medication therapy: analgesics for pain relief

7. Planning and implementation

  a. Prepare client for diagnostic studies

  b. Once diagnosis is confirmed or likely, prepare client for emergency surgery

  c. After surgery for detorsion of the testicle and fixation of the scrotum, which usually requires a small, midline incision in the scrotum: apply cold packs and scrotal support to minimize pain; observe incision for redness or purulent drainage; provide analgesics as needed

8. Client education

  a. Reinforce knowledge concerning the effect of surgery on sexuality

  b. Teach the signs and symptoms of complications; bleeding, gaping incision, purulent drainage from incision

NCLEX!

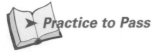

Practice to Pass

Why is testicular torsion considered a medical emergency?

c. Teach methods to control pain, such as ice bags and scrotal support

d. Remain at home for about 5 days and avoid driving for 1 week

e. Avoid strenuous physical activity for 3 weeks

f. Follow healthcare provider's instructions for resuming sexual activity

9. Evaluation: client describes importance of wearing scrotal support; demonstrates changing wound dressing; verbalizes reason for elevating scrotum; and lists symptoms to be reported

I. Testicular cancer

1. Description: unregulated growth of abnormal cells within the testicles

2. Etiology and pathophysiology

    a. Exact cause is unknown, but risk factors include cryptorchidism (undescended testicles at birth), maternal treatment with DES during pregnancy, mumps orchitis, trauma, environmental factors, and age

    b. Testicular cancer is the most common cancer among males age 15 to 35

    c. 90 percent of cancers arise from germ cell epithelium of the testes

    d. Testicular cancer is usually slow-growing and localized, with a good prognosis

3. Assessment

    a. Clinical manifestations

        1) Presenting sign is most often a painless, hardened area or lump found during self-examination

        2) Dull ache in pelvis or scrotum

        3) Testicular pain may occur with associated infection, necrosis, or hemorrhage

        4) Weight loss and fatigue

        5) Metastatic signs such as respiratory symptoms, GI disturbances, lumbar back pain, lymphadenopathy, and gynecomastia

    b. Diagnostic and laboratory tests

        1) Scrotal ultrasound; CT or MRI scan of chest, abdomen and pelvis to rule out metastasis

        2) Intravenous pyelogram

        3) Alpha fetoprotein (AFP) and beta unit of human chorionic gonadotropin (HCG) are markers that are helpful in monitoring therapeutic responses; elevated levels provide strong evidence of testicular cancer; markers are measured after surgery to help determine presence of residual disease, possibly in lymph nodes

        4) Serum lactic acid dehydrogenase (LDH) is elevated with testicular cancer

4. Therapeutic management

    a. Orchiectomy and exploration of the adjacent area to identify the cancer cell type and stage the disease (see Box 15-2)

Box 15-2

Staging of Testicular Cancer

Stage A (I) Tumor confined to the testis
Stage B1 (IIa) A few lymph nodes affected in the retroperitoneum, usually detected at time of node dissection
Stage B2 (IIb) Nodes greater than 2 to 6 cm
Stage B3 (IIc) Nodes greater than 6 cm
Stage C (III) Spread above the diaphragm, especially to the lungs or abdominal solid organs

    b. Radiation therapy

    c. Chemotherapy

    d. Lymphadenectomy

5. Priority nursing diagnosis: Risk for disturbed body image; Risk for ineffective health maintenance; Knowledge deficit; Ineffective individual and/or family coping

6. Planning and implementation

    a. Prepare client for screening tests to determine type of cancer and stage

    b. Provide emotional support for client and family; respond to questions and encourage client to express his feelings

    c. Prepare client for surgery if indicated

    d. Prepare client for chemotherapy after surgery and possible radiation therapy, if cancer has spread to lymph nodes

    e. After surgery: provide analgesics, ice packs, and scrotal support to control; monitor for complications, such as bleeding or infection

7. Medication therapy: chemotherapy with platinum-based combination of drugs

8. Client education

    a. Reinforce explanation of the type of cancer found, extent of the disease, and plans for treatment

    b. Stress importance of monthly testicular examination, because malignancy may develop in the remaining testis

    c. Discuss the possibility of preserving sperm in a bank before surgery to help relieve client's fears about infertility

    d. Instruct client that orchiectomy should have no lasting effects on client's sexual or reproductive function

    e. Teach the signs of complications: bleeding, gaping incision, or purulent drainage from incision

    f. Teach methods to control pain, such as ice bags and scrotal support

    g. Remain at home for about 5 days and avoid driving for 1 week

    h. Avoid strenuous physical activity for 3 weeks

    i. Follow healthcare provider's instructions for resuming sexual activity

NCLEX!

NCLEX!

NCLEX!

NCLEX!

NCLEX!

NCLEX!

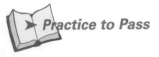

Practice to Pass

What is the survival rate for testicular cancer?

j. Stress importance of follow-up, especially if retroperitoneal lymph nodes were not surgically explored; client will need periodic physical examinations, tumor markers, and CT scans of retroperitoneal nodes for 5 to 10 years after surgery

9. Evaluation: client reports that postoperative pain is decreased or no longer present; describes realistically the effects of surgery on his appearance and function; resumes self-care activities; describes the plan of treatment; demonstrates care of incision; describes importance of monthly self-examination; demonstrates testicular self-examination; states date and time of first postoperative follow up visit and importance of frequent appointments

J. Benign prostatic hyperplasia (BPH)

1. Definition: overgrowth of cells in the prostate gland

2. Etiology and pathophysiology

   a. Appears to be a normal part of aging, but exact cause is unknown; occurs only in aging men with normal testicular function

   b. Usually occurs as nodules in lateral or middle lobes of the prostate; nodules grow and compress the normal prostatic tissue

   c. Nodular enlargement also presses against the urethra and reduces its diameter

      1) Bladder muscles hypertrophy (enlarge) to compensate for resistance to urination; fibromuscular bands or cords form, along with bladder diverticula; client has increased risk for bladder calculi and urinary retention

      2) Ureters may dilate because of increased voiding pressure

      3) Kidneys may become distended, leading to renal insufficiency

3. Assessment

   a. Clinical manifestations

      1) Many men have no symptoms

      2) Classic symptoms: urinary frequency, nocturia, difficulty starting and stopping urine stream, a weak stream, overflow dribbling, and feeling of being unable to completely empty the bladder

      3) Signs of cystitis, which may develop due to retained urine: painful urination, pyuria, and fever

      4) Digital rectal examination will reveal an enlarged prostate gland

   b. Diagnostic and laboratory tests

      1) Routine urinalysis and culture

      2) Acid phosphatase and prostate-specific antigen (PSA) to rule out prostatic cancer

      3) Urodynamic studies to determine degree of urinary obstruction

      4) Post-voiding catheterization; residual urine of more than 100 mL is considered high

      5) Ultrasound

      6) Cystoscopy

4. Therapeutic management

    a. Pharmacologic (see section to follow)

    b. Nonsurgical invasive management

        1) Application of heat

        2) Balloon dilation: balloon-tipped catheter is inserted through the urethra and then is inflated to stretch the urethra where it is narrowed by the prostate

        3) Laser ablation

        4) Application of stents or coils in the prostatic urethra

    c. Surgical intervention

        1) Transurethral resection of the prostate (TURP): this is the most common approach for partial removal of the prostate; no surgical incision is made; the approach is through a resectoscope inserted through the urethra

        2) Transurethral incision of the prostate (TUIP): incision is made through the bladder neck

        3) Suprapubic resection: the surgical approach involves an abdominal incision and cutting through the bladder to the anterior aspect of the prostate

        4) Retropubic resection: a low midline abdominal incision is made to approach the prostate

        5) Perineal resection: this is used commonly in cases of prostatic cancer; incision to approach the prostate is made between the anus and the scrotum

5. Priority nursing diagnoses: Urinary retention; Risk for infection; Risk for disturbed body image; Risk for ineffective health maintenance

6. Planning and implementation

    a. Client's treatment is based on severity of symptoms, degree of prostate enlargement, and presence of complications (urinary retention leading to urinary tract infections, pyelonephritis, and sepsis)

    b. Monitor medication therapy if indicated

    c. Encourage fluids (2,000 to 3,000 mL per day) to reduce risk of infection

    d. Suggest diet high in minerals: calcium, magnesium, zinc, and manganese

    e. Avoid drugs that could cause urinary retention (anticholinergics)

    f. Provide postoperative care following prostatectomy

    g. The client who undergoes a TURP will have a three-way urinary catheter and CBI; the care of a client with CBI was discussed previously in this chapter

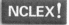

    h. For the client with a retropubic prostatectomy, assess the abdominal incision for signs of infection; urine in the dressing is not a normal finding since the bladder is not accessed in this type of surgery

NCLEX!

NCLEX!

NCLEX!

    i. For the client with a suprapubic prostatectomy, monitor outputs from both the suprapubic and urethral catheters

    j. For the client with a perineal prostatectomy, preventing infection is vital since the incision is in close proximity to the anus; avoid rectal temperatures or enemas

    k. Monitor urine character following prostatectomy

        1) Clear to pale pink: normal during entire hospital course

        2) Light red to red: normal or expected on day of surgery and first postoperative day

        3) Very dark red: could indicate venous bleeding or inadequate CBI flow; check flow rate and vital signs and tell the surgeon

        4) Bright red: could indicate arterial bleeding; check CBI flow rate, check vital signs and notify surgeon

        5) Blood clots: are normal if they are only occasional, but increase CBU flow rate to prevent catheter obstruction

7. Medication therapy: finasteride (Proscar) reduces hypertrophy by inhibiting an enzyme which blocks uptake of androgens and reduces size of gland, but has severe side effects (impotence); alpha-blockers inhibit alpha-adrenergic mediated contraction of prostatic smooth muscle to decrease straining on urination

8. Client education

    a. Engaging in regular prostatic massage and sexual intercourse helps decrease prostatic congestion

    b. Limit the amount of fluids taken at one time to avoid distending the bladder

    c. Increase fluid intake to 2,000 to 3,000 mL daily to decrease risk for bladder infection

    d. Urinate at the first urge

    e. Avoid drugs that can cause urinary retention, such as anticholinergics, antidepressants, decongestants, and tranquilizers

9. Evaluation: client voids without difficulty and reports steady stream of urine; free of signs of urinary tract infection; verbalizes use, purpose, and potential adverse effects of medications; verbalizes usefulness of regular prostatic massage; increases fluid intake to 2,000 to 3,000 mL per day; and lists classes of drugs that cause urinary retention

K. Prostatitis

1. Definition: inflammation of the prostate gland caused by an infectious agent

2. Etiology and pathophysiology

    a. Bacterial infection usually ascends from urinary tract or comes from the blood or lymph nodes; *Escherichia coli* most common organism

    b. Chronic bacterial prostatitis may follow an acute episode

    c. Nonbacterial prostatitis is most common type; cause is unknown

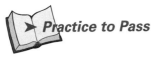

Practice to Pass

What symptoms would alert you to a possible enlarged prostate gland?

NCLEX!

NCLEX!

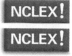

    d. Prostatodynia: symptoms of prostatitis without physical findings; possibly caused by muscle spasms of the urethral sphincter

3. Assessment

    a. Clinical manifestations

        1) Client complains of urinary burning, urgency, or frequency

        2) Urethral discharge

        3) Low back pain or perineal pain

        4) Generalized pain or pain associated with ejaculation or voiding

        5) If acute, client may have sudden onset of fever, chills, and pain

        6) Symptoms of acute cystitis including cloudy and malodorous urine

        7) Tender, swollen prostate; in chronic prostatitis, the prostate may be irregular, firm, and tender on manual examination

    b. Diagnostic and laboratory tests

        1) WBC elevated

        2) Urine positive for WBCs and bacteria

        3) Prostatic secretions may be cultured to determine presence and type of blood cells and bacteria

4. Therapeutic management

    a. Antibiotic therapy

    b. Anti-inflammatory agents in nonbacterial prostatitis

    c. Prostatic massage

5. Priority nursing diagnoses: Pain; Risk for infection; Risk for urinary retention; Risk for disturbed body image; Risk for ineffective health maintenance

6. Planning and implementation

    a. Administer antibiotic therapy as prescribed

    b. Maintain client on bedrest to decrease swelling and pain of prostate until symptoms subside

    c. Promote comfort with analgesics, antispasmodics, sedatives

    d. Offer sitz baths and rectal irrigation for pain relief

    e. Reassure client that sexual and reproductive functions are not damaged

7. Medication therapy: antibiotics to treat infection; analgesics for discomfort; NSAIDs for inflammation; anticholinergic drugs to facilitate voiding; stool softeners; alpha-blocking agents for prostatodynia to relax perineal muscles; and stool softeners to promote comfort

8. Client education

    a. Instruct in purpose, use, and potential adverse effects of medications

    b. Encourage normal sexual activity during prostatodynia

NCLEX!

c. Provide instructions on use of sitz baths to control pain and spasms

d. Drink 2,000 to 3,000 mL of water daily to dilute urine and keep feces soft; high-fiber diet helps soften stools

e. Instruct clients with chronic bacterial prostatitis that periodic prostate massage may be helpful to release pus cells and bacteria

NCLEX!

f. Instruct that alcohol, caffeine, and foods containing hot spices may increase symptoms

9. Evaluation: client states that pain intensity has decreased or pain is gone; reports that urinary symptoms have decreased or disappeared; verbalizes the need to restrict certain foods and beverages; describes measures to prevent recurrence; and verbalizes correct use of medications

L. **Prostate cancer**

1. Description: Unregulated growth of abnormal cells in the prostate gland

2. Etiology and pathophysiology

a. Adenocarcinoma is most common type; high levels of testosterone may play a role

b. Usually begins in peripheral tissue on back and sides of the gland

NCLEX!

c. Metastasis via lymph and venous channels is common; bony tissue is major site of distant metastasis—especially pelvic bones and spine

d. Is seen predominantly over 40 years of age

3. Assessment

a. Clinical manifestations

NCLEX!

1) Clients in early stages often show no symptoms; tumor may be found during digital prostate exam

NCLEX!

2) Genitourinary: dysuria, frequency, reduced force of stream, hematuria, nocturia, abnormal prostate found on digital rectal exam

3) Musculoskeletal: back pain, migratory bone pain, bone or joint pain

4) Neurologic: nerve pain, muscle spasms, bowel or bladder dysfunction, bilateral weakness of lower extremities

5) Systemic: fatigue and weight loss

b. Diagnostic and laboratory tests: prostate-specific antigen (PSA) levels, transrectal ultrasonography (obtained if PSA results are abnormal), tissue biopsy, bone scan; MRI, or CT scans to detect metastasis

4. Therapeutic management

a. Hormone therapy

b. Radiation therapy

c. Brachy therapy (radioactive seeds implanted in the prostate)

d. Prostatic cryosurgery

    e. Surgery

        1) Orchiectomy decreases androgen production

        2) Radical procedures include removal of gland, capsule, ampulla, vas deferens, seminal vesicles, adjacent lymph nodes, and cuff of bladder neck

        3) Suprapubic prostatectomy: abdominal and bladder incisions to remove prostate tissue

        4) Retropubic prostatectomy: low abdominal incision without opening bladder

        5) Perineal prostatectomy: incision between scrotum and anus (perineal area)

        6) Homium laser: laser treatment; less bleeding, fewer complications, and shorter hospital stay

5. Priority nursing diagnoses: Altered urinary elimination; Sexual dysfunction; Pain; Disturbed self-esteem; Disturbed body image

6. Planning and implementation

    a. Treatment is complex and depends on stage of cancer, client's age and general health

    b. Encourage annual prostate examination for men 40 years old and above

    c. Preoperative and postoperative care of the client undergoing prostatic surgery

7. Medication therapy: estrogen therapy or luteinizing hormone antagonist (Lupron) given to slow rate of growth and extension of tumor

8. Client education

    a. Assess client's knowledge about his illness and treatment plan; reinforce knowledge and option questions

    b. Teach methods to deal with urinary incontinence, which occurs temporarily after surgery, although it could be permanent if bladder sphincters have been permanently damaged

    c. Care of the urinary catheter

    d. Teach methods of pain control

    e. Instruct about the impact of therapy on sexual function (temporary or permanent impotence, permanent infertility after radical prostatectomy)

    f. Refer client to support groups, such as the American Cancer Society

    g. Stress the importance of follow-up tests for recurrence of the disease

    h. Teach signs of spinal cord compression (back pain and lower extremity weakness), because of high incidence of metastasis to spinal cord

    i. Instruct in activity levels as prescribed

9. Evaluation: client verbalizes knowledge of disease and treatment plan; states importance of follow-up visits, understands signs of spinal cord compression, and verbalizes activity limitations following surgery

VI. Sexually Transmitted Diseases (STDs)

A. Pelvic inflammatory disease (PID)

1. Description: inflammatory condition of the pelvic cavity that may involve the ovaries, fallopian tubes, vascular system, or pelvic peritoneum

2. Etiology and pathophysiology

   a. Usually caused by more than one microbe (polymicrobial)

   b. Microorganisms enter vagina and travel to uterus during sexual activity, childbirth, abortion, or surgery

   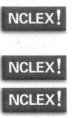

   c. Infection spreads to uterine tubes and obstructs them with scar tissue; may cause abscesses on the ovaries and spread to blood stream through lymphatic system

   d. PID is a major cause of female infertility

   e. Prognosis depends on number of episodes, prompt treatment, and modification of risk factors by the client

3. Assessment

   a. Clinical manifestations

      1) Fever

      2) Nausea, malaise, severe lower abdominal pain, and dysuria; moving or walking may also aggravate the pain

      3) Nausea and vomiting

      4) Tenderness in both lower abdominal quadrants

      5) Purulent, foul-smelling vaginal discharge

      6) Dyspareunia

   b. Diagnostic and laboratory tests

      1) Vaginal examination

      2) Elevated leukocyte and erythrocyte sedimentation rate

      3) Cultures from the vagina or cervix

      4) Ultrasound to detect abscess

4. Therapeutic management

   a. Antibiotic therapy

   b. Application of heat to relieve pain

   c. Surgical excision of abscess if present

5. Priority nursing diagnoses: Pain; Noncompliance; Sexual dysfunction; Impaired social interaction

6. Planning and implementation

   a. Place client in semi-Fowler's position to facilitate drainage

   b. Apply warmth to abdomen for comfort

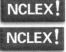
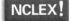

   c. Administer warm douches to improve circulation

   d. Monitor vital signs, especially temperature

   e. Administer antibiotics as prescribed

   f. Note nature and amount of vaginal discharge

   g. Use infection control techniques (standard precautions)

7. Medication therapy: combination antibiotic therapy with broad-spectrum antibiotics to treat infection; analgesics for discomfort; and antipyretics for fever

8. Client education

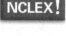

   a. Teach risk factors for PID: use of IUDs, history of sexually transmitted disease, multiple sexual partners, and previous PID

   b. Teach importance of completing treatment regime and keeping follow-up appointments, even if symptoms resolve (noncompliance is common)

   c. Instruct in proper perineal care, especially wiping from front to back

   d. Caution client about using tampons; change tampons at least every 4 hours

   e. Provide information about safe sexual practices and family planning

   f. Instruct client to report unusual vaginal discharge or odor

9. Evaluation: client reports abdominal pain and abnormal vaginal discharge resolves; body temperature returns to normal limits; verbalizes causes and risk factors for PID; states importance of completing treatment regime and follow-up visits; and verbalizes proper perineal care

B. Syphilis

1. Description: a systemic STD, caused by a spirochete, which may infect almost any body tissue or organ

2. Etiology and pathophysiology

   a. Caused by the spirochete *Treponema pallidum,* transmitted from open lesions during any type of sexual contact (oral-genital, anal-genital, or genital)

   b. Organism can survive for days in fluids; average incubation period is 10 to 90 days

   c. Course of disease varies and is prolonged; 30 to 40 years may pass between initial infection and late clinical signs; many clients experience a latency period when no symptoms are present (see Table 15-1)

   d. Primary syphilis: stage 1, occurs 3 to 4 weeks after infection; disease is highly infectious at this stage, but often goes unrecognized; chancres (painless indurated lesions) are seen in this stage

   e. Secondary syphilis: stage 2, occurs 2 weeks to 6 months after initial chancre appears; signs disappear within 2 to 6 weeks and latency period begins; highly infectious (latent syphilis: begins 2 or more years after initial infection and can last up to 50 years; disease not transmitted by sexual contact during this stage

Table 15-1	Primary Syphilis	Secondary Syphilis	Latent Syphilis	Tertiary Syphilis
Stages and Clinical Signs of Syphilis	Appearance of chancre at site of inoculation	Skin rash, especially on palms of hands or soles of feet	No apparent symptoms Disease not transmitted by sexual contact	Benign late syphilis: localized tumors in skin, bones, liver
	Lymphadenopathy	Mucous patches in oral cavity, sore throat, general lymphadenopathy	Occurs 2 or more years after initial infection; may last for 50 years	Diffuse inflammatory syphilis: involves CNS and cardiovascular system
	Highly infectious but onset often goes unnoticed	Onset any time from 2 weeks to 6 months after original chancre appears Highly infectious		

NCLEX!

  f. Tertiary syphilis: spirochetes enter internal organs and cause irreversible damage, especially to cardiovascular system (aorta and aortic valve) and central nervous system (meningitis, general paresis, progressive mental deterioration leading to insanity)

 3. Assessment

  a. Clinical manifestations: refer again to Table 15-1

NCLEX!

  b. Diagnostic and laboratory tests: VDRL becomes positive about 4 to 6 weeks after infection, but is nonspecific; FTA-ABS is specific for syphilis and can confirm the diagnosis; once a client has positive serology test, it will remain positive indefinitely

 4. Therapeutic management: parenteral penicillin G

 5. Priority nursing diagnoses: Risk for ineffective health maintenance; Noncompliance; Sexual dysfunction; Impaired social interaction; Ineffective individual coping; Deficient knowledge

 6. Planning and implementation

  a. Education is the primary nursing intervention for syphilis (see client education section)

NCLEX!

  b. Administer penicillin as prescribed and monitor client periodically to see that adequate treatment has occurred; treatment is based on length of illness and stage of the disease

  c. Create an environment where client feels safe to discuss questions and concerns

  d. Encourage all clients with syphilis to be tested for HIV

NCLEX!

  e. Encourage client to refer sexual partners for evaluation and treatment

NCLEX!

  f. Report all cases of syphilis to health authorities for treatment of contacts

 7. Medication therapy: penicillin G, given intramuscularly

 8. Client education

  a. Teach client to recognize signs of syphilis

b. Instruct client to seek immediate treatment if exposure occurs

c. Advise client to abstain from sex for 1 month after treatment

d. Educate client about need for simultaneous treatment of partner

e. Instruct client about need for follow-up testing in 3 and 6 months

9. Evaluation: client states the cause of syphilis; describes symptoms and primary mode of transmission; verbalizes treatment regime; takes medications as prescribed; returns for follow-up visits; serologic tests are negative; and identifies ways to prevent reinfection

C. **Gonorrhea**

1. Description: infection caused by *Neisseria gonorrhoeae,* leading to inflammation of mucous membranes of the genitourinary tract

2. Etiology and pathophysiology

a. *Neisseria gonorrhoeae* is a Gram-negative diplococcus; resistance to antibiotics is an increasing concern

b. Incidence is of epidemic proportion in the United States

c. Incubation period is 2 to 8 days after exposure

d. Transmitted by direct sexual contact; organism targets cervix and male urethra, spreads to other organs (such as rectum, joints, oral mucosa) unless treated

e. May lead to sterility in males, PID and other infections in women, and blindness and other serious problems for neonates exposed in the birth canal

3. Assessment

a. Clinical manifestations

1) Male clients: dysuria; signs of urethritis, serous, milky, or purulent urethral discharge, and lymphadenopathy; may be asymptomatic

2) Female clients: dysuria, abnormal vaginal discharge, and urinary frequency; many women have no symptoms

3) Proctitis (transmitted through anal intercourse or contamination)

4) Pharyngitis (transmitted through orogenital sex)

b. Diagnostic and laboratory tests

1) Culture (urethra, throat, and rectum) isolates the organism

2) Gram stain smear of the urethral discharge

3) Polymerase chain reaction (PCR)

4. Therapeutic management: medication therapy (see below)

5. Priority nursing diagnoses: Risk for ineffective health maintenance; Noncompliance; Sexual dysfunction; Impaired social interaction

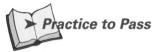

Practice to Pass

List two reasons why client education is so important in treating syphilis.

6. Planning and implementation

   a. Teaching is an important nursing intervention (see Client Education section below)

   b. Administer antibiotics as prescribed

   c. Arrange treatment for sexual partner

   d. Evaluate client's response to treatment and allow time to discuss concerns

7. Medication therapy: broad-spectrum antibiotic therapy; many strains of *N. gonorrhoeae* are now penicillin-resistant; ceftriaxone (Rocephin) single dose intramuscularly and doxycycline for uncomplicated cases

8. Client education

   a. Teach client to recognize signs of gonorrhea

   b. Instruct client to seek immediate treatment if exposure occurs

   c. Advise client to abstain from sex until cure is achieved; sexual intercourse can spread the disease and also delays healing because of the vascular congestion resulting from the activity

   d. Advise client to refrain from alcohol for 2 to 4 weeks; alcohol interrupts in the healing of the urethral walls

   e. Educate client about need for simultaneous treatment of partner

   f. Instruct client about need for follow-up visit 4 to 7 days after completing treatment

   g. Teach importance of taking medication exactly as prescribed

   h. Report all cases of gonorrhea to health authorities for treatment of contacts

9. Evaluation: client states the cause of gonorrhea; describes symptoms and primary mode of transmission; verbalizes treatment regime; takes medications as prescribed; returns for follow-up visits; follow-up tests are negative; and identifies ways to prevent reinfection

D. Genital herpes

1. Description: infection with the herpes simplex virus (HSV), usually type 2

2. Etiology and pathophysiology

   a. Spread by oral-genital, vaginal, or anal contact; incubation period is 3 to 7 days; virus enters body through mucous membranes or small breaks in the skin

   b. Lesions are small, painful blisters in the genital area; blisters contain virus particles, which can spread to other parts of the body

   c. A chronic, often asymptomatic, disease; may cause periodic recurrences

   d. First episode lasts about 12 days; recurrent infections lasts 4 to 5 days; period between outbreaks is called latency (virus is dormant)

   e. 45 million diagnosed cases in the United States

   f. May be lethal to fetus if exposed during delivery

3. Assessment

   a. Clinical manifestations

      1) Localized: herpetic lesions, tender swollen regional lymph nodes, dysuria, urinary retention, vaginal discharge (females), urethral discharge (males)

      2) Systemic: general malaise, fever, headache

      3) Factors that may trigger a recurrent outbreak: heat, intercourse, stress, anxiety, emotional upset, menstruation, or ovulation

   b. Diagnostic and laboratory tests

      1) Tissue culture isolates the virus

      2) Anti-HSV antibodies; is an unreliable for differentiating HSV1 from HSV2 antibodies

4. Therapeutic management

   a. Symptomatic treatment

   b. Pain management of lesions

   c. Medication therapy (see below)

5. Priority nursing diagnoses: Pain; Sexual dysfunction; Risk for infection; Anxiety; Risk for ineffective health maintenance

6. Medication therapy: anti-viral drug acyclovir (Zovirax) to reduce length and severity of first episode and recurrences; some strains becoming resistant to Acyclovir, so foscarnet (Foscavir) is used; and acetylsalicylic acid (aspririn) or acetaminophen (Tylenol) for pain; valcyclovir (Valtrex) is also used

7. Planning and implementation

   a. Cleanse genital area with warm water several times daily; dry with hair dryer or air dry

   b. Avoid lubricants and cream, which can prolong healing time

   c. Apply drying agents to relieve pain and itching

   d. Use soaks and compresses to promote drying and comfort

   e. Provide supportive, nonjudgmental environment; encourage client to ask questions and express feelings

8. Client education

   a. Instruct female clients to pour water over genitals while voiding to dilute acidity of urine during outbreak

   b. Wear loose clothing and cotton underwear to promote drying and reduce pressure

   c. Keep lesions and surrounding areas clean and dry

   d. Instruct on symptoms and factors that trigger recurrences

   e. Teach abstinence from sexual activity from time prodromal symptoms appear until 10 days after all lesions are healed

NCLEX!

NCLEX!

NCLEX!

NCLEX!

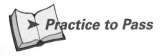

Practice to Pass

How would you reply to a client who asks how you plan to cure her genital herpes?

      f. Offer information about support groups and other resources

      g. Instruct client to avoid touching or scratching the lesions

      h. Discuss need to inform sexual partners about the disease, in order to plan prevention of transmission

      i. Instruct on the need for special precautions with pregnancy

  9. Evaluation: client describes prodromal symptoms and potential causes of recurrences; states that pain is diminished or absent; able to carry out normal daily activities; signs of secondary infection are absent; performs skin care as instructed; and describes health practices to reduce risk of infection and transmission

E. Genital warts

  1. Description: warts that appear in the anogenital area, caused by human papillomavirus (HPV)

  2. Etiology and pathophysiology

      a. Also called condyloma acuminatum, or venereal warts; more than 20 subtypes

      b. Virus infects nuclei of epithelial cells, causing them to proliferate

      c. May occur anywhere in the genital area: cervix, vagina, vulva, penis, urethra, scrotum, or anus

      d. Transmitted by direct skin-to-skin contact, usually through sexual activity; nonsexual transmission is possible

      e. Incubation period ranges from 6 weeks to 8 months, with an average of 3 months

      f. Warts may resolve spontaneously within 1 to 2 years

  3. Assessment

      a. Clinical manifestations

         1) Small to large wart-like growths on genitals (only symptom); warts are usually multiple and may form large masses; may spread internally to vagina and anus

         2) Bleeding and infection of warts may occur

      b. Diagnostic and laboratory tests: pap smear to assess for cervical cell changes—cervical cancer is often associated with genital warts

  4. Therapeutic management

      a. Medication therapy

      b. Cryotherapy, electrocautery, or surgical excision

  5. Priority nursing diagnoses: Risk for sexual dysfunction; Risk for infection; Anxiety; Risk for ineffective health maintenance; Fear; Impaired tissue integrity

  6. Planning and implementation

      a. Suggest annual pap test for female clients to detect cancer

      b. Administer antibiotics to treat infection

    c. Apply podophyllin (a cytotoxic agent), as ordered, to surfaces of warts, avoiding normal skin surfaces; treatment repeated every 7 days for up to 4 weeks

    d. Provide emotional support and education for client

7. Medication therapy: Podophyllin (cytotoxic agent) applied topically; trichloracetic and dichloroacetic acids applied topically to external warts

8. Client education

    a. Instruct female clients about increased risk for genital malignancy and need for annual gynecologic exams

    b. Keep lesions and surrounding areas clean and dry; instruct in signs of infection (pain, drainage, tenderness)

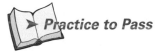

    c. Use condoms to prevent spread of genital warts

    d. Instruct client to avoid touching or scratching the lesions

    e. Instruct client to notify sexual partners to plan for prevention of transmission

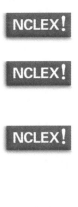

Practice to Pass

How are genital warts spread?

9. Evaluation: client states cause, symptoms, and mode of transmission of genital warts; identifies ways to decrease risk of infection; uses medications as prescribed; performs skin care techniques as instructed; and verbalizes need for annual gynecologic exams

F. Trichomoniasis

1. Description: vaginal protozoan infection caused by *Trichomonas vaginalis*

2. Etiology and pathophysiology

    a. One of most common sexually transmitted infections; often found with other STDs

    b. Overgrowth of protozoan normally present in vaginal tract

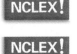

    c. May be carried by asymptomatic male partners, but is difficult to isolate in men

3. Assessment

    a. Clinical manifestations

        1) Malodorous and profuse vaginal discharge that may cause discomfort; discharge is greenish gray and watery, may appear frothy

        2) Burning with urination and itching; red and inflamed genitals

        3) Hemorrhagic spots on cervix or vaginal walls

    b. Diagnostic and laboratory tests: saline microscopic examination

4. Therapeutic management: medication therapy (see below)

5. Priority nursing diagnoses: Pain; Risk for ineffective health maintenance; Anxiety

6. Planning and implementation

    a. Administer Flagyl as prescribed

    b. Give soothing compresses, colloidal baths

c. Apply medicated creams

d. Treat sexual partners concurrently

7. Medication therapy: metronidazole (Flagyl), single dose

8. Client education

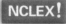

a. Instruct client to abstain from sexual intercourse during active infection, or to use condoms

b. Explain how infection is transmitted, including by towels and other personal items

c. Suggest use of cool compresses, sitz baths, and vinegar-water douches to relieve discomfort and itching

d. Suggest pouring water over genitals while voiding to ease dysuria

e. Instruct about genital hygiene practices and need to maintain normal vaginal flora

9. Evaluation: client states itching and pain are diminished or absent; able to carry out normal daily activities; signs of secondary infection are absent; carry out recommended hygiene practices; and recognizes cause and symptoms of trichomoniasis

G. Chlamydia

1. Description: bacterial infection of vulva or vagina caused by *Chlamydia trachomatis*

2. Etiology and pathophysiology

a. Most common STD; contracted by 3 to 4 million Americans each year; leading cause of pelvic inflammatory disease (PID)

b. Incubation period is 1 to 2 weeks after initial exposure

c. *Chlamydia trachomatis* is a bacterium, but behaves like a virus because it reproduces only within the host cell; takes over a cell and uses its energy

d. Chlamydia trachomatis conjunctivitis causes blindness; common cause of blindness in undeveloped countries; may also cause blindness or pneumonia in newborns exposed during birth

e. Asymptomatic infection is common; symptoms usually don't occur until infection invades the uterus and uterine tubes

f. Spread by any form of sexual contact

g. Risk factors: personal or partner history of STD, pregnancy, adolescent sexual activity, oral contraceptive use, unprotected sex, and multiple sexual partners

3. Assessment

a. Clinical manifestations

1) Vaginal or urethral discharge, white or mucous in males, purulent yellow or green cervical discharge in females

2) Signs and symptoms of urethritis (dysuria, urethral discharge), epididymitis (fever, scrotal pain), proctitis (rectal discharge and pain) in men

3) Signs and symptoms of PID may be the first symptom the female client notices (refer back to earlier discussion of PID)

   b. Diagnostic and laboratory tests

   1) A tissue sample for direct-slide monoclonal antibody test is the fastest and least expensive diagnostic test

   2) For definitive diagnosis, tissue samples for culture are obtained, which may take up to 7 days; treatment often begun on a presumptive basis

4. Therapeutic management: medication therapy (see below)

5. Priority nursing diagnoses: Pain; Disturbed body image; Risk for ineffective health maintenance; Risk for infection; Risk for noncompliance; and Anxiety

6. Planning and implementation

   a. Administer antibiotics as prescribed

   b. Provide privacy and confidentiality

   c. Treat client's sexual partner(s)

7. Medication therapy: antibiotics, such as doxycycline and azithromycin

8. Client education

   a. Instruct in importance of taking any and all prescribed medication

   b. Teach client the symptoms, cause, and potential complications of chlamydia

   c. Ask client to refer sexual partners for evaluation and treatment

   d. Instruct client to abstain from sexual activity for 1 month after treatment

   e. Instruct in need to use condoms to prevent future infections

9. Evaluation: client verbalizes symptoms and complications of chlamydial infections; lists ways to reduce risk of reinfection or transmission; verbalizes risk factors; takes medications as ordered and verbalizes actions, schedule, and adverse effects; and sexual contacts seek medical consultation and evaluation

VII. Infertility

A. Description: infertility is an inability to conceive after 1 year of regular intercourse with no contraceptive measures, or inability to deliver a live fetus after three consecutive conceptions

B. Etiology and pathophysiology

1. Approximately 8 to 10 percent of couples in the United States are infertile; 10 to 20 percent of these have no physical basis for infertility

2. Approximately 40 to 50 percent of infertility is attributed to female disorders

3. Female causes of infertility

   a. Hormonal dysfunction leading to insufficient gonadotropin secretions

   b. Ovarian, uterine, tubal, peritoneal, or cervical abnormalities

   c. Psychological problems

   d. Immunologic reaction to partner's sperm

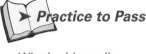

NCLEX!

Practice to Pass

Why is chlamydia difficult to diagnose based on physical examination findings alone?

NCLEX!

    4. Male causes of infertility

       a. Semen disorders: volume, motility, density; abnormal or immature sperms

       b. Systemic disorders, such as diabetes mellitus

       c. Genital infection

       d. Disorders of the testes

       e. Structural abnormalities

       f. Genetic defects

       g. Immunologic disorders

       h. Chemicals, drugs, and environmental factors

       i. Psychological problems

       j. Sexual problems

C. Assessment

    1. Clinical manifestations: none apparent; client reports inability to conceive or carry a fetus to term

    2. Diagnostic and laboratory tests

       a. Female clients

          1) Basal body temperature graph

          2) Endometrial biopsy

          3) Progesterone blood levels

          4) Tests to determine structural integrity of tubes, ovaries, and uterus

       b. Male clients

          1) Semen analysis (most conclusive test)

          2) Other laboratory tests: gonadotropin assay, serum testosterone levels, and urine 17-ketosteroid levels

          3) Testicular biopsy

D. Therapeutic management

    1. Female clients

NCLEX!

       a. Identify and correct underlying abnormalities or problems

       b. Hormone therapy

       c. Surgical restoration

       d. Medication therapy (female hormones)

    2. Male clients

NCLEX!

       a. Identify and correct underlying abnormalities or problems

       b. Counseling for sexual dysfunction

       c. Hormone supplements

E. Priority nursing diagnoses: Anxiety; Disturbed self esteem; Knowledge deficit

F. Planning and implementation

1. Assist in improving the general health of the couple

2. Teach stress reduction techniques

3. Discuss intrauterine insemination

4. Discuss and assist in in-vitro fertilization

5. Provide emotional support

6. Refer the couple to a support group

G. **Medication therapy:** testosterone or chorionic gonadotropin hormone therapy for male clients; female hormones for female clients

H. **Client education**

1. Inform couple about diagnostic and treatment techniques

2. Teach about reproductive and sexual function and factors that may interfere with fertility

3. Encourage questions; encourage couple to discuss their frustrations and other feelings

4. Explore alternatives, such as adoption

I. **Evaluation:** clients verbalize feelings and concerns about infertility; identify reproductive functions and factors that interfere with fertility; verbalize purpose of all diagnostic tests; verbalize reason for infertility and possible treatments; and discuss alternatives, such as adoption

VIII. Disorders of the Female Reproductive System

A. **Premenstrual syndrome (PMS)**

1. Definition: group of symptoms preceding the monthly menses that regress or disappear during menstruation

2. Etiology and pathophysiology

a. Affects women of all ages, races, and cultures

b. Believed to be related to hormonal changes such as altered estrogen–progesterone ratios, increased prolactin levels, and rising aldosterone levels during luteal phase of menstrual cycle (7 to 10 days before onset of flow)

c. Increased aldosterone causes sodium retention and edema

d. Decreased monamine oxidase in brain causes depression

e. Decreased serotonin causes mood swings

f. Produces multisystem effects that vary with each client and from month to month

3. Assessment

a. Clinical manifestations

1) See Figure 15-4 for multisystem effects of premenstrual syndrome

2) Clinical manifestations appear only during the luteal phase of the menstrual cycle (7 to 10 days before menstrual flow)

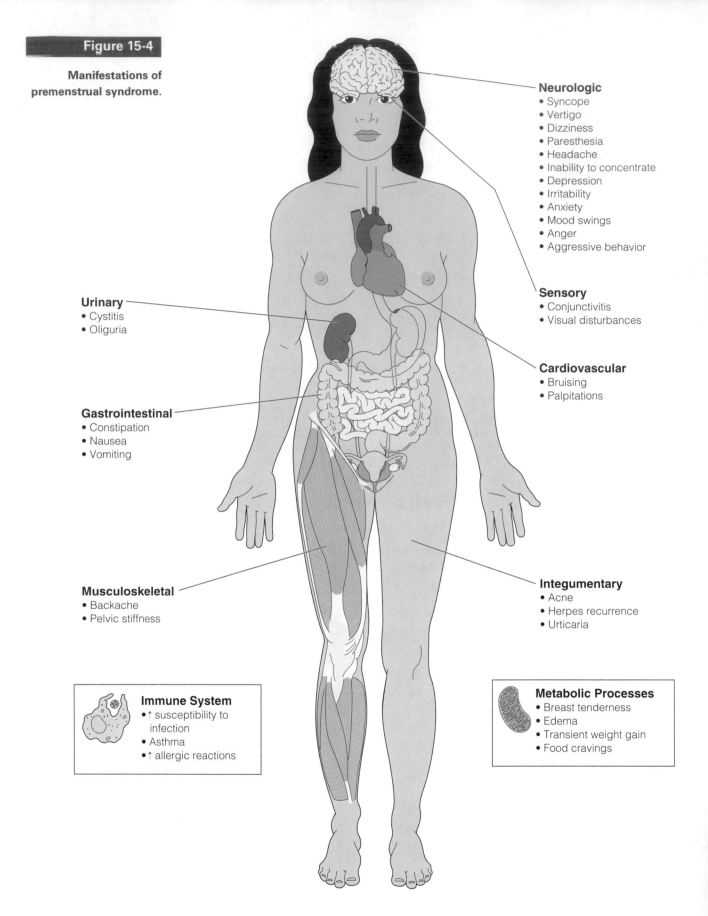

Figure 15-4

Manifestations of premenstrual syndrome.

Neurologic
- Syncope
- Vertigo
- Dizziness
- Paresthesia
- Headache
- Inability to concentrate
- Depression
- Irritability
- Anxiety
- Mood swings
- Anger
- Aggressive behavior

Sensory
- Conjunctivitis
- Visual disturbances

Cardiovascular
- Bruising
- Palpitations

Urinary
- Cystitis
- Oliguria

Gastrointestinal
- Constipation
- Nausea
- Vomiting

Musculoskeletal
- Backache
- Pelvic stiffness

Integumentary
- Acne
- Herpes recurrence
- Urticaria

Immune System
- ↑ susceptibility to infection
- Asthma
- ↑ allergic reactions

Metabolic Processes
- Breast tenderness
- Edema
- Transient weight gain
- Food cravings

    b. Diagnostic and laboratory tests

        1) Organic causes are ruled out first; there are no definitive diagnostic tests for PMS

  4. Therapeutic management

    a. Pharmacologic management

    b. Nonpharmacological management includes modifications in diet (see below), establishing an exercise plan, and stress management

  5. Priority nursing diagnoses: Pain; Ineffective individual coping

  6. Planning and implementation

    a. Nursing care focuses on teaching self-care and relieving symptoms

    b. Ask client to keep menstrual log on a daily basis for 1 to 4 months, recording symptoms and their relationship to the menstrual cycle

    c. Evaluate severity of symptoms and their effects on client's life

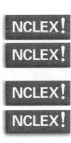

    d. Reduce sodium intake to minimize fluid retention

    e. Diet should be high in complex carbohydrates with limited simple sugars and alcohol to minimize reactive hypoglycemia

    f. Restrict caffeine to reduce irritability

    g. Increase intake of calcium, magnesium, and vitamin B_6

  7. Medication therapy: oral contraceptives to suppress ovulation in severe cases; NSAIDs to relieve cramping; diuretics to relieve bloating; and selective serotonin reuptake inhibitors, such as fluoxetine (Prozac), sertraline (Zoloft), paroxetine (Paxil) to manage mood swings

  8. Client education

    a. Teach measures to relieve pain

    b. Instruct client to use relaxation techniques, get regular physical exercise, and eat a well-balanced diet

    c. Encourage client to keep a diary of PMS symptoms and methods that produce relief

    d. Explore self-care measures to help with mood alterations, including stress identification

  9. Evaluation: client identifies personal symptoms of PMS; verbalizes ways to cope with each symptom; demonstrates use of menstrual log; identifies sources of stress and ways to reduce stress; verbalizes need for adequate rest and exercise; and verbalizes dietary interventions to prevent PMS symptoms

B. Dysmenorrhea

  1. Description: pain associated with menstruation

  2. Etiology and pathophysiology

    a. In primary dysmenorrhea, excess prostaglandins cause uterine muscle fibers to contract, producing uterine ischemia and painful cramps

    b. Onset is just before or at beginning of first menstrual flow—lasts from a few hours to several days

    c. Childbirth tends to reduce severity

    d. Secondary dysmenorrhea is related to underlying conditions that cause scarring or injury to reproductive tract (endometriosis, fibroid tumors, PID, and ovarian cancer)

3. Assessment

    a. Clinical manifestations

        1) Sharp pain located in lower abdomen, radiating to lower back, groin, or thighs

        2) Headache, nausea, anorexia, bloating, diarrhea, faintness, or fatigue

    b. Diagnostic and laboratory tests

        1) Pelvic examination to determine structural abnormalities

        2) FSH and LH levels to assess pituitary gland function

        3) Progesterone and estradiol levels to assess ovarian function

        4) Thyroid function tests

        5) CT or MRI

        6) Laparoscopy

        7) Dilatation and curettage (D&C) to obtain tissue samples for analysis

4. Therapeutic management

    a. Pharmacologic management

    b. Stress reduction, exercise, dietary counseling

5. Priority nursing diagnoses: Pain; Ineffective role performance; Disturbed sleep pattern; Ineffective individual coping

6. Planning and implementation

    a. Provide information on use of relief measures, including medication, heat, relaxation, and exercise

    b. Recommend reducing intake of sodium, sugar, caffeine, and alcohol

    c. Ask client to describe type, degree, time of onset, and duration of pain

    d. Assess characteristics of menstrual cycle, such as length of cycle, age at onset, type of flow usually experienced

    e. Assess for presence of underlying problems, such as STD, PID, fibroid tumors, ovarian cancer

    f. Ask client about relief measures she has tried

    g. Note physical factors that may contribute: poor posture, poor hygiene, and lack of exercise

7. Medication therapy: either nonprescription prostaglandin inhibitors or nonsteroidal anti-inflammatory drugs (NSAIDs) for pain relief and oral contraceptives in severe cases to inhibit ovulation

8. Client education

   a. Provide information that in most cases the disorder is benign in nature

   NCLEX!

   b. Teach relief measures, such as regular exercise, good posture, balanced diet and good hygiene; waist-bending exercises before onset of menstruation can help

   c. Instruct client to avoid constipation, which creates abdominal pressure

   d. Use a heating pad to help reduce pain

   NCLEX!

   e. Instruct client that increased intake of protein, calcium, magnesium, and vitamin B_6 may help relieve symptoms

9. Evaluation: client describes use of nonpharmacologic interventions; identifies and complies with taking prescribed medications; and explains the relationship of good posture, exercise, balanced diet, and good hygiene in preventing dysmenorrhea

C. **Abnormal uterine bleeding**

1. Description: vaginal bleeding that is painless but abnormal in amount, duration, or time of occurrence

2. Etiology and pathophysiology

   a. Primary **amenorrhea:** absence of menstruation; caused by structural abnormalities, hormonal imbalances, polycystic ovary disease, or imperforate hymen

   b. Secondary amenorrhea: absence of menstruation in a previously menstruating client; caused by anorexia nervosa, excessive athletic activity, hormonal imbalance, or ovarian tumors

   c. **Oligomenorrhea:** scant menses; usually related to hormonal imbalance

   d. **Menorrhagia:** excessive or prolonged menstruation; related to thyroid disorders, endometriosis, PID, ovarian cysts, or uterine fibroids

   e. **Metrorrhagia:** bleeding between menstrual periods; caused by hormonal imbalance, PID, cervical or uterine polyps or cancer; early evaluation for cancer is important with metrorrhagia

   f. Postmenopausal bleeding: caused by endometrial polyps, endometrial hyperplasia, or uterine cancer; early evaluation for cancer is important

3. Assessment

   a. Clinical manifestations: abnormal amount of vaginal bleeding

   b. Diagnostic and laboratory tests

      1) CBC to rule out other causes

      2) Endocrine studies, including thyroid hormones, to rule out cause

      3) hCG levels

      4) Pelvic ultrasound

      5) Hysteroscopy to detect uterine abnormalities

      6) Endometrial biopsy

4. Therapeutic management

   a. Hormonal therapy

   b. Therapeutic dilation and curettage, or scraping the uterine wall to correct excessive bleeding

   c. Endometrial ablation, destroying endometrial layer of uterus with laser surgery, which ends menstruation and reproduction

   d. Hysterectomy, or removal of the uterus

5. Priority nursing diagnoses: Ineffective individual coping; Sexual dysfunction; Disturbed self-esteem

6. Planning and implementation

   a. Assess characteristics of client's menstrual cycle

   b. Evaluate symptoms, including type and duration of menstrual bleeding, absence of bleeding, pain, mood changes, breast tenderness, nausea, headache, and bloating

   c. Assess client's coping strategies and psychosocial support system

   d. Assist client in dealing with self-esteem disturbances and anxiety

   e. Assist client through the diagnostic and treatment processes

7. Medication therapy: hormonal agents used to correct many menstrual irregularities; oral iron supplements to replace iron lost through excessive bleeding

8. Client education

   a. Teach the physiology of normal menstruation; answer questions about myths and cultural beliefs

   b. Instruct client in purpose, benefits, and risks of diagnostic tests and treatments

   c. Discuss results of all tests and examination and encourage questions

   d. Educate client about normal hygiene during menstruation (use of tampons, importance of cleanliness, and normal activities

   e. Teach measures to reduce discomfort associated with menstruation or treatments (see Dysmenorrhea)

   f. Emphasize the need to report episodes of excessive bleeding or postmenopausal bleeding due to the risk for cancer

9. Evaluation: client verbalizes understanding of diagnosis and treatment plan; identifies prescribed medications and their correct use; understands importance of follow-up visits to evaluate progress, and reports normal menstrual cycle at follow-up visit

D. Uterine prolapse

1. Description: downward displacement of the uterus into the vaginal canal

   a. First-degree prolapse: less than half of uterus extends into vagina

   b. Second-degree prolapse: descent of entire uterus into vaginal canal

      c. Third-degree prolapse (procidentia): complete prolapse of uterus outside the body, with inversion of vaginal canal

  2. Etiology and pathophysiology

      a. May be congenital or acquired

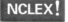

      b. Usually related to weakened pelvic musculature caused by stretching of supporting ligaments during pregnancy and childbirth

      c. Risk factors: unrepaired lacerations from childbirth, rapid deliveries, multiple pregnancies, congenital weakness, loss of elasticity and muscle tone with aging, and chronic coughing

      d. Prolapse is often accompanied by cystocele or rectocele

  3. Assessment

      a. Clinical manifestations

         1) Lump protruding from vagina; typically painless and has increased in size for months or years; usually worse with standing or straining

         2) Discomfort in lower abdomen, or pressure and heaviness in vaginal area; client may complain of low backache with standing

         3) Difficulty in defecation due to rectocele

         4) Difficulty urinating due to cystocele

         5) Urinary incontinence

         6) Pain with intercourse

         7) Signs of infection, chafing, ulceration, and bleeding from exposed uterus in third-degree prolapse

      b. Diagnostic and laboratory tests: pelvic examination

  4. Therapeutic management

      a. Kegel exercises

      b. Insertion of a vaginal pessary, a donut-shaped ring placed in the vagina to provide uterine support

      c. Vaginal hysterectomy

  5. Priority nursing diagnoses: Disturbed body image; Risk for infection; Anxiety; Stress incontinence

  6. Planning and implementation

      a. Advise client about nonsurgical techniques to manage prolapse, i.e., Kegel exercises to strengthen pelvic muscles

      b. Discuss use of pessary, device inserted into vagina to provide temporary support

      c. Discuss treatment options and prepare client for hysterectomy, which is treatment for third-degree prolapse

      d. Teach ways to deal with stress incontinence, which may accompany uterine prolapse

7. Medication therapy: none

8. Client education

   a. Teach Kegel exercises to strengthen pelvic muscles

   b. Instruct in the use of pessary: insertion and cleaning

   c. Instruct on perineal care and the importance of good hygiene to prevent infection

   d. Dietary counseling if obesity is a factor

   e. Encourage questions from client and explain treatment options

9. Evaluation: client verbalizes purpose and technique of Kegel exercises; verbalizes importance of good hygiene to prevent infection; and verbalizes understanding of treatment options

E. Cystocele and rectocele

1. Description

   a. **Cystocele:** herniation of the bladder into the vagina

   b. **Rectocele:** herniation of the rectum into the vagina

2. Etiology and pathophysiology

   a. Both conditions are usually related to weakened pelvic musculature caused by stretching of supporting ligaments during pregnancy and childbirth

   b. With cystocele, client may experience stress incontinence and difficulty emptying bladder, leading to retention and infection

   c. Risk factors: unrepaired lacerations from childbirth, rapid deliveries, multiple pregnancies, congenital weakness, loss of elasticity and muscle tone with aging, chronic coughing

3. Assessment

   a. Clinical manifestations

      1) Bearing-down sensation in pelvic area, constipation, hemorrhoids, urinary incontinence, and fecal incontinence

      2) With rectocele, client reports she has to press on rectocele from inside of vagina in order to defecate

      3) With cystocele, signs of urinary tract infection, urinary retention, and stress incontinence

      4) Cystocele and rectocele can sometimes be seen on inspection, but usually recede when client is lying down; diagnosis is made by asking client to bear down

      5) Bulging just below urethral orifice

   b. Diagnostic and laboratory tests

      1) Cystography is performed to determine if there is bladder herniation

      2) Measurement of residual urine

      3) Urinalysis and culture

4. Therapeutic management

    a. Kegel exercises

    b. Surgical correction

        1) Posterior colporrhaphy is surgical treatment for rectocele, to shorten pelvic muscles and provide tighter support for rectum

        2) Anterior colporrhaphy is surgical treatment for cystocele, to shorten pelvic muscles and provide tighter support for bladder

        3) Marshall-Marchetti-Krantz procedure suspends the bladder in correct anatomic position to help correct cystocele

5. Priority nursing diagnoses: Disturbed body image; Risk for infection; Stress incontinence; Disturbed self-esteem; Risk for sexual dysfunction

6. Planning and implementation

    a. Advise client about available treatments, which often involve surgery

    b. Provide emotional support

    c. Pre- and postoperative care of the client undergoing surgery

7. Medication therapy: none

8. Client education

    a. Instruct client in Kegel exercises to reduce stress incontinence

    b. Discuss treatment options and prepare client for surgery, which is main treatment for rectocele and cystocele

    c. Describe what to expect in the postoperative period

    d. Explain to client that both colporrhaphy procedures shorten the overall length of the vagina and may result in discomfort during sexual intercourse

9. Evaluation: client verbalizes understanding of diagnosis and treatment plan; understands importance of follow-up visits to evaluate progress; reports normal voiding and defecation at follow-up; verbalizes procedure for Kegel exercises to strengthen pelvic muscles

F. Vulvitis

1. Definition: inflammation or infection of the vulva

2. Etiology and pathophysiology

    a. Skin of the vulva is prone to inflammation from mechanical or chemical irritation, due to its location

    b. Causes include: tight-fitting clothes; exposure to urine, fecal material, vaginal discharge, and glandular secretions; chemical irritants, such as soap, feminine hygiene spray, powder, vaginal lubricants, etc.

3. Assessment

    a. Clinical manifestations

        1) Assess for itching, the cardinal symptom

        2) Burning sensation aggravated by urination or defecation

3) Tissues appear red and swollen; there may be abrasions where client has scratched

4) Vaginal discharge may be present with vaginitis

b. Diagnostic and laboratory tests

1) Culture of the discharge

2) KOH analysis, wet smear analysis, and Gram stain

3) Urinalysis and urine culture

4) Serologic testing

4. Priority nursing diagnoses: Pain; Risk for ineffective health maintenance

5. Planning and implementation

a. Ask client about personal habits that could contribute to inflammatory process: type of undergarments, allergies, use of perfumed soap and powder, overuse of feminine hygiene products such as sprays or douches

b. Identify type of infection through observation or cultures

c. Provide appropriate pharmacologic treatment for infection and inflammation

d. Give soothing compresses or colloidal baths

e. Apply medicated creams

6. Medication therapy: topical creams to relieve inflammation and antibiotics if infection is present

7. Client education

a. Teach client how to properly clean the vulva: don't use soap between the labia, rinse thoroughly to remove soap residue, dry area completely

b. Teach client to avoid tight-fitting clothes, wear 100 percent cotton underpants, and wear knee-high or thigh-high stockings instead of pantyhose when possible

c. Avoid strong laundry soaps, talcum powder, perfumed soap, scented toilet paper, and deodorant sprays

d. To kill yeast in underwear, soak in half-strength bleach for 20 minutes before washing

e. Instruct in use of comfort measures, such as sitz baths, cool or warm compresses, and topical creams

8. Evaluation: client reports that pruritus is relieved; vulvar tissue free of redness and edema; lists ways to prevent vulvitis; and describes proper techniques for cleaning the vulva

G. Candidiasis

1. Definition: fungal vaginal infection caused by *Candida albicans* (yeast)

2. Etiology and pathophysiology

a. 500,000 Americans get this infection yearly—usually seen in women

b. Widespread use of antibiotics increases incidence, because antibiotics destroy normal vaginal flora

c. Vaginal flora is normally acidic; changes in flora allow yeast to proliferate

d. Candida thrives on sugar-carbohydrate rich environment

e. Risk factors: tampons; sexual intercourse; chemical irritation; fecal contamination; infestation with parasites, such as pinworms; sexually transmitted organisms, frequent or prolonged use of antibiotics

3. Assessment

   a. Clinical manifestations

      1) Scant white cottage cheese-like vaginal drainage

      2) Itching of vulva and burning with urination

      3) Vulva and vaginal area red and swollen

      4) Inflamed cervix

   b. Diagnostic and laboratory tests

      1) Wet mounts (direct microscopic examination of vaginal discharge)

      2) Vaginal, urethral, or cervical cultures

      3) Gram stain

4. Therapeutic management: medication therapy (see below)

5. Priority nursing diagnoses: Pain; Risk for ineffective health maintenance; Knowledge deficit

6. Planning and implementation

   a. Identify type of infection through observation or cultures

   b. Provide appropriate pharmacologic treatment for infection and inflammation

   c. Give soothing compresses or colloidal baths

   d. Apply medicated creams

7. Medication therapy: miconazole (Monistat), clotrimazole (Lotrimin), or terconazole (Terazol7 or Terazol3) creams or suppositories; povidone-iodine or vinegar douches

8. Client education

   a. Teach client how to properly clean the vulva: don't use soap between the labia; rinse thoroughly to remove soap residue; dry area completely

   b. Teach client to avoid tight-fitting clothes, wear 100 percent cotton underpants, and wear knee-high or thigh-high stockings instead of pantyhose when possible

   c. To protect vaginal flora, avoid strong laundry soaps, talcum powder, perfumed soap, scented toilet paper, and deodorant sprays

   d. To kill yeast in underwear, soak in half-strength bleach for 20 minutes before washing

   e. Instruct in use of comfort measures, such as sitz baths, cool or warm compresses, and topical creams

NCLEX!

      f. Instruct client to consume 8 ounces of yogurt containing live active cultures daily to help restore normal vaginal flora

      g. Teach client how infection is transmitted and that sexual partner will also need treatment; infection may be asymptomatic in one partner

   9. Evaluation: client reports that pruritus and discharge have resolved; vaginal tissue free of redness and edema; states ways to prevent candidiasis; describes proper techniques for cleaning the vulva; sexual partner presents for treatment; and verbalizes need for safe-sex practices

H. Cervical cancer

   1. Description: unregulated growth of abnormal cells in the cervix

   2. Etiology and pathophysiology

NCLEX!

NCLEX!

      a. Most common cancer of the reproductive system

      b. Usually seen in clients between ages of 30 and 50

      c. May become invasive and spread to tissue outside cervix, fundus of the uterus, and the lymph glands

      d. Treatment depends on extent of disease

      e. Squamous cell carcinoma accounts for 90 percent of cervical cancers; they have gradual onset; spread by direct invasion of accessory structures

   3. Assessment

      a. Clinical manifestations

         1) Thin, watery, blood-tinged vaginal discharge, which may go unnoticed by client

         2) Painless bleeding between periods, often seen after intercourse, douching, or other contact

         3) Late symptoms occur as cancer progresses to other organs, including referred pain in back and thighs, hematuria, bloody stools, anemia, and weight loss

NCLEX!

         4) Early diagnosis is critical, because cervical cancer can be cured in early stages

      b. Diagnostic and laboratory tests

         1) Cervical pap test; abnormal results call for repeat test, colposcopic exam of cervix, and tissue biopsy; diagnosis is based on biopsy results

   4. Therapeutic management: chemotherapy, radiation therapy, and surgery

   5. Priority nursing diagnoses: Fear; Anxiety; Knowledge deficit; Risk for impaired tissue integrity; Ineffective individual coping

   6. Planning and implementation

      a. Assist client in dealing with psychologic effects of illness; provide information and emotional support

      b. Explore treatment options with client and family

      c. Develop strategies for pain control

d. Maintain skin and tissue integrity during radiation treatment and following surgery

e. Observe for fistula formation between vagina and the bladder or rectum, a possible complication of radiation therapy

f. Recommend a high-carbohydrate, high-protein diet

7. Medication therapy: chemotherapy for tumors not responsive to other therapy, tumors that cannot be removed, or as adjunct therapy for metastasis; and analgesics for pain control

8. Client education

a. Explain and discuss all diagnostic tests and treatments, allowing client time to express her feelings and ask questions

b. Teach wound and skin care if surgery or radiation therapy are performed

c. Explain that 66 percent of all women with cervical cancer survive for 5 years or more

d. Emphasize the importance of regular screening exams and follow-up after treatment is completed

9. Evaluation: client makes informed decisions about treatment options; develops strategies for pain control; expresses feelings about fear of cancer and death; and maintains skin and tissue integrity during treatment

I. Ovarian cancer

1. Description: unregulated growth of abnormal cells in the ovaries

2. Etiology and pathophysiology

a. The most lethal of gynecologic cancers; etiology not understood

b. Is often asymptomatic, leading to late diagnoses; usually detected by chance, not through screening

c. Risk increases after age 40

d. May involve one or both ovaries; staged according to tissue involvement

e. Four stages of ovarian cancers: Stages: I—limited to ovaries; II—pelvic extension; III—metastasis outside pelvis or positive lymph nodes, and IV—distant metastasis

3. Assessment

a. Clinical manifestations

1) Symptoms are rare until extensive tumor growth is present

2) Feeling of pelvic pressure or heaviness, vague abdominal discomfort, dyspepsia, bloating, constipation, urinary frequency, and increased abdominal size

3) Palpable hard, fixed, firm mass in the area of the ovaries during pelvic exam

b. Diagnostic and laboratory tests

1) No definitive diagnostic tool is available; diagnosis is made during surgery (exploratory laparotomy)

NCLEX!

2) CA125 antigen level is sometimes useful in detecting ovarian cancer; CA125 is a tumor marker

4. Therapeutic management: surgery, radiation therapy, and chemotherapy

5. Priority nursing diagnoses: Fear; Anxiety; Impaired skin integrity; Constipation; Diarrhea; Ineffective Individual Coping

6. Planning and implementation

NCLEX!

   a. Explore treatment options with client and family; surgery is treatment of choice, radiation is used for palliative purposes to shrink tumor

   b. Assist client in dealing with psychologic effects of illness; provide information and emotional support

   c. Develop strategies for pain control

   d. Maintain skin and tissue integrity during radiation treatment and following surgery

7. Medication therapy: chemotherapy may be used to achieve remission, but is not a cure

8. Client education

   a. Explain and discuss all diagnostic tests and treatments, allowing client time to express her feelings and ask questions

NCLEX!

   b. Teach wound and skin care if surgery or radiation therapy is performed

   c. Emphasize the importance of regular screening exams and follow-up after treatment is completed

   d. Teach client not to ignore vague symptoms, such as indigestion, nausea, or urinary frequency

9. Evaluation: client makes informed decisions about treatment options; develops strategies for pain control; expresses feelings about fear of cancer and death; maintains skin and tissue integrity during treatment; and verbalizes need for follow-up visits after treatment

J. Breast cancer

1. Definition: unregulated growth of abnormal cells in breast tissue

2. Etiology and pathophysiology

   a. Cause unknown, but many risk factors influence development

      1) Female gender and white/Caucasian race

      2) Family history of mother or sister with breast cancer

      3) Medical history of cancer of other breast, endometrial cancer, or atypical hyperplasia

      4) Menarche before age 12 (early) or menopause after age 50 (late)

      5) First birth after 30 years of age, oral contraceptive use (early or prolonged), prolonged use of estrogen replacement therapy

      6) Lifestyle factors: high-fat diet, obesity, high socioeconomic status, breast trauma, smoking, ingesting more than 2 alcoholic drinks daily

      7) Exposure to radiation through chest X-ray, fluoroscopy

b. Begins as a single transformed cell and is hormone-dependent; does not develop in women without functioning ovaries who never received hormone replacement therapy

c. Most often occurs in ductal areas of breasts

d. Noninvasive: does not penetrate surrounding tissues; may be ductal or lobular; usually diagnosed through mammogram or nipple discharge

e. Invasive: penetration of tumor into surrounding tissue; five types of invasive cancers, with only slight differences in prognosis

f. Staging depends on size of tumor, lymph node involvement, and metastasis to distant sites

g. 70 percent of clients with Stage I tumors survive for ten years with therapy

3. Assessment

   a. Clinical manifestations

      1) Lump in upper outer quadrant of breast, usually nontender, but may be tender

      2) Dimpling of breast tissue surrounding nipple, or bleeding from the nipple

      3) Asymmetry, with affected breast being higher

      4) Regional lymph nodes swollen and tender

   b. Diagnostic and laboratory tests: mammography, ultrasonography, MRI, PET, tissue biopsy, sentinel node biopsy (uses radionuclides to locate sentinel node for removal and analysis rather than a chain of nodes)

4. Therapeutic management: surgery, radiation therapy, chemotherapy, and hormonal therapy

5. Priority nursing diagnoses: Anxiety; Fear; Decisional conflict; Anticipatory grieving; Risk for injury; Risk for infection; Risk for disturbed body image

6. Planning and implementation

   a. Explore treatment options with client and family; prepare client for treatment, which is based on stage of disease

   b. Radiation therapy is used to destroy remaining cancer cells after surgery, or to shrink tumor prior to surgery

   c. Various types of mastectomy may be performed

      1) Segmental mastectomy or lumpectomy: removes the tumor and a margin of breast tissue surrounding the tumor

      2) Simple mastectomy: removal of the complete breast but no other structures

      3) Modified radical mastectomy: removal of the breast and axillary lymph nodes, but chest wall muscles are not resected

      4) Radical mastectomy: removal of the breast, axillary lymph nodes, and underlying chest wall muscles

5) Breast reconstruction: may be performed at the time of mastectomy or may be done at a later time; can be accomplished through submuscular breast implant, placing an implant after using a tissue expander, using muscles with intact blood supply from the back or abdomen, or creating a free muscle flap with the gluteus maximus muscle

d. Assist client in dealing with psychologic effects of illness; provide information and emotional support, including information about breast reconstruction surgery

e. Maintain skin and tissue integrity during radiation treatment and following surgery

NCLEX!

7. Medication therapy: tamoxifen (Novadex) interferes with estrogen activity for treating advanced breast cancer, and chemotherapy when axillary nodes are involved

8. Client education

a. Explain and discuss all diagnostic tests and treatments, allowing client time to express her feelings and ask questions

b. Review information about mastectomy surgery and what to expect afterward

NCLEX!

c. Teach wound care if surgery is performed, including care of short-term wound drains

NCLEX!

d. Teach techniques for proper skin care if radiation therapy is performed

e. Encourage client to meet other women who've undergone treatment, if appropriate

f. Teach client how to protect affected arm and hand from infection and injury if lymph nodes are removed during mastectomy (refer back to client care following mastectomy earlier in chapter)

NCLEX!

g. Teach postoperative exercises and self breast-examination

h. Teach self-care during radiation and chemotherapy treatments

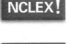

i. Emphasize the importance of regular screening exams and follow-up after treatment is completed

9. Evaluation: client makes informed decisions about treatment options; develops strategies for pain control; expresses feelings about fear of cancer and death; maintains skin and tissue integrity during treatment; verbalizes need for follow-up visits and breast self-examination after treatment; demonstrates care of affected arm and hand; and demonstrates postoperative exercises

Case Study

M. S., a 48-year-old married client, is scheduled for an incisional biopsy to evaluate a lump in her left breast. You are the nurse in the ambulatory care center where the procedure will take place.

❶ How will you describe the surgery to M. S. when she arrives at the clinic?

❷ If the biopsy is malignant, list three nursing diagnoses for M. S.

❸ How could breast cancer treatment affect sex and intimacy for M. S.?

❹ What steps would you take when helping M. S. decide what treatment to undergo for breast cancer?

❺ How would you describe a modified radical mastectomy to M.S.?

For suggested responses, see page 739.

Posttest

1 A client asks the nurse what causes syphilis. The nurse answers correctly that syphilis is caused by a:

(1) Bacterial infection.
(2) Spirochete.
(3) Fungal infection.
(4) Yeast infection.

2 A client with syphilis exhibits flu-like symptoms, a skin rash on the palms of the hands, and hair loss. The nurse develops a plan of care based on which stage of the disease?

(1) Primary syphilis
(2) Secondary syphilis
(3) Tertiary syphilis
(4) Latent syphilis

3 Which of the following nursing diagnoses is the top priority during a client's first outbreak of genital herpes?

(1) Pain
(2) Sexual dysfunction
(3) Anxiety
(4) Risk for infection

4 The nurse is teaching a group of men about testicular cancer. Which of the following statements would the nurse include about this type of cancer?

(1) It's usually painless, and therefore hard to detect.
(2) It causes severe pain in the early stages.
(3) Testicular self-examination doesn't help detect it.
(4) It rarely affects young men.

5 The nurse working in an urgent care center would consider it a surgical emergency if a client presented with which of the following conditions?

(1) Hydrocele
(2) Spermatocele
(3) Testicular torsion
(4) Varicocele

6 A client is admitted for treatment of hydrocele. The nurse understands this results from which of the following?

(1) A fluid-filled mass within the scrotum
(2) A mass containing dead spermatozoa
(3) Dilated veins within the spermatic cord
(4) Twisting of the testes and spermatic cord

7 The nurse anticipates that a client being evaluated for erectile dysfunction may receive a prescription for which of the following medications?

(1) Propranolol (Inderal)
(2) Diazepam (Valium)
(3) Sildenafil (Viagra)
(4) Progesterone

8 The nurse is teaching a male client about the use of sildenafil (Viagra). Which of the following instructions is correct?

(1) "Take the drug after a high-fat meal to avoid GI upset."
(2) "You may combine the drug with your vacuum constriction device."
(3) "It's acceptable to use the drug several times a day."
(4) "Don't use the drug if you take nitrate medications, such as nitroglycerin."

9 The nurse is teaching about sexually transmitted diseases. Which of the following is the greatest concern with chlamydial infection that the nurse should emphasize?

(1) It causes severe pain and burning with urination.
(2) There is lack of symptoms until infection invades the uterus.
(3) It is caused by yeast infection that spreads easily.
(4) Older women are at highest risk in contracting the disease.

10 When teaching a male client about prostate cancer, the nurse explains that the survival rate for prostate cancer is:

(1) Excellent when diagnosed early.
(2) Poor, no matter when diagnosed.
(3) Best for men under 40.
(4) Best for African-American men.

See page 625 for Answers and Rationales.

Answers and Rationales

Pretest

1 Answer: 3 *Rationale:* Various relationships between BPH and diet, obesity, sexual activity, and racial origins have been explored; however, none of these provide insight into its etiology.
Cognitive Level: Application
Nursing Process: Implementation; *Test Plan:* HPM

2 Answer: 1 *Rationale:* Priapism is considered a medical emergency, because continued erection may lead to tissue fibrosis and impotence. Immediate treatment involves ice packs, not warm soaks. Options 2 and 4 do not apply.
Cognitive Level: Application
Nursing Process: Implementation; *Test Plan:* PHYS

3 Answer: 1 *Rationale:* Propranolol, a beta adrenergic blocker, and many other antihypertensive medications can contribute to erectile dysfunction. Other examples include clonidine (Catapres) and benazepril (Lotensin). The medications listed in options 2, 3, and 4 aren't known to have this effect.
Cognitive Level: Application
Nursing Process: Analysis; *Test Plan:* PHYS

4 Answer: 2 *Rationale:* Because painless vaginal bleeding is often the only symptom of cervical or uterine cancer, this client should be tested for cancer. Options 1 and 4 are not probable given the client's

age. Hormonal imbalances (option 3) may cause bleeding but are less urgent than the threat of cancer.
Cognitive Level: Application
Nursing Process: Planning; *Test Plan:* PHYS

5 Answer: 3 *Rationale:* NPTR monitoring helps differentiate between psychogenic and organic causes of erectile dysfunction. The other options are not assessed using NPTR monitoring.
Cognitive Level: Application
Nursing Process: Analysis; *Test Plan:* PHYS

6 Answer: 4 *Rationale:* Third-degree uterine prolapse is visible outside the body as the uterus inverts the vaginal canal. Rectocele is prolapse of the rectum. Cystocele is prolapse of the urethra. A vaginal infection would not cause tissue protrusion from the vagina, although the vaginal tissues would be reddened and/or edematous.
Cognitive Level: Application
Nursing Process: Assessment; *Test Plan:* PHYS

7 Answer: 3 *Rationale:* The Pap smear test is used to screen women for cervical cancer, assess hormonal status, and identify the presence of sexually transmitted diseases, such as HPV infection. Infertility and AIDS are not diagnosed with the Pap test. Sterility is a male reproductive problem.
Cognitive Level: Application
Nursing Process: Assessment; *Test Plan:* SECE

8   Answer: 4 *Rationale:* Early menstruation, before the age of 12, is a risk factor for breast cancer. Use of foam contraceptives is not a factor. Late menopause increases the risk for breast cancer, but not early menopause. A first birth after the age of 30 is a risk factor, but first birth before age 20 is not.
Cognitive Level: Application
Nursing Process: Assessment; *Test Plan:* HPM

9   Answer: 2 *Rationale:* Breast examinations should be done monthly, at the same time each month to aid in remembering to do it regularly. A post-menopausal woman would select the same date each month, while premenopausal women should do BSE at completion of the menstrual cycle. Breast examination during menstrual flow is not the best time, because of hormonal influences on the breasts.
Cognitive Level: Application
Nursing Process: Implementation; *Test Plan:* HPM

10   Answer: 2 *Rationale:* Syphilis is transmitted from open lesions during any sexual contact: genital, oral-genital, or anal-genital. Kissing, sharing eating utensils, and shaking hands do not transmit the disease.
Cognitive Level: Application
Nursing Process: Analysis; *Test Plan:* HPM

Posttest

1   Answer: 2 *Rationale:* The spirochete *Treponema pallidum* causes syphilis. The other responses are incorrect.
Cognitive Level: Comprehension
Nursing Process: Implementation; *Test Plan:* PHYS

2   Answer: 2 *Rationale:* The client's symptoms are consistent with secondary syphilis, which occurs 2 weeks to 6 months after the initial chancre disappears. Latent syphilis produces no symptoms, and tertiary syphilis is the final stage of the illness. Tertiary syphilis is characterized by the development of infiltrating tumors and involvement of the central nervous and cardiovascular systems.
Cognitive Level: Application
Nursing Process: Planning; *Test Plan:* PHYS

3   Answer: 1 *Rationale:* Herpetic lesions are very painful, so the first priority is to provide comfort measures for the client. The other diagnoses do not address the client's most immediate concern.
Cognitive Level: Analysis
Nursing Process: Planning; *Test Plan:* PHYS

4   Answer: 1 *Rationale:* A painless, hard nodule is the classic presenting symptom of testicular cancer. Testicular self-examination can help detect this sign. Testicular cancer is the most common cancer in men between the ages of 15 and 35, and is the third-leading cause of cancer death in young men.
Cognitive Level: Application
Nursing Process: Implementation; *Test Plan:* PHYS

5   Answer: 3 *Rationale:* Testicular torsion, or twisting of the testes and spermatic cord, is a potential emergency, because compromised blood flow to the testicle may lead to ischemia and necrosis. The other conditions usually don't require emergency intervention.
Cognitive Level: Application
Nursing Process: Analysis; *Test Plan:* PHYS

6   Answer: 1 *Rationale:* Hydrocele is a fluid-filled mass within the scrotum. Option 2 describes spermatocele. Option 3 describes varicocele. Option 4 describes testicular torsion.
Cognitive Level: Comprehension
Nursing Process: Planning; *Test Plan:* PHYS

7   Answer: 3 *Rationale:* Sildenafil is an oral medication used to treat erectile dysfunction in men. The other medications may worsen the client's condition.
Cognitive Level: Application
Nursing Process: Planning; *Test Plan:* PHYS

8   Answer: 4 *Rationale:* Clients who take nitrates may experience severe hypotension when using sildenafil. Taking the drug after a high-fat meal will delay its onset. The drug should not be combined with other treatments for erectile dysfunction, and should not be taken more often than once daily.
Cognitive Level: Application
Nursing Process: Implementation; *Test Plan:* PHYS

9   Answer: 2 *Rationale:* Chlamydial infection may be present for months or years without producing symptoms in women. The disease may invade the uterus, resulting in devastating complications. It is caused by *Chlamydia trachomatis,* a bacterium that behaves like a virus. Young women using oral contraceptives have the highest risk.
Cognitive Level: Application
Nursing Process: Implementation; *Test Plan:* SECE

10   Answer: 1 *Rationale:* When diagnosed early and confined to the prostate gland, prostate cancer is curable and the 5-year survival rate is 100 percent. Men under the age of 40 rarely have prostate cancer. African-American men have a higher incidence of prostate cancer and a higher mortality rate.
Cognitive Level: Application
Nursing Process: Implementation; *Test Plan:* HPM

References

Berger, K. J. & Williams, M. (1999). *Fundamentals of nursing: Collaborating for optimal health* (2nd ed.). Upper Saddle River, NJ: Prentice Hall, Inc., pp 427–430.

Christensen, B. L. & Kockrow, E. O. (1999). *Adult health nursing.* St. Louis, MO: Mosby, pp. 478–539.

Ignatavicius, D. & Workman, L. (2002). *Medical-surgical nursing: Critical thinking for collaborative care* (4th ed.). Philadelphia: Saunders, pp. 1707–1727, 1730–1749, 1751–1803, 1807–1822.

Illustrated manual of nursing practice (2nd ed.) (1999). Springhouse: Springhouse Corporation, pp. 981–1032; 1157–1202.

Kozier, B., Erb, G., Berman, A., & Burke, K. (2003). *Fundamentals of nursing: Concepts, process, and practice* (7th ed.). Upper Saddle River, NJ: Prentice Hall, Inc., pp. 923–947; 849–887.

LeMone, P. & Burke, K. (2003). *Medical-surgical nursing: Critical thinking in client care* (3rd ed.). Upper Saddle River, NJ: Prentice-Hall, Inc., pp. 1951–2076

Monahan, F. & Neighbors, M. (1998). *Medical-surgical nursing: Foundations for clinical practice* (2nd ed.). Philadelphia: W.B. Saunders, pp. 1693–1840.

North American Nursing Diagnosis Association. (2000). *Nursing diagnosis: Definitions and classification, 2001–2002.* Philadelphia: NANDA.

Olds, S., London, M., & Ladewig, P. (2000*). Maternal-newborn nursing: A family and community-based approach.* Upper Saddle River, NJ: Prentice Hall, Inc., pp. 38–77; 177–206.

Phipps, W., Monahan, F., Sands, J., Marek, J, & Neighbors, M. (2003). *Medical-surgical nursing: Health and illness perspectives* (7th ed.). St. Louis, MO: Mosby, pp. 1717–1739, 1747–1786, 1823–1871.

Thibodeau, G. A. & Patton, K. T. (1999). *Anatomy and physiology* (4th ed.). St. Louis, MO: Mosby, pp. 772–786, 787–809.

Zaret, B. (1998). *The Yale University School of Medicine patient's guide to medical tests.* New York: Houghton Mifflin Company, pp. 229–244, 245–272, 537–554.

CHAPTER 16

Eye and Ear Disorders

Mary Ann Hogan, RN, CS, MSN

CHAPTER OUTLINE

OBJECTIVES

▌ Identify basic structures and functions of the eye and ear.

▌ Describe the pathophysiology and etiology of common eye and ear disorders.

▌ Discuss expected assessment data and diagnostic test findings for selected eye and ear disorders.

▌ Identify priority nursing diagnoses for selected eye and ear disorders.

▌ Discuss therapeutic management of selected eye and ear disorders.

▌ Discuss nursing management of a client experiencing an eye or ear disorder.

▌ Identify expected outcomes for the client experiencing an eye or ear disorder.

[**Media Link**]

Use the CD-ROM enclosed with this text, or log onto the address given to access the free, interactive Companion Website created for this series. The CD-ROM and Companion Website accompanying this book offer additional practice opportunities and information—NCLEX Review, Case Studies, Glossary, In Depth with NCLEX, and more.

www.prenhall.com/hogan

REVIEW AT A GLANCE

cataract *a progressive and gradual development of opacity in the lens or lens capsule that results in loss of vision*

conjunctivitis *inflammation of the conjunctiva of the eye caused by infection, allergen, toxin, or other irritant*

cycloplegic *referring to the ability to paralyze the ciliary muscle of the eye*

glaucoma *an eye disorder characterized by an imbalance between aqueous humor production and drainage, leading to increased intraocular pressure*

gonioscopy *measurement of the angle of the anterior chamber of the eye*

labyrinthectomy *complete removal of labyrinth that destroys cochlear function, relieving vertigo but causing loss of any minimal remaining hearing as well*

Meniere's disease *a disorder of the inner ear in which there is excessive accumula-*

tion of endolymphatic fluid in the membranous labyrinth

miotic *refers to the ability to constrict the pupil of the eye*

mydriatic *refers to the ability to dilate the pupil*

myringotomy *surgically performed perforation of tympanic membrane to allow drainage of middle ear secretions and relieve pain and pressure of otitis media*

nystagmus *involuntary rhythmic, oscillating movement of the eyes that can be horizontal, vertical, rotary, or a mixture of these*

presbycusis *an age-related change in the ear that results in a decreased ability to hear high-frequency sounds*

presbyopia *an age-related decrease in the elasticity of the lens of the eye, mak-*

ing it more difficult to focus on objects at a short distance

proprioception *sensation about the body's position in space that is transferred to the brain after changes in body position trigger fluid movement and bending of hair cells in vestibular structures*

otosclerosis *hereditary disorder of the labyrinthine capsule in which abnormal bone growth occurs around the ossicles and causes fixation of the stapes, leading to conductive hearing loss*

tonometry *a diagnostic test for glaucoma that measures intraocular pressure by determining resistance of the eyeball to an applied force*

tympanoplasty *surgical reconstruction of ossicles and tympanic membrane of the middle ear to help restore hearing*

Pretest

1 A client who has undergone a visual acuity test has results of 20/120 in the right eye. When explaining this finding to the client, which of the following statements would be most appropriate?

(1) The client is nearsighted.
(2) The client is farsighted.
(3) The client's vision is normal.
(4) The client is legally blind in that eye.

2 A client being prepared for an ocular examination has an order for a topical eye medication. The nurse prepares to administer which of the following medications?

(1) Carbachol (Carboptic)
(2) Latanoprost (Xalatan)
(3) Glycerin (Ophthalgan)
(4) Cyclopentolate (Cyclogyl)

3 A client has just been diagnosed with glaucoma. The nurse should place highest priority on teaching the client which of the following pieces of information?

(1) Fluid restriction is needed to reduce intraocular pressure.
(2) The disorder often has no symptoms.
(3) Adherence to medication therapy is essential to reduce risk of vision loss.
(4) The disorder is typically diagnosed after an episode of eye infection.

4 The nurse notes a slight cloudy appearance to the lens of a 64-year-old client's eye. Which of the following symptoms should the nurse question the client about?

(1) Sense of a curtain falling over vision
(2) Blurring of vision
(3) Slight but constant eye pain
(4) Double vision

5 A client admitted to the hospital has a notation on the medical record that reads "legally blind." The nurse interprets that the client's best corrected vision in the better eye must be no better than which of the following?

(1) 20/200
(2) 20/120
(3) 20/360
(4) 20/100

6 A client with a suspected impaction of cerumen has an order for an otic irrigation. The nurse should take which of the following essential actions before beginning the irrigation?

(1) Draw up no more than 120 mL of solution for use at one time
(2) Make sure the client is seated comfortably in the bathroom
(3) Make sure the irrigant is at room temperature
(4) Examine the tympanic membrane to be sure it is intact

7 A client has been treated for acute otitis media. The nurse would evaluate whether the client obtained relief from which of the following primary symptoms associated with this disorder?

(1) Dizziness
(2) Headaches
(3) Ear pain
(4) Nausea

8 The nurse working in an ambulatory surgery center would plan to instruct the client that which of the following activities is acceptable following ear surgery?

(1) Blowing the nose
(2) Talking
(3) Sneezing
(4) Doing push-ups

9 The nurse is performing an otic examination on a client with otosclerosis. Then nurse documents that the tympanic membrane is:

(1) Reddish or pinkish-orange.
(2) Light, pale pink.
(3) Ecchymotic.
(4) Pearly white.

10 The nurse has conducted discharge teaching for a client diagnosed with Meniere's disease. The nurse evaluates that the client understood the instructions given if the client states to refrain from eating which of the following favorite foods?

(1) Granola bars
(2) Baked eggplant
(3) Sherbet
(4) Salted pretzels

See pages 659–660 for Answers and Rationales.

I. Overview of Anatomy and Physiology of the Eye

A. Eye structures

1. Outer protective layer, also referred to as fibrous coat

   a. Sclera: white and opaque in color, made of fibrous connective tissue

   b. Cornea: clear fibrous covering that continues anteriorly from sclera; is avascular, and is part of refractive media of the eye

2. Middle vascular layer, also referred to as uveal tract

   a. Iris: thin, pigmented muscle with a central aperture called the pupil; responsible for constriction and dilation of pupil to regulate amount of light entering the eye

   b. Ciliary body: circular structure that surrounds lens and connects anteriorly to iris and posteriorly to choroids; maintains intraocular pressure by producing aqueous humor (a watery refractive medium) that flows from posterior to anterior chamber before draining through trabecular meshwork into Schlemm's canal

   c. Choroid: thin membrane that contains blood vessels to supply eye tissues, attaches to both ciliary body and optic nerve

      3. Inner layer, the retina: thin, semitransparent layer containing rods and cones, responsible for vision in dim light and for perception of fine details, respectively

B. Eye functions

      1. Eye receives light waves through cornea; waves are refracted by aqueous humor, the lens, and vitreous humor as they are transmitted to retina; retinal images formed by light rays are inverted and reversed by the biconvex lens

      2. Rods and cones of retina translate light waves into neural impulses for relay to optic nerve, and then to the brain's occipital lobes for interpretation as vision

      3. The fusing of images in the brain from each eye into a single image is called binocular vision

NCLEX!

C. Age-related changes of the eye that affect vision

      1. Decreased ability of pupil to dilate, which reduces night vision and increases light needed for reading and small motor tasks, such as sewing

      2. Development of **presbyopia,** a decreased elasticity of the lens that makes focusing for near vision more difficult, and results in farsightedness

      3. Lens becomes discolored and opacified, which reduces color perception (especially green, blue, and violet)

      4. Decreased eye motility and senile enophthalmos (sinking in) of eyes, limits peripheral vision upward, downward, and to the sides

      5. Degenerative changes to choroid, retina, and optic nerve reduce depth perception and ability to see lines of demarcation (stair edges, doorframes)

II. Diagnostic Tests and Assessments of the Eye

A. Fluorescein angiography: injection of sodium fluorescein into arm vessel, followed by serial imaging and recording to detect disorders in retinal vessels, such as with diabetic retinopathy and eye tumors

      1. Preprocedure care

         a. Assess for allergies and/or history of reactions to dye

         b. Ensure client has given informed consent

NCLEX!

         c. Give prescribed mydriatic medication 1 hour prior to test to dilate pupil

      2. Postprocedure care

         a. Encourage rest and increased fluid intake (fluids aid in dye excretion)

         b. Teach client that dye causes temporary skin discoloration in injected area and temporary green discoloration of urine

NCLEX!

         c. Teach client to avoid sunlight or other bright light sources for some hours until pupil dilation returns to normal

B. Corneal staining: instillation of dye into conjunctival sac to highlight irregularities caused by trauma, abrasions, or ulcers; damaged corneal epithelium appears green when viewed through a blue filter

      1. Ensure that contact lenses are removed prior to procedure, if worn

2. Tell client to blink to distribute dye evenly over cornea

3. Wipe excess dye from cheeks and instruct client not to rub eyes

C. **Tonometry:** measurement of intraocular pressure (IOP) to detect glaucoma, by determining resistance of the eyeball to an applied force

1. Normal IOP ranges from 12 to 21 mmHg

2. Eye may be anesthetized, and client stares forward

3. Applanation: most accurate method, measures force needed to flatten a small area of cornea; eye is anesthetized

4. Indentation: measures change in form of globe after standard weight (Schiøtz tonometer) is applied to cornea; eye is anesthetized

5. Noncontact: calculates IOP by measuring deflection of a puff of air applied to cornea; no anesthetic needed

6. Tell client not to rub eyes after test if anesthetic was used to avoid possible corneal scratches or injury

D. **Physical assessment of eye and vision**

1. Acuity of distance vision: measures vision using Snellen chart hung 20 feet away

   a. Client reads chart lines with one eye covered, moving downward from row that is most clear, until unable to cite more than one half of characters in a line

   b. Record findings as a fraction: the numerator being the client's distance from chart (20 feet), and the denominator being the number identified at the end of the smallest line read, which corresponds to distance at which the normal eye can read that line; normal vision is 20/20; a larger denominator indicates myopia (nearsightedness)

   c. Repeat process for other eye

   d. Test eyes of clients with corrective lenses both with and without correction, noting *sc* (sine correctio, without correction) and *cc* (cum correctio, with correction)

2. Acuity of near vision: measures vision using a Rosenbaum chart or a card with newsprint 12 to 14 inches from client's eyes; impairment indicates hyperopia (farsightedness) in a young client, or presbyopia in an adult after approximately 45 years of age

3. Refraction test

   a. Uses Snellen chart to assess visual acuity while client reads through various strengths of corrective lenses

   b. Used to measure and prescribe correction for errors in visual focus with *myopia* (nearsightedness), *hyperopia* (farsightedness), and *astigmatism* (irregularity or indentation of the corneal surface that inhibits light rays from focusing clearly on the retina)

4. Visual fields: measures peripheral vision, often called confrontation test

   a. Client and examiner sit facing each other with client looking into examiner's eyes

   b. Client covers right eye and examiner covers left eye

   c. Examiner raises a finger or other small object at arm's length midway between client and examiner, and brings it in from the periphery into the line of vision; procedure is repeated from above and below on the same side

   d. Client states "now" when able to see the object; examiner should see object at about the same time (test assumes examiner has normal peripheral vision)

   e. Test is repeated on the other eye

5. Color vision

   a. Tested for driver's license, employment requiring color discrimination, or with history of difficulty distinguishing colors; sensitive for red/green blindness, but not for blue

   b. Involves picking colored numbers or letters out of plates with multiple colors in background (such as an Ishihara chart)

   c. Results recorded as a fraction of the number of plates identified correctly and the total number shown

6. Extraocular muscle movements

   a. Client holds head still and follows a small object with the eyes through six cardinal positions of gaze: to the right (lateral), upward and right (temporal), down and right, left (lateral), upward and left (lateral), and down and left

   NCLEX!

   b. Client should have parallel eye movement and absence of **nystagmus,** involuntary rhythmic oscillating eye movements (vertical, horizontal, rotary, or mixed)

   c. As last step, client follows finger as it moves in to bridge of nose; eyes should sustain convergence to within 5 to 8 centimeters

7. Outer eye structures

   NCLEX!

   a. Sclera white in color, although in dark-skinned client may appear slight yellow cast or have pigmented dots; yellow discoloration (or heightened yellow) can indicate jaundice

   b. Cornea normally transparent, smooth, and shiny; opacities (cloudy areas) or specks may indicate prior injury

   c. Pupils should be round, equal in size, and constrict in response to direct light or to light shone in opposite pupil (consensual response); pupils should constrict and converge when looking at object over examiner's shoulder and then shifting gaze to an object 4 to 6 inches from own nose (accommodation)

8. Ophthalmoscopy

   a. Used to examine retina, optic disk, optic blood vessels, fundus, and macula

   b. Client sits in darkened room to heighten pupil dilation, stares straight ahead

   c. Examiner holds ophthalmoscope in right hand and uses own right eye when examining client's right eye and vice versa

   d. Examiner approaches client from 12 to 15 inches away and 15 degrees lateral to client's line of vision

NCLEX!

e. As light shines on pupil, reflection of light on retina causes a red glare (red reflex); absence of red reflex may indicate lens opacity

III. Common Nursing Techniques and Procedures for the Eye

A. Ocular medications

1. Eye drops

NCLEX!

   a. Ensure that medication is sterile and treat each eye separately, if both being medicated, to prevent cross-contamination

   b. Tilt client's head back slightly, having client look up with eyes open

   c. Expose lower conjunctival sac by gently pulling down skin of cheekbone with gloved hand

   d. Hold bottle like a pencil and rest wrist on client's forehead or cheek for stability, to prevent bottle from touching eye and causing injury

   e. Instill correct number of drops into conjunctival sac

NCLEX!

   f. Have client close eye gently (not squeezing) and move eye inside closed lid to evenly distribute medication; apply pressure to nasolacrimal duct (tear duct, at inner canthus) with tissue or cotton ball to prevent systemic drug absorption

   g. Wipe away excess from cheek with tissue or cotton ball if needed

NCLEX!

   h. Wait 2 to 5 minutes between drops as per manufacturer's directions

2. Eye ointments

   a. Use same client positioning as for eye drops

   b. Squeeze a thin bead of ointment along inside of conjunctival sac, moving from inner to outer canthus

   c. Have client close eye gently and move eyeball to evenly distribute ointment

NCLEX!

   d. Instruct client that the ointment may blur the vision temporarily

3. Medicated eye disk

   a. Open package and press tip of index finger of gloved hand against convex part of disk

   b. Position client as for eye drops/ointment and expose lower conjunctival sac

   c. Place disk horizontally in sac between iris and lower eyelid

   d. Pull lower eyelid out and up over disk and ask client to blink a few times until disk is not visible

   e. Have client press fingers against closed lids without moving eyes or disk to secure disk in position

   f. To remove disk, expose lower conjunctival sac and use thumb and index finger to pinch and lift disk from sac; if positioned in upper eye, stroke closed eyelid gently in long circular motions; once disk moves to corner of eye, slide to lower lid and remove as described

B. Ocular irrigation

1. Position client with head tilted toward side to be irrigated and place waterproof pad and curved basin under affected side

2. Cleanse eyelids and lashes with gloved hand and moistened cotton ball, discarding each cotton ball after one wipe

3. Draw up ordered irrigant into sterile irrigation set or bulb syringe

4. Use nondominant hand to hold eyelids open

5. Hold syringe 1 inch above eye and push fluid gently into conjunctival sac (fluid flows across eye from inner to outer canthus)

NCLEX!

6. Avoid flushing directly onto eyeball to avoid damage to cornea

7. Eyelid speculum or irrigating contact lens may be used if ordered in special circumstances, topical anesthetic may be used

C. Eye patches and shields

1. Have client close both eyes during application of patch or shield

2. Position patch and secure with two strips of tape extending from midforehead to lateral cheekbone (medial top to lateral bottom) on same side

NCLEX!

3. Do not use pressure unless specifically ordered, and then use two to three pads and extra tape

4. Change only with physician order

5. Apply shield alone or over an eye patch to protect eye from pressure or other type of irritation

6. Place shield on bony prominences of cheek, nose, and brow; secure with transparent tape in same manner as for eye patch

D. Eye prosthesis (artificial eye) care

1. Allow client to perform own artificial eye care if preferred; some prostheses are permanently implanted while others are removable

2. Remove prosthesis by retracting lower eyelid and exerting pressure just below eye to break suction and lift it from socket; can also use rubber bulb syringe or medicine dropper bulb to create suction effect

3. Cleanse with normal saline or tap water according to client's routine

4. Irrigate eye socket with normal saline using aseptic technique if ordered (such as for infection)

5. Cleanse edges of eye socket and surrounding area with moistened gauze

6. Reinsert by retracting upper and lower eyelids and slipping prosthesis into eye socket comfortably under upper eyelid

7. When prosthesis is stored, place in labeled container with saline or tap water

IV. Nursing Management of Client Having Eye Surgery

A. Preoperative period

1. Reduce anxiety through preoperative teaching about procedure and postoperative course and care

NCLEX!

2. Assess client's support systems and ability to care for self after surgery, including assessment of environmental safety (such as hand rails, absence of throw rugs)

3. Complete shampoo or scrub around eyes if ordered; remove eye makeup; store contact lens or eyeglasses (needed to aid vision in other eye) so they are available upon completion of surgery

4. Administer preanesthetic medications and eyedrops as ordered, which commonly include **mydriatic** eye drops (to dilate pupils) and **cycloplegic** eye drops (to paralyze ciliary muscles); see Table 16-1 (pp. 638–640) for overview of commonly ordered eye medications

B. Postoperative period

1. Perform baseline assessments as for all postoperative clients (vital signs, level of consciousness, status of dressing); changes may be minimal if surgery done under local anesthesia

2. Maintain eye patch or eye shield in place to prevent injury to eye, and instruct client not to rub or touch the area

3. Elevate head to 30 to 45 degrees and have client lie on back or unaffected side (to reduce intraocular pressure) after surgery done to treat cataracts or glaucoma; use small pillows at sides of head to immobilize head when lying on back

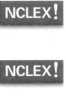

4. Position client with repair of detached retina as prescribed so that area of detachment is dependent/inferior (to maintain pressure on the repaired retinal area and improve its contact with choroid)

5. Instruct and assist the client to avoid activities that increase IOP, such as coughing, sneezing, vomiting, or straining at stool; if it is necessary to cough or sneeze, client should do so with mouth open

6. Maintain client safety: orient to environment, keep articles and call bell on unaffected side, use side rails with bed in low position, and assist with ambulation

7. Give antibiotic, antiinflammatory, and other prescribed topical (eye) or systemic medications

8. Give analgesics as ordered, avoiding or using caution with opioids to prevent postoperative nausea, vomiting, and constipation; discomfort may be described as achy or scratching; avoid morphine, which can cause miosis

9. Assess for possible surgical complications that should be reported immediately to preserve sight:

   a. Sudden sharp eye pain, possibly indicating hemorrhage, sudden rise in intraocular pressure, or other ocular emergency

   b. Hemorrhage, with blood noted in anterior chamber of eye

   c. Retinal detachment, noted by client sensations of flashes of light, floaters, or a curtain being drawn over the eye

   d. Corneal edema, noted by a cloudy appearance to cornea

10. Teach the client and family about post-discharge care (see Box 16-1)

11. Refer to community health agency for assistance with post-discharge home care if needed

Box 16-1

**Client Education
Following Eye Surgery**

The following points should be included in discharge instructions given to the client and family after eye surgery:

- Leave eye shield in place until the surgeon's office visit on the day after surgery; then use eye shield at night during sleep for eye protection as prescribed
- Avoid rubbing, scratching, touching, squeezing, or putting pressure on surgical eye
- Avoid activities that increase intraocular pressure, such as sneezing, coughing, vomiting, straining, moving rapidly, bending, or lifting more than 5 pounds
- Maintain sedentary lifestyle for approximately 2 weeks or as prescribed by surgeon; avoid heavy work, such as gardening, mowing the lawn, or moving furniture
- Avoid reading until allowed by surgeon, and then read in moderation during healing
- Use measures to prevent constipation, such as adequate fiber and fluid intake, maintaining mobility as able, and possible use of stool softener
- Wear sunglasses with side shields when out of doors (photophobia commonly occurs)
- New corrective lenses (if needed) will not be prescribed until vision stabilizes, which may take several weeks; make and keep all recommended follow-up appointments with physician
- Proper techniques for use of eye patch or shield and/or instillation of eye drops
- Medication names, dose, schedule, side effects, purpose, and anticipated duration of use
- Symptoms to report to physician: new, increased or severe eye pain or pressure, decreased vision, redness, cloudiness, drainage, floaters or light flashes, halos around brightly lit objects

V. Glaucoma

A. Description

    1. Imbalance between aqueous humor production and drainage, leading to increased IOP; it affects 2 percent of those over age 40 and is a leading cause of blindness worldwide

    2. Can be of two types: open-angle or angle closure (narrow angle, closed angle)

B. Etiology and pathophysiology

    1. Usually exists as a primary condition without identified precipitating cause; most frequent in adults over 60 years of age

    2. Open-angle glaucoma: most frequent form with unknown cause although heredity suspected; the angle of the anterior chamber between the iris and cornea is normal; the flow of aqueous humor through trabecular network to Canal of Schlemm is obstructed; it is usually a bilateral process

    3. Angle-closure (narrow angle, closed angle) glaucoma: less common form, is often unilateral, although the other eye can be affected at a later time

        a. Anterior chamber narrows due to corneal flattening or bulging of iris

        b. When iris thickens (pupil dilation) or lens thickens (during visual accommodation), angle can close completely, blocking outflow and causing sudden elevation of IOP

        c. Damage to neurons in retina and optic nerve can occur, rapidly lead to loss of vision if not treated quickly

C. Assessment

    1. Open-angle

a. Loss of peripheral vision, mild headaches, difficulty adapting to the dark, seeing halos around lights, and difficulty focusing on near objects

      b. Symptoms may be vague with client unaware of them for a time; visual acuity deteriorates over time with rising IOP

    2. Angle-closure

      a. Triggered by pupil dilation, such as with high emotions and darkness, among others

      b. Symptoms include severe eye and face pain, nausea and vomiting, malaise, colored halos around lights, and episodes of sudden decline in vision; possible reddened eye, cloudy cornea from edema, and pupil fixed at midpoint.

    3. Diagnosed by history; presenting symptoms; tonometry; ophthalmoscopy; **gonioscopy** (measurement of anterior chamber angle, differentiates open-angle from angle-closure glaucoma)

D. Priority nursing diagnoses: Disturbed sensory perception: visual; Risk for injury; Pain; Anxiety; Deficient knowledge

E. Planning and implementation

    1. Acute glaucoma: medical emergency; vision loss can occur within 1-2 days if untreated; provide information to client and administer ordered therapies such as osmotic diuretics or carbonic anhydrase inhibitors to lower IOP (see Table 16-1); surgical intervention may be needed

    2. Chronic glaucoma: interventions primarily consist of medication therapy and client education

    3. Provide pre-and postoperative care as previously outlined in section IV B; if eye surgery is needed; surgical procedures to facilitate drainage of aqueous humor can include trabeculectomy, laser trabeculoplasty, iridectomy, or laser iridotomy

F. Medication therapy: miotic drugs that constrict pupils, carbonic anhydrase inhibitors to decrease production of aqueous humor, and beta-adrenergic blockers to constrict pupils and reduce production of aqueous humor (refer again to Table 16-1)

G. Client education

    1. Drug therapy is needed for life; noncompliance can lead to loss of vision that cannot be regained

    2. Avoid mydriatic medications such as atropine that dilate pupils

    3. Obtain Medic-Alert card or bracelet specifying type of glaucoma

    4. Use safety precautions at night (lighting, hand rails) to compensate for reduced ability of pupils to dilate because of miotics, and remove obstacles in environment for safety

    5. Follow general instructions following eye surgery (see Section IV B)

    6. Review specific drug information and procedures for self-administration

H. Evaluation: client verbalizes medication understanding and demonstrates their use correctly, utilizes safety measures, identifies measures to prevent increases in IOP, has relief of eye pain, maintains existing vision, and complies with postoperative instructions

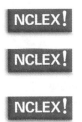

➤ Practice to Pass

A client who has just been diagnosed with glaucoma states that she is not worried about the condition because she has no symptoms. How should you respond?

NCLEX!

NCLEX!

NCLEX!

NCLEX!

NCLEX!

NCLEX!

Table 16-1	Medications Commonly Used to Treat Eye Disorders		
Drug Class and Name: Generic (Trade)	**Therapeutic Use(s)**	**Mechanism of Action**	**Nursing Responsibilities**
Ophthalmic Antiinfectives idoxuridine (Herplex) natamycin (Natacyn) sulfacetamide (AK-Sulf, Cetamide) trifluridine (Viroptic)	Local treatment of bacterial or viral infections	Interfere with reproduction or growth of microorganism	Assess eye lesions daily during therapy Assess for allergy to sulfonamides prior to use (sulfacetamide) Implement and teach careful handwashing to prevent spread of infection Use aseptic technique during administration Teach client to: use caution with activities if drug causes temporary blurred vision, wear sunglasses, and avoid bright light to prevent photophobic reactions, use exactly as prescribed
Ophthalmic Beta-adrenergic Blocking Agents betaxolol (Betoptic) carteolol (Ocupress) levobunolol (Betagan) metipranolol (OptiPranolol) timolol (Timoptic)	Treatment of glaucoma	Decrease the formation of aqueous humor to lower intraocular pressure	Use aseptic technique during administration Use cautiously in clients with asthma or bronchospasm, heart failure, other cardiovascular disease, or diabetes mellitus Monitor intake and output, daily weight, lung crackles, peripheral edema, pulse, and blood pressure Teach diabetic client that tachycardia and increased blood pressure that accompany hypoglycemia may be masked by this drug Teach client to: use exactly as prescribed follow instructions precisely if changing from one drug to another expect transient stinging or burning with instillation, but report if severe wear sunglasses to minimize risk of photophobia keep appointments for follow-up eye exams
Ophthalmic and Non-ophthalmic Carbonic Anhydrase Inhibitors acetazolamide (Diamox) dichlorphenamide (Daranide) dorzolamide (Trusopt) methazolamide (Neptazane)	Treatment of glaucoma	Inhibits carbonic anhydrase to reduce secretion of aqueous humor in the eye, causes self-limiting excretion of sodium, potassium, bicarbonate, and water	May be given PO, IM, IV, or topically to eye to lower IOP Assess for contraindications to therapy: allergy to sulfa drugs, severe liver or kidney disease, existing electrolyte or acid-base imbalances Assess for eye discomfort, reduced visual acuity, or local adverse effects such as conjunctivitis or lid reactions Assess for anorexia, malaise, metallic or bitter taste, paresthesias, electrolyte or acid-base imbalances, nephrolithiasis Monitor intake and output, daily weight, vital signs for possible fluid volume deficit Give in A.M. to prevent diuresis from disrupting sleep

(continued)

Table 16-1	Medications Commonly Used to Treat Eye Disorders (*Continued*)		
Drug Class and Name: **Generic (Trade)**	**Therapeutic Use(s)**	**Mechanism of Action**	**Nursing Responsibilities**
			Teach client to avoid driving or other activities requiring alertness if drowsiness occurs, use sunscreen to avoid photosensitivity reactions, and keep appointments for follow-up eye exams

Ophthalmic Cholinergic Agents
 Direct-Acting Cholinergics
 carbachol (Carboptic)
 pilocarpine (Pilocar, Ocusert-Pilo, others)
 Cholinesterase Inhibitors
 demecarium (Humorsol)
 echothiophate (Phospholine Iodide)
 isoflurophate (Floropryl)
 physostigmine (Isopto Eserine)
 Prostaglandin
 latanoprost (Xalatan)
	Miotics used in treatment of glaucoma	Facilitate the outflow of aqueous humor to lower intraocular pressure	Use aseptic technique during administration
			 Avoid concurrent use of anticholinergic drugs, such as atropine, that block drug action
			 Monitor blood pressure, pulse, and lung sounds; report hypotension, bradycardia, bronchospasm
			 Assess for and report symptoms of systemic absorption: shortness of breath, increased sweating or salivation, nausea, vomiting, diarrhea, abdominal cramps, increased urge to urinate
			 Avoid concurrent use of drugs that block drug effects, including many OTC sleep and cough preparations
			 Teach client that:
			    pupil size will decrease (miosis)
			    blurred vision, eye or brow ache, and reduced night vision can occur; use safety precautions such as nightlights and avoid night driving
			    it is important to keep follow-up eye appointments
			    latanoprost can cause or increase brown pigmentation to eye

Ophthalmic Cycloplegic Mydriatics cyclopentolate (Cyclogyl, others) homatropine (Isopto Homatropine) tropicamide (Opticyl, others) atropine (Ocutropine)	Local therapy before eye surgery or ophthalmic examination, treatment of inflammatory disorders of the iris	Dilates the pupil (anticholinergic, mydriatic effect) and paralyzes ciliary muscle for accommodation (cycloplegic effect)	Use aseptic technique during administration These drugs are contraindicated with sensitivity to belladonna alkaloids and are either contraindicated or must be used cautiously in clients with glaucoma Assess for and report signs of systemic absorption: drowsiness, confusion, tachycardia, dry mouth, flushed face Assess for hallucinations and psychotic reactions as adverse CNS effects Teach client to use caution because drug may temporarily impair ability to judge distances, and to wear dark glasses because pupil(s) cannot constrict in bright light

(continued)

Table 16-1	Medications Commonly Used to Treat Eye Disorders (*Continued*)		
Drug Class and Name: Generic (Trade)	**Therapeutic Use(s)**	**Mechanism of Action**	**Nursing Responsibilities**
Ophthalmic Sympathomimetics apraclonidine (Iopidine) dipivefrin (Propine) epinephrine	Reduction of intraocular pressure during laser eye surgery (apraclonidine) or due to open-angle glaucoma	Decreases aqueous humor formation (apraclonidine) or increases aqueous outflow (epinephrine, dipivefrin)	Use aseptic technique during administration Monitor for increased pulse and BP, and CNS effects such as nervousness, muscle tremors, and anxiety Teach client to: wear dark glasses and use caution in bright light because pupillary dilation will occur keep appointments for follow-up eye exams report signs of hypersensitivity reaction: itching, lid edema, and eye discharge report changes in visual acuity or eye pain; eye pain could indicate an attack of angle-closure glaucoma avoid OTC sinus and cold medications that contain sympathomimetics (pseudoephedrine, phenylephrine) and could increase side effects
Osmotic Diuretics glycerin (Ophthalgan) mannitol (Osmitrol) urea	Short-term reduction of edema of the cornea prior to ophthalmic exam or surgery (glycerin) and short-term reduction of intraocular pressure (all)	Increases osmotic pressure of glomerular filtrate, thus inhibiting reabsorption of electrolytes and water	Administer 60 to 90 minutes before surgery as ordered Ophthalmic solution of glycerin may cause eye pain and irritation; precede with local anesthetic as ordered Monitor intake and output, assess for signs of dehydration Avoid infusing hypotonic fluids following administration, because this will offset the osmotic effect of glycerin

VI. Cataracts

A. Description

1. Progressive and gradual development of opacity in the lens or lens capsule that results in loss of vision

2. Incidence increases with age (found to some extent in 50 to 70 percent of adults over 65 years of age), called "senile cataracts"

B. Etiology and pathophysiology

1. Other risk factors besides age include long-term exposure to ultraviolet light (UV-B rays), cigarette smoking, heavy alcohol use, eye injury or inflammation, congenital defect, diabetes mellitus, and some medications (such as systemic corticosteroids, chlorpromazine [Thorazine], busulfan [Myleran])

2. Fibers and proteins of lens degenerate with age or following insult; opacity often begins at periphery of lens and moves to center

3. Partial opacity is termed "immature cataract"; opacity of entire lens is termed "mature cataract"

4. Opacity tends to occur bilaterally but is asymmetric in development, with one maturing faster than the other

C. Assessment

NCLEX!

1. Decline in close and distance vision, blurred vision, changes in color vision (loss), glare, halos around lights, object distortion, white or cloudy gray pupil

2. Diagnosed by history and physical exam, results of visual acuity tests and slit-lamp exam; absence of red reflex with ophthalmoscopy

D. Priority nursing diagnoses: Disturbed sensory perception: visual; Risk for injury; Deficient knowledge

E. Planning and implementation

1. Provide emotional support since impaired vision is anxiety-producing for clients

NCLEX!

2. Identify safety concerns in the environment related to impaired vision and correct them

3. Surgical removal of lens is sole treatment option and is accompanied by lens implant or is treated with corrective lenses

NCLEX!

4. Assist client in decision making about surgery, which is indicated when vision or activities of daily living are affected, or if causing secondary problems such as uveitis or glaucoma

5. Reinforce explanations about surgical extraction of lens

   a. Cryoextraction: forceps or supercooled probe used to extract lens after making small incision in cornea

   b. Phacoemulsification: ultrasound vibrations break lens into fragments that are aspirated (suctioned) from the eye

   c. Intracapsular extraction: removal of entire lens and surrounding capsule (see Figure 16-1a)

   d. Extracapsular extraction: removal of lens nucleus and cortex, leaving posterior capsule intact to support lens implant; currently most popular method (see Figure 16-1b)

6. Surgery is done on one eye at a time, usually on an outpatient basis and using local anesthesia

7. Lens implant rapidly restores binocular vision and depth perception

8. If lens implant is not used, a thick convex corrective lens or contact lens is needed to provide light refraction and restore visual acuity to the surgical eye

9. Provide preoperative and postoperative care as outlined in previous section

F. Medication therapy

1. Indicated for temporary use after surgery

NCLEX!

2. Generally includes antibiotic and anti-inflammatory agents

Figure 16-1

Cataract removal with lens implant. A. Intra-capsular cataract extraction removes entire lens and capsule, with lens implantation in anterior chamber. B. Extra capsular catar-act extraction removes lens and anterior cap-sule, with lens implanta-tion within the intact posterior capsule.

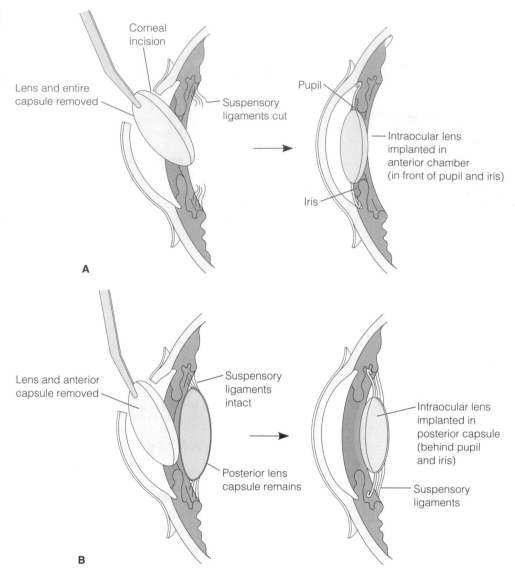

G. Client education

1. Include adaptive strategies to compensate for changes in vision and depth per-ception if surgery not currently indicated or desired

2. Instruct postoperative client as outlined in previous section on eye surgery

3. Teach client to leave eye patch or shield in place until changed or removed by surgeon at postoperative visit, usually within 24 to 48 hours

4. Eye protection may include use of sunglasses during day in bright light and use of eye shield at night

5. Teach client information and procedures for medication use after surgery, such as acetaminophen for general discomfort, combination steroid (anti-inflamma-tory) and antibiotic eye drops, and others as needed by individual client (refer back to Table 16-1)

6. Teach client about insertion and care of postoperative contact lenses if prescribed

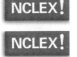

7. Teach client that when convex corrective lenses are worn postoperatively, visual field is narrowed by thick convex lens, so client must move head side to side (rather than just look side to side) to compensate; depth perception may also be affected, requiring attention to safety

8. Permanent eyeglasses will be prescribed several weeks after surgery when healing is complete and vision has stabilized

H. **Evaluation:** client exhibits behavior changes as needed to adapt to vision changes, remains free of injury, and demonstrates understanding of pre- and post-operative eye care

VII. **Detached Retina**

A. **Description**

1. Separation of the sensory layer of retina from the choroid, the pigmented vascular layer

2. Retina may tear and fold back onto itself, or remain intact and be pulled away from choroid by shrinking of vitreous humor

B. **Etiology and pathophysiology**

1. Most frequently occurs due to aging with shrinkage of vitreous humor, which pulls on retina at points of attachment, such as the optic disk, macula, and periphery of eye

2. Can also be caused by trauma, inflammation, tumor, or complication of eye surgery (lens removal)

3. With a retinal break or tear, fluid enters defect, possibly leading to further rapid tearing and separation due to pressure

4. Incomplete area of detachment can progress slowly or can enlarge quickly and become complete

5. Will lead to permanent blindness if untreated, so is considered a medical emergency

C. **Assessment**

1. Initial: presence of floating spots (floaters) and/or flashing lights

2. Progressive blurring of vision, visual field deficits corresponding to area of damage, sense of curtain or veil coming down, up or across field of vision, painless

3. Ophthalmic exam shows area of gray opaque retina, with possible accompanying tears, holes, or folds

D. **Priority nursing diagnoses:** Disturbed sensory perception: visual; Risk for injury; Anxiety or fear; Deficient knowledge

E. **Planning and implementation**

1. Preoperative care

a. Protect eye from further damage: bedrest, cover both eyes with eye patches to limit movement and prevent eye stress, instruct client not to bend forward or make sudden or jerking head movements

NCLEX!

NCLEX!

b. Position client with detached area dependent/inferior so gravity pushes detachment closer to choroid (e.g., with left eye superior temporal detachment, keep client supine with head turned toward left)

c. Protect client from injury keeping bed low, side rails up, call bell within reach; talk to client before approaching bed, assist with self-care

d. Reinforce explanations about surgical repair

1) Laser photocoagulation or cryotherapy (cold probe): creates a local inflammation that will locally adhere retina onto the choroid

2) Scleral buckling: holds retina and choroid together with an implant or encircling strap or "buckle"

3) Pneumatic retinopexy: injects air/gas into vitreous with adjustment of client's head position to push detached portion of retina back into contact with choroid

4) Surgical instrument manipulation to move detached segment of torn retina into place, followed by laser therapy or injection of gas or silicone oil to create a bond

e. Provide psychological support to alleviate anxiety associated with sudden loss of vision; reassure client most detachments are successfully treated (often on outpatient basis)

f. Provide preoperative care as described in section IV, A

2. Postoperative care

a. Provide standard postoperative care as described in section IV, B

b. Stress the importance of maintaining prescribed position (affected eye inferior or dependent to maintain contact between retina and choroid)

F. **Medication therapy:** usually includes antibiotic, anti-inflammatory, and analgesic medications

G. **Client education:** as previously described in Box 16-1

H. **Evaluation:** client demonstrates understanding of pre- and postoperative eye care, exhibits behavior changes as needed to promote surgical healing, and remains free of injury

VIII. Macular Degeneration

A. **Description**

1. Defined as degeneration of the macular area (center area) of the retina, which normally receives light from the center of the visual field and has the greatest visual acuity

2. The most common type is age-related macular degeneration (ARMD), currently the leading cause of legal blindness in the United States for those over 65 years of age

B. **Etiology and pathophysiology**

1. The causes of age-related macular degeneration are unknown, although heredity, smoking, injury, inflammation, and nutritional factors are suspected to play a role; males and females are affected equally

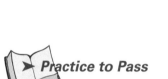

Practice to Pass

A client tells you that "all of a sudden" it seems like a window shade is being pulled down over one eye. What are your immediate assessments and interventions?

2. In ARMD, there is gradual failure of the outer layer of the retina (the pigmented epithelium that attaches the retina to the choroid layer and removes cellular wastes); in this process, photoreceptor cells are lost, metabolic wastes accumulate in the subretinal space, leading to cell death

3. There are two types of macular degeneration

   a. Atrophic ("dry") form: bilateral and gradual but progressive loss of vision occurs because of atrophy and degeneration of the macula (90 percent of cases)

   b. Exudative ("wet") form: there is accumulation of serous fluid or blood in the subretinal space, which leads to more rapid, severe loss of vision; scar tissue forms and leads to cell death and vision loss (10 percent of cases but responsible for 90 percent of the cases of legal blindness)

C. Assessment

NCLEX!

1. Clinical manifestations include loss of central vision while peripheral vision remains intact), appearance of pale yellow spots on the macula called "drusen," visual distortion of images (i.e., straight lines may appear wavy) and difficulty with activities requiring focused and close central vision (i.e., sewing, needlepoint, reading)

2. Diagnostic tests: vision testing, fundoscopy (examination of fundus of eye); fluorescein angiography (for wet form only); and electroretinography (ERG) to measure retinal responses to light

D. Priority nursing diagnoses: Disturbed sensory perception: visual; Risk for injury; Anxiety; Knowledge deficit

E. Planning and implementation

1. Currently there is no treatment for dry macular generation and no curative therapy for either wet or dry macular degeneration

2. Wet macular degeneration may be treated by:

   a. Laser photocoagulation

   b. Photodynamic therapy, in which a light-activated drug is injected into the vein and circulates to the retinal blood vessels; a low-intensity laser light is shone on the retina; this activates the drug to eventually occlude the blood vessel and stop the leakage; note that it is possible for the process to recur in another area

3. Nursing measures

NCLEX!

   a. Standard nursing interventions to prevent falls and other injuries stemming from impaired vision

   b. Standard measures to assist those with impaired vision (see also section XI, D, planning and implementation for legal blindness)

NCLEX!

   c. Obtain home safety evaluation prior to discharge to minimize risk of injuries and falls in the home setting

F. Medication therapy: no medications are available to treat this condition

G. Client education

1. Need for regular eye examinations to determine disease progression

2. Use of Amsler grid for self-monitoring of central vision (available from eye care professionals or on the Internet)

3. Measures to maintain safety at home and adapt to visual changes

    a. Obtain aids to enhance vision and promote safety (i.e., magnification devices, enhanced lighting)

    b. Determine availability of large print books and newspapers and audio books

4. Post-procedure self-care for photodynamic therapy includes use of dark glasses and protective clothing as well as avoiding bright indoor light for a few days

H. Evaluation: client is free of injury; adapts to vision changes effectively; verbalizes an understanding of importance of continued monitoring of sight; and verbalizes adaptation to changing vision

IX. Eye Infections or Inflammations

A. Description and assessment findings

1. Blepharitis (inflammation of the eyelid margin glands and lash follicles): red-rimmed eyes; irritation, burning, itching of eyelid margins; mucous discharge with crusting and scaling of lid margins

2. Hordoleum or sty (infection of sebaceous glands of eyelid): raised area of lid, pain, redness, tenderness, possible photophobia, tearing, and sensation of foreign body in the eye

3. Chalazion (gramulomatous eyelid cyst or nodule): hard swelling, painless, reddened local conjunctival tissue, possibly due to inadequately treated hordoleum

4. **Conjunctivitis** (infection of conjunctiva, or inflammation caused by allergen, toxin, other irritant): eye redness and itching; possible scratchy, burning, or gritty sensation; photophobia, tearing, discharge (watery, purulent, or mucoid); usually not painful; if severe, possible conjunctival edema, hemorrhage, or perforation

5. Corneal ulcer (local necrosis of cornea): caused by infection, trauma, or misuse of contact lenses; manifested by: photophobia, discomfort ranging from gritty sensations to severe pain, excessive tearing; possible discharge; decreased visual acuity, inability to open eye or spasm of eyelid, visible area of ulceration

6. Keratitis (inflammation of cornea): similar to conjunctivitis, can lead to ulceration and blindness

7. Uveitis (inflammation of uveal tract, e.g., vascular layer): pupillary constriction, erythema around limbus, severe eye pain, photophobia, blurred vision

B. Collaborative management

1. Medication therapy with topical or systemic antibiotics or antiviral agents, antihistamines, and corticosteroids

2. Promote infection control through diligent handwashing and proper care of contact lenses; teach the client that conjunctivitis can be highly contagious

3. Reduce pain or discomfort with warm compresses, dark sunglasses, and analgesics (acetaminophen and/or codeine)

4. If corneal perforation is suspected, have client lie supine, close the eye, and cover with dry, sterile dressing to avoid loss of eye contents until surgery is done

X. Eye Injury

A. Description and assessment findings

1. Corneal abrasion (disruption of superficial cornea from drying, contact lenses, eyelashes, or foreign bodies such as dust, dirt, or fingernails): pain, photophobia, tearing

2. Burns (from chemicals, heat, radiation, explosion): eye pain, decreased vision, swollen eyelids, burns, reddened and edematous conjunctiva, possible corneal haziness or cloudiness, ulcerations

3. Blunt trauma (caused by sports injuries, motor vehicle accidents, falls, physical assault): includes lid ecchymosis (black eye), conjunctival hemorrhage (painless erythema), hyphema (bleeding into anterior chamber with eye pain, decreased vision, and seeing a reddish hue), and orbital fractures (diplopia/double vision, pain with upward eye movement, limited eye movements, sunken appearance to eye, and decreased sensation on affected cheek)

B. Collaborative management

1. If chemical burn present, irrigate the eye with copious amounts of normal saline (preferred) or water (if necessary), until pH of eye is in range of 7.2 to 7.4; use topical anesthetic to make irrigation easier; then evaluate vision with and without any corrective eyeglasses

2. If no chemical burn injury is present, first evaluate vision with and without eyeglasses to provide data about extent of injury and for use as a baseline

3. Remove loose foreign bodies quickly using a sterile moistened cotton-tipped applicator or by irrigation to prevent corneal abrasion

4. Apply eye patches or sterile gauze dressings over both eyes if severe or penetrating eye injury occurs to reduce eye movements; stabilize any penetrating objects until surgery is done to help preserve vision; institute bedrest

5. Provide follow-up client education about purpose, effects, and use of medications, use of eye patch or shield, avoidance of activities that increase intraocular pressure during healing (lifting, bending, straining), and how to avoid future injury

XI. Legal Blindness

A. Description: visual acuity that is no better than 20/200 even with correction in the better eye, or a visual field of less than 20 degrees (instead of 180 degrees)

B. Etiology

1. In the United States, the two most common causes are glaucoma and cataracts, followed by other retinal disorders (macular degeneration, diabetic retinopathy, congenital disorders)

2. Worldwide, the causes include cataracts, glaucoma, trauma, eye infections, and nutritional deficiencies; two-thirds of worldwide cases are preventable and result from lack of access to care, fear or ignorance about treatment or its need, poor sanitation, and poor nutrition

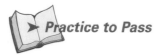

Practice to Pass

You are admitting a client who is legally blind to the nursing unit. How would you orient this client to the bedside unit?

NCLEX!

NCLEX!

NCLEX!

C. **Priority nursing diagnoses:** Disturbed sensory perception: visual; Self-care deficit: bathing, hygiene, dressing, grooming, feeding; Knowledge deficit; Grieving; Disturbed self-esteem; Hopelessness

D. **Planning and implementation**

1. Assist the client to move through the grieving process that accompanies vision loss, not only because of loss of sight, but because of its interference with mobility, self-sufficiency, and possibly financial status

2. Support the client who is experiencing changes in roles and relationships, communication patterns (through loss of ability to perceive nonverbal cues), and possibly sexual expression

3. Foster independence in the hospital environment

   a. Verbally and physically orient the client to the room using the bed as a reference point

   b. Keep room and hallway free of clutter

   c. Introduce yourself when entering the client's room and state when you are leaving

   d. Use increased verbal communication: describe activities in the environment and provide stimuli such as radio or television; ask client what assistance is needed

   e. Ensure that call bell and other needed articles are within easy reach of the client and that the client knows where they are located

   f. Describe the location of food on the plate using a clock face description (for a client who was previously sighted and knows what a clock face is)

   g. Assist with ambulation, walking slightly ahead and allowing client to hold your arm (not the reverse); describe the environment that lies ahead, such as turns or stairs

E. **Client education:** teach client and family measures to minimize risk of injury in the home setting and adapt to performing ADLs with impaired vision

F. **Evaluation:** client exhibits adaptation to vision loss by moving purposefully within the environment without injury, providing self-care for ADLs, and coping verbally and behaviorally with the loss of vision

XII. Overview of Anatomy and Physiology of the Ear

A. **Ear structures**

1. External ear: outer visible ear or auricle and external auditory canal

2. Middle ear: tympanic membrane; malleus, incus, and stapes bones; and window membranes

3. Inner ear: semicircular canals, cochlea, distal portion of cranial nerve VIII (vestibulocochlear nerve)

B. **Ear functions**

1. Hearing: sound is transferred from tympanic membrane to malleus, incus, and stapes and through cochlea; vibrations are changed by transduction into action potentials that are sent to the brain as neural impulses

2. Proprioception (balance): sensation about the body's position in space that is transferred to the brain after changes in body position trigger fluid movement and bending of hair cells in vestibular structures

3. Age-related changes of the ear that affect hearing

   a. External auditory canal narrows; cerumen glands atrophy and produce thicker, drier cerumen

   b. Tympanic membrane is less flexible, and ossicle joints calcify

   c. Cochlear hair cell degeneration and loss of auditory neurons in the organ of Corti lead to **presbycusis,** an age-related sensorineural hearing loss, characterized by decreased ability to hear high-frequency sounds and results in difficulty hearing and localizing normal speech

XIII. Diagnostic Tests and Assessments of the Ear

A. Otoscopic examination

1. Hold speculum with handle downward if client is cooperative, or with handle upward if uncooperative; rest the hand holding the otoscope against the client's head for support if needed while handle is upward

2. Tilt the client's head slightly away, pull the pinna up and back in an adult (down and back in a child) to straighten the external auditory canal, and insert the speculum while visualizing the canal

3. Normal findings

   a. Pink, intact external canal with no lesions and variable amount of cerumen and fine hairs; absence of inflammation, deviations, or foreign bodies

   b. Tympanic membrane that is transparent, opaque, pearly gray, slightly concave, intact, and free of lesions or perforations

B. Whisper test

1. Have client occlude one ear at a time with a finger, and stand 1 to 2 feet away from the client on the side of the unoccluded ear

2. Whisper numbers or a statement and ask client to repeat; repeat for other ear

3. Note whether it is necessary to stand closer or raise the voice to be heard

4. A similar test is the watch test, in which a ticking watch is held 5 inches from each ear and hearing is assessed

C. Rinne test

1. Hold a tuning fork by the stem and strike the tines softly on the back of the hand to activate it; place the stem on the mastoid bone and ask client to signal when the sound is no longer heard

2. Quickly place the vibrating end of the tuning fork in front of the ear close to the ear canal; ask the client if the sound is heard; if yes, have client indicate when sound is no longer heard

3. With no conductive hearing loss, the sound is heard twice as long by air conduction as by bone conduction

4. With conductive hearing loss, bone conduction is greater than air conduction in the affected ear

D. **Weber test**

1. Is especially valuable when hearing in one ear is reported as better than the other

2. Place the stem of the vibrating tuning fork on the midline of the forehead or the vertex of the head (skull) and ask whether the sound is heard equally in both ears or if one side is better than the other

NCLEX!

3. Sound that lateralizes to one ear indicates conductive hearing loss in that ear or sensorineural hearing loss in the opposite ear

E. **Audiometry:** quantifies hearing deficits by presenting various sound frequencies to each ear by either sound or bone conduction; client sits in soundproof room wearing earphones, and is asked to signal when tones are heard

F. **Speech audiometry:** identifies the intensity at which speech is identifiable

G. **Tympanometry:** indirectly monitors compliance and impedance of the middle ear to sound transmission after neutral, positive, and negative air pressure is applied to the external auditory meatus

H. **Tests of vestibular function**

1. Test for falling: assure client that a fall will be prevented; then ask client to close the eyes while feet are together and arms are hanging at sides; observe for a normal slight sway; significant sway is called a positive Romberg test

2. Past pointing test

   a. Have client sit facing examiner, close the eyes, and point both index fingers at examiner

   b. Place own index fingers under the client's to provide a reference point, then ask client to raise both arms and then lower them to original location with eyes closed

   c. With normal response, the client can return to reference point easily; with vestibular dysfunction, fingers deviate to the left or the right

3. Gaze nystagmus test: observe the client's eyes as they look straight ahead, 30 degrees to each side, upward, and downward; with vestibular problems the eyeballs exhibit nystagmus, an involuntary, constant, and cyclical movement of the eyeballs in any direction

4. Hallpike maneuver: have client lie supine and rotate head to side for one minute; the test is positive for positional vertigo or induced dizziness if nystagmus occurs

XIV. **Common Nursing Techniques and Procedures for the Ear**

A. **Otic medications**

NCLEX!

1. Use clean technique unless tympanic membrane is damaged, then use sterile technique

2. Assist the client to a side-lying position with the ear being medicated uppermost

3. Clean the pinna of the ear and the opening of the external ear canal with solution and cotton-tipped applicators as needed

4. Warm the medication container in your hand or in warm water for comfort; partially fill the ear dropper with medication

5. Straighten the auditory canal by pulling the pinna up and back in the adult or older child, or down and back in an infant or young child

6. Hold the bottle or dropper 1/2-inch above the ear canal and instill the correct number of drops along the side of the ear canal

7. Apply gentle pressure with your finger to the tragus of the ear to enhance flow of medication into the ear canal

8. Have the client maintain a side-lying position for 2 to 5 minutes for even medication dispersion

9. Before the client arises, loosely place a cotton ball at the meatus and leave in place for 20 to 30 minutes to prevent medication loss

B. Otic irrigation

1. Assist the client to a sitting or lying position with the head tilted toward the affected ear; place a waterproof pad and drainage receptacle under the affected ear

2. Check that the temperature of the irrigant is 37°C or 98°F

3. Determine that the tympanic membrane is intact before beginning an otic irrigation

4. Straighten the ear canal and gently insert the syringe tip into the auditory meatus; direct the solution slowly and steadily along the wall of the canal (not the center, which could damage the tympanic membrane); use no more than 50 to 70 mL at one time

5. After the solution drains, dry the outside of the ear with cotton balls and place a dry one in the auditory meatus lightly to absorb remaining excess fluid

6. Assist the client to a side-lying position on the affected side for further drainage, and assess client for discomfort

C. Hearing aid prosthesis care

1. There are several types of hearing aids: behind-the-ear (BTE, postaural), in-the-ear (ITE, intra-aural), in-the-canal (ITC), eyeglasses aid, and body hearing aid; hearing aids are useful to improve quality of hearing with conductive hearing loss but only intensify the distortions heard with sensorineural hearing loss (they may be useful in signaling client of danger, i.e., able to hear alarms)

2. Wash hands before handling an external hearing aid

3. Make sure battery is working properly and is inserted correctly; keep an extra battery on hand

4. Do not drop the hearing aid or twist the cord

5. To insert a hearing aid: inspect to ensure it is intact, turn down the volume, insert the ear mold first into the ear canal, then secure the rest of the device according to its design; once in place, turn up volume slowly until comfortable, and check for structural problems or placement problems if feedback occurs

6. Remove a hearing aid after turning it off and lowering the volume; remove the earmold by rotating it forward slightly and pulling outward

7. After removal of a hearing aid, clean a detachable earmold with mild soap and water, rinse and dry well, and avoid excessive wetting or use of alcohol, which can damage the aid; wipe nondetachable earmolds with a damp cloth

8. Avoid using aerosol sprays, oils, or cosmetic products near the hearing aid, because the earmold opening could become clogged

9. Remove the battery to prevent battery corrosion and leakage if the aid will not be used for more than 24 hours; store in a safe place away from moisture and heat

XV. Nursing Management of Client Having Ear Surgery

A. Preoperative period

1. Reduce anxiety through preoperative teaching about procedure and postoperative course and care

2. Complete a baseline assessment of client's hearing ability to use as a comparison postoperatively

3. Assess client's support systems and ability to care for self after surgery, including assessment of environmental safety (such as hand rails, absence of throw rugs)

4. Complete shampoo or scrub around ear if ordered; complete usual preoperative activities and checklist; administer preanesthetic medications as ordered

B. Postoperative period

1. Perform baseline assessments as for all postoperative clients (vital signs, level of consciousness, bleeding or drainage from dressing, pain, recovery from anesthesia)

2. Implement standard interventions for care of the postoperative client (pain control, mobility, prevention of postoperative complications)

3. Keep client on bedrest for 24 hours with the head of bed either elevated or flat (depending on surgeon's order) and lying on nonoperative side (operative ear upward) for 12 to 24 hours

4. Change internal or external dressings if ordered; wipe away discharge from ear with dry sterile dressing material

5. Assess for nausea and vomiting; medicate with antiemetics p.r.n. to avoid vomiting, which can disrupt the surgical site by increasing pressure in middle ear

6. Assess for dizziness and vertigo postoperatively; avoid unnecessary movements or turning in bed; provide antivertigo medications; and provide assistance when allowed to ambulate to reduce falls

7. Assess client's hearing postoperatively and compare to baseline; use alternate communication means as needed

8. Remind client that decreased hearing immediately after surgery may be due to edema and drainage at operative site; permanent hearing loss may be expected if cochlea is involved or no middle ear reconstruction is done

9. Teach the client and family about post-discharge care (see Box 16-2)

Box 16-2

Client Education Following Ear Surgery

The following points should be included in discharge instructions given to the client and family after ear surgery:

- Keep the outer ear dressing clean and dry; change it as ordered if needed; do not remove inner ear dressing until allowed by surgeon; do not insert small objects to clean external ear canal

- Whenever possible, avoid activities that increase middle ear pressure, such as blowing nose, sneezing, coughing, straining

- If it is necessary, cough or sneeze with mouth open; blow nose one nostril at a time with mouth open; avoid drinking through a straw for 2 to 3 weeks; avoid air travel until allowed by surgeon

- Use measures to prevent constipation, such as adequate fiber and fluid intake, maintaining mobility as able, and possible use of stool softener

- Do not shower or shampoo hair until allowed by surgeon (usually for 1 or more weeks)

- Keep ear dry for 6 weeks with use of petrolatum-coated cotton ball placed in external auditory canal as ordered, if used change it daily; do not swim or dive until allowed by surgeon (when full healing occurs)

- Reduce risk of infection by avoiding those with respiratory infections

- Medication names, dose, schedule, side effects, purpose, and anticipated duration of use (antibiotics, antiemetics, antivertigo agents)

- Symptoms to report to physician: persistent postoperative headache, increased drainage or bleeding from site, fever, new or increased ear pain or dizziness, decreasing hearing

XVI. Ear Infections

A. Description and etiology

1. Otitis externa: infectious, inflammatory, or allergic response in the external auditory canal or auricle; also called "swimmer's ear"; more frequent in warm, humid areas

2. Otitis media: infection or inflammation of the middle ear; often a consequence of upper respiratory infection when organisms travel from nose and throat via Eustachian tube; may be acute or chronic

3. Mastoiditis: infection of the mastoid process (temporal bone adjacent to middle ear), usually a consequence of untreated or inadequately treated otitis media

B. Assessment

1. Otitis externa: redness, swelling, and exudate in external auditory canal, earache, itching, sensation that ear is "plugged" or "blocked," hearing loss in affected ear

2. Otitis media

   a. Acute: severe earache or ear pain (classic), ear pressure, fever, malaise, diminished hearing, dizziness or vertigo, nausea and possible vomiting, possible tinnitus, presence of fluid behind a bulging tympanic membrane

   b. Chronic: slight fever, diminished hearing, chronic ear discharge

3. Mastoiditis: fever, malaise, possible tinnitus and headache, persistent throbbing ear pain worsened by head movement, tenderness behind the ear (over

mastoid process), local cellulitis of skin, drainage from ear, diminished hearing in affected ear

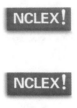

C. Priority nursing diagnoses: Pain; Disturbed sensory perception: Auditory; Risk for injury; Risk for falls (if vertigo present)

D. Planning and implementation

1. Apply local heat three times per day for 20 minutes at a time as prescribed

2. Encourage bedrest as applicable to reduce head movements and pain

3. Administer prescribed antibiotics (otic or systemic), decongestants, antihistamines, analgesics (acetaminophen or aspirin), and antivertigo agents

4. Teach client to use caution while hearing is diminished

5. Provide care to clients undergoing ear surgery as per section XIV

E. Surgical procedures

1. **Myringotomy:** surgically performed perforation of tympanic membrane to allow drainage of middle ear secretions and relieve pain and pressure (otitis media)

2. Tympanocentesis: insertion of a 20-gauge spinal needle through inferior portion of tympanic membrane to drain secretions, possibly to obtain culture, and relieve pain and pressure (otitis media)

3. Mastoidectomy: surgical removal of infected mastoid air cells, bone, and pus; radical mastoidectomy involves removal of middle ear structures such as incus and malleus as well as diseased tissue (conductive hearing loss then occurs unless reconstructive surgery is done as well)

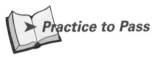

Practice to Pass

A client is being discharged to home following myringotomy. What would you include in postoperative discharge teaching?

4. **Tympanoplasty:** surgical reconstruction of ossicles and tympanic membrane of the middle ear to help restore hearing

F. Evaluation: resolution of signs and symptoms of infection

XVII. Otosclerosis

A. Description: hereditary disorder of the labyrinthine capsule in which abnormal bone growth occurs around the ossicles and causes fixation of the stapes, leading to conductive hearing loss

B. Etiology and pathophysiology

1. Is an autosomal dominant hereditary disorder most common in Caucasians and females; onset is in adolescence or early adulthood; pregnancy exacerbates the condition

2. Stapes do not vibrate as easily due to stiffening, thus reducing sound transmission to inner ear

C. Assessment

1. Bilateral conductive hearing loss that is progressive and asymmetrical, tinnitus, possible retention of bone conduction (so client has difficulty in ordinary conversation but can use the telephone adequately)

2. Reddish or pinkish-orange tympanic membrane from increased vascularity (Schwartz's sign)

3. Rinne test results: bone sound conduction equal to or longer than air conduction (abnormal finding) if hearing loss greater than 25 decibels (dB)

4. Weber test results: lateralization to ear with greater conductive hearing loss

D. Priority nursing diagnoses: Disturbed sensory perception: auditory; Impaired verbal communication; Risk for falls; Risk for social isolation

E. Planning and implementation

1. Encourage use of a hearing aid(s) to augment sound

2. Administer sodium fluoride as ordered to slow bone resorption and overgrowth

NCLEX!

3. Implement strategies to enhance communication with a hearing-impaired client

   a. Approach the client from within the client's line of vision or tap client lightly on the shoulder to get attention before beginning to speak

   b. Reduce background noise, such as radio or TV, before beginning to speak

   c. Avoid covering mouth with hands or other objects while speaking

   d. Face the client and speak slowly and clearly—pronounce words clearly without over-articulating them; speak using low pitch and normal loudness

   e. Use nonverbal cues and written messages to enhance communication

   f. Repeat sentences using different words if client has difficulty understanding

   g. Ask client to repeat directions or teaching that was done to ensure the client's understanding

4. Surgical intervention

   a. Stapedectomy with fenestration: microsurgical removal of diseased stapes, with drill or laser creation of a hole in the footplate, followed by insertion of a steel or synthetic prosthesis to restore hearing

   b. Stapedotomy: insertion of a wire or platinum ribbon prosthesis into a small hole created in the stapes footplate

> ➤ *Practice to Pass*
>
> A client has just been given a diagnosis of otosclerosis. How would you explain the disorder? What communication strategies will you use?

F. Client education: referral to appropriate community agencies; postoperative care as outlined in section XV

G. Evaluation: client uses alternate communication means as needed, indicates improved hearing postoperatively or with use of aids, does not suffer injury, and maintains social contacts

XVIII. Meniere's Disease

A. Description: Meniere's disease is a disorder of the inner ear in which there is excessive accumulation of endolymphatic fluid in the membranous labyrinth; also called idiopathic endolymphatic hydrops

B. Etiology and pathophysiology

1. Unknown etiology, possibly heredity, viral influence, and immune dysfunction play a role; affects men and women equally; highest risk between ages 35 to 60

2. Impaired reabsorption of endolymph leads to dilation of lymph channels, which causes the symptoms

C. **Assessment and diagnostic findings**

1. Recurrent severe attacks of vertigo accompanied by sense of fullness in the ears, roaring or ringing tinnitus, nausea, headache, and gradual but progressive sensorineural hearing loss (often unilateral)

2. Attacks may last minutes to hours with possible associated symptoms of hypotension, diaphoresis, and nystagmus

3. Attacks may be triggered by increased sodium intake, vasoconstriction, premenstrual fluid retention, stress, or allergies, although sometimes no trigger is identified

4. Diagnosis is by electronystagnography (including caloric testing), Rinne and Weber tests, X-ray, CT scan, evaluation of response to a test dose of an osmotic or loop diuretic

D. **Priority nursing diagnoses:** Risk for injury/trauma; Disturbed sleep pattern; Disturbed sensory perception: auditory

E. **Planning and implementation**

1. Low-sodium diet and, if symptoms are severe, fluid restriction

2. Avoid use of alcohol, caffeine, nicotine

3. Bedrest to control vertigo; assist with ambulation for safety

4. Medication therapy: atropine (to reduce parasympathetic response) or CNS depressant as an alternative to atropine, diuretics, antihistamines (if allergy present), antivertigo and antiemetic drugs

5. Surgical procedures (postoperative care as per section XV)

   a. Endolymphatic decompression: relieves pressure in labyrinth and creates shunt between membranous labyrinth and subarachnoid space for fluid drainage (preserves hearing in most cases, relieves vertigo approximately 70 percent of cases, relieves tinnitus and sensations of ear fullness in 50 percent of cases)

   b. Vestibular neurectomy: severing of portion of eighth cranial nerve that controls balance and sensation of vertigo (relieves vertigo in up to 90 percent of cases)

   c. **Labyrinthectomy:** complete removal of labyrinth, destroying cochlear function, relieving vertigo but causing loss of any minimal remaining hearing as well ("last resort")

   d. Cochlear implant: for sensorineural hearing loss two types of procedures available depending on whether there are remaining auditory neurons capable of being excited

      1) A device is implanted in the ear for use in receiving and transmitting sound; two types of devices are available

      2) An electrode that is implanted in the cochlea receives stimuli from a processor worn on the body; used for a client with intact neurons capable of stimulation (see Figure 16-2)

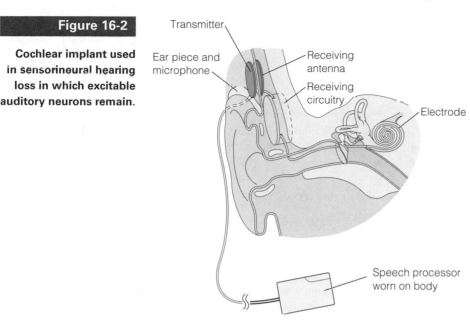

Figure 16-2

Cochlear implant used in sensorineural hearing loss in which excitable auditory neurons remain.

Transmitter

Ear piece and microphone

Receiving antenna

Receiving circuitry

Electrode

Speech processor worn on body

3) A second type of device, used for clients with no excitable auditory fibers, amplifies and transmits a signal to a receiver implanted in the brainstem

4) Devices do not restore normal hearing but allow perception of sound to alert a client to conversation or dangers in the environment

e. Complications of all inner ear surgical procedures include infection and cerebrospinal fluid leakage

F. Client education

1. Follow restrictions in sodium, fluid, nicotine, alcohol, and caffeine

2. Take medications as prescribed

3. Learn signs of an impending attack: fullness in affected ear, increasing tinnitus, headache; lie down in bed in a dark quiet room if at home when an attack begins, or pull off the road for safety if driving

4. Avoid sudden movements or position changes; move the head slowly, and do not get up unassisted during an attack

5. Wear a Medic-Alert bracelet or necklace to indicate the condition

6. Learn stress reduction techniques of choice to help reduce severity of attacks

7. If tinnitus persists between attacks, use white noise or ambient sound machine to mask tinnitus and promote sleep; consider use of medication most commonly effective—oral antidepressant nortriptyline (Pamelor) taken at bedtime

8. Practice balance training exercises to help the brain learn to compensate for damage to vestibular system; these consist of moving the head up and down, side to side, and tilting the head to the left and right; repeated 10 times each twice a day

NCLEX!

NCLEX!

G. **Evaluation:** client identifies how to prevent injury during an attack, complies with measures to reduce frequency of attacks, maintains normal sleep patterns and daily interactions with others

---

Case Study

P. M., a 65-year-old female client, is scheduled for cataract surgery this morning. You are the nurse working in the ambulatory surgery center where the client's ophthalmic surgery will be performed.

❶ What questions will you ask of P. M. when she arrives prior to surgery?

❷ What assessments will you make before the procedure begins?

❸ What are the priorities of care for P. M. immediately after the procedure?

❹ What discharge instructions will you give to P. M.?

❺ When P. M. asks you about what to expect regarding vision changes after surgery, how would you respond?

For suggested responses, see pages 739–740.

Posttest

1 A client comes to the ambulatory clinic seeking care with a complaint of "getting something in my eye." Which of the following actions should the nurse take first?

(1) Provide copious irrigation with normal saline
(2) Get a detailed health history
(3) Evaluate the client's vision
(4) Swab the cornea several times using a cotton-tipped applicator

2 A client is being admitted to the post-anesthesia recovery area following lens removal and replacement in the left eye for a cataract. The nurse places the client into which of the following most appropriate positions?

(1) On the left side with the head of bed elevated 30 degrees
(2) On the right side with the head of bed elevated 30 degrees
(3) Supine with the head of bed flat
(4) Upright with the head and neck turned to the right

3 A client who has developed impaired vision because of previously undiagnosed glaucoma asks the nurse if the lost vision will return. Which of the following replies by the nurse is most accurate?

(1) "Vision that is lost will not return, but compliance with therapy can help to maintain current vision."
(2) "It will take at least 2 to 3 months for vision to return to baseline."
(3) "It is difficult to answer that question with accuracy. Some clients experience return of vision, while others do not."
(4) "Vision will return to normal within a week or so if intraocular pressure is reduced quickly."

4 A client is admitted with a newly diagnosed detached retina. The nurse should place highest priority on doing which of the following?

(1) Limiting visitors and providing clear liquids
(2) Allowing the client to get out of bed but keeping the room darkened
(3) Giving eye drops every hour and allowing bathroom privileges only
(4) Placing the client on bedrest and patching the eyes

5 The nurse who is planning care for a client who is legally blind should do which of the following as most important to ensure the client's safety?

(1) Leave doors partially closed
(2) Orient the client verbally and physically to the room
(3) Provide radio and television for stimulation
(4) Describe the weather and community events for the client

6 The nurse is performing the Rinne test on a client with a suspected hearing impairment. The nurse places the base of the tuning fork in which of the following locations?

(1) On the forehead in the midline
(2) On the tip of the nose
(3) On the vertex of the skull
(4) On the mastoid bone

7 The nurse is providing instructions to a client who has been diagnosed with hearing impairment and has just received a hearing aid. The nurse would include which of the following statements in discussion with the client?

(1) Immerse the hearing aid daily in warm water for 15 minutes to clean it.
(2) Leave the hearing aid on at all times to keep the battery charged.
(3) Avoid use of aerosol sprays near the aid, because particles can clog the receiver.
(4) Adjust the volume control to the maximum setting for efficient use.

8 A nurse is providing care to a client who just underwent a stapedectomy. The nurse checks the client's medical record, noting that this client had which of the following diagnoses prior to surgery?

(1) Otitis externa
(2) Otosclerosis
(3) Meniere's disease
(4) Foreign body obstruction of the auditory canal

9 A 72-year-old client reports to the nurse during a health history that the physician previously diagnosed an age-related loss of hearing. The nurse documents in the medical record that the patient reports which of the following disorders?

(1) Otosclerosis
(2) Meniere's disease
(3) Presbycusis
(4) Otalgia

10 The nurse would prioritize that which of the following nursing diagnoses has highest priority for a client experiencing an attack of Meniere's disease?

(1) Risk for injury
(2) Risk for disturbed sleep pattern
(3) Sensory perception: auditory
(4) Risk for ineffective individual coping

See pages 660–661 for Answers and Rationales.

Answers and Rationales

Pretest

1 **Answer: 1** *Rationale:* A result of 20/120 means that this client can read at a distance of 20 feet what another individual with normal vision can read at a distance of 120 feet. This means that the client is nearsighted in that eye. The other responses are incorrect.
Cognitive Level: Application
Nursing Process: Analysis; *Test Plan:* PHYS

2 **Answer: 4** *Rationale:* Cyclopentolate is a mydriatic and a cycloplegic medication that is used to dilate the pupil and paralyze the ciliary muscles before an eye exam. Carbachol and latanoprost are miotics that con-

strict the pupil and are used to treat glaucoma. Glycerin is an osmotic diuretic used to treat acute angle-closure glaucoma.
Cognitive Level: Application
Nursing Process: Planning; *Test Plan:* PHYS

3 **Answer: 3** *Rationale:* It is important to share with the client that lifelong medication therapy is needed to preserve vision. The statement in option 2 is correct also but is not as critical as option 3, since the client has just been diagnosed. Options 1 and 4 are false statements.
Cognitive Level: Analysis
Nursing Process: Implementation; *Test Plan:* HPM

4   Answer: 2 *Rationale:* A cloudy-appearing lens is characteristic of cataract development. Early symptoms of cataract formation include blurred vision and a loss of ability to see colors. A sense of a curtain falling across the field of vision characterizes detached retina. Eye pain and double vision are not symptoms associated with cataracts.
Cognitive Level: Analysis
Nursing Process: Assessment; *Test Plan:* PHYS

5   Answer: 1 *Rationale:* A client who is legally blind has either visual acuity no better than 20/200 in the better eye with optimal correction, or has a visual field of 20 degrees rather than 180 degrees.
Cognitive Level: Application
Nursing Process: Analysis; *Test Plan:* PHYS

6   Answer: 4 *Rationale:* It is essential to determine that the tympanic membrane is intact before completing an otic irrigation. No more than 50 to 70 mL of solution should be drawn up at one time, and the fluid should be at body temperature. The client may be positioned wherever it is comfortable, and needs only a receptacle to hold the drainage, and a waterproof pad to protect clothing.
Cognitive Level: Application
Nursing Process: Implementation; *Test Plan:* PHYS

7   Answer: 3 *Rationale:* Ear pain is a primary or classic symptom associated with otitis media. Secondary manifestations could include dizziness, vertigo, and diminished hearing in the affected ear.
Cognitive Level: Application
Nursing Process: Evaluation; *Test Plan:* PHYS

8   Answer: 2 *Rationale:* Following ear surgery, clients should avoid activities that could result in increased pressure in the middle ear. These include blowing the nose, sneezing, coughing, or doing any activities that involve holding the breath or bearing down. Talking is an acceptable activity.
Cognitive Level: Application
Nursing Process: Planning; *Test Plan:* HPM

9   Answer: 1 *Rationale:* Otosclerosis is characterized by Schwartz's sign, a tympanic membrane that is reddish or pinkish-orange because of increased vascularity. It would not be pearly white or pale (options 2 and 4), nor would it have a bruised appearance (option 3).
Cognitive Level: Application
Nursing Process: Assessment; *Test Plan:* PHYS

10   Answer: 4 *Rationale:* The client with Meniere's disease should limit intake of salty foods that could cause an increase in endolymphatic fluid in the inner ear. The other foods listed pose no problem.
Cognitive Level: Application
Nursing Process: Evaluation; *Test Plan:* HPM

Posttest

1   Answer: 3 *Rationale:* The nurse should evaluate the client's vision first to provide a baseline, and then treat the injury. Irrigation is often used to remove foreign bodies from the eye, followed by application of an eye patch.
Cognitive Level: Analysis
Nursing Process: Implementation; *Test Plan:* PHYS

2   Answer: 2 *Rationale:* Following eye surgery, the head of bed should be elevated 30 to 45 degrees and the client should lie on back or unaffected side to reduce intraocular pressure. Small pillows may be used at the sides of the head to immobilize the head when lying on the back.
Cognitive Level: Application
Nursing Process: Implementation; *Test Plan:* PHYS

3   Answer: 1 *Rationale:* Glaucoma is characterized by a gradual loss of vision that is irreversible because of the effects of increased intraocular pressure on the optic neurons. Compliance with medication therapy is important to preserve the current level of vision, although vision that is lost cannot be regained.
Cognitive Level: Analysis
Nursing Process: Implementation; *Test Plan:* PSYC

4   Answer: 4 *Rationale:* The client with a detached retina should have activity restricted with eyes patched to reduce eye movement and prevent worsening of the detachment. The client may be prepared for surgery quickly, and thus may be placed on NPO status rather than clear liquids.
Cognitive Level: Analysis
Nursing Process: Planning; *Test Plan:* SECE

5   Answer: 2 *Rationale:* The nurse should orient the client to the room for safety, using both words and a physical walking tour for best effect. Options 2 and 4 are helpful, but do not ensure client safety. Leaving doors partially closed (option 1) is hazardous because the client could inadvertently walk into the door during ambulation. Pathways should be free of obstacles.
Cognitive Level: Analysis
Nursing Process: Planning; *Test Plan:* SECE

6   Answer: 4 *Rationale:* The nurse places the base of the tuning fork on the client's mastoid bone to perform the Rinne test. When the sound is no longer

heard, it is quickly repositioned in front of the client's ear, and hearing is again assessed. The tuning fork may be placed at the top of the forehead or the vertex of the skull in the midline to perform the Weber test. The bridge of the nose is not used as a reference point for assessing hearing.
Cognitive Level: Application
Nursing Process: Assessment; *Test Plan:* PHYS

7 **Answer: 3** *Rationale:* The client should avoid the use of aerosol sprays, cosmetics, or other hair or facial products near the hearing aid. The aid should not get excessively wet. The hearing aid should be turned off when not in use, and should be maintained on the lowest setting that is comfortable and effective.
Cognitive Level: Application
Nursing Process: Implementation; *Test Plan:* HPM

8 **Answer: 2** *Rationale:* A stapedectomy is a common surgical procedure used to treat the hearing loss that

is associated with otosclerosis. It is not performed for the other conditions listed.
Cognitive Level: Application
Nursing Process: Analysis; *Test Plan:* PHYS

9 **Answer: 3** *Rationale:* Presbycusis is an age-related decline in hearing. Otosclerosis is a familial disorder characterized by hearing loss. Meniere's disease is a disorder of the inner ear that results in vertigo. Otalgia is an earache.
Cognitive Level: Application
Nursing Process: Assessment; *Test Plan:* PHYS

10 **Answer: 1** *Rationale:* Meniere's disease is characterized by bouts of vertigo, which place the client at risk for falls and injury. The client may have manifestations of the other nursing diagnoses as well, but the highest priority is on preventing injury.
Cognitive Level: Analysis
Nursing Process: Planning; *Test Plan:* PHYS

References

Ebersole, P., & Hess, P. (1998). *Toward healthy aging: Human needs and nursing response* (5th ed.). St. Louis: MO: Mosby-Year Book, Inc., pp. 98–100.

Gutierrez, K. (1999). *Pharmacotherapeutics: Clinical decision-making in nursing.* Philadelphia: W.B. Saunders, pp. 1286–1310.

Harkreader, H. & Hogan, M. (2003). *Fundamentals of nursing: Caring and clinical judgment.* (2nd ed.). Philadelphia: W.B. Saunders, pp. 583–589.

Jarvis, C. (2000). *Physical examination and health assessment* (3rd ed.). Philadelphia: W.B. Saunders, pp. 329–334, 360–366.

Kozier, B., Erb, G., Berman, A., & Burke, K. (2003). *Fundamentals of nursing: Concepts, process, and practice* (7th ed.). Upper Saddle River, NJ: Prentice Hall, Inc., pp. 735–737.

Lehne, R. (2001). *Pharmacology for nursing care* (4th ed.). Philadelphia: W.B. Saunders., pp. 1141–1150.

LeMone, P., & Burke, K. (2003). *Medical-surgical nursing: Critical thinking in client care* (3rd ed.). Upper Saddle River, NJ: Prentice-Hall, Inc., pp. 1876–1897, 1898–1950.

Malkiewicz, J. (2002). Assessment of the ear and hearing. In D. Ignatavicius, & M. Workman (Eds.), *Medical-surgical nursing: Critical thinking for collaborative care* (4th ed.). Philadelphia: W.B. Saunders, pp. 1048–1060.

Martin, J. (2002). Interventions for clients with ear and hearing problems. In D. Ignatavicius, & M. Workman (Eds.), *Med-*

ical-surgical nursing: Critical thinking for collaborative care (4th ed.). Philadelphia: W.B. Saunders, pp. 1209–1226.

Meadows, C. (2003). Assessment of the auditory system. In W. Phipps, F. Monahan, J. Sands, J. Marek, & M. Neighbors (Eds.), *Medical-surgical nursing: Health and illness perspectives* (7th ed.). St. Louis, MO: Mosby, Inc., pp. 1909–1918.

Meadows, C. & Monahan, F. (2003). Problems of the ear. In W. Phipps, F. Monahan, J. Sands, J. Marek, & M. Neighbors (Eds.), *Medical-surgical nursing: Health illness perspectives* (7th ed.). St. Louis, MO: Mosby, Inc., pp. 1919–1933.

Smith, C. (2003). Problems of the eye. In W. Phipps, F. Monahan, J. Sands, J. Marek, & M. Neighbors (Eds.). *Medical-surgical nursing: Health and illness perspectives* (7th ed.). St. Louis, MO: Mosby, Inc., pp. 1885–1908.

Smith, S.C. & Wilbur, M.E. (2000). Nursing assessment: visual and auditory systems. In S. Lewis, M. Heitkemper, & S. Dirksen. *Medical-surgical nursing: Assessment and management of clinical problems* (5th ed.). St. Louis, MO: Mosby, Inc., pp. 417–441.

Smith, S.C. & Wilbur, M.E. (2000). Nursing management: visual and auditory problems. In S. Lewis, M. Heitkemper, & S. Dirksen (Eds). *Medical-surgical nursing: Assessment and management of clinical problems* (5th ed.). St. Louis, MO: Mosby, Inc., pp. 442–481.

Wilson, B., Shannon, M., & Stang, C. (2003). *Nurses drug guide 2003.* Upper Saddle River, NJ: Prentice Hall, pp. 1484–1491.

Workman, M. (2002). Assessment of the eye and vision. In D. Ignatavicius, & M. Workman (Eds.), *Medical-surgical nursing: Critical thinking for collaborative care* (4th ed.). Philadelphia: W.B. Saunders, pp. 1011–1022.

Workman, M. (2002). Interventions for clients with eye and vision problems. In D. Ignatavicius, & M. Workman (Eds.), *Medical-surgical nursing: Critical thinking for collaborative care* (4th ed.). Philadelphia: W.B. Saunders, pp. 1167–1194.

CHAPTER 17

Common Problems Encountered in Emergency and Critical Care Nursing

Deborah Jane Schwytzer, RN, MSN, CEN

CHAPTER OUTLINE

OBJECTIVES

▪ Describe the pathophysiology and etiology of common problems seen in the emergency and critical care settings.

▪ Discuss expected assessment data and diagnostic findings for common problems seen in the emergency and critical care settings.

▪ Identify priority nursing diagnoses for common problems seen in the emergency and critical care settings.

▪ Discuss therapeutic management of common problems seen in the emergency and critical care settings.

▪ Discuss nursing management of common problems seen in the emergency and critical care settings.

▪ Identify expected outcomes for common problems seen in emergency and critical care settings.

[Media Link]

Use the CD-ROM enclosed with this text, or log onto the address given to access the free, interactive Companion Website created for this series. The CD-ROM and Companion Website accompanying this book offer additional practice opportunities and information—NCLEX Review, Case Studies, Glossary, In Depth with NCLEX, and more.

www.prenhall.com/hogan

REVIEW AT A GLANCE

asphyxiation *effects of decreased amount of oxygen and increased carbon dioxide in the body and blood*

autotransfusion *therapeutic method of transfusing the client's own shed and filtered blood back to him or her*

cardiac index *a measurement of cardiac performance which considers client surface area; cardiac output divided by body surface area*

defibrillation *asynchronous external application of electrical charge to depolarize the myocardial cells and terminate abnormal cardiac activity to re-establish a normal rhythm*

dysrhythmia *abnormal cardiac activity*

emergent *immediate care required; condition presents a threat to life or limb*

Glascow coma scale *assessment tool that evaluates the client's level of consciousness through the eye opening, best motor response, and best verbal response*

isoelectric *showing no variation in electrical activity; the baseline between each cardiac complex on an EKG strip*

morbidity *illness*

mortality *death*

non-urgent *routine care is required; may delay care for a period of time*

phlebostatic axis *the point where the fourth intercostal space and midaxillary line meet, which serves as the reference point for the right atrium*

primary assessment *assessment of the airway, breathing, circulation, and brief neurological status*

secondary assessment *a head-to-toe assessment of the client to identify all injuries*

triage *method of determination of priority of clients cared for in emergency care*

urgent *condition requires care as soon as possible; condition may deteriorate if care is not provided*

Pretest

1 The client you are caring for has severe continuous bleeding from a self-inflicted wrist laceration. While applying direct pressure to the area with a dry, sterile dressing, your next action would to be to do which of the following?

(1) Call for a psychiatric evaluation since this was a self-inflicted injury.
(2) Apply ice to lower the body temperature to slow circulation.
(3) Lower the extremity to below heart level.
(4) Assess for signs of shock.

2 You have assessed a client and suspect that the client has developed a tension pneumothorax. Which of the following assessment findings would support this conclusion?

(1) Decreased tidal volume and normal respiratory rate
(2) Hypertension
(3) Respiratory alkalosis and hypoxemia
(4) Mediastinal shift toward uninjured side

3 Your client is exhibiting signs of an allergic reaction to a bee sting. Which of the following symptoms would you find?

(1) Normal respiratory rate
(2) Prolonged expiratory phase
(3) Wheezing on inspiration
(4) Decreased respiratory rate

4 Prior to performing tracheal suctioning for a client with a tracheostomy, the nurse should do which of the following?

(1) Instill 10 ml of normal saline to loosen secretions.
(2) Preoxygenate with 100 percent oxygen.
(3) Inflate tracheostomy cuff to the maximum inflation pressure.
(4) Apply negative pressure to the suction catheter as it is being inserted.

5 A nurse in the triage area of the emergency unit would prioritize and assist in the treatment of which of the following clients first?

(1) A client with a closed fracture of the femur
(2) A client in ventricular fibrillation
(3) A client with a penetrating wound to the abdomen
(4) A client with an eye injury

6 A nurse caring for a client with a human bite to the hand anticipates that the physician will order which of the following?

(1) Antibiotics to prevent infection from oral bacteria
(2) Application of a tourniquet to prevent the spread of the microorganisms
(3) Administration of anti-venom
(4) A pressure dressing to control swelling and pain

7 The client is being weaned from a ventilator. Arterial blood gases drawn prior to extubation reveal: pH 7.32; PaO_2 90 mmHg; $PaCO_2$ 56 mmHg; HCO_3 26 mEq/L. The nurse calls the physician with these results because they indicate that the client is in a state of:

(1) Metabolic alkalosis.
(2) Respiratory alkalosis.
(3) Respiratory acidosis.
(4) Metabolic acidosis.

8 The nurse assesses that a client is at risk for developing disseminated intravascular coagulopathy. Which of the following laboratory findings should be reported to the physician immediately?

(1) Hemoglobin 15 g/dL
(2) Partial thromboplastin time (PTT) of 80 seconds
(3) Fibrinogen level 110 mg/dL
(4) Prothrombin time (PT) 11 seconds

9 The nurse is walking past a client's room and hears a visitor calling for help. Upon entering the room, the client is noted to be choking. The first nursing intervention should be to:

(1) Call a code.
(2) Ask him if he can speak.
(3) Give him a back blow.
(4) Begin cardiopulmonary resuscitation (CPR).

10 A client is brought to the triage area unresponsive and in acute respiratory distress with a respiratory rate of 44/min and labored. He is cyanotic, and you note multiple missing and loose teeth along with facial trauma. The most appropriate nursing diagnosis for this client would be:

(1) Decreased cardiac output.
(2) Ineffective tissue perfusion.
(3) Ineffective airway clearance.
(4) Ineffective coping.

See pages 721–722 for Answers and Rationales.

I. Introduction to Emergency Nursing

A. Emergency nursing

1. The practice of *episodic* (as needed), primary, critical, and acute nursing care of clients of all ages who experience physical, emotional, or psychological alterations in health; this care may be given in a variety of practice settings; care ranges from minimal intervention to life support

2. The emergency nurse is a licensed professional who systematically utilizes the components of the nursing process to ensure that optimal care is provided to the client and family experiencing health status alterations based upon established standards of care and collaboration with other healthcare providers

3. Emergency nursing requires a vast knowledge of pathophysiology and diverse disease processes, disease and injury prevention, life-saving measures, cultural characteristics, legal and ethical issues, mental health issues, and age-specific healthcare requirements to meet the individualized health-care needs of the client and their families

B. Care of the client presenting to an Emergency Department

1. **Triage:** the classification of all clients presenting to the emergency department for the purpose of prioritizing treatment

   a. It is utilized to promptly identify those clients requiring immediate, life-saving treatment and those who would receive more efficient and effective care in another area, such as an outpatient clinic, walk-in center, or minor trauma area/fast track area

b. Triage also begins the process of identifying emotional and psychosocial needs of the client and family

c. Triage requires a brief, thorough interview and assessment of the client's reason for presenting to the emergency department, determination of acuity, and initiation of care

d. Triage rating systems frequently include three categories:

    1) **Emergent:** those conditions that require immediate care and intervention because of increased risk of **mortality** (death) or threat to life, limb, or vision; pre-hospital care providers usually transport these clients; however, families or friends may also bring them to the hospital; examples of emergent conditions include major burns, cardiac arrest, chest pain, respiratory distress, major blunt or penetrating trauma, or hemorrhage secondary to ectopic pregnancy

    2) **Urgent:** those conditions that require care as soon as possible and generally within 1 hour because the condition has the potential for causing the deterioration of health state if not treated as soon as possible; these clients will have stable vital signs but have acute illness and must be treated to prevent increased **morbidity** (illness); examples of urgent conditions include fever (including rectal temperature > 101°F in an infant less than 3 months old), abdominal pain, stable fractures, headache, lacerations with controlled bleeding, or dehydration

    3) **Non-urgent:** those conditions that require routine care that can be delayed for greater than 2 hours without the possibility of deterioration; clients presenting with non-urgent conditions frequently utilize the emergency department because they do not have a primary care physician; examples of non-urgent conditions include colds, sore throat, toothache, rashes, or abrasions

2. Disaster management plan: a community-wide, hospital-wide, or emergency department plan to handle mass casualty incidents that may occur at any time

    a. It involves the coordinated planning of how each unit will respond to the prevention of a disaster occurrence, care of victims following the disaster, and recovery of the victims and staff following the incident

    b. It requires planning, mock drills, and refinement of the plan for optimal preparedness

C. Assessment of the client presenting to the Emergency Department

1. Primary assessment: the rapid initial assessment of the client's presenting symptoms to determine the presence of life-threatening conditions while simultaneously intervening

    a. A = Airway with C-spine (cervical spine) immobilization

        1) Assess the client's airway and maintain a patent airway; assessment includes determining the client's ability to speak, checking for foreign body in the airway, and evaluating chest expansion

        2) If the airway appears compromised, observe for possible causes such as: foreign body (tongue, teeth, dentures, food, vomitus), airway or facial trauma, edema of the face, neck, or trachea, or smoke inhalation as appropriate

3) Possible interventions to maintain a patent airway include chin lift/jaw thrust, suctioning, oropharyngeal or nasotracheal intubation, cricothyroidotomy or tracheostomy

NCLEX!

4) During this evaluation and all interventions, the cervical spine must remain in an anatomically neutral position and may be immobilized with cervical collar or manually stabilized to prevent morbidity due to potential spinal cord injury

b. B = Breathing

1) Assess the client's effectiveness of breathing and ventilation ability

2) Normally, the client should exhibit spontaneous, unlabored respirations with full bilateral equal chest expansion and bilateral breath sounds

NCLEX!

3) Abnormal findings on assessment of breathing are: apnea; weak, shallow, or labored respirations; diminished or absent breath sounds; unequal chest expansion; retractions or paroxysmal chest wall movement; tracheal deviation; distended neck veins; open chest wound or signs of chest trauma; and subcutaneous emphysema

NCLEX!

4) Possible interventions for ineffective breathing pattern include application of supplemental oxygen by face mask or bag-valve mask device, assisting with chest tube insertion or intubation, covering of open chest wound with a three-sided occlusive dressing, and use of a pressure dressing on a flail segment of the ribs

c. C = Circulation/controlled hemorrhage

1) Assess the client for the presence of adequate circulation to maintain cellular tissue perfusion

2) Findings of adequate perfusion include: full, regular, and normal pulse rate; pink, warm, and dry skin with capillary refill < 3 seconds; absent external uncontrolled bleeding; and client's ability to respond appropriately

NCLEX!

3) Indications of decreased circulation include: bradycardia or tachycardia; hypotension; cool, pale and diaphoretic skin, obvious uncontrolled external bleeding; or decreased level of consciousness

4) Signs of hypovolemia, pericardial tamponade, or cardiac arrest indicate that an immediate life threatening condition exists

5) Possible interventions to enhance circulation include: direct pressure to control external bleeding; insertion of intravenous (IV) access device; fluid volume replacement with normal saline, blood or blood products; cardiopulmonary resuscitation (CPR), *pericardiocentesis* (aspiration of blood from pericardial sac); or **autotransfusion** (transfusion of one's own blood)

d. D = Disability

1) Complete a brief neurological assessment to determine baseline functioning, potential life-threatening complications, and level of consciousness

2) The **Glasgow Coma Scale** assesses the arousal component of responsiveness; it measures eye opening, best verbal response, and best motor response; minimum score is 3 and maximum score is 15

3) Normal findings include: the client is alert and responding appropriately to questioning; pupils equal and reactive to light; and appropriate motor and sensory functioning are demonstrated

4) A client who is unresponsive, demonstrating an alteration in level of consciousness, loss of sensory/motor function, pupillary response abnormalities, or fixed pupils indicates possible neurological dysfunction; these findings require more extensive assessment during the secondary assessment and the need to assist in the maintenance of a patent airway

e. E = Expose: remove all clothing from the client to facilitate a thorough complete secondary assessment examination

2. **Secondary assessment:** a brief systematic head-to-toe assessment that identifies all injuries; cervical immobilization is maintained at all times during the secondary assessment as well as the continual assessment of hemodynamic and oxygenation status

a. F = Fahrenheit: it is also important to provide measures to prevent body heat loss at this time through the use of warmed IV fluids, warmed blankets, or heating lamps

b. G = Get vital signs: obtain a full set of vital signs (with rectal temperature if possible); and other assessment aids such as cardiac monitor, pulse oximeter, urinary catheter, nasogastric tube; laboratory studies can be drawn, commonly included are complete blood count (CBC), electrolytes, coagulation studies including fibrin degradation products (FDP), amylase, lactate, hepatic and renal studies, arterial blood gas, urinalysis, and a blood type and cross-match; in some cases, toxicology studies may be indicated

c. H = History and head-to-toe assessment: obtain from the client, family, or pre-hospital care provider a thorough history of the mechanism of injury, client presentation at the time of injury, pre-hospital vital signs and treatment, and past medical history, allergies, and medications; then complete a head-to-toe assessment to assess for all injuries

1) Head and face: inspect for bleeding, deformities, ecchymosis, wounds, drainage from ears, eyes, or nose, and eyes for pupil for size, reaction to light, accommodation, and extraocular movement; palpate head and face for bony deformities, tenderness, crepitus, or swelling

2) Neck: carefully remove the anterior portion of the cervical collar while another team member maintains cervical spine stabilization; inspect neck for wounds, bleeding, swelling, or tracheal deviation; palpate neck for pain, tenderness, and crepitus; auscultate carotid arteries for the presence of bruits

3) Chest: inspect for breathing pattern, depth, chest symmetry, ecchymosis, wounds, paradoxical movement, or use of accessory muscles; palpate for tenderness, bony crepitus or deformities, or subcutaneous emphysema; auscultate breath and heart sounds

4) Abdomen and flanks: inspect for wounds, bleeding, distension, ecchymosis, or scars; auscultate bowel sounds and vessels for bruits; palpate in all four quadrants for tenderness, guarding, masses, and pulses

5) Pelvis and perineum: inspect for wounds, deformities, ecchymosis, blood at urinary meatus or perineum, or priapism; palpate pelvis for tenderness, stability, or fractures; assess sphincter tone

6) Extremities: inspect for wounds, bleeding, deformities, and movement; palpate for pulses, temperature, sensation, tenderness, deformities or bony crepitus

7) Posterior surfaces: while maintaining cervical spine stabilization, logroll the client to inspect back for wounds, bleeding, ecchymosis, or deformities; palpate for tenderness or deformities

II. Common Problems Seen in Emergency Settings

A. Airway obstruction

1. Description: the partial or complete obstruction of the airway

2. Etiology and pathophysiology

   a. Facial and neck trauma can cause the presence of foreign bodies such as teeth, tongue, or vomitus to block the airway

   b. Mechanical obstruction can also occur from the loss of structural support or the development of a narrowed airway due to the accumulation of fluid or blood in the airway tissues

   c. Allergic reactions, infection, exposure to chemical irritants, or burns can cause bronchospasm, laryngospasm, and laryngeal edema

   d. Medical and neurological conditions such as stroke, seizures, drug and alcohol intoxication, or mental retardation can predispose the client to the potential for airway obstruction

3. Assessment

   a. Clinical manifestations: depend on the etiology of the obstruction

   1) Airway obstruction can be manifested by the inability of the client to speak, breathe, or cough

   2) Stridor, wheezing, choking, gagging, or drooling indicate a partial obstruction

   3) Late manifestations of airway obstruction include: cyanosis, shortness of breath, altered mental status, bradycardia, hypotension, and cardiopulmonary arrest

   4) Diminished or absent breath sounds or adventitious breath sounds may be present as a result of decreased airflow into the lungs

   b. Diagnostic and laboratory tests

   1) Radiographic studies of the neck may show altered tissue densities or foreign body in the airway

    2) Arterial blood gases will show respiratory acidosis in the later stages of airway obstruction and are rarely used

4. Therapeutic management

    a. Allow conscious clients with partial airway obstruction to attempt to clear their own airway

    b. Clients may require suctioning assistance for removal of foreign bodies such as blood or vomitus as a result of trauma; suctioning with a hard suction catheter should be attempted with care to avoid further obstruction of the airway or stimulation of vomiting

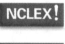

    c. Unconscious clients with partial or complete airway obstruction must receive immediate life-saving measures; perform the chin-lift or jaw-thrust maneuver; if the airway remains obstructed, endotracheal intubation, cricothoratomy, or tracheostomy must be performed

5. Priority nursing diagnoses: Ineffective airway clearance, Ineffective breathing pattern

6. Planning and implementation

    a. The goal of nursing care for the client with ineffective airway clearance would be to maintain airway patency; this can be accomplished by monitoring respiratory pattern, rate, and increasing evidence of further airway obstruction such as stridor, hoarseness, cough, increased edema or swelling

    b. Keep suction equipment available to remove blood, vomitus, or foreign bodies

    c. Maintain cervical spine immobilization until fractures have been ruled out

    d. Provide emotional support and provide alternative communication methods if intubation should be required

    e. Supplemental humidified oxygen will also be used

    f. Collaborate with the continued treatment of the underlying cause of the airway obstruction

7. Medication therapy: antibiotics may be ordered if edema caused by bacterial infection is present; bronchodilators may be given to reduce bronchospasm; if intubation and mechanical ventilation are required, sedation and muscle relaxant agents will be used

8. Client education

    a. Discuss ways to prevent specific cause of the airway obstruction

    b. Explain procedures during course of treatment to the client and family to allay anxiety

9. Evaluation: the client maintains a patent airway with adequate oxygenation and ventilation; oxygen saturation is greater than 90 percent; breathing pattern is regular and unlabored and ABGs and vital signs are appropriate for the client

B. Tension pneumothorax

1. Description: a tension pneumothorax occurs when air enters the pleural space through a tear during inspiration and accumulates because it cannot escape during expiration

NCLEX!

2. Etiology and pathophysiology

   a. Tension pneumothorax can be caused by blunt or penetrating trauma, fractured ribs which penetrate the pleura, barotrauma, injury to the tracheobronchial tree, infection, or can be a result of a ruptured bleb or positive-pressure mechanical ventilation

   b. The increased intrathoracic pressure is caused by a "one-way value effect" that leads to hyperinflation, lung collapse on the injured side, increased mediastinal pressure and shift towards the uninjured side

   c. This mediastinal shift causes compression of the vena cava, decreased cardiac output and a potentially life-threatening condition due to circulatory failure if not corrected

3. Assessment

NCLEX!

   a. Clinical manifestations: labored respirations, dyspnea, tachypnea, hypoxia, decreased or absent breath sounds on the side of injury, tracheal deviation away from the injured side, distended neck veins caused by impedance of blood flow return to the heart, and decreased cardiac output are all signs of a tension pneumothorax

   b. Diagnostic and laboratory findings: a diagnosis is usually made by noting clinical manifestations and mechanism of injury; an upright posterior-anterior (PA) chest film will confirm the diagnosis, but no upright films should be done unless there is no spinal injury

4. Therapeutic management: administer high-flow oxygen and prepare for a needle thoracostomy or chest tube placement; a needle thoracostomy involves the insertion of a large bore (16- or 18-gauge) needle above the third rib in the mid-clavicular line to allow for the release of pressure; a chest tube of appropriate size for client may also be placed using sterile technique and attached to waterseal drainage

5. Priority nursing diagnoses: Ineffective breathing pattern; Decreased cardiac output; and Impaired gas exchange

6. Planning and implementation

   a. The goal of nursing care would be that the client demonstrates a respiratory rate of 12 to 20/min, client's arterial blood gases would be within normal parameters, and that the client remains hemodynamically stable

NCLEX!

   b. To achieve these outcomes, administer supplemental oxygen, assist with chest tube insertion or needle thoracostomy, closely monitor for signs of hypoxia such as restlessness, anxiety and mental status changes, and monitor the patency and functioning of the closed chest-drainage system, especially monitoring for signs of resolution of the air leak

   c. Encourage the client to take deep breaths and to change position every 2 hours to promote full lung expansion and prevent atelectasis

7. Medication therapy: analgesics to promote comfort during chest tube insertion and during deep-breathing exercises

8. Client education

   a. Teach deep-breathing exercises

b. Teach client to report increasing shortness of breath

c. Discuss the purpose of therapeutic interventions

9. Evaluation: the client maintains an effective breathing pattern and adequate gas exchange, remains hemodynamically stable, and has pain that is controlled to a tolerable level

C. Flail chest

1. Description: the force of impact to the chest wall during injury causes the fracture of three or more contiguous ribs in two or more places, resulting in a "floating" segment

2. Etiology and pathophysiology

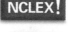

a. The development of a flail chest is usually as a result of blunt trauma to the chest wall as when striking the steering wheel, falls, etc.

b. Because the rib cage is no longer intact, as the intrathoracic pressure increases with normal inspiration, the flail segment is drawn inward and conversely bulges outward with expiration

c. Pain, pulmonary contusion (which frequently coexist) and the increased work of breathing cause the clinical manifestations observed

3. Assessment

a. Clinical manifestations: dyspnea, poor air movement, chest wall pain, ecchymosis, splinting respirations, hypoxia, pain on inspiration, paradoxical chest wall movement, or palpable subcutaneous emphysema

b. Diagnostic and laboratory findings: chest radiography will confirm multiple rib fractures; arterial blood gases may reveal the extent of hypoxemia

4. Therapeutic management: initial stabilization will include supplemental oxygen application, IV access, pulse oximetry monitoring, and arterial blood gases; if severe hypoxia is present, the client may require endotracheal intubation to prevent respiratory failure; adequate pain management is essential; stabilize chest wall with elastoplast

5. Priority nursing diagnosis: Ineffective breathing pattern; Impaired gas exchange; Pain; Impaired tissue integrity

6. Planning and implementation

a. The goal of nursing care is to assure an effective breathing pattern and perfusion with tolerable pain management

b. Because of the increased incidence of concurrent pulmonary tissue damage, assessment for pulmonary contusion and measures to ensure the ABCs (airway, breathing, and circulation) are essential

c. Administer supplemental oxygen as tolerated by the client to maintain oxygen saturation > 90%

d. Maintain IV access and titrate fluids to avoid overhydration, which may exacerbate interstitial pulmonary edema if present from the damage

e. Pain management is essential and should be utilized to avoid splinting, hypoventilation, and atelectasis

f. Splinting, such as positioning the client on the affected side, may assist with pain control as well, but is not necessary for treatment

7. Medication therapy: pain management with opioid analgesics such as morphine sulfate, hydromorphone, fentanyl, or acetaminophen/oxycodone; intercostal nerve blocks, epidural or patient-controlled analgesia (PCA) may also be utilized, particularly for the hospitalized client

8. Client education

   a. Teach client about client controlled analgesia if used

   b. Teach splinting techniques

   c. Discuss treatment approaches utilized

9. Evaluation: client achieves an effective breathing pattern; arterial blood gases are within normal limits, pain management is effective

D. Uncontrolled hemorrhage

1. Description: uncontrolled bleeding

2. Etiology and pathophysiology

   a. Hemorrhage can be the result of blunt or penetrating trauma, gastrointestinal (GI) or genitourinary (GU) bleeding, or hemoptysis

   b. The clinical manifestations of uncontrolled bleeding are due to the lack of adequate circulating blood volume causing decreased tissue perfusion

   c. Decreased tissue perfusion and metabolism results in hypoxia, vasoconstriction, and shunting of the available circulating blood volume to the vital organs (brain and heart)

   d. Sympathetic nervous system (SNS) stimulation, hormonal release of antidiuretic hormone (ADH) and the angiotensin-renin mechanisms, and neural responses attempt to compensate for the loss of circulating volume, but over time these mechanisms fail

   e. Eventually metabolic acidosis, multi-organ system failure occurs, respiratory failure and cardiac arrest occur

3. Assessment

   a. Clinical manifestations: cool, clammy, pale skin and distal extremities, delayed capillary refill (> 3 seconds), weak, rapid pulses, decreased blood pressure (systolic pressure < 90 mmHg), rapid, shallow respirations > 28/min or respiratory rate < 10/minute, restless, anxious, or decreased level of consciousness, cardiac **dysrhythmias** (abnormalities of cardiac rhythm), and decreased urinary output

   b. Diagnostic and laboratory findings

      1) Evidence of bleeding from thorocostomy or a thorocostomy that indicates bleeding from chest area

      2) Abdominal or pelvic CT scan, abdominal ultrasound, or peritoneal lavage indicate intra-abdominal bleeding

      3) Endoscopy indicates upper or lower GI bleeding

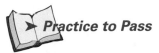

Practice to Pass

A client involved in a motor vehicle accident (MVA) has experienced multiple contiguous fractured ribs. What are the goals for your nursing care?

NCLEX!

4) Angiography procedures diagnose severe vascular damage

5) Extremity radiographs show long bone fractures are suspected

6) Hemoglobin and hematocrit from the CBC are decreased due to blood loss

7) Elevated serum lactate if bleeding continues and client becomes acidotic

8) ABGs show metabolic acidosis as blood loss continues

9) Baseline coagulation studies should be reviewed; initial PT/PTT and platelet counts will be within normal limits but as coagulation factors become depleted, clotting times will increase and platelet counts will decrease

10) Other laboratory tests would include serum electrolytes to assess renal function and intravascular volume states; these values will vary based upon level of fluid loss and length of time of blood depletion

4. Therapeutic management

   a. Perform initial stabilization of uncontrolled bleeding simultaneously with assuring an effective patent airway

   b. Cervical spine immobilization

   c. Use respiratory adjuncts to establishing effective breathing pattern for oxygen delivery to circulating volume

 d. Stop obvious bleeding with direct pressure and find a hidden source of bleeding quickly; if bleeding cannot be stopped immediately, surgical intervention may be necessary

 e. Initiate IV fluid resuscitation with warmed balanced salt solutions such as lactated Ringers or normal saline solution

 f. Initiate blood replacement therapy as needed; blood replacement should be with typed and cross-matched blood if time permits, however, type-specific packed red blood cells (PRBCs) or low titer, type O-negative red blood cells may be utilized until type specific blood becomes available; transfuse platelets and coagulation factors as indicated by laboratory results; one unit of PRBCs are needed for each three liters of crystalloid solution to prevent hemodilution

 g. Monitor cardiac rhythm, vital signs, central venous pressure (CVP) if available, mental status, and urinary output to evaluate the effectiveness of therapeutic interventions

5. Priority nursing diagnoses: Impaired tissue perfusion, Deficient fluid volume, Decreased cardiac output

6. Planning and implementation

   a. The goals of the nursing interventions for uncontrolled bleeding are to assist in the reestablishment of adequate tissue perfusion and to prevent tissue damage

   b. After successfully establishing an adequate airway, breathing pattern, and applying supplemental oxygen, give priority to interventions to control external bleeding, such as direct pressure to the wound site, or assisting with surgical interventions

c. Establish IV access with two large-bore (14-, 16-, or 18-gauge) catheters and begin fluid replacement with crystalloid solutions such as lactated Ringers or normal saline at a rate of 3 mL crystalloid solution for every 1 mL estimated blood loss

d. Draw blood specimens as ordered to assist in the evaluation of hemoglobin, hematocrit, electrolyte, oxygenation, and hydration status

e. Insert an indwelling urinary catheter and nasogastric (NG) tube to assist in accurate recording of fluid balance status

f. Perform and document continuous serial assessments of hemodynamic parameters such as vital signs, capillary refill, CVP, cardiac rhythm, LOC, urinary output and laboratory findings

g. Keep the client warm to prevent hypothermia

7. Medication therapy: crystalloids and blood products to maintain adequate circulating volume status; sodium bicarbonate to correct acidosis state; vasopressor medications such as dopamine if necessary (only after providing appropriate fluid resuscitation)

8. Client education

a. Explain procedures to the client

b. Support the family by explaining emergency measures and interventions

9. Evaluation: there is improved and adequate tissue perfusion, as noted by improved LOC; vital signs return to within normal limits; hemodynamic parameters are within normal limits; urinary output is >30 mL/hr, and capillary refill < 3 sec; bleeding is controlled; client is normothermic; ABGs are within normal limits; client has an adequate breathing pattern and tissue oxygenation

E. Motor vehicle accidents (MVAs): blunt and multiple trauma

1. Description: injuries sustained from MVA, including blunt injuries and multiple trauma

2. Etiology and pathophysiology

a. The high incidence of morbidity and mortality in MVAs is because of blunt trauma

b. Three types of forces commonly occur with blunt MVA trauma

1) Acceleration/deceleration forces occur when there is an increase in velocity of a moving object followed by a decrease in velocity either from the speed of a vehicle, speed of the occupant, or speed of the internal organs

2) Compression forces occur when organs or body parts are pressed against immovable objects; this can result in explosive injury to air-filled organs (such as bowel) or crush injury to solid organs such as liver or spleen

3) Shearing forces occur when there is a rotational force exerted around a fixed site

    c. Type of impact, speed at impact, point of impact, restraint systems utilized, organ systems involved, and the client's preexisting conditions also affect the results of these forces in motor vehicle or multiple trauma incidents

    d. Blunt trauma injuries can involve fractures, lacerations, contusions, rupture or tearing of solid and hollow organs, as well as major blood vessels

3. Assessment

    a. Clinical manifestations: in general, the clinical manifestations seen in an MVA or blunt trauma depend on the organ system impacted

      1) Signs of hypovolemia (tachycardia, mental status change, pale, cool skin, hypotension, etc.), respiratory distress or inadequate breathing pattern may be due to the bruising of lung tissue, pneumothorax, hemothorax, or the loss of the functional structure of the thoracic cage as with flail chest or rib fractures

      2) Blunt trauma to the head, neck or spinal column may result in an altered LOC, loss of sensation or decreased motor ability due to fracture of the spine or damage to the central nervous system; it may also result in impaired respiratory function caused by swelling or loss of integrity of the upper airway

      3) Blunt abdominal trauma may result in signs of hypovolemia from bladder, liver, or spleen rupture as well as damage to the GI tract

      4) Blunt trauma to the extremities may cause fractures, pain, swelling, loss of large quantities of blood into the surrounding cavities, as well as loss of function

    b. Diagnostic and laboratory findings: the effects of blunt trauma are usually more difficult to diagnose because of their frequent lack of external signs of injury

      1) Based on the physical assessment and mechanism of injury, radiological procedures such as x-ray, CT scans, ultrasounds, and MRIs may be utilized to assess the various injuries

      2) Diagnostic peritoneal lavage may be useful in detecting abdominal injury or intra-abdominal bleeding; abdomen can contain red blood cells, white blood cells, bile, feces, or food products if rupture has occurred in the abdominal cavity or GI tract

      3) An electrocardiogram (ECG) will determine myocardial damage

      4) Laboratory tests such as a CBC, electrolytes, urinalysis, serum amylase and lactate, liver enzymes, cardiac enzymes, type and cross/screen, clotting studies, ABGs, and toxicology studies will establish baseline or detect abnormal findings

4. Therapeutic management

    a. Initially assess and stabilize airway, breathing and circulation while assuring immobilization of the cervical spine region; depending upon injury pattern, intubation may be necessary

    b. Provide supplemental oxygen

c. Place the client in modified Trendelenburg position if shock symptoms are present; control any obvious bleeding with direct pressure

d. Insert two large-bore IV lines and infuse lactated ringers or normal saline as ordered; aggressively manage signs or symptoms of shock while diagnostic procedures and preparation takes place

e. Complete NGT and indwelling urinary catheter insertion, radiological procedures, and ECG to determine what injury management will be required

f. Positioning, splinting, ice, and elevation may be useful for closed fractures

g. Preparation for surgery may be needed

5. Priority nursing diagnoses: Ineffective airway clearance; Ineffective breathing pattern; Impaired gas exchange; Fluid volume deficit; Decreased cardiac output; Impaired tissue perfusion; Anxiety; Pain

6. Planning and implementation

a. Care goals are focused on adequate oxygenation, tissue perfusion, comfort, and supportive measures

b. Manage the airway management with the least invasive yet most effective method; nasopharyngeal, oropharyngeal, or endotracheal intubation may be needed to maintain a patent airway, especially in clients who have sustained blunt trauma to the face or neck

c. Immobilize the cervical spine with a cervical collar and keep the collar in place until cervical spine has been cleared by radiography

d. Continuously observe the client's breathing pattern to assure effective oxygenation and gas exchange for tissue perfusion

e. Be prepared to assist with chest tube insertion and then continuously monitor the drainage device for quantity and character of the drainage, if present, and the presence of any air leak

f. Assist with diagnostic procedures as ordered and continually monitor the client's response during procedures

g. Perform serial assessment of vital signs, LOC, characteristics and location of pain, which are essential; initiate pain management as soon as possible

h. Initiate measure to provide psychological support to the client and family as soon as possible; advise the client and family of the plan of care and offer information about tests to be performed

7. Medication therapy: immediate fluid resuscitation with normal saline or ringers lactate if shock is present; stable clients may receive tetanus immunization, antibiotics, analgesics, and vasopressors if necessary to maintain adequate perfusion pressures after hydration has been completed

8. Client education

a. Explain all procedures to the client

b. Provide explanations of resuscitative procedures to families of clients with trauma

9. Evaluation: client demonstrates a patent airway, effective breathing pattern, and is hemodynamically stable; all injuries are identified and appropriate interventions are completed; pain is controlled within a tolerable level and client and family are aware of plan of care and extent of injury as appropriate

F. **Penetrating injuries (stab wounds, gunshot wounds)**

1. Description: penetrating injuries are those caused by an object or missile set in motion that penetrates the body

   a. The extent of the penetration and damage to the body will depend upon the velocity of the missile, the energy created by the missile, the area of the body penetrated, and the characteristics of the missile

   b. Low-velocity missiles such as knives, pencils, forks, etc. generally will create tissue damage only along the path of the weapon because of the low energy force of the weapon

   c. Penetrating injuries from high-velocity, high-energy missiles such as from guns, rifles, or high-pressure injection devices such as paint guns, cause damage to the tissue immediately in the path of the missile but also tissue damage caused by stress and strain to surrounding tissues and the toxins of any chemicals injected

2. Etiology and pathophysiology

   a. Low-velocity missiles or those weapons with low kinetic energy have little energy to be dissipated as it penetrates the body

      1) The damage caused by these weapons can be calculated by many factors, including the weapon used, the structure of the weapon (length, shape, etc), the position of the victim when struck, and the position of the attacker

      2) The gender of the attacker is also appropriate in estimating penetrating injury damage; men usually stab with an upward motion and women usually stab with a downward motion since this is how they generate most of their power

      3) The assessment of possible injuries must take into consideration the possibility of more extensive internal injury than the entrance wound indicates because of victim movement; a low-velocity weapon can be life-threatening if it strikes a highly vascular or vital organ

   b. High-velocity, high-kinetic energy missiles cause a great deal more damage to the tissues directly effected by the missile and also those tissues affected by the cavitation, shock wave, and heat of the missile

      1) The severity of the wound can be predicted by knowing the caliber (diameter), type of missile (potential to fragment or deform, *yaw* [veer from a straight path], or tumble), distance from the victim, and the trajectory into the body

      2) High-pressure injection missile injuries, such as from paint guns, usually appear as a minor puncture wound; however, the major damage is caused by the injection of toxic, foreign substances into the surrounding tissues, which causes infection, pain, swelling, and potential compartment syndrome

NCLEX!

3. Assessment

   a. Clinical manifestations

      1) An open wound is present

      2) Symptoms of shock exist, such as hypotension, tachycardia, dyspnea, pallor, cool and clammy skin, and changes in mental status

   b. Diagnostic and laboratory findings: generally the extent of the wound and damage to surrounding tissues are diagnosed by direct assessment, radiographic studies (determine the presence of blood, air or fluid in body compartments; the location of the missile, and the integrity of organ systems); soft tissue damage is usually diagnosed by ultrasound studies; CBC, electrolytes, cardiac and hepatic enzymes, amylase, and ABG are useful to determine the extent of damage to the various organ systems

4. Therapeutic management

   a. The extent of the organ and tissue damage will determine the therapeutic management of the wound

   b. Initial stabilization of the airway, breathing, and circulation must be established

   c. Penetrating trauma to the lung tissue may require the placement of a chest tube to reinflate a lung

   d. Penetrating trauma to the heart may require surgical exploration and repair; usually leads to traumatic full arrest and open cardiac massage

   e. Penetrating trauma to the bowel or GI tract will require surgical intervention (probable bowel resection or ostomy) to prevent the development of peritonitis caused by leakage of GI contents into the peritoneal cavity

   f. Bladder rupture or tears will also require surgical intervention for repair

   g. The management of penetrating trauma to the head, neck, and face may also require surgical repair or intervention to determine extent of injury

   h. Penetrating trauma of high velocity to soft tissue such as in the leg may be monitored for complications, whereas trauma to the firm tissues such as bone may require surgical intervention or amputation to prevent the development of infection or further neurovascular damage

5. Priority nursing diagnoses: Ineffective airway clearance; Ineffective breathing pattern; Impaired gas exchange; Deficient fluid volume; Decreased cardiac output; Impaired tissue perfusion; Impaired skin integrity; Risk for infection; Anxiety; Pain; Disturbed body image

6. Planning and implementation

   a. Care goals will be focused on adequate oxygenation, tissue perfusion, prevention of further alterations in body systems affected, comfort and supportive measures

   b. Airway management may be necessary if trauma has occurred to the face or neck; the least invasive but effective management device should be utilized; if an effective breathing pattern has been disrupted because of loss of integrity of the lung, diaphragm or because of pain, assisting with intubation and mechanical ventilation may be necessary

c. Non-invasive methods of splinting area and coughing and deep-breathing should be initiated if the chest has been the site of trauma

d. Excessive blood loss, whether overt or covert, will be assessed by initial and serial vital signs; the administration of fluids and blood products as ordered should be performed as quickly as possible to avoid inadequate tissue perfusion

e. The disruption of the skin integrity will present a potential for the development of infection; sterile dressing changes, monitoring of the puncture site for drainage, redness, and signs of healing, and administration of antibiotics as ordered are essential

f. Provide pain management as necessary to encourage mobility as well as for psychological well-being

g. Keep the client and family informed of the plan of care and prognosis as much as possible

NCLEX!

7. Medication therapy: tetanus immunization, antibiotics for infection control, and analgesics for pain

8. Client education: provide explanations of all procedures done; families usually require emotional support and honest discussions about therapeutic interventions and plans

9. Evaluation: client maintains a clear airway, effective breathing pattern, and adequate tissue perfusion; client remains free of signs of infection; pain and anxiety are minimized; client and family are aware of plan of care and prognosis as appropriate

G. Hypothermia

1. Description: a condition where the core body temperature is 36°C (96.8°F) or less

2. Etiology and pathophysiology

a. Exposure to extreme cold causes a decrease in the basal metabolic rate after a period of compensatory mechanism attempts to increase the body temperature

b. As the body utilizes all of its energy stores, decreased circulation and cellular perfusion causes a state of acidosis, which causes further metabolic cellular dysfunction and eventual death

3. Assessment

a. Clinical manifestations

NCLEX!

1) Core body temperature of 36°C (96.8°F) or less

2) In mild hypothermia (33° to 36°C or 91.4 to 96.8°F), the client will appear lethargic, shivering, mildly confused, ataxic, and demonstrate diminished fine motor skills

3) In clients with moderate hypothermia (28° to 32°C or 82.4 to 91.3°F), shivering will cease, level of consciousness will decrease to coma, bradycardia and bradypnea will be present, and pupils will be dilated; cardiac rhythm will show atrial and ventricular dysrhythmias

4) With a core body temperature below 28°C (82.4°F), the client will have severely depressed respiratory, cardiovascular, and neurological function and appear dead; the client's ECG may show asystole, and there will be muscle rigidity; may defibrillate once but then must rewarm to 85°F before second attempt

b. Diagnostic and laboratory findings: core temperature is decreased; ABGs show level of acidosis

4. Therapeutic management

NCLEX!

a. Initially stabilize airway and breathing with administration of supplemental oxygen; mechanical ventilation may be necessary if there is ineffective or no respiratory effort present

b. Observe cardiac monitor continuously for dysrhythmia development

c. Faster rewarming is generally more effective than slow rewarming, particularly in clients with a core body temperature <32°C; active rewarming involves the use of heated humidified oxygen delivered at 40 to 44°C, heated IV solutions delivered at 40 to 42°C, heated gastric lavage if airway has been secured, heated peritoneal lavage at 40 to 45°C, and heated pleural irrigation through inserted chest tube at 40 to 42°C if no cardiac activity is present; cardiopulmonary bypass may also be utilized in clients with severe hypothermia

NCLEX!

d. If CPR and defibrillation attempts were unsuccessful initially, they should be retried after rewarming; monitor ABGs and electrolytes for hyperkalemia caused by cellular damage

5. Priority nursing diagnoses: Hypothermia; Decreased cardiac output; Ineffective airway clearance; Ineffective breathing pattern; Impaired gas exchange; Deficient fluid volume

6. Planning and implementation

a. Assist with establishing an effective airway and breathing

b. Initiate cardiac monitoring and monitor for development of dysrhythmias

NCLEX!

c. Assist with rewarming measures

d. Monitor urine output with indwelling urinary catheter insertion

e. Frequently assess pulmonary status for development of pulmonary edema

f. Monitor ABGs and electrolytes and assist in treatment of acidosis and electrolyte imbalances, which may contribute to cardiac dysrhythmias

g. Keep client and family informed of plan of care and prognosis

7. Medication therapy: Dextrose 50% 50 mL IV to correct hypoglycemia, and amiodarone (Cardarone) 300 mg IV push; repeat 150 mg every 3 to 5 minutes as needed with maximum 2.2 grams IV over 24 hours to correct ventricular dysrhythmias, followed by IV drip at 15 mg/minute

8. Client education: the families of client in severe hypothermia should be given emotional support; explain treatments and interventions; teach prevention techniques related to cold exposure when client is stable

9. Evaluation: body temperature has returned to >36°C; effective airway and breathing pattern is established with ABGs within normal limits; cardiac

output is adequate for perfusion, and dysrhythmias are absent; LOC is improved; urinary output is > 30 mL/h; client and family verbalize understanding of plan of care

H. Frostbite

1. Description: injury caused by exposure to cold environment and conditions

2. Etiology and pathophysiology

   a. Exposure to cold results in loss of body heat and vasoconstriction to preserve core body heat

   b. As the vasoconstriction occurs at the periphery, tissue ischemia occurs

   c. As the tissue freezes, ice crystals form in the extravascular space, causing edema and mechanical damage to the cells

   d. This cellular damage causes clumping of platelets and erythrocytes when thawing is attempted and the potential for progressive ischemic damage occurs

3. Assessment

   a. Clinical manifestations: pain, loss of sensation and paresthesia of affected body parts; area may be edematous, red, blistered, white, hard and cold to the touch, or necrotic depending upon extent of exposure and stage of frostbite; the client may describe the pain as stinging, burning or aching

   b. Diagnostic and laboratory findings: diagnosis is based on clinical findings; in the case of severe frostbite, baseline CBC, electrolytes, BUN, creatinine, and glucose may be drawn to determine organ systems status; a urinalysis may be done to determine the presence of myoglobinuria (seen in muscle damage)

4. Therapeutic management

   a. The client should be removed from the cold environment before thawing is attempted because refreezing after thawing can increase the risk of permanent loss of the affected extremity

   b. Immerse the areas in warm water (100° to 106°F), gently circulating the water around the extremity

   c. The area should not be rubbed but the client may move the affected extremity during the warming process; mechanical friction to area can cause increased tissue damage

   d. Monitor the client's core temperature to prevent hypothermia caused by the return of cold blood into the central circulation

   e. After thawing, gently wrap the extremity and elevate it to prevent edema formation

   f. Blisters may or may not be debrided based upon physician preference

   g. Amputation of affected extremities will not be considered until the extent of permanent tissue damage is determined, which may take several months

5. Priority nursing diagnoses: Impaired peripheral tissue perfusion; Impaired skin integrity; Risk for infection; Pain; Deficient knowledge

6. Planning and implementation

   a. Assist with the thawing process and monitor for signs of further tissue ischemia

   b. Remind the client not to rub the areas but that gentle movement is appropriate

   c. Antibiotics and sterile bulky dressings will be utilized to prevent infection

   d. The newly thawed areas will be very painful and pain should be managed at a tolerable level

   e. Since the client is expected to undergo an extended period of care, the client and family should understand the plan of care and expected outcomes

7. Medication therapy: aloe vera (topical) can be utilized because of its thromboxane-inhibiting effect, which inhibits platelet aggregation; tetanus prophylaxis may be indicated based upon the client's immunization status; both topical and parenteral antibiotics may be ordered to prevent infection; pain should be controlled with parenteral and oral analgesics

8. Client education

   a. Teach client about pain management

   b. Teach client signs and symptoms of infection to observe

   c. Emphasize the importance of adhering to follow-up care

   d. Teach preventive techniques for future cold-related injuries

   e. Discuss the importance of maintaining circulatory integrity by avoiding nicotine

9. Evaluation: function and sensation is restored to the affected area; pain and infection are minimized; client verbalizes understanding of all follow-up care needs

H. Heat exhaustion

1. Description: vasomotor collapse sustained from prolonged exposure to heat

2. Etiology and pathophysiology

   a. Dehydration occurs because of increased sweating through evaporation; this results in the loss of salt and water

   b. The symptoms associated with heat exhaustion are the result of these losses

   c. The condition usually results from exercising vigorously in hot weather

   d. Predisposing factors include advanced age, use of diuretics, and a preexisting fluid disorder such as diarrhea

3. Assessment

   a. Clinical manifestations

      1) Client reports nausea, vomiting, headache, lightheadedness, malaise, or myalgia

      2) Pale, warm, and moist skin

3) Core body temperature ranges from 39 to 41°C (103 to 105°F)

4) The client may have impaired judgment and be slightly confused

b. Diagnostic and laboratory findings

1) Serum electrolytes show a decrease in potassium level

2) Decrease in serum sodium (depletes in 2 hours with excessive perspiration)

3) Increased hematocrit from hemoconcentration

NCLEX!

4. Therapeutic management: rest in cool, shaded area; sponge with tepid water and direct fans toward client; fluid and electrolyte replacement orally and intravenously, if needed

5. Priority nursing diagnoses: Deficient fluid volume; Risk for hyperthermia; Deficient knowledge

6. Planning and implementation

a. Prevention of further fluid and electrolyte loss and increasing body temperature will direct implementation

b. Fluid and electrolyte replacement for rehydration and assisting the client to rest in a cool environment is essential

c. The client may be sponged with tepid water and evaporation allowed to occur

NCLEX!

d. Attempts should be made to prevent shivering, which may raise temperature

7. Medication therapy: fluid and electrolyte solutions

8. Client education

a. Teach prevention of future exposure to heat

NCLEX!

b. Encourage oral fluids containing electrolytes prior to and after engaging in strenuous exercise; can also teach client to mix 1 teaspoon of salt in 1/2 liter of water and drink to maintain sodium level

c. Teach client regarding signs and symptoms of electrolyte abnormalities

d. Teach measures to maintain fluid balance in hot environments

9. Evaluation: body temperature returns to normal; serum electrolytes are within normal limits and adequate hydration status is maintained; client and family verbalize understanding of preventive measures

J. Heat stroke (hyperthermia)

1. Description: an extremely elevated core body temperature caused by a failure of the hypothalamus' perspiration-regulating mechanism; carries 70% mortality rate

2. Etiology and pathophysiology

a. Most serious heat-related emergency; results in death if untreated

b. Common predisposing factors include elderly clients, high humidity and temperature, preexisting illnesses such as diabetes, cardiovascular disease, previous stroke, obesity, medications such as phenothiazines, tricyclic antidepressants, diuretics, and beta-blockers

   c. Street drugs such as alcohol, amphetamines, and phencyclidine can also predispose to development of heat stroke

   d. The person who is exposed to hot environments normally perspires, but as the person progressively loses fluid through evaporation, he or she eventually is unable to produce enough perspiration to normalize the body temperature

   e. When sweating stops the core body temperature increases, resulting in cardiac collapse

   f. If heat stroke is left untreated serious brain injury and nervous system damage results

  3. Assessment

    a. Clinical manifestations

      1) Core body temperature > 42°C (105°F)

      2) Ataxia, stupor, delirium, seizures, coma, tachycardia, tachypnea, hypotension, dysrhythmia, nausea, vomiting, and diarrhea

      3) Dry, hot, flushed skin

    b. Diagnostic and laboratory findings

      1) CBC to rule out contributory factors causing the high temperature, such as infection

      2) Serum electrolytes reveal hypernatremia, hypokalemia, and hypoglycemia

      3) Liver function tests may reveal liver failure; rhabdomyolysis may also be present

      4) Prothrombin time (PT) or partial thromboplastin time (PTT) may indicate clotting abnormalities

      5) Arterial blood gases indicate metabolic acidosis

  4. Therapeutic management: institute aggressive cooling measures, including full body exposure and cooling by evaporation; prevent shivering because it raises body temperature; utilize cardiac monitoring to assess for dysrhythmias; assist with ice water gastric and peritoneal lavage; continually monitor core temperature to prevent over-correction and hypothermia

  5. Priority nursing diagnoses: Hyperthermia; Ineffective thermoregulation

  6. Planning and implementation

    a. Ensure establishment of stable airway

    b. Monitor breathing pattern

    c. Maintain circulatory status with IV access and infusion of normal saline (NS) or D_5 1/2 NS; do not use lactated Ringer's solution because liver is unable to metabolize lactate

    d. Insert urinary catheter to maintain accurate output

e. Initiate cooling measures with iced solutions and cooling by evaporation; cold packs may be placed in areas of large blood volume such as groin, axilla, neck, and head

f. Continually monitor cardiac rhythm for dysrhythmias

g. Prevent shivering, acidosis, and cerebral edema

7. Medication therapy: chlorpromazine (Thorazine) 10 to 25 mg to prevent shivering (do not use aspirin or acetaminophen [Tylenol] because they will have no effect); benzodiazepines to prevent seizures; mannitol (Osmitrol) and methylprednisolone (Solu-Medrol) to decrease cerebral edema

8. Client education

a. Teach client about prevention of this type of injury

b. Inform clients who are at risk (elderly, those receiving phenothiazines) to take extra precautions in avoiding prolonged heat exposure

9. Evaluation: client's body temperature returns to normal; effective airway, breathing pattern, and gas exchange are maintained; cardiac dysrhythmias are recognized and treated; the client and family verbalize understanding of treatment regime and preventive measures

K. Drowning and Near-drowning

1. Description: drowning is death caused by asphyxia and aspiration after submersion in water; near-drowning is risk of death occurring within 24 hours after submersion in water

2. Etiology and pathophysiology

a. **Asphyxiation** (suffocation) can be caused by laryngotracheal spasm from a small amount of water entering the larynx or large amounts of water swallowed and then vomited and aspirated into the lungs, filling with water

b. In most cases, water enters the lungs from aspiration, which cause drowning or near-drowning symptoms

c. Depending upon the type of fluid aspirated, water entering the lungs will cause removal or displacement of surfactant and increased alveolar surface tension, decreasing oxygen perfusion

d. Chlorinated swimming pool water will cause a chemical pneumonitis as well because of chemical destruction of the alveolar membrane

e. Salt water, because of its hypertonic state, will cause pulmonary edema because it will cause a fluid shift from the vascular space into alveoli space

f. A serious chain of events occurs as alveolar ventilation decreases; inflammation, obstruction, and collapse of smaller alveolar and capillary membranes cause pulmonary edema, decreased lung capacity, hypoventilation, oxygen desaturation, and eventually cardiac arrest

g. Although victims of near-drowning events do not expire immediately, the severe hypoxia, alveoli membrane damage, possible aspiration of gastric secretions, and acidosis will produce cardiac, renal, hepatic, metabolic, and neurological dysfunction

3. Assessment

   a. Clinical manifestations: hypoxia, dyspnea, wheezing, crackles, rhonchi, cough with pink, frothy sputum, tachycardia, cyanosis, mental confusion, seizures, cardiac or respiratory arrest

   b. Diagnostic and laboratory findings: arterial blood gas reveals acidosis; CBC reveals hemodilution; serum sodium level may be elevated or decreased depending upon the type of fluid aspirated (in freshwater drowning, serum electrolytes will be reduced; in saltwater drowning, serum sodium and chloride will be elevated); serum osmolality is elevated in saltwater drowning; chest x-ray reveals bilateral infiltrate

4. Therapeutic management

   a. Establish a patent airway and effective breathing pattern

   b. Endotracheal intubation and mechanical ventilation with PEEP may be needed for adequate ventilation in the presence of pulmonary edema and low lung compliance

   c. Use CVP monitoring, pulmonary capillary wedge pressure monitoring, and arterial line monitoring to monitor fluid resuscitation and fluid volume status

   d. Correct hypoxia and correct acidosis with sodium bicarbonate

   e. If near-drowning occurred in cold water, undertake rewarming measures

   f. Initiate CPR and advanced cardiac life support (ACLS) measures until client's body temperature has returned to normal

   g. Developing pulmonary infections as a result of near-drowning incidents must be managed aggressively with appropriate antibiotics

5. Priority nursing diagnoses: Impaired gas exchange; Ineffective airway clearance; Ineffective breathing pattern; Decreased cardiac output; Anxiety

6. Planning and implementation

   a. Adequate ventilation and perfusion measures provide the basis for nursing care interventions; ABCs must be ensured

   b. Frequent suctioning and supplemental oxygen are necessary to enhance ventilatory efforts

   c. Provide IV infusion of lactated ringers for saltwater drowning and normal saline solutions for freshwater drowning to prevent hypervolemia or hypovolemia

   d. Use cardiac monitoring to diagnose and appropriately treat developing dysrhythmias

   e. Insert a urinary catheter to maintain accurate intake and output recording

   f. Assist with correction of acidosis and rewarming if immersion occurred in cold water

   g. Close monitoring of cardiac, respiratory, and neurological status must be performed, recorded, and reported as changes occur

   h. Assist client and family to understand the prognosis and plan of care

7. Medication therapy: epinephrine 1 mg IV push (IVP), lidocaine 1 to 1.5 mg/kg IVP, amiodarone 150 mg IVP, atropine 1 mg IVP per ACLS protocol for cardiac arrest; sodium bicarbonate to correct acidosis; steroids, bronchodilators, and isoproterenol to counter the effects of edema and bronchospasm; antibiotics for respiratory infections because of aspiration

8. Client education

   a. Teach clients and families strategies to prevent drowning; life jackets/vests should be worn when engaging in water activities; learn to swim; never swim alone; keep gates locked in swimming pools to prevent accidental drowning of children; and never swim immediately after a meal

   b. Teach clients the importance of knowing CPR; refer clients to agencies where they could be trained in the life-saving technique

9. Evaluation: client exhibits effective breathing pattern with adequate gas exchange; acidosis is corrected; complications involving the respiratory, cardiac, and neurological systems are avoided; family and client verbalize understanding and agreement with plan of care

L. **Bites (dog, cat, rodent, human, insect/bee, spider, tick, snake)**

1. Description: a break in the continuity of the skin caused by a bite from an animal, insect, or human

2. Etiology and pathophysiology

   a. It is assumed that all bites that break the skin's surface will potentially inoculate the area with bacteria or virus

   b. The presence of bacteria is most common in human, dog, and cat bites

   c. Venom from poisonous spiders and snakes have substances which are capable of causing localized tissue damage because of their enzyme effects, as well as cardiotoxic, neurotoxic, and hematological effects

   d. Inoculation with toxins from bee stings and venomous bites can cause an anaphylactic reaction

3. Assessment

   a. Clinical manifestations

      1) Initial presentation will reveal a break in the skin integrity caused by bite from animal, human, or insect

      2) Pain and tenderness are usually seen with fresh bites

      3) Further underlying damage such as bruising or swelling from crush injury to surrounding tissues, fractures of bone, tendon or nerve damage may also be found, particularly with large animal or human bites

      4) If the wound occurred several hours or days prior to presentation for care, redness, swelling or cellulitis symptoms may be observed

      5) Bites from insects, spiders and snakes may present with a local reaction of itching, swelling, and local inflammation; however, some spider and snakebites will cause a systemic reaction as severe as nausea, vomiting, respiratory difficulty and seizures; that is why it is very important to assess the nature of the bite, time of injury, location of the wound, and

what interventions have been completed prior to presentation for treatment

   b. Diagnostic and laboratory findings: there are no specific laboratory tests; diagnosis is based upon clinical findings; cultures of injury sites may be sent for antibiotic sensitivity testing; baseline electrolyte and CBC may be drawn; in the case of "old" bites, white blood counts will be elevated indicating the presence of infection

4. Therapeutic management

   a. For most human and animal wounds, the most important factor in the treatment of bite wounds is meticulous wound care

   b. The wound should be thoroughly cleansed and irrigated with copious amounts of solution

   c. Devitalized tissue should be debrided and a topical antibiotic ointment applied

   d. The wound should be left open and a bulky dressing applied

   e. For most human bites and severe, high-risk animal bites, IV antibiotics will be ordered

   f. Rabies prophylaxis is based upon the type of animal bite and the likelihood of the animal carrying rabies

   g. All carnivores have the potential for carrying rabies, so bites from bats, raccoons, and most wild animals should be considered contaminated unless proven otherwise

   h. Herbivores, such as mice and other rodents, usually do not carry rabies; in most communities, the local public health department should be contacted for regional information

   i. Venomous bites such as those from black widow spiders and poisonous snakes will require antivenom treatment as well as methods such as a constricting band or ice to slow the circulation and spread of the venom throughout the circulatory system

   j. Allergic reactions and systemic allergic reactions will be treated with epinephrine and diphenhydramine (Benadryl) quickly to avoid system-wide vascular collapse and histamine response

5. Priority nursing diagnoses: Impaired skin integrity; Risk for infection; Knowledge deficit; Risk for ineffective breathing pattern; Risk for decreased cardiac output

6. Planning and implementation

   a. Priority nursing care for the client with a bite injury is to prevent further tissue damage

   b. Generally, the wound should be thoroughly cleansed, left open, and an antibiotic topical ointment applied

   c. A dry and sterile dressing may be applied and the area monitored for signs of infection or wound healing

   d. Rabies prophylaxis should be given, if appropriate, based upon information obtained from the local public health department

     e. Antibiotics, either intravenous or oral, should be administered as ordered

     f. Spider bites, such as from a black widow spider require symptomatic care

     g. Ice should be applied to the bite area to decrease absorption while antivenom therapy is being administered

     h. The client should be observed for signs of neurotoxicity and muscle relaxants should be administered as ordered

     i. An effective airway and breathing pattern must be maintained at all times and interventions completed to assure the prevention of hypoxia

     j. Bites from poisonous snakes should also be treated aggressively and closely monitored for signs of systemic reaction such as syncope, paralysis, paresthesia or seizures

     k. Because snake venom can also affect the clotting factors, the nurse should monitor for signs of hemorrhage such as excessive bleeding or hematuria

     l. Nursing interventions will include the prevention of further systemic spread of the venom through the use of a constricting band to the extremity and ice while antivenom therapy is initiated

     m. Continuous monitoring of vital signs, cardiac rhythm and neurological status should be performed

7. Medication therapy: the most common intervention for all bites is tetanus prophylaxis based upon immunization history; topical, oral and IV antibiotics should be considered based upon the type of bite and clinical signs; rabies prophylaxis may be indicated as well; species-specific anti-venom will be utilized for poisonous snake and spider bites and will frequently need to be obtained from a local public health department source

8. Client education

     a. Methods to avoid reinjury if appropriate

     b. Need to notify animal control for animal bite and impound animal for 10 days to evaluate for rabies; notify police for human bites if occurred during an altercation

9. Evaluation: in all bite cases, further tissue damage is absent; there is reduced infection potential, and client understands the plan of care; client is aware of the need for strict follow-up if rabies and tetanus prophylaxis are started; clients exposed to venomous bites maintain effective cardiorespiratory function and remain neurologically intact

M. Poisonings

1. Description: substances that are harmful to humans that are inhaled, ingested (food, drug overdose) or acquired by contact (insecticides)

2. Etiology and pathophysiology

     a. Carbon monoxide inhalation signs and symptoms are caused by cellular toxicity and tissue hypoxia that result from the formation of carboxyhemoglobin, which replaces oxygen on the hemoglobin molecule; as a result, oxygen is not released to the tissues and cellular destruction occurs; the organ systems most critically affected are those that require the most oxygen (cardiovascular and CNS); because of tissue hypoxia, lactic acid also builds up causing a metabolic acidosis

   b. Food poisoning is most often caused by *Staphylococcus aureus, Salmonella, Escherichia coli, Clostridium perfringens,* or *Bacillus ceruns;* these bacteria release a toxin into the body; the symptoms are generally self-limiting and non-life-threatening except in the debilitated client

   c. Drug overdose: the etiology and pathophysiology of a drug overdose depends upon the type and amount of medication/drug ingested and the speed of medical intervention; pathophysiological changes are usually caused by the toxic effect of the medication; some examples include the following:

      1) Salicylate overdose symptoms result from overstimulation of the respiratory center and metabolic acidosis, which cause hyperventilation, hyperthermia, and hyperglycemia

      2) Narcotic/opiate overdoses generally cause a depression of the CNS, hypotension, nausea/vomiting, and respiratory depression

      3) Excessive acetaminophen will cause hepatic damage because of the increased amounts of toxic metabolites that are hepatotoxic

   d. Insecticide surface absorption: both organophosphates and carbamates are cholinesterase inhibitors and allow acetylcholine to accumulate and can cause a cholinergic crisis

3. Assessment

   a. Clinical manifestations

      1) Carbon monoxide inhalation: mild exposure—nausea, vomiting, mild throbbing headache, flu-like symptoms; moderate exposure—dyspnea, dizziness, confusion, increased severity of mild symptoms; severe/prolonged exposure—seizures, coma, respiratory arrest, hypotension and dysrhythmias

      2) Food poisonings: nausea, vomiting, diarrhea, abdominal cramps, fever, chills, dehydration, headache

      3) Drug overdose: depends upon the substance ingested; symptoms may include nausea, vomiting, CNS depression or agitation, altered pupil response, respiratory changes such as tachypnea or bradypnea, alterations in temperature control, seizures, or cardiac arrest

      4) Surface absorption of insecticides (organophosphates or carbamates): nausea, vomiting, diarrhea, headache, dizziness, weakness or tremors, mild to severe respiratory distress, slurred speech, seizures, and cardiopulmonary arrest

   b. Diagnosis and laboratory findings: the diagnosis of many poisonings is based on a thorough client history and clinical manifestations; laboratory toxicology screens (serum and urine) determine the extent of the absorption; baseline blood work such as CBC, electrolytes, renal and hepatic studies enable future determination of organ and tissue damage

4. Therapeutic management

   a. Generally, airway, breathing, and circulation interventions should take priority

b. Initiate IV access and infused ordered fluids

NCLEX!

c. Give antagonists such as naloxone (Narcan) for respiratory depression caused by narcotic overdose and flumazanil (Romazicon) for benzodiazepine ingestions; dose for Narcan is 0.4 mg in 10 mL normal saline and give 0.5 mL every 2 minutes as needed; dose for flumazanil is 0.2 mg IV, repeating with 0.3 mg IV every 30 seconds as needed to maximum dose of 3 mg

d. Treatment of any life-threatening dysrhythmias, seizures or shock should be initiated

NCLEX!

e. To decrease the amount of drug ingested from further absorption and to hasten elimination, vomiting may be induced, or charcoal and a cathartic can be administered either orally or by NG tube

f. Gastric lavage (irrigation of stomach using large volumes of solution) is controversial in many cases

NCLEX!

g. Vomiting is contraindicated in cases of decreased levels of consciousness, absence of gag reflex, and ingestions of corrosive materials

h. Antidotes if available should be administered such as physostigmine for anticholinergic medications such as antidepressants, tricyclics, or antihistamines or atropine for cholinergic crisis due to insecticide absorption

NCLEX!

5. Priority nursing diagnoses: Risk for ineffective airway clearance; Risk for decreased cardiac output; Deficient fluid volume; Ineffective breathing pattern; Impaired tissue perfusion; Risk for injury; Anxiety; Risk for self-directed violence; Hopelessness

6. Planning and implementation

a. Nursing interventions should be directed to decreasing further damage to organ systems, assisting with the treatment of life-threatening conditions, and client and family education

b. Assist with the management of an effective airway, breathing pattern, and circulatory status

NCLEX!

c. Give treatment of life-threatening dysrhythmias and conditions as ordered; continual monitoring of vital signs, cardiac rhythm, and neurological status and supportive care is essential

d. Assist in the hastening in the elimination of the medication or poison, decrease the amount of absorption, and administer antidotes as ordered

e. Assist the client and family in seeking the appropriate referrals and provide client education to prevent further complications or incidence of overdose

f. It is particularly important to ensure that the client and family understand discharge instruction for follow-up care or reason for admission

NCLEX!

7. Medication therapy: antidotes will vary with medication ingested; generally, syrup of ipecac 30 mL PO followed by 240 mL water is used for adults; activated charcoal powder slurry 30 to 100 g PO or per NG tube; and magnesium citrate will be used for GI evacuation; other medications needed for supportive care may be utilized

8. Client education: varies depending on nature of the poisoning

9. Evaluation: client maintains effective oxygen and perfusion status as seen in regular respiratory rate and normal ABGs; has incurred no further organ system damage or injury; absorption has been minimized and toxic by-products have been reduced; client and family verbalize understanding of preventive measures for further occurrences and need for follow-up care or admission

N. Electrocution

1. Description: injury sustained by electric current

2. Etiology and pathophysiology

   a. Electrical energy converts to heat energy as it passes through the body

   b. This heat energy, which increases with the amperage of the current, causes extensive underlying tissue damage

   c. Entrance and exit wounds may be small; however, the current can cross blood vessels, nerves, and muscles as it passes through the body

   d. Damage to the myocardium occurs as a result of heat transfer as well as damage to the electrical conduction system of the heart causing ventricular fibrillation

   e. Smaller body parts (such as fingers, hands, toes, and feet), because of their smaller surface area and ability to dissipate heat, will suffer extensive damage if in the path of the current

3. Assessment

   a. Clinical manifestations

      1) Are related to the strength of electrical current encountered, type of current, path of the current through the body, and duration of contact

      2) Cardiac dysrhythmias may include sinus tachycardia, artrial tachycardias, premature ventricular contractions, ventricular fibrillation, or asystole

      3) Respiratory arrest may occur as a result of inhibition of respiratory center, tetany of chest muscles or diaphragm, or paralysis of respiratory muscles

      4) Neurological symptoms may include altered level of consciousness, amnesia, seizures, coma, and paresthesia

      5) Musculoskeletal injuries may include fractures, compartment syndrome, corneal burns, and thermal burns

   b. Diagnostic and laboratory findings: ECG may demonstrate cardiac conduction alterations; cardiac isoenzyme of creatinine phosphokinase (CK-MB) will be elevated with myocardial tissue damage; hyperkalcmia will indicate cellular damage; metabolic acidosis will be seen in clients with extensive tissue and organ system damage; the presence of myoglobin in the urine will indicate significant muscle damage

4. Therapeutic management

   a. Stabilize and ensure an adequate airway, breathing pattern, and effective circulation

b. Initiate spinal immobilization due to the possibility of a fall

c. Fluid resuscitation measures to maintain a urine output of 1 mL/kg/hr will be required because of the third-spacing of fluids to the injured muscles; an adequate urinary output will also decrease the complications of renal failure due to myoglobinuria

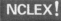

d. Immobilize fractures of extremities to prevent further tissue damage until definitive care can be provided

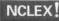

e. Local wound care to external thermal burns will require cleansing, possible debridement, and dressing to prevent infection

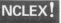

f. Tetanus prophylaxis should be initiated based upon the client's immunization history

5. Priority nursing diagnoses: Impaired tissue integrity; Decreased cardiac output; Pain; Risk for infection

6. Planning and implementation

a. Assist with the stabilization of the airway, breathing and circulation measures

b. Initiate continuous cardiac monitor and administer antiarrhythmic medications as ordered

c. Continuously monitor vital signs, breath sounds for development of pulmonary edema, neurovascular status of extremities, and urinary output

d. Elevate affected limbs to decrease edema and monitor for signs of compartment syndrome, which may develop due to potential extensive internal muscle and tissue damage

e. Provide support to family and client; answer questions appropriate and advise of plan of care and procedures being completed

7. Medication therapy: bicarbonate is added to IV solutions to maintain a urinary pH >7.45 to increase myoglobin solubility in the urine; mannitol is given to increase urinary output; tetanus prophylaxis 0.5 mL IM should be administered based upon immunization status of client; antiarrhythmic medications such as lidocaine, amiodarone, and epinephrine may be needed in cases of cardiac arrest

8. Client education: focused on prevention of future injury

9. Evaluation: client is hemodynamically stable with dysrhythmias appropriately treated; risk of infection is minimized with administration of topical and IV antibiotics as needed; further tissue damage is minimized; client and family verbalize understanding of plan of care

III. Common Problems Seen in the Critical Care Setting

A. Critical care nursing

1. Description

a. The critical care nurse is a licensed professional who provides care to meet the client's individualized needs in response to potentially life-threatening conditions

NCLEX!

    b. Care is provided in an environment supportive of highly technological, collaborative, and holistic care

    c. The critical care nurse serves as a client advocate, provider of comprehensive care, and coordinator of interdisciplinary care aimed at the achievement of the optimum outcome to life-threatening conditions

B. Problems encountered by the client in a critical care setting

    1. Anxiety

        a. In the critical care setting, anxiety is related to the fear of death and the unknown in both the client and the family

NCLEX!

        b. Clients are experiencing a change in health status that is frequently an unexpected and unfamiliar stressor; their usual coping mechanisms are often ineffective initially

        c. Anxiety is also present because of the unfamiliar surroundings, care providers, and the technology to which they are exposed

        d. Overt and covert symptoms that the client may exhibit can include: verbalization of feelings of fear and excessive concern for their family, restlessness, irritability, preoccupation with the surroundings and the asking of many questions, rapid speech, physiologic symptoms of increased heart rate, hyperventilation, nausea, vomiting, and palpitations

NCLEX!

        e. To alleviate anxiety, encourage the client to discuss concerns about the current situation and perceived outcomes

        f. An introduction of all interdisciplinary care providers involved in the client's care and a thorough discussion of the plan of care with the client and family is important to alleviate anxiety in both the family and client

        g. Allow the family to participation in the care as appropriate, encourage the use of touch, relaxation, and imagery therapies and manage physiologic symptoms as ordered

    2. Impaired communication

        a. Many clients in the critical setting will experience communication difficulties because of physical barriers such as endotracheal intubation, new tracheostomy, or as a sequellae of trauma

        b. Cultural and language differences may also make communication difficult and anxiety producing

        c. Preexisting conditions such as inability to read or write or new sensory, motor, and neurological conditions such as hearing or visual impairment or new onset stroke, may also make it very difficult for the client and family to express their needs and concerns

NCLEX!

        d. The nurse must first acknowledge the client's communication concern

        e. Use reassurance and attempt to alleviate communication difficulties with such measures as translators, word cards, paper and pencil, picture cards, or facial or hand gestures

        f. Family feedback may also be an excellent source of information about usual communication methods utilized by the client

    g. The client and nurse should collaboratively determine method to be utilized

    h. Communication between healthcare providers coordinating methods of communication utilized is also essential to successful care of the client

3. Sleep deprivation

    a. The client in the critical care setting will experience periods of sleep deprivation due to the alteration in usual sleeping pattern, lack of consistent periods of rapid eye movement (REM) and non-REM (NREM) sleep, care interventions and treatments, anxiety, and some medications

    NCLEX!

    b. Clinical signs of sleep deprivation may be restlessness, increased irritability or sensitivity to pain, confusion, hallucinations, decreased ability to concentrate or apparent excessive sleepiness

    c. All healthcare providers must be aware of the potential and presence of this condition and reasonable attempts should be made to decrease the causative factors

    d. The nurse should attempt to determine the client's usual sleeping patterns such as body position, favorite bedtime routine, and sleeping pattern

    NCLEX!

    e. If possible, nursing interventions, treatments, assessments, and family visits should be scheduled to allow for several 90-minute periods of rest in a 24-hour period

    NCLEX!

    f. Although the critical care environment is inherently a source of noise and activity, attempts should be made to decrease stimulation by dimming the lights, decreasing alarm limits within a safe range, providing soft music, providing ear plugs or eye covers

    g. Staff should be discouraged from loud talking or activity in the immediate vicinity of the client's bed

    h. Provide pain relief as needed; non-pharmaceutical methods such as relaxation exercises, guided imagery and audiotapes may also be helpful to enhance rest

4. ICU psychosis

    NCLEX!

    a. An acute confusional state, called ICU psychosis, may develop in the critical care environment as a result of many factors

    b. Medications commonly utilized such as narcotics, anticholinergics, CNS stimulants and depressants, and steroids may cause a state of confusion

    c. Sleep deprivation, sensory overload, fluid and electrolyte imbalances, inadequate oxygenation, infection, head trauma, and underlying preexisting conditions such as confusion or chronic brain disorders also contribute to this condition

    NCLEX!

    d. Symptoms of loss of orientation, ability to reason, concentrate, or follow directions develop abruptly

    e. The client may attempt to remove all monitoring lines, catheters, and dressing in a state of confusion

    f. Visual and auditory hallucinations may be observed

    g. Nursing management of this condition involves a multidiscipline approach

h. Collaboration with other healthcare providers to communicate with the client is essential

i. Treatment for physiological conditions should be aggressively pursued

NCLEX!

j. Frequent orientation to person, place, and time, reality orientation, reason for presence in the ICU, rationale and process of treatment is necessary from all persons who interact with the client

k. Frequent explanations of noises and activities within the ICU environment are important

l. Measures to prevent or minimize sleep deprivation should be assured

m. Provide medications as ordered and monitor for and report any undesirable effects

C. Common nursing procedures in the critical care setting

1. Hemodynamic monitoring

   a. Concepts important in hemodynamic monitoring

   1) *Cardiac output* (CO) is the volume of blood that is ejected from the heart in 1 minute; it is determined by the heart rate times the stroke volume (milliliters of blood expelled per heartbeat); the normal CO is 4 to 8 liters/minute

   2) *Preload* is the amount of stretch in the left ventricle just before ventricular contraction at the end of diastole; it is also the result of the volume of blood in the left ventricle, which is influenced by the venous return or amount of blood returned to the ventricles; it is measured by the CVP on the right side of the heart and the pulmonary artery wedge pressure (PAWP) on the left side of the heart

   3) *Afterload* is the tension the ventricles must overcome to eject the blood into the arterial systems (pulmonary and aortic); it is measured by the systemic vascular resistance (SVR) on the left side of the heart and the pulmonary vascular resistance (PVR) on the right side of the heart

   NCLEX!

   4) **Cardiac index** is the CO divided by the body surface area; it is a better indicator of the body's ability to perfuse the tissues effectively than CO; the normal cardiac index is 2.5 to 4.0 liters/minute/meters^2

   b. Types of hemodynamic monitoring

   1) Arterial lines

      a) Purpose: to provide a direct, intra-arterial measurement of blood pressure; it assists in the continuous measurement of the client's systolic, diastolic, and mean arterial pressure

      b) Methods/equipment: a 20-gauge arterial catheter is inserted into the radial, brachial or femoral artery and connected to high-pressure tubing leading to a pressure transducer and amplifier; the transducer converts the mechanical physiologic waves to electrical energy, which are displayed on a monitor screen as pressure waves and digitally read in mm/Hg; the patency of the arterial catheter is maintained by a flush infusion of heparinized saline (contained within a pressure bag at 300 mm Hg connected to IV tubing and a three-way

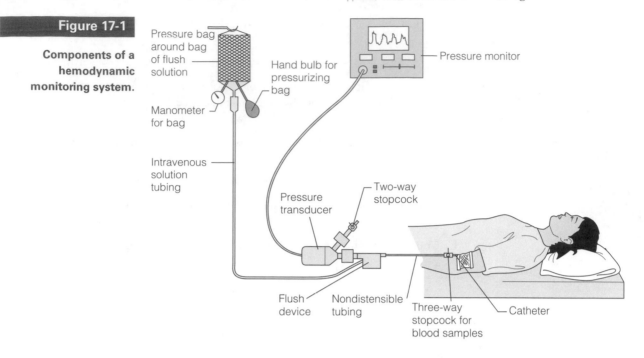

Figure 17-1

Components of a hemodynamic monitoring system.

Pressure bag around bag of flush solution

Hand bulb for pressurizing bag

Pressure monitor

Manometer for bag

Intravenous solution tubing

Pressure transducer

Two-way stopcock

Flush device

Nondistensible tubing

Three-way stopcock for blood samples

Catheter

stopcock); the site is covered and maintained with a sterile dressing (see Figure 17-1)

c) Indications for use: clients requiring accurate perfusion pressures, such as those with low cardiac output, excessive vasocontriction, unstable conditions requiring vasopressor or vasodilator medication titration, or clients requiring frequent ABG analysis

NCLEX!

d) Nursing management: level and calibrate or "zero" the system (normalize the system to a built-in constant) at the beginning of each shift to accurate trending of readings; using a level, align the transducer with the client's right atrium; ensure no air is in the transducer tubing to prevent distortion, dampened waveforms, and inaccurate readings; compare arterial pressure readings and indirect sphygmomanometer pressures each shift for correlation; observe the waveform at eye-level and assess for a sharp normal waveform frequently throughout the shift; draw arterial blood samples through the three-way stopcock after aspirating approximately 5 mL of blood and discarding specimen to prevent contamination of heparinized solution; flush arterial line with valve flush device after blood collection is completed to allow return of a sharp arterial waveform; change sterile dressings and IV solution and tubing as needed or per hospital policy; usually tubing and IV solution are changed every 48 to 72 hours with dressing changes every 24 to 48 hours

Practice to Pass

Your client is to have an arterial line placed prior to surgery. What is the preferred site for placement?

e) Removal of the arterial catheter should take place per physician order; utilizing sterile technique, remove the catheter from the artery with one smooth motion while direct pressure is applied to the site with a dry sterile dressing for at least 5 minutes; then observe the site for oozing or swelling at the site and pressure continued as needed; after oozing has been controlled, apply a new dry sterile dressing and check the site frequently for rebleeding; check distal pulses and motor and sensory function frequently for complications caused by thrombosis

f) Possible complications: bleeding from insertion site, hemorrhage, infection at insertion site or systemic, air embolus, thrombus formation; occlusion of circulation with loss of circulation distal to insertion site may occur; performance *Allen test* prior to radial artery insertion and frequently monitor distal pulses to decrease adverse effects

g) Priority nursing diagnoses: Risk for impaired tissue perfusion; Risk for infection; Risk for decreased cardiac output

2) Swan-Ganz (pulmonary artery balloon flow) catheter

a) Purpose: to provide indirect measurement of left ventricular function for detection and treatment of cardiac and pulmonary changes

b) Methods/equipment: a five-lumen, balloon-tipped, flow-directed catheter connected to a pressure transducer and pressurized heparin flush system is inserted through a percutaneous or cutdown venous site and directed into the right atrium; the subclavian vein is usually utilized; however, peripheral veins may be used; arterial inflation of the balloon tip allows for normal circulatory blood flow to carry the catheter tip through the tricuspid valve, the right atrium, pulmonary valve and into the pulmonary artery; once in the pulmonary artery, the balloon is deflated and pulmonary artery systolic, diastolic and mean pressures are recorded; the balloon is again inflated fully with approximately 1.5 mL of air and the pulmonary artery wedge pressure reading is recorded; the balloon is completely deflated and locked to prevent accidental wedging and pulmonary infarction; cardiac monitoring is performed throughout this procedure because of the potential for PVCs to develop as a result of myocardial irritation during insertion; the catheter is sutured in place and a dry sterile occlusive dressing is applied; a chest x-ray is completed to check placement and absence of pneumothorax

c) Indications for use: when there is a need to monitor pulmonary artery pressure and/or pulmonary capillary wedge pressure (PCWP) that indirectly reflects left ventricular function; provide information about cardiac output, tissue perfusion, and blood volume; obtain venous blood specimens; and the proximal ports can be used for continuous fluid or medication infusion

d) Nursing management: level and secure the transducer at the **phlebostatic axis** (the point at the fourth intercostal space, mid-axillary line that serves as the reference point for the right atrium); to ensure accurate readings ensure that the system is free of air bubbles that will dampen the waveform and digital measurement; zero and calibrate the system at least once a shift; maintain sterility with dressing and line changes; notify physician if waveforms or evidence of a permanent wedge form develops; because the line is present in the client's heart, he or she is at risk for microshock and the development of ventricular fibrillation

e) Taking readings: record the pulmonary artery systolic and diastolic pressures (usually about 25/10 mmHg); to obtain a PCWP or left ventricular end-diastolic (LVEDP) reading, inflate the catheter balloon slowly and watch for waveform changes (dampening) that indicate wedging (normal ranges from 5 to 12 mmHg); after reading has been recorded, allow the balloon to fully deflate passively and lock it to prevent accidental wedging; take all readings at the end of expiration

f) Potential complications: dysrhythmias, infection, air embolism, pneumothorax, catheter occlusion or thrombus formation

g) Priority nursing diagnoses: Risk for impaired tissue perfusion; Risk for infection; Decreased cardiac output; Risk for impaired gas exchange; Deficient knowledge

2. Circulatory assist device (intra-aortic balloon pump, or IABP)

   a. Purpose: a counterpulsation device that assists to augment cardiac output and to provide adequate tissue perfusion, while allowing the myocardium to rest and recover

   b. Methods/equipment: the IABP is a mechanical circulatory support device that consists of a 30 to 40 mL balloon catheter and a console that is set to mechanically inflate and deflate the balloon; the balloon is placed into the descending aorta distal to the subclavian artery through the femoral artery and sutured in place; the console is set to trigger balloon inflation during diastole and deflation during systole to decrease the afterload and workload of the heart; initially, it is set to trigger with every client heartbeat (1:1) and, as the strength of the myocardium improves, it can be decreased to a 1:2, 1:4, or 1:8 interval; the inflation and deflation sequence is triggered by the client's ECG pattern that is displayed on the console

   c. Indications for use: cardiogenic shock, heart failure, support before heart transplantation, unstable angina and/or failure to wean from cardiopulmonary bypass after coronary artery bypass surgery

   d. Nursing management

     1) Assist with placement as needed and maintain sterility with dressing changes

     2) Monitor and record effectiveness as indicated by increased cardiac output, increased blood pressure, increased urinary output, increased level of consciousness, palpable peripheral pulses, improved ischemic EKG changes

     3) Monitor and record ECG rhythm, vital signs, heart and lung sounds, and IABP settings

     4) Monitor circulation, sensation, and motor function in leg of insertion; keep the affected leg straight at all times

     5) Keep head of bed elevated at least 30 degrees to prevent migration of the balloon

     6) Because the client will be receiving anticoagulants, monitor for signs of hematuria, excessive oozing from insertion or hemodynamic catheter sites, positive stool guiac, or abnormal PT, PTT, or platelet counts

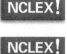

e. Potential complications: air or foreign body embolus if balloon should rupture; thrombus formation at insertion site and loss of distal circulation; migration of catheter; dissection of the aorta; sepsis; complications of immobility

f. Priority nursing diagnoses: Risk for impaired tissue perfusion; Risk for infection; Risk for decreased cardiac output; Impaired skin integrity; Deficient knowledge

3. Airway maintenance adjuncts

a. Endotracheal tube (ET)

1) Purpose: to assist in the maintenance of a patent airway when the client is unable to maintain an airway or who requires mechanical ventilation

2) Methods/equipment: a laryngoscope and blade are utilized to visualize vocal cords and trachea for insertion of endotracheal tube; after insertion, the cuff of the tube is inflated to ensure minimal occlusion and the presence of bilateral breath sounds is checked; the position of the tube is marked at the client's mouth and secured with twill or adhesive tape to prevent tube displacement; supplemental oxygen delivered by t-piece or ventilator is attached; tube placement is confirmed with a chest x-ray

3) Indications: clients who are unable to maintain an effective airway for oxygenation; clients who have experienced facial or neck trauma where swelling may cause potential airway obstruction; clients with altered level of consciousness; or absence of gag or swallowing reflex

4) Nursing management

a) Gather equipment

b) Check oxygen saturation, color, dysrhythmias, and hypoventilation prior to initiating 30-second attempt to place ET tube

c) Assist with intubation by providing cricoid pressure during insertion of ET tube

d) Evaluate lung sounds prior to inflating cuff to determine tube placement above carina (not in right mainstem bronchus)

e) Monitor for cuff pressure, that tube placement remains as initially marked, and continued presence of bilateral breath sounds

f) Provide oral and tracheal suctioning, good mouth care, and observe for development of pressure areas or ulceration around mouth

g) Provide alternative communication means and emotional support for client

5) Potential complications: migration of tube causing airway obstruction; laryngeal damage due to prolonged intubation; accidental extubation; aspiration from inadequate cuff inflation

6) Priority nursing diagnoses: Risk for impaired tissue perfusion; Risk for infection; Risk for impaired gas exchange; Risk for injury; Anxiety; Deficient knowledge; Impaired verbal communication

b. Tracheostomy

   1) Purpose: to assist in the maintenance of an effective airway in clients who are unable maintain their airway or for clients who will require prolonged mechanical ventilation

   2) Method/equipment: placement of a tracheostomy requires surgical intervention to create a stoma into the trachea; a sterile tracheal tube with obturator is inserted into the incisional area and the obturator is removed to allow for air passage; the client is hyperoxygenated and suctioned using sterile technique; the tracheostomy tube area is then cleansed and secured with twill tape

   3) Indications: upper-airway trauma or obstruction; facial or neck trauma with the potential for airway obstruction; head or neck surgery that may impair the maintenance of an effective airway; or need for long-term mechanical ventilation

   4) Nursing management

      a) Explain procedure and rationale to the client and assist as needed with placement

      b) Following placement, keep the area clean with frequent dressing changes and suctioning to prevent infection

      c) Maintain appropriate tracheal cuff inflation to prevent aspiration and prevent tracheal pressure necrosis

      d) Monitor respiratory status and monitor for signs of hemorrhage with new tracheostomy

      e) Perform routine cleansing of inner cannula and ostomy site as needed

   5) Potential complications: accidental extubation; airway obstruction from dried secretions; hemorrhage from tracheostomy site; excessive secretions requiring frequent suctioning; tracheal necrosis due to elevated cuff pressure

   6) Priority nursing diagnoses: Ineffective airway clearance; Impaired tissue perfusion; Risk for infection; Deficient knowledge; Anxiety

c. Mechanical ventilation

   1) Purpose: to assist with breathing to provide for adequate gas exchange for tissue perfusion

   2) Method/equipment: mechanical ventilation requires a ventilator to be connected to an artificial airway, either endotracheal tube or tracheostomy

   3) Types of ventilators

      a) Positive-pressure volume-cycled, which exerts a positive pressure on the airway delivering a predetemined volume of gas; this type allows for pressure and time limits to be set and is the most common ventilator used

b) Positive-pressure time-cycled ventilator, which exerts a positive pressure on the airway, delivering a set volume of gas over a preset time

c) Positive-pressure pressure-cycled ventilator, which exerts positive pressure on the airway within pressure limits set to stop inspiration of that pressure is exceeded

d) Positive-pressure jet ventilators, which exert a positive pressure on the airway and deliver small volumes of gas at a very high rate

e) Negative-pressure ventilators, which exert a negative pressure on the external chest and do not require intubation; an iron lung used for polio clients is an example of this type of ventilator

4) Modes of ventilation

a) Intermittent mandatory ventilation (IMV): delivers a preset tidal volume at a preset rate despite client breathing spontaneously at his/her own rate and tidal volume

b) Assist control ventilation (ACV): delivers a preset volume for every breath set on the machine as well as those initiated by the client; allows for hyperventilation when needed

c) Controlled mandatory ventilation (CMV): delivers a preset volume at a preset rate and is most frequently utilized for those clients with no ventilatory effort

d) Synchronized intermittent mandatory ventilation (SIMV): delivers a preset, mandatory volume that is synchronized to the client's inspiratory effort; this is the most common ventilation currently used

5) Key ventilator settings

a) Rate: number of breaths per minute that the ventilator delivers; is a number that is combined with the mode oftentimes in clinical practice (e.g., SIMV of 6/min)

b) FiO_2: fraction of inspired oxygen or oxygen percent; is the amount of oxygen in the inhaled air via the ventilator; is expressed as a decimal instead of a percentage (e.g., FiO_2 of .40 versus 40%)

c) Tidal volume: the amount of air delivered with each breath; often expressed in milliliters or liters (e.g., 700 mL or 0.7 L)

d) PEEP: abbreviation for positive end expiratory pressure; is the amount of positive pressure set in the system at the end of exhalation; serves to keep the alveoli open during exhalation to increase opportunity for gas exchange to occur; is expressed in terms of centimeters of pressure (e.g., 5 cm)

6) Indications: physical findings of ineffective breathing pattern or hypoxia (e.g., dyspnea, cyanosis, altered mental status, absent breath sounds, tachycardia with no underlying cardiac disease); oxygen saturation levels of <80 mmHg, pH <7.35, $PaCO_2$ >50 mmHg; tidal volumes < 5 mL/kg, or minute volumes <10 L/min

7) Nursing management

a) Position client for maximum alveolar ventilation and comfort; maintain soft restraints to avoid accidental extubation

b) Monitor for any changes in respiratory status or effort

c) Maintain ventilator settings as ordered and remain knowledgeable about how to troubleshoot ventilator alarms (high pressure frequently indicates need for suctioning or kinking/compression of ET; low pressure indicates leak or disconnection); manually bag the client should the alarms sound without apparent cause

d) Monitor ABGs and maintain continuous oxygen saturation monitoring

e) Complete a thorough physical assessment with emphasis on cardiac, neurological, and respiratory areas

f) Administer antibiotics, neuromuscular blocking agents, and sedatives as ordered

g) Maintain nasogastric suction to prevent aspiration

h) Supply nutritional support as ordered

i) Perform frequent oral care and suctioning to maintain airway patency

j) Provide emotional support to client and family and alternate communication method

8) Potential complications: pneumothorax, GI stress ulcers, hypotension caused by decreased venous return from increased intrathoracic pressure, increased intracranial pressure, infection

9) Priority nursing diagnoses: Impaired gas exchange; Ineffective breathing pattern; Ineffective airway clearance; Risk for infection; Anxiety

D. Common complications seen in the critical care setting

1. Sepsis

   a. Description: a diffuse inflammatory systemic response to a chemical, mechanical, bacterial, or microbial assault; if untreated it can lead to shock

   b. Etiology and pathophysiology

   1) A bodily insult leads to an inflammatory response, which is intended to protect the body from further injury and promote healing

   2) The vascular response to the assault causes a massive release of histamine, prostaglandin, bradykinin, and other mediators which cause vasodilatation and increased capillary, membrane permeability and initiating of the clotting cascade

   3) This maldistribution of circulating blood volume causes decreased cellular oxygen supply, impaired tissue perfusion and impaired cellular metabolism

   4) Severe sepsis, which is characterized by hypoperfusion, organ dysfunction, and hypotension, can lead to septic shock and death caused by multiple organ system failure

5) In the early stages of sepsis, the hyperdynamic phase, the body attempts to compensate for the decreasing oxygenation at the cellular level; the heart rate and respiratory rate increase and urine output decreases because of shunting of blood to the vital organ systems; the body temperature increases as the metabolic activity increases, and the skin becomes warm and flushed because of vasodilatation

6) In the late stage of sepsis, compensatory mechanisms begin to fail; SNS compensatory mechanisms cause extreme tachycardia but CO is low because of vasoconstriction and poor stroke volume; peripheral pulses become weak or absent and skin becomes cool, pale, and cyanotic (vasoconstriction); respirations become labored and decreased because of toxin accumulation and hypoxia in the CNS; the LOC decreases to coma because of severe hypoxia

c. Assessment

NCLEX**!**

1) Clinical manifestations: early signs of sepsis are signs of inflammation such as fever >38°C (100.4°F) or <36°C (96.8°F), tachypnea, hypocarbia, tachycardia, restlessness, hyperglycemia; late signs will include diminished LOC, coma, respiratory failure, heart failure, and oliguria

2) Diagnostic and laboratory findings

a) WBCs increase initially because of inflammatory process and later decrease because of bone marrow exhaustion

b) Glucose levels are high in early sepsis from glucogenesis and decrease in later sepsis because of hepatic failure

c) Serum lactate levels are elevated because of cellular hypoxia, and renal, hepatic and cardiac enzymes show abnormalities as organ systems begin to fail

NCLEX**!**

d) Blood cultures done early will usually show the causative agent for the sepsis and should direct the antibiotic therapy regime

e) ABGs will demonstrate increasing metabolic acidosis and respiratory acidosis as respiratory failure occurs

f) Clotting studies will show increasing clotting times as clotting factors begin to be utilized beyond available reserves

g) Chest and other radiographic studies may be utilized to determine the site of the underlying cause of infection

d. Therapeutic management

NCLEX**!**

1) Is directed toward supportive measures of vital organ systems with supplemental oxygen, mechanical ventilation, and fluid administration to maintain an adequate cardiac output

2) Positive inotropic medications such as dopamine (Intropin) and dobutamine (Dobutrex) may be utilized to increase cardiac contractility; they can be combined with vasodilators such as nitroglycerine (Tridil) or sodium nitroprusside (Nipride) to decrease preload and after load to decrease the work of the myocardium

3) Nutritional support will be administered to enhance tissue rebuilding

4) Cooling blankets or antipyretics will be utilized to normalize body temperature

5) All of these measures are supportive while appropriate antibiotic therapy is initiated in an attempt to treat the causative agent

e. Priority nursing diagnoses: Impaired tissue perfusion; Deficient fluid volume; Decreased cardiac output; Impaired gas exchange; Imbalanced nutrition: less than body requirements; Ineffective thermoregulation; Anxiety

f. Planning and implementation

1) The goal of nursing care is to provide collaborative supportive measures while antibacterial therapy is being administered

2) Assist with establishing and managing the ABCs; IV solutions of NS or lactated ringers should be infused to maintain a systolic blood pressure above 100 mmHg and a CVP of 5 to 10 mmHg

3) Use continuous cardiac monitoring and 12-lead ECG to detect and manage dysrhythmias caused by hypoxia, acidosis, or endotoxin effect on the myocardium

4) Use aseptic technique at all times to prevent further infective processes and administer organism-specific antibiotics as ordered

5) Keep the client comfortable and begin attempts to reduce fever, such as use of antipyretics and hyperthermia measures

6) Keep the client and family informed of the plan of care and rationale for procedures

g. Medication therapy: antibiotics based upon determination of the causative agent; antiarrhythmics such as lidocaine to control cardiac dysrhythmias; positive inotropic medications such as dopamine and dobutamine, vasodilators such as nitroglycerine, and vasopressors such as epinephrine to control myocardial and vascular functioning

h. Evaluation: client is hemodynamically stable, normothermic, and free of dysrhythmias; antibiotic therapy is effective and no additional organ system injury has occurred; client and family verbalize understanding of follow-up plan of care and preventive measures

2. Multiple organ system failure (MOSF)

a. Description: failure of one or more body systems after a major insult to the body, such as from infection, trauma, or severe illness

b. Etiology and pathophysiology

1) The cause of MOSF is some type of inflammatory response or infection, persistent hypotension, and hypoxia

2) In general, as the body responds to an uncontrolled inflammatory response, damage at the organ system level becomes the result of hypoperfusion, hypoxia, and necrosis of tissue

3) The four major organ systems effected by MOSF are the pulmonary, renal, cardiovascular and coagulation

4) Pulmonary dysfunction and the development of adult respiratory distress syndrome (ARDS) are the result of pulmonary vascular endothelium and alveolar epithelial damage with resultant surfactant deficiency, mild pulmonary hypertension, and pulmonary edema and hypoxia

5) Renal dysfunction is the direct result of prolonged hypovolemia, hypoperfusion and acute tubular necrosis; the use of nephrotoxic medications in resuscitation efforts also intensify renal damage

6) Cardiovascular dysfunction is the result of prolonged compensation efforts to increase cardiac output and vasoconstriction to enhance organ perfusion; during resuscitation efforts, cardiac function becomes vasopressor dependent and eventually becomes unresponsive even to the vasopressor; another influence on the myocardium is the release of myocardial depressant factor from the pancreas

7) The coagulation system failure is seen in the development of disseminated intravascular coagulopathy (DIC), an uncontrolled excessive consumption of coagulation factors

c. Assessment

1) Clinical manifestations: general symptoms observed in MOSF are related to the organ system effected; all symptoms are a result of decreased oxygen supply, increased oxygen demands, and circulating toxins.

a) The GI tract will demonstrate signs of abdominal distention, paralytic ileus, diarrhea, and GI bleeding

b) Pulmonary assessment will reveal tachypnea, pulmonary hypertension and acute respiratory distress syndrome (ARDS)

c) The renal system will show increasing renal failure as oliguria, anuria and increasing BUN and creatinine

d) Cardiovascular assessment will reveal early compensatory signs of tachycardia, increased cardiac output and decreased systemic vascular resistance; in the later stages of MOSF there is increased systemic vascular resistance, decreased cardiac output and absent or weak peripheral pulses

e) Decreasing level of consciousness to coma will be seen

f) Excessive bleeding and fibrinolysis will be observed as well

2) Diagnostic and laboratory findings

a) ABG results reveal a severe acidotic state with a pH < 7.35 and pCO_2 < 32 mmHg

b) WBC counts will be decreased and platelet counts will be < 80,000/mm^3

c) Fibrinogen levels will be decreased

d) PT and PTT will increase and hemoglobin and hematocrit levels will show severe anemia

NCLEX!

    e) Creatinine levels and BUN will increase

    f) Cardiac and hepatic enzymes will be elevated

    g) Serum potassium will be severely elevated as a result of cellular damage

    h) ECG findings will show ST-segment changes indicating ischemia

    i) Chest x-ray will show interstitial edema and hypoperfusion

d. Therapeutic management

1) The goals of management are to support tissue oxygenation, reduce oxygen consumption, reduce organ system damage, and control the causative agent; specifically, the client will receive supplemental oxygen and mechanical ventilation as the symptoms of ARDS develop

2) Fluid resuscitation is given to maintain circulatory volume and maintain a CVP of at least 8 to 10 mmHg in most clients

3) Blood and blood products such as platelets and clotting factors are often be required to control bleeding and to enhance the oxygen-carrying capacity of the circulating volume

4) Hemodialysis or hemofiltration can be utilized to filter waste products and excessive fluid volume

5) Nutritional support is given to enhance tissue regeneration and provide glucose stores

6) Antibiotic therapy is utilized based upon causative agent

e. Priority nursing diagnoses: Impaired gas exchange; Impaired tissue perfusion; Risk for deficient or excess fluid volume; Imbalanced nutrition: less than body requirements; Risk for infection; Anxiety

f. Planning and implementation

1) Nursing interventions are directed to facilitating tissue perfusion, decreasing oxygen consumption, promoting nutritional support, providing comfort and emotional support to client and family, and carefully monitoring effectiveness of treatment plan

2) Assess perfusion by monitoring level of consciousness, vital signs, peripheral circulation and urinary output and titrate medications as ordered

3) Provide hydration and nutritional support as ordered with assessment of intestinal status, weight, and ability to tolerate supplemental feedings

4) Carefully assess respiratory status, including adventitious breath sounds, effectiveness of mechanical ventilation and supplemental oxygen administration methods, provide meticulous oral care and suction as needed

5) Institute continuous cardiac monitoring to assess and treat cardiac dysrhythmias that may develop

6) Monitor for signs of coagulation dysfunction; to reduce bleeding potential, avoid procedures that may cause a break in skin integrity (such as IV starts, invasive procedures, or aggressive turning)

7) Implement emotional and comfort measures such as limiting activities, providing a calm environment, reducing external stimuli as possible, and providing client and family teaching about condition and plan of care

g. Evaluation: client is hemodynamically stable; respiratory status is improved and mechanical ventilation is no longer needed; signs of increased tissue perfusion and organ system healing are present; bleeding is controlled and urinary output is returning to normal; the client and family verbalize understanding of follow-up plan of care and preventive measures

3. Shock

a. Description: a state of imbalance between oxygen supply and demand in the body that leads to inadequate blood flow to organs, poor tissue perfusion, and possibly fatal cellular dysfunction

b. Etiology and pathophysiology

1) The etiology of shock can be classified as due to loss of circulation volume (hypovolemic), decreased pump function (cardiogenic), spinal cord injury (neurogenic) or an overwhelming presence of endogenous mediators which cause an overwhelming inflammatory response (septic)

2) All forms of shock cause reduction in oxygenation and tissue perfusion, which lead to cellular damage and eventual organ system failure because of hypoxia

3) Compensatory mechanisms in the SNS and the endocrine system attempt to compensate for the loss of oxygenation capability

a) A decrease in circulating volume in the right atrium and in the area of the baroreceptors in carotid arteries and the aorta stimulates a massive release of norepinephrine, which then stimulates the SNS to increase heart and respiratory rate, increase glycolysis, decrease urinary output, shunt blood from less vital organs such as the GI tract, liver and kidneys, and cause vasoconstriction

b) The endocrine system attempts to increase circulating blood volume and oxygen carrying capacity by secreting high levels of ADH for water reabsorption; the decreased blood flow to the kidneys also stimulates release of angiotensin II which causes vasoconstriction and water reabsorption to augment water and sodium reabsorption

c) If these initial compensatory responses do not restore homeostasis, further hypoperfusion and hypoxia lead to cellular death, which ultimately leads to multiple organ system failure and death

c. Assessment

1) Clinical manifestations will be varied

a) In the early stages of shock, the body is attempting to compensate for a decreased perfusion and oxygenation state

b) Generally findings will reveal a normal blood pressure, slightly increased pulse rate, normal or slightly decreased urinary output, slight restlessness, anxiety, and thirst

NCLEX!

c) During the next stage, the progressive shock state, classic shock symptoms will be seen, including cool, clammy, and pale skin, decreased capillary refill, tachycardia, tachypnea, decreased blood pressure, decreased cardiac output, decreased temperature, decreased urinary output, altered level of consciousness and mental status; metabolic acidosis will begin to develop

d) During the later stages of shock, signs of specific organ failure will be seen such as anuria, slow, thready pulse, ARDS, bleeding and coagulation dysfunction, and coma

2) Diagnostic and laboratory findings

a) Hemoglobin and hematocrit are decreased

b) ABGs show an acidotic state

c) Serum lactate and potassium levels are elevated

d) Cardiac, hepatic and GI enzymes are elevated

e) Increased creatinine and BUN levels will indicate renal failure

f) Serum glucose levels initially increase and then decrease as glucose stores are depleted

g) Urine specific gravity is increased

h) Clotting studies show depletion in fibrinogen, platelets, and other clotting factors; PT/PTT and fibrinogen split/degradation products (FSP/FDP) are elevated

i) ECG shows ST ischemic changes

d. Therapeutic management

1) The goal is to restore oxygenation delivery and decrease oxygen consumption

2) First establish an effective airway and breathing pattern with supplemental oxygen and possible mechanical ventilation

3) Next, establish adequate circulating volume with IV infusion of NS, lactated ringers, or blood products if needed

4) Use vasopressor, vasodilating, and positive inotropic medications to enhance cardiac output and systemic perfusion

5) Correct acidotic state and provide treatment of specific causative agent in the case of anaphylactic reaction or sepsis

e. Priority nursing diagnoses: Impaired gas exchange; Impaired tissue perfusion; Deficient or excess fluid volume; Decreased cardiac output; Risk for infection; Anxiety

f. Planning and implementations

1) Nursing interventions are directed to facilitating tissue perfusion, decreasing oxygen consumption, providing comfort and emotional support to client and family, and carefully monitoring effectiveness of treatment plan

2) Assess perfusion by monitoring LOC, vital signs, peripheral circulation, and urinary output; titrate medications as ordered

3) Complete careful respiratory assessment, including adventitious breath sounds, effectiveness of mechanical ventilation and supplemental oxygen administration methods; provide meticulous oral care and suctioning as needed

4) Institute continuous cardiac monitoring to assess and treat cardiac dysrhythmias that may develop

5) Monitor for signs of coagulation dysfunction; maintain strict intake and output records

6) Document continual serial assessments of vital signs, LOC, hemodynamic status, and response to treatments and report changes to physician as needed

7) Provide emotional and comfort measures such as limiting activities, providing a calm environment, reducing external stimuli as possible, providing client and family teaching about condition and plan of care

g. Evaluation: the client has adequate tissue perfusion as measured by hemodynamic stability, improved level of consciousness, and urinary output; bleeding is controlled; effective breathing pattern is established and gas exchange is appropriate as measured by resolution of acidosis; the client and family verbalize understanding of plan of care and follow-up care needed

4. Acute respiratory distress syndrome (ARDS)

a. Description: a syndrome characterized by a non-cardiac type of pulmonary edema and increasing hypoxemia despite administration of treatment measures; formerly known as adult respiratory distress syndrome

b. Etiology and pathophysiology (see Figure 17-2)

1) Injury to the alveolar and capillary membranes of the lungs can be caused by aspiration of gastric contents or water, inhalation agents, embolism, endotoxins, or multiple trauma

2) This damage causes fluid and protein shifts into the alveoli and interstitial tissue

3) With the increase in edema, terminal bronchioles collapse and the alveoli space fills with fluid

4) Lung compliance and functional residual capacity decrease, dead space increases in the lung, and the work of breathing begins to increase oxygen consumption while oxygen perfusion capability has decreased

c. Assessment

1) Clinical manifestations: labored respirations, restlessness, and dry, nonproductive cough are early symptoms of ARDS; cyanosis, pallor, adventitious breath sounds and use of accessory muscles with retraction are late findings

2) Diagnostic and laboratory findings: chest x-ray will initially appear normal and then progress to complete "white out" due to bilateral diffuse infiltrates; pulmonary function tests will show a decrease in com-

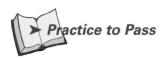

Practice to Pass

Medical and nursing management of the client exhibiting signs of shock are directed towards what three concerns?

NCLEX!

NCLEX!

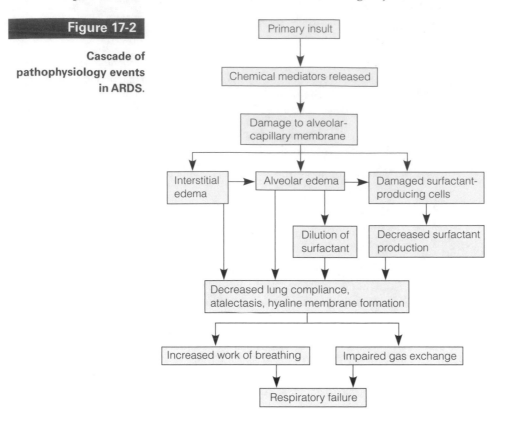

Figure 17-2

Cascade of pathophysiology events in ARDS.

pliance, lung capacity and elevated peak inspiratory pressures; ABGs initially show respiratory alkalosis due to hyperventilation and then progress to respiratory acidosis; hemodynamic monitoring shows elevated pulmonary artery systolic and diastolic pressures with a normal PCWP/LVEDP

d. Therapeutic management

1) Provide oxygen therapy and mechanical ventilation in the late stages to assure adequate oxygen delivery and decrease the work of breathing

2) Neuromuscular blocking agents and sedation may be necessary to allow client to tolerate mechanical ventilation

3) Fluid therapy will consist of crystalloids and colloids to maintain intravascular volume

4) Use hemodynamic monitoring to assess pulmonary and cardiac functioning

5) Treat the underlying cause of the ARDS (antibiotics must be used if an infective process is present)

6) Provide nutritional support with a positive protein balance, which is essential for healing

7) Administer steroid therapy as ordered to stabilize cellular membranes and decrease fluid shifts

8) Initiate support of other body systems to prevent further damage

NCLEX!

NCLEX!

NCLEX!

NCLEX!

e. Priority nursing diagnoses: Ineffective airway clearance; Impaired tissue perfusion; Activity intolerance; Risk for infection; Imbalanced nutrition: less than body requirements

f. Planning and implementation

1) The goal of care is to maintain tissue oxygenation and ventilation, assist in the treatment of underlying cause, and to prevent further organ system damage

2) Assist and maintain mechanical ventilation

3) Monitor oxygen saturation; provide thorough suctioning, oral care, and sedation as needed to tolerate mechanical ventilation

4) Administer diuretic therapy and nutritional support as ordered

5) Monitor effectiveness of treatment plan through serial assessments of vital signs, heart, lung and bowel sounds, EKG rhythm, urinary output, and neurological status

6) Position the client for comfort, turn frequently, and elevate head of bed to enhance respiratory effort

7) Schedule activities to conserve energy

8) Provide client and family education concerning plan of care and prognosis

g. Evaluation: client demonstrates improved oxygenation and gas exchange; further organ system failure is decreased; family and client verbalize understanding of prognosis and plan of care

IV. Cardiopulmonary Resuscitation

A. Basic cardiac life support (BCLS)

1. Purposes

    a. To recognize cardiac or respiratory arrest

    b. To reestablish or provide an effective airway, breathing pattern, and effective circulation until the client responds or until another type of life support is initiated

NCLEX!

2. ABCs of resuscitation

    a. Establish unresponsiveness and lack of respiratory effort

    b. A = open *airway* by lifting the jaw and tilting the head back (head-tilt/chin-lift) or thrust jaw forward by placing the fingers of both hands at the angle of the jaw and pushing forward while keeping the head in a neutral position (jaw thrust)

    c. B = restore *breathing* by artificial ventilation with mouth-to-mouth, bag-valve mask (Ambu bag), or other asssistive device; remember to maintain a tight seal to ensure maximum air exchange

    d. C = restore *circulation* by delivering closed chest compressions

3. Management of foreign body airway obstruction

    a. It is necessary to remove any airway obstruction prior to initiation of artificial ventilation

  b. If the air does not go into the lungs when ventilations are attempted, reposition the head and try again

  c. Open the mouth and see if any obstruction is visible; frequently the tongue is obstructing the airway or dentures, which can be removed easily

 4. Airway obstruction

  a. Conscious adult

   1) Ask the client if he or she is choking and whether he/she can speak

   2) If the client answers "yes" to these questions, the airway is only partially obstructed; allow the client to attempt to cough or clear the obstruction on own

   3) If unable to speak, tell client that you are going to help

   4) Position yourself behind the client and give abdominal thrusts until obstruction clears or client becomes unresponsive

  b. Unconscious adult

   1) Establish unresponsiveness and call the emergency medical services (EMS) system

   2) Open the airway and check for breathing; if breathing is absent or ineffective, attempt to ventilate the client

   3) If breaths do not cause chest to rise, reposition airway and try again; if unsuccessful, perform five abdominal thrusts with the client supine

   4) Open the airway and gently sweep the mouth to attempt to remove the obstruction

   5) Attempt to ventilate again; if successful, give two slow full breaths and assess for need for chest compressions

   6) If unable to ventilate after mouth sweep, continue with five abdominal thrusts, mouth sweep, and attempts to ventilate until obstruction is successfully removed, or until further assistance arrives

 5. Adult one-rescuer CPR

  a. Establish that the victim is unresponsive and activate the EMS system

  b. Open the airway utilizing the head-tilt/chin-lift maneuver or jaw thrust maneuver; check for signs of breathing (see chest rise, hear air movement with mouth open, feel breath on check)

  c. If no spontaneous breathing, give two slow breaths (each over 2 seconds); observe for chest rising and for chest falling (exhalation) between breaths

  d. Check for signs of circulation (cough, breathing, carotid pulse palpable); if no signs of circulation are present, begin chest compressions; compress lower one-third sternum 1 1/2 to 2 inches at a rate of 100 times per minute; perform 15 chest compressions and then 2 more slow breaths

  e. Repeat this 15:2 ratio cycle for 4 cycles (about 1 minute) and then recheck carotid pulse and other signs of circulation; continue this cycle until additional help arrives to take over

Practice to Pass

What assessment findings indicate a need for cardiopulmonary resuscitation?

NCLEX!

6. Adult two-rescuer CPR

   a. The first rescuer establishes unresponsiveness and activates the EMS system

   b. The first rescuer initiates one-rescuer CPR

   c. When the second rescuer arrives and identifies that he/she knows CPR, the first rescuer completes the current cycle of chest compressions, gives 2 breaths and checks for signs of circulation; the second rescuer establishes position to begin chest compressions when it is established that no circulatory signs are present and the two rescuers perform compressions and give breaths at a 15:2 ratio until other helps arrives

B. **Advanced cardiac life support (ACLS)**

   1. Airway management

      a. After establishing unresponsiveness and the presence of an unobstructed airway, the ACLS provider will manage the airway through endotracheal intubation or use of an advanced airway device

      b. The effectiveness of breathing and ventilation is assessed by checking for appropriate endotracheal tube placement (chest rising and falling bilaterally and presence of bilateral breath sounds)

      c. Respirations are given by positive pressure ventilation with a bag-valve device attached to a supplemental oxygen supply

   2. Venous access

      a. A peripheral IV is started to provide a route for medications to be administered (large-bore 16- or 18-gauge catheter preferred); two lines may be needed

      b. Care should be taken to ensure that the IV is secured and IV fluid is infusing without difficulty

   3. Medication therapy

      a. Ventricular fibrillation/pulseless ventricular tachycardia (ventricular contraction absent/ineffective)

         1) Epinephrine (Adrenalin) 1 mg (1:10,000) IV push, repeat every 3 to 5 minutes; tracheal administration 2.0 to 2.5 mg diluted in 10 mL NS (up to 0.04 mg/kg weight)

         2) Vasopressin (Pitressin) 40 U IV or ET, single dose, 1 time only

         3) Amiodarone (Cordarone) 300 mg IV, repeat in 3 to 5 minutes 150 mg IV to a maximum cumulative dose of 2.2 gm IV in 24 hours

         4) Lidocaine (Xylocaine) 1 to 1.5 mg/kg IV, repeat in 5 to 10 minutes 1 to 1.5 mg/kg to a maximum dose of 3 mg/kg; tracheal administration is 2 to 4 mg/kg followed by 10 mL NS and manual ventilation with Ambubag to dispense drug

         5) Lidocaine drip 1 to 4 mg/min for maintenance infusion

         6) Procainamide 20 mg/min to 50 mg/minute IV infusion to a maximum total dose of 17 mg/kg

7) Sodium bicarbonate 1 mEq/kg IV bolus, may repeat half-dose every 10 minutes to correct acidosis but should be used with caution and with ABG analysis to avoid precipitating alkalosis

b. Asystole/pulseless electrical activity (PEA): "flat line"/electrical activity not accompanied by carotid pulse

1) Epinephrine (Adrenalin) 1 mg (1:10,000) IV, may repeat every 3 to 5 minutes

2) Atropine sulfate 1 mg IV, repeat every 3 to 5 minutes if asystole persists to a maximum dose of 0.03 to 0.04 mg/kg; use in PEA if rate is slow on monitor

c. Bradycardia (ventricular rate < 60/minute)

1) Atropine sulfate 0.5 to 1.0 mg IV every 3 to 5 minutes, may not exceed a total dose of 0.04 mg/kg; tracheal administration: 2 to 3 mg diluted in 10 mL NS

4. Recognition and treatment of cardiac dysrhythmias

a. Ventricular fibrillation

1) Rapid, disorganized depolarization of the ventricles

2) ECG pattern shows:

a) Rate: unable to determine

b) Rhythm: rapid, chaotic, irregular

c) P wave: unable to identify

d) PR interval: unable to identify

e) QRS complex: unable to identify

f) ST segment: unable to identify

g) T wave: unable to identify

NCLEX!

3) Treatment includes oxygen, **defibrillation** (electrical shock therapy to the heart) with stacked shocks of 200–300–360 joules, CPR, and pharmacological treatment with epinephrine and antiarrhythmic agents such as amiodarone and lidocaine

b. Ventricular tachycardia

1) Rapid, ventricular contractions at a rate greater than 100 beats/minute

2) ECG pattern shows:

a) Rate: slightly irregular

b) Atrial rhythm: unable to identify

c) Ventricular rhythm: often 150 to 250 beats/minute

d) P wave: unable to identify

e) PR interval: unable to identify

f) QRS complex: wide (>0.12 sec), bizarre

g) ST segment: unable to identify

h) T wave: unable to identify

NCLEX!

3) Treatment includes:

a) If client is hemodynamically stable, oxygen and antiarrhythmic agents such as lidocaine and amiodarone to decrease ventricular irritability

b) If client is hemodynamically unstable, oxygen, defibrillation with stacked shocks of 200–300–360 joules, CPR, and the pharmacological treatment with epinephrine and antiarrhythmic agents such as amiodarone and lidocaine

c) Note: client may be a candidate for automatic internal cardioverter defibrillator (AICD) if this is a frequent occurrence

c. Asystole

1) Total absence of ventricular electrical activity

2) ECG characteristics

a) Rate: none; may see a rare, wide, bizarre QRS

b) Rhythm: none

c) P wave: may be an occasional P-wave

d) PR interval: unable to identify

e) QRS complex: none

f) ST segment: none

g) T wave: none

NCLEX!

3) Treatment includes: oxygen, CPR, Epinephrine 1 mg (1:10,000) IV, may repeat every 3 to 5 minutes; atropine sulfate 1 mg IV, may repeat every 3 to 5 minutes; if asystole persists, repeat up to a maximum dose of 0.03 to 0.04 mg/kg; consider transcutaneous pacing or defibrillation if rhythm could be fine ventricular fibrillation

d. Electromechanical dissociation (EMD)/Pulseless electrical activity (PEA)

NCLEX!

1) Absence of palpable pulse and blood pressure with normal EKG pattern on cardiac monitor

2) ECG pattern shows:

a) Rate: normal sinus rate

b) Rhythm: regular

c) P wave: normal configuration

d) PR interval: <.20 sec

e) QRS complex: <.10

f) ST segment: **isoelectric** (on baseline)

g) T wave: normal configuration

3) Treatment includes CPR, oxygen, consideration of possible causes (hypovolemia, hypoxia, cardiac tamponade, tension pneumothorax, drug overdose, massive MI, acidosis); correct possible cause; epinephrine 1 mg IV, may repeat every 3 to 5 minutes

e. Bradydysrhythmias

1) Dysrhythmia in which atrial rate is <60 beats/minute

2) ECG pattern shows:

a) Rate: less than 60 beats for atrial and ventricular

b) Rhythm: regular

c) P wave: normal

d) PR interval within normal limits for sinus bradycardia; prolonged for A-V heart blocks

e) QRS complex: within normal limits

f) ST segment: normal

g) T wave: normal

3) Treatment includes the following:

a) Assess ABCs; provide oxygen, IV access, cardiac monitor

b) Assess if client is symptomatic, i.e., decreased blood pressure, short of breath, chest pain

c) If client is asymptomatic, monitor and consider transcutaneous pacer if rhythm is Type II AV block or third-degree heart block because of potential for symptom development

d) If client is symptomatic, use Atropine 0.5 to 1.0 mg IV, transcutaneous pacer, Dopamine 5 to 20 μg/kg/min, epinephrine 2 to 10 μg/min

e) In all cases, consider eventual transvenous pacemaker

f. Premature ventricular contractions (PVC)

1) Ectopic beats that occur earlier than expected; is usually followed by a compensatory pause

2) ECG pattern:

a) Rate: regular; may be slow if frequent PVCs occur

b) Rhythm: atrial and ventricular rate irregular

c) P wave: absent in the premature beat, present and normal in underlying rhythm

d) PR interval: absent in the premature beat

e) QRS complex: bizarre and wider (>.12) in the premature beat; underlying rhythm, ORS complex normal

f) ST segment: normal in underlying rhythm

g) T wave: deflection in the opposite direction of the PVC and followed by a long compensatory pause

NCLEX!

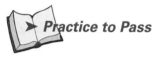

3) They are of concern because they indicate ventricular irritability; they are most dangerous when they occur more frequently than 6 per minute, occur in pairs, are multifocal (have differing shapes) or fall on the T wave of the preceding normal complex (R-on-T) because they could lead to ventricular tachycardia or ventricular fibrillation

4) Treatment includes: monitor number of PVCs in 1 minute; assess for possible cause, i.e., hypoxia, electrolyte imbalance (potassium), or bradycardia; if client is symptomatic with frequent PVCs, administer oxygen, correct cause if known, administer Lidocaine 1 mg/kg and maintain the client on a continuous IV drip at 2 to 4 mg/min to decrease myocardial irritability

g. Supraventricular tachycardia

1) Dysrhythmia with a rate greater than 100 beats/min originating above the ventricle but not in the sinus node

2) ECG pattern

a) Rate: atrial rate >140 beats/min; ventricular rate depends on degree of block

b) Rhythm: regular

c) P wave: may or may not be identifiable

d) PR interval: not measurable

e) QRS complex: within normal limits

f) ST segment: unidentifiable

g) T wave: unidentifiable

3) Treatment includes: attempt vagal nerve stimulation, i.e., cough, Valsalva's maneuver; administer adenosine 6 mg rapid IV push, may repeat 12 mg after 1 to 2 min and then repeat once more; if client is asymptomatic, verapamil (Isoptin) 2.5 to 5.0 mg IV over 2 minutes and repeated at 5 to 10 mg IV after 15 to 30 minutes; to a maximum of 20 mg if medications are ineffective, synchronized cardioversion may be attempted

C. Nursing role during a code

1. Call code: upon finding client for confirming need for assistance, initiate calling of the code team per hospital or agency protocol

2. Assure appropriate CPR procedure is done

3. Once team and equipment has arrived, assure the placement of the backboard under the client and effective placement of cardiac monitor, defibrillator, medication and supply cart or "code cart"

4. Determine who is the team leader so that all will know who is responsible for code management

5. Assist as needed with airway management and IV access and provide for the timely administration of medications, treatments, and transportation of labs as ordered

6. Assist with dysrhythmia recognition, defibrillation, and treatment as needed

Practice to Pass

Your client's monitor is showing ventricular tachycardia. The client is unresponsive, and has no pulse or blood pressure. What would your immediate response be?

7. Continue making serial assessments of the client

8. Document in a thorough and concise manner all actions and responses during the code process

9. Crowd control: all persons not actively participating in the code should be excluded from the vicinity

10. Assist with the psychosocial needs of family, roommates, and staff following the code

---

Case Study

A client presents to the emergency department with a chief complaint of "accidental overdose" of acetaminophen. You are working in the department.

❶ What would the triage category be for this client?

❷ What are the priorities in treating this client?

❸ What methods could be utilized to decrease absorption of this medication?

❹ What would be three priority nursing diagnoses for this client?

❺ What would be three evaluation criteria indicative for successful treatment of this client?

For suggested responses, see pages 740–741 .

Posttest

1 The nurse observes that a client being monitored is in ventricular fibrillation. The first action should be to do which of the following?

(1) Administer sodium bicarbonate for developing acidosis.
(2) Initiate cardiopulmonary resuscitation (CPR).
(3) Immediately defibrillate the patient with 200 joules.
(4) Administer oxygen.

2 The nurse is caring for a client with a tracheostomy. While performing tracheostomy care, the nurse makes sure that the cuff of the tracheostomy tube:

(1) Is never deflated.
(2) Creates a very tight seal between the cuff and the trachea.
(3) Is deflated for 5 minutes every hour.
(4) That the cuff is inflated to allow a slight air leak at the height of inspiration.

3 The nurse prepares a client for insertion of a pulmonary artery catheter. Preprocedural teaching for this client will include which of the following statements?

(1) "The catheter will assist in directly monitoring your arterial pressure."
(2) "The catheter will provide information about your cardiac output."
(3) "The catheter will provide information about your left ventricular function."
(4) "The catheter will provide information about your cardiac index."

4 The nurse suspects that the client is in cardiogenic shock based upon which of the following findings?

(1) Decreased or muffled heart sounds
(2) Cardiac index >2.2 L/min/m^2
(3) Bounding pulses
(4) Increased cardiac output

5 A nurse observes a client who is on mechanical ventilation to be fighting the ventilator. Pancuronium bromide is ordered for the client. This medication is classified as a(n):

(1) Psychotropic.
(2) Neuromuscular blocking agent.
(3) Antihistamine.
(4) Immunosuppressant.

6 During the insertion of a Swan-Ganz catheter, the client complains of shortness of breath and assessment findings of labored respirations, decreased breath sounds on the side of the insertion, and asymmetrical chest movement. The nurse should suspect:

(1) Pulmonary embolism.
(2) Myocardial infarction.
(3) Pneumothorax.
(4) Anxiety.

7 A client presents in acute respiratory distress after an automobile collision. The nurse observes that the client has facial trauma. The most urgent nursing diagnosis for this client would be:

(1) Impaired gas exchange.
(2) Ineffective airway clearance.
(3) Decreased cardiac output.
(4) Anxiety.

8 A client presents with circumferential burns to the chest and shortness of breath following an electrical burn injury. The nurse identifies that the priority nursing diagnosis for *this* injury would be:

(1) Deficient fluid volume.
(2) Risk for injury.
(3) Ineffective breathing pattern.
(4) Decreased cardiac output.

9 A client is brought to the emergency department after being found with a body temperature of 106°F. The client is unresponsive, hypotensive, and tachypneic. A medical diagnosis of heat stroke is made. What would be the nurse's priority nursing intervention in the care of this client?

(1) Obtain a complete health assessment
(2) Obtain an oral temperature to monitor effectiveness of treatment
(3) Contact next of kin for any advanced directives
(4) Remove all clothing, wrap in wet sheets and cool with fans

10 You have just given charcoal to your client for a drug overdose. You explain to the client that the purpose of the charcoal is to:

(1) Induce vomiting and removal of pill remnants.
(2) Absorb toxins from the GI tract.
(3) Decrease the present serum drug level.
(4) Cause diarrhea and quick evacuation of pill fragments.

See pages 722–723 for Answers and Rationales.

Answers and Rationales

Pretest

1 Answer: 4 *Rationale:* Excessive blood loss will result in the development of shock symptoms such as tachycardia, cool, clammy skin, and changes in mental status, because hypovolemia leads to vasoconstriction and shunting of blood to the central circulation. Applying ice to lower the body temperature would not be appropriate since the body temperature is usually decreased with hypovolemia. Measures to decrease circulation to the affected extremity, such as elevation of that extremity to heart level would be appropriate, although elevating it further could lead to ischemia. A psychiatric evaluation would be appropriate after the client has become hemodynamically stable.
Cognitive Level: Application
Nursing Process: Implementation; *Test Plan:* PHYS

2 Answer: 4 *Rationale:* Tracheal and mediastinal shifting will occur to the uninjured side because of increased intrathoracic pressure on the side of the injury. The client will exhibit hypotension caused by the decreased cardiac output (option 2), respiratory acidosis caused by hypoxemia (option 3), and tachypnea (option 1). Mediastinal shift is always a late sign and requires immediate treatment to relieve the buildup of trapped air to prevent death.
Cognitive Level: Analysis
Nursing Process: Assessment; *Test Plan:* PHYS

3 Answer: 2 *Rationale:* The expiratory phase is prolonged caused by the air trapping and alveoli distention that occurs as a result of the anaphylactic response. Wheezing occurs during expiration because

of edematous constricted bronchi, and the respiratory rate is usually within normal limits.
Cognitive Level: Analysis
Nursing Process: Assessment; *Test Plan:* PHYS

4 **Answer: 2** *Rationale:* Suctioning produces hypoxia as its primary complication. Preoxygenation for 1 to 2 minutes with 100 percent oxygen will reduce the risk of hypoxia. A tracheostomy cuff should have minimal occlusive pressure applied to reduce the occurrence of tracheal necrosis. Only 3 to 5 mL of normal saline should be instilled in a tracheostomy tube to loosen secretions (if needed), and the negative pressure on the suction catheter should only be applied while the catheter is being withdrawn from the tube. Additionally, suctioning should be limited to 10 seconds for each pass and the suction catheter should be rotated during withdrawal.
Cognitive Level: Application
Nursing Process: Implementation; *Test Plan:* PHYS

5 **Answer: 2** *Rationale:* A client in ventricular fibrillation is exhibiting a life-threatening dysrhythmia that will cause irreversible brain injury within minutes because of a lack of effective circulation. Immediate CPR and defibrillation should be completed. The other conditions are serious but are not immediately life-threatening. The client with the penetrating wound is the second priority because of possible disruption to circulation, followed by the client with an eye injury (possible vision loss) and the client with the fractured femur.
Cognitive Level: Analysis
Nursing Process: Assessment; *Test Plan:* PHYS

6 **Answer: 1** *Rationale:* Human bites are considered highly contaminated wounds, and antibiotics are ordered prophylactically. Antibiotics are usually begun by the IV route prior to discharge. A sterile dressing may be applied to the site after cleaning and application of triple antibiotic ointment. Neither administration of anti-venom nor application of a tourniquet is an appropriate intervention for a human bite.
Cognitive Level: Analysis
Nursing Process: Analysis; *Test Plan:* PHYS

7 **Answer: 3** *Rationale:* Evaluate the pH first to determine acidosis or alkalosis. Then evaluate $PaCO_2$ as the respiratory component and HCO_3^- as the metabolic component. The client's pH <7.35 and $PaCO_2$ > 45mm Hg indicate a state of respiratory acidosis and indicates that the client is not tolerating the weaning process. Metabolic alkalosis would be indicated by a pH > 7.45 and a HCO_3^- >26 mEq/L. Respiratory alkalosis would be seen in a client with a pH >7.45 with a

PCO_2 <35 mmHg. Metabolic acidosis would be indicated in a client with a pH <7.35 with a HCO_3^- <21 mEq/L.
Cognitive Level: Analysis
Nursing Process: Assessment; *Test Plan:* PHYS

8 **Answer: 3** *Rationale:* A normal fibrinogen level is 200 to 400 mg/dL in adults. A decreased fibrinogen level indicates excessive usage of fibrinogen during the clotting process. All of the other laboratory findings are within normal limits.
Cognitive Level: Analysis
Nursing Process: Analysis; *Test Plan:* PHYS

9 **Answer: 2** *Rationale:* Asking the client if he can speak establishes that the client has something in his airway and does not have a patent airway. The ability to speak indicates that the airway is clear or only partial obstructed. Calling a code, beginning CPR, or providing back blows would not be appropriate initial interventions.
Cognitive Level: Application
Nursing Process: Assessment; *Test Plan:* PHYS

10 **Answer: 3** *Rationale:* The unresponsiveness and loose teeth indicate a possible airway obstruction. The airway should be opened and cleared immediately. Labored respirations, cyanosis, and tachypnea are the result of an obstructed airway and hypoxia.
Cognitive Level: Analysis
Nursing Process: Analysis; *Test Plan:* PHYS

Posttest

1 **Answer: 3** *Rationale:* Defibrillation is the definitive treatment for this life-threatening arrhythmia when a defibrillator is immediately accessible. CPR would be used if defibrillation is not successful in converting this arrhythmia. Oxygen should be administered but does not take priority over defibrillation; sodium bicarbonate is used to treat acidosis that may develop with prolonged CPR but also does not take priority.
Cognitive Level: Analysis
Nursing Process: Implementation; *Test Plan:* PHYS

2 **Answer: 4** *Rationale:* The cuff should be inflated to allow a minimal seal on inspiration so as not to cause tracheal tissue necrosis from circulatory obstruction. The cuff should not provide a tight seal, which may cause necrosis. It may be deflated to allow suctioning of secretions which are above the cuff but do not require routine deflation throughout the shift.
Cognitive Level: Analysis
Nursing Process: Assessment; *Test Plan:* PHYS

3 Answer: 3 *Rationale:* A pulmonary artery catheter will provide information about the function of the left ventricle when the balloon is wedged. The pulmonary artery catheter does not directly determine the cardiac output and cardiac index. An arterial line is used to directly monitor the client's arterial pressure.
Cognitive Level: Application
Nursing Process: Implementation; *Test Plan:* HPM

4 Answer: 1 *Rationale:* Cardiogenic shock is caused by a decrease in pumping ability of the myocardium. The decrease can be caused by a weakened myocardium or restriction of the myocardium by fluid or blood. Decreased or muffled heart sounds would be indicative of a fluid restriction in the pericardial sac, causing restriction of the heart's ability to pump effectively. Decreased pumping ability would cause a decrease in the cardiac index, thready, weak pulses, and decreased cardiac output.
Cognitive Level: Analysis
Nursing Process: Assessment; *Test Plan:* PHYS

5 Answer: 2 *Rationale:* Pancuronium bromide (Pavulon) is a neuromuscular blocking agent because it acts to prevent acetylcholine from activating nicotinic receptors on the skeletal muscles thus causing muscle relaxation. Medications classified as psychotropic, antihistamine, and immunosuppressant do not cause skeletal muscle relaxation.
Cognitive Level: Comprehension
Nursing Process: Planning; *Test Plan:* PHYS

6 Answer: 3 *Rationale:* The anatomical proximity of the apex of the lung and the subclavian vein increases the possibility of the development of a pneumothorax caused by accidental puncture of the lung. The client was demonstrating classic signs of pneumothorax. Pulmonary embolism, myocardial infarction, and anxiety do not cause asymmetrical chest movement.
Cognitive Level: Analysis
Nursing Process: Assessment; *Test Plan:* PHYS

7 Answer: 2 *Rationale:* Facial trauma can prevent the client from having a patent airway and lead to subsequent respiratory distress. Impaired gas exchange will occur as a result of the client's inability to maintain a patent airway. Decreased cardiac output can be a result of tissue hypoxia. Anxiety may be an appropriate diagnosis for this client but is not the most life-threatening.
Cognitive Level: Analysis
Nursing Process: Planning; *Test Plan:* PHYS

8 Answer: 3 *Rationale:* Circumferential burns to the chest wall will decrease chest expansion and ventilation and will compromise breathing. An ineffective breathing pattern is evident as a result of this injury. There is potential for further tissue damage, decreased cardiac output, and fluid volume deficit caused by hypoxia and edema formation for burn with third-spacing of fluids. However, breathing and airway are priorities in this case.
Cognitive Level: Analysis
Nursing Process: Analysis; *Test Plan:* PHYS

9 Answer: 4 *Rationale:* Heat stroke is a life-threatening situation, and interventions to cool the body must be accomplished quickly. Removing the clothing and cooling by evaporation is the most effective intervention to accomplish cooling quickly. A complete health assessment and documentation are important but after the cooling process has begun. Core body temperatures will be utilized to monitor effectiveness of treatment.
Cognitive Level: Application
Nursing Process: Implementation; *Test Plan:* PHYS

10 Answer: 2 *Rationale:* Activated charcoal will absorb toxins from the GI tract. Its primary action is not to cause vomiting or diarrhea. The use of charcoal can potentially decrease future serum drug levels but not current ones.
Cognitive Level: Application
Nursing Process: Implementation; *Test Plan:* SECE

References

American Heart Association (2000). *Basic life support: Instructor manual.* Dallas, TX: American Heart Association.

Black, J., Hawks, J., & Keene, A. (2000). *Medical surgical nursing: Clinical management for positive outcomes* (6th ed.). Philadelphia: W. B. Saunders.

Christensen, B. L. & Kockrow, E. O. (1999). *Adult health nursing.* St. Louis: Mosby, Inc.

Emergency Nurses Association (2000). *Trauma nursing core course* (5th ed.). Des Plaines, IL: Emergency Nurses Association.

Ignatavicius, D. & Workman, M. (2002). *Medical-surgical nursing: Critical thinking for collaborative care* (4th ed.). Philadelphia: W. B. Saunders.

Kee, J. (2001). *Handbook of laboratory and diagnostic tests with nursing implications.* (4th ed.). Upper Saddle River, NJ: Prentice-Hall, Inc.

Kidd, P. & Wagner, K. (2001). *High acuity nursing* (3rd ed.). Upper Saddle River, NJ: Prentice Hall, Inc.

Kozier, B., Erb., G., Berman, A., & Burke, K. (2003). *Fundamentals of nursing: Concepts, process, and practice* (7th ed.). Upper Saddle River, NJ: Prentice Hall, Inc.

Lehne, R.A. (2002). *Pharmacology for nursing care* (4th Ed.). Philadelphia: W.B. Saunders, Co.

LeMone, P. & Burke, K. (2003). *Medical-surgical nursing: Critical thinking in client care* (3rd ed.). Upper Saddle River, NJ: Prentice Hall, Inc.

Lewis, S. M., Heitkemper, M. M., & S. R. Dirksen. (2000). *Medical-surgical nursing: Assessment and management of clinical problems* (5th ed.). St. Louis, MO: Mosby, Inc.

McKenry, L. & Salerno, G. (2001). *Mosby's pharmacology in nursing* (21st ed.). St. Louis, MO: Mosby, Inc.

Newberry, L. (Ed) (1998). *Sheehy's emergency nursing principles and practice* (4th ed.). St. Louis, MO: Mosby-Year Book, Inc.

North American Nursing Diagnosis Association. (2001). *Nursing diagnosis: Definitions and classification 2001–2002.* Philadelphia: Author.

Phipps, W., Monahan, F., Sands, J., Marek, J., & Neighbors, M. (2003). *Medical-surgical nursing: Health and illness perspectives.* St. Louis, MO: Mosby.

Porth, C. (1998). *Pathophysiology: Concepts of altered health states* (5th ed.). Philadelphia: Lippincott.

Schell, H. M. & Puntillo, K. A. (2001). *Critical care nursing secrets.* Philadelphia: Hanley & Belfus, Inc.

Smith, S., Duell, D., & Martin, B. (2000). *Clinical nursing skills: Basic to advanced skills* (5th ed.). Upper Saddle River, NJ: Prentice Hall, Inc.

Swearinger, P. L. & Keen, J. H. (2001). *Critical care nursing: Nursing interventions and collaborative management* (4th ed.). St. Louis: Mosby, Inc.

Urden, L. D. & Stacy, K. M. (2000). *Priorities in critical care nursing* (3rd ed.). St. Louis, MO: Mosby, Inc.

Wilson, B., Shannon, M., & Stang, C. (2003). *Prentice Hall nursing drug guide 2003.* Upper Saddle River, NJ: Prentice Hall, Inc.

Youngkin, E., Sawin, K., Kissinger, J., & Israel, D. (1999). *Pharmacotherapeutics: A primary care guide.* Upper Saddle River, NJ: Prentice Hall, Inc.

Appendix

➤ Practice to Pass Suggested Answers

Chapter 1

Page 10: Solution—To increase the ability to obtain an accurate health history, the nurse should do the following:

1. Determine if the client uses any sensory aids such as a hearing aid, reads lips, utilizes sign language, communicates in writing, or uses a companion for communication purposes; and utilize those methods as much as possible.
2. Convey presence in the room by approaching from the front or by a gentle touch to the shoulders.
3. Face the client at all times and speak in a normal tone and amplitude of voice. Increased volume and exaggerated articulation can cause distortion and misinterpretation of information.
4. Validate all information.

Page 13: Solution—The questions should be directed to obtain the following information:
- When did the nausea begin (i.e., time, setting)?
- What were you doing at the time and what had you recently eaten?
- Is pain associated with the nausea and, if so, where is the pain located?
- If there is pain, does it radiate anywhere?
- Are there foods, medications, and activities that aggravate or alleviate the nausea?
- How disruptive is the nausea to your normal activities?

Page 15: Solution—In general, the physical examination should proceed as usual with the following exceptions. Inspection of the abdomen will include an assessment of the status of the incisional area (drainage, redness, approximation, etc.). Auscultation should be completed next since palpation and percussion can cause activation of bowel activity and distort assessment findings. Percussion and palpation should be done in all quadrants as usual; however, it is advisable to assess the area of an incisional wound or an area of discomfort at the end of the exam to prevent an extended period of discomfort.

Page 30: Solution—Coumadin is an oral anticoagulant that serves as an antagonist of vitamin K. Because it increases clotting time, it is essential that the PT be measured frequently. Usually clotting times with Coumadin are controlled at 1.5 to 2.0 times the normal clotting time of 10 to 13 seconds. It is important to remind the client to advise the physician of any changes in other medications and the use of any herbal remedies that may affect the client's clotting times. The client must also be advised to report any signs of bleeding to the physician immediately.

Page 33: Solution—The RPR test is a screening test for syphilis. A positive finding can be the result of syphilis; however, certain chronic diseases or exposure to many other diseases can also cause reactivity. Diseases such as TB, mononucleosis, chickenpox, smallpox, recent vaccinations, systemic lupus erythematosus, and pneumonia can cause reactivity of the test. Review with the client possible sexual history exposures and a history of any of the other identified diseases. The client should also be informed that the positive results can be verified with additional testing to eliminate false-positive results.

Chapter 2

Page 60: Solution—Ventilation and perfusion are gravity-dependent, so when the client is lying on one side, gravity accounts for greater ventilation and perfusion to the dependent lung. Since pneumonia produces excess secretions and possible obstructed airways, ventilation and perfusion will be optimized when the client is placed in a position with the good lung in a dependent position.

Page 60: Solution—Carbon dioxide level in the blood is a major stimulus for breathing. Clients with COPD retain carbon dioxide and typically have higher than normal blood levels of carbon dioxide and development of a hypoxic drive. Administration of high concentration of oxygen lowers or removes this stimulus for breathing. Initial oxygen supplementation for clients with suspected or known COPD should be low concentration, 1 to 2 L/min via nasal cannula to avoid respiratory depression or arrest.

Page 62: Solution—The priority for the client with a tracheostomy is maintenance of a patent airway. Equipment for suctioning, tracheostomy cannula, supplemental oxygen, and a call signal should be available at the client's bedside at all times. Additionally, a note should be placed near the call light console in the nurses' station indicating that the client cannot speak, and that calls must be answered in person.

Page 66: Solution—The main nursing measure to prevent recurrence of pneumothorax is to maintain water seal of the chest tube. This means that the chest tube should not be clamped. The physician should be notified immediately of a suspected obstruction of a chest tube such as might occur from a blood clot. Chest tubes should not be milked except by specific order for a specific reason, since this can cause tissue damage inside the chest.

Page 66: Solution—In the postoperative pneumonectomy client, positioning includes lying on the back and turning toward the operative side. The client may be turned temporarily slightly toward the non-operative side, but should not remain in this position. Turning the client with the operative side in the dependent position promotes desired consolidation of fluid in the pleural space previously occupied by the removed lung and prevents the heart and remaining lung from shifting into the operative side. The client should not be positioned in a completely lateral position on the operative side, however, to avoid shifting of mediastinal contents.

Page 67: Solution—Emphysema is a chronic disease with progressive destruction of alveoli and loss of alveolar area available for gas exchange. Paralysis of respiratory muscles, airway obstructions, and pleural effusion would diminish ventilatory capacity that could ultimately lead to decreased oxygen supply.

Page 71: Solution—The primary cause of chronic bronchitis is cigarette smoking, so smoking cessation is the priority lifestyle change to enhance wellness. Clients who utilize multiple approaches to smoking cessation, such as nicotine withdrawal medications and social support, are usually more successful at achieving and maintaining smoking cessation than those without a support system.

Page 75: Solution—Chylothorax is the abnormal accumulation of lymph fluid within the pleural cavity. Chylothorax can be caused inadvertently during a surgical procedure by disruption of lymph vessels. Disease or traumatic processes that erode into lymph vessels can also produce chylothorax. Clients with chy-

lothorax are unable to absorb lipids from the intestinal tract, so they may need intravenous administration of lipids to prevent fatty acid deficiency until the chylothorax is resolved.

Page 77: Solution—Tension pneumothorax is the accumulation of free air within the pleural cavity. When there is no mechanism for this air to escape into the atmosphere, the pressure caused by this air continues to increase. Increasing pressure on the great vessels within the chest can progress until the vessels actually collapse and interrupt blood supply to the heart and lungs, thereby causing the clinical condition known as cardiovascular collapse. This condition is life-threatening within a few seconds to a few minutes.

Page 79: Solution—The primary cause of atelectasis is diminished breathing activity such as occurs with anesthesia or immobility. The easiest maneuver to prevent atelectasis is to encourage, teach, and assist the client to cough and deep breathe frequently (every hour). Enhancing mobility as soon as feasible is also beneficial in preventing atelectasis.

Page 81: Solution—

	Bacterial	*Viral*
Temp	High	Normal or low-grade
Cough	Productive	Nonproductive
Chest x-ray	Diffuse infiltrates	Often normal
Clinical course	More severe	Less severe

Page 83: Solution—Antibiotic prophylaxis for individuals exposed to clients with active disease includes Isoniazid as the drug of choice for 6 months if there is no clinical evidence of disease. Among clients with an abnormal chest x-ray, or high-risk population such as clients with HIV or drug-induced immunosuppression, Isoniazid is the drug of choice for 12 months.

Page 86: Solution—The primary cause of pulmonary emboli is immobility. Therefore, optimizing mobility as soon as feasible is beneficial. Among clients who are immobilized due to severe illness, the use of passive range of motion, antiembolism devices, and anticoagulation may be indicated to prevent pulmonary emboli.

Chapter 3

Page 110: Solution—A priority for a client with new atrial fibrillation is the prevention of thrombus formation due to blood pooling in the atria. The client should be instructed to report calf tenderness or pain and not to massage the calf. If warfarin (Coumadin) is prescribed, instruct the client about the importance of getting blood tests for prothrombin time (PT) and INR at regular intervals, and not to vary the amount of vitamin K–rich foods in the diet (green leafy vegetables), because vitamin K decreases the effectiveness of warfarin (Coumadin).

Page 119: Solution—The nurse assessing a client for signs of MI should make frequent assessments of the level and type of client's pain, continuous ECG monitoring for dysrhythmias or ST elevations, blood pressure and pulse, oxygen saturation, and cardiac enzymes levels.

Page 121: Solution—The nurse should explain that although frequent urination poses difficulties, diuretic therapy is essential in preventing fluid overload on the heart and preventing acute episodes of heart failure. The nurse should work with the client to determine a diuretic schedule for the client that maintains the prescribed dosage at a time of the day that allows optimal activity.

Page 122: Solution—The nurse should explain that once a client has SBE, he or she has increased risk for repeat infections. In order to prevent future episodes, the client needs to be taught symptoms to report to the physician, and always remember to obtain a prescription for prophylactic antibiotics prior to invasive procedures including all dental work.

Page 125: Solution—The client who is taking warfarin (Coumadin) for valve repair should receive an explanation that this therapy will be a lifelong treatment. The nurse should explain the routine management of warfarin (Coumadin) therapy including blood tests for prothrombin time (PT) and INR. Dietary teaching regarding the high vitamin K content of green leafy vegetables should be included. Inconsistent intake of these foods reduces the effect of warfarin and can alter the effectiveness of the anticoagulant therapy.

Page 126: Solution—Restrictive cardiomyopathy is associated with right-sided failure, and the nurse would expect to see peripheral edema and possible abdominal tenderness or ascites.

Page 128: Solution—Cardiac tamponade is a serious complication of pericarditis. The nurse would expect to see jugular venous distention (JVD) with clear lungs, high CVP, narrowing pulse pressure, decreased BP or urine output (signs of decreased cardiac output), and muffled heart sounds.

Chapter 4

Page 143: Solution—The DASH (Dietary Approaches to Stop Hypertension) diet is based on findings of several research studies that demonstrated lowered blood pressure through dietary modification. The diet is rich in fruits and vegetables and low in saturated and total fat. The DASH eating plan is based on a 2,000-calorie diet, although it can be modified if weight loss is also required. The client must be reminded to center the meal around carbohydrates, such as pasta, rice, beans, or vegetables. Meat is part of the meal, not the focus. The DASH diet should be used in combination with foods lower in salt, keeping a healthy weight, being physically active, and engaging in smoking cessation and stress reduction behaviors.

Page 149: Solution—Explain to the client that angiography allows for visualization of arteries to determine if there is occlusion or an aneurysm present. A local anesthetic will be used, so minimal discomfort will be felt. A catheter will be inserted, usually into the femoral artery, although a subclavian, axillary,

brachial, or translumbar approach may be used. Contrast dye will be injected and then serial x-rays will be taken. After the catheter is removed, direct pressure is placed on the site. Nursing implications include:

- Assess for bleeding
  - Bed rest for several hours post-procedure
  - Assess puncture site frequently and remind client to report any wetness, warmth or pressure at the site
  - Conduct neurovascular checks q 1 to 2 h on the extremities
- Assess for embolism
  - Neurovascular checks of both extremities q 1 to 2 h. Have client report any feelings of pain, numbness, coolness, or tingling of the feet immediately
  - Administer anticoagulants as ordered
- Assess for pseudoaneurysm
  - Observe puncture site for pulsatile mass
  - Neurovascular checks of lower extremities q 1 to 2 h

Page 151: Solution—Arterial thrombosis is usually due to arterial obstruction from a blood clot that formed *within* an artery damaged by atherosclerosis. An embolus is a clot that has traveled—the wall of the artery may be healthy and the thrombus most likely originated from the heart. Most of these emboli lodge in the legs with a small percentage lodging in the arms.

Surgical management of arterial thrombosis usually involves revascularization of the extremity by bypass grafting. Arterial emboli may be removed by an embolectomy. Emboli and thrombi may be treated medically with thrombolytic agents if ischemia is not present.

Page 155: Solution—Monitor graft site and report any signs of possible leakage evidenced by:

- decreased CVP, pulmonary artery pressure or pulmonary artery wedge pressure
- oliguria (output less than 30 mL/hr)
- ecchymoses of the scrotum or perineum
- new or enlargement of incision site hematoma
- increasing abdominal girth
- diminishing/absent peripheral pulses
- decreasing blood pressure and increasing pulse
- sudden pain in the abdomen, back, or groin

Prevent hemovolemic shock by:

- administering IV fluids as ordered
- recording accurate intake and output
- assessing blood pressure, pulse, and level of consciousness
- monitoring incision site and assessing for graft leakage
- monitoring lab values

Page 156: Solution—Your client is most likely experiencing a pulmonary embolism. Most pulmonary emboli arise from clots in the legs. Symptoms include dyspnea, tachpnea, tachycardia, cough, chest pain, fever, and hypoxia.

Nursing interventions include:

- apply oxygen immediately
- assess pulse oximetry to determine oxygen saturation
- call physician and report findings

* establish an IV line if not present
* maintain bedrest
* encourage cough and deep-breathing exercises to prevent atelectasis
* prepare client for a lung scan
* provide preoperative teaching for an embolectomy if pulmonary artery obstruction is greater than 50 percent

Page 161: Solution—The pain of varicose veins is due to prolonged interruption of blood flow back to the heart and pooling of blood in the lower extremity. This poor blood flow and pooling deprives the tissues of oxygen and nutrients, which results in pain. Over time, tissue necrosis and ulceration may occur.

Chapter 5

Page 177: Solution—Acute confusion and chronic confusion differ in a number of ways:

* Onset: acute confusion begins abruptly over hours to days, while chronic confusion develops slowly over a number of years.
* Memory: acute confusion results in limited immediate and recent memory, while chronic confusion can affect recent and remote memory.
* Timing: in acute confusion, alertness can fluctuate during the day and often occurs at night; in chronic confusion, there is no cycling that coincides with the time of day or night.
* Awareness: acute confusion presents with decreased alertness and awareness that is interspersed with lucid intervals; in chronic confusion there is no change in level of consciousness.
* Attention: acute confusion limits the client's attention, while chronic confusion does not.
* Language: acute confusion often leads to incoherent speech because of disorganized thinking, while chronic confusion often leads to aphasia.
* Perception: acute confusion can be marked by hallucinations, dreams, and vivid but frightening misperceptions, while chronic confusion is not marked by hallucinations until late in the disease process.
* Sleep cycle: acute confusion disturbs and may even reverse a client's sleep-wake cycle, while in chronic confusion, sleep may be interrupted but is not characterized by reversal in the day/night cycle.

Page 188: Solution—Signs of meningitis include the following:

* Restlessness, agitation, and irritability
* Abdominal and back pain
* Nausea and vomiting
* Severe headaches
* Signs of meningeal irritation, nuchal rigidity (stiff neck), Brudzinski's sign (pain, resistance and hip and knee flexion occur with flexion of the neck to the chest in the supine position) and Kernig's sign (pain and/or resistance occurs with flexion of the knee and hip and straightening of the knee in the supine position) and photophobia

* Chills and high fever
* Confusion, altered LOC
* Seizures
* Signs and symptoms of increasing ICP

Page 192: Solution—While supportive nursing care is similar for clients who have had a stroke or CVA, the differences can be attributed to the pathophysiology of the stroke. In hemorrhagic CVA, bleeding into the ventricles or brain tissue has occurred, resulting in a subarachnoid hemorrhage or an intracerebral bleed. In these clients, it is important to ensure that rebleeding does not occur, making it important to institute subarachnoid or aneurysm precautions, which limit environmental and physiological stimuli. It is also important to recognize or prevent blood vessel spasm in the area of the bleed, which can trigger a rebleed. In contrast, a client with an ischemic stroke has suffered either thrombus formation or embolus. In these cases, the client may be treated with a thrombolytic agent to dissolve the clot, or may at least be given heparin, an anticoagulant, to prevent propagation of existing thrombus. These clients need the typical precautions used with any client receiving anticoagulant therapy.

Page 194: Solution—The client is likely to have need for physical therapy, occupational therapy, a medical social worker, nursing staff, and possibly a psychologist and a vocational counselor.

Page 198: Solution—

* This medication may cause drowsiness or dizziness, so tasks requiring alertness should be avoided until medication response is known.
* Carry medical identification stating disorder and the name of anticonvulsant used.
* Take exactly as prescribed; call prescriber if doses are missed for 2 consecutive days; if one dose is missed, take within 4 hours if multiple doses are taken each day, or when remembered when once daily dosing is done (time of regular administration may need to be changed).
* Avoid using OTC products or alcohol while taking phenytoin.
* See dentist regularly for cleanings to prevent gingival hyperplasia, gum tenderness, or bleeding.
* Do not switch brands of medication; bioavailability may be different.
* Phenytoin may change the color of urine to pink, red, or reddish brown, but this is insignificant.
* Do not take medication within 3 hours of antacids or 2 hours of antidiarrheals for best absorption.
* Use an additional nonhormonal contraceptive method (females) while taking phenytoin; notify prescriber if pregnant or plan to become pregnant.

Chapter 6

Page 234: Solution—The client may be having urinary retention with overflow. Since urine stasis becomes a good medium for bacterial growth, the client is at risk for developing urinary tract infection. In addition, decreased urinary output may also indicate other medical conditions such as dehydration. The client should be advised that an evaluation by a healthcare practitioner is necessary.

Page 236: Solution—The involuntary flow of urine from the bladder is incontinence. This client describes stress incontinence, an incontinence characterized by incompetence of the bladder outlet allowing for urine to escape involuntarily. The involuntary escape of urine is caused by increased intra-abdominal pressure, which occurs with laughing, sneezing, coughing, lifting, or Valsalva maneuver. This client should be advised to see a urologist because pharmacologic and surgical intervention, such as a vesicourethropexy, have successfully improved the lives of clients with stress incontinence.

Page 236: Solution—Anatomical differences between females and males predispose females to urinary tract infections. The female has a shorter urethra and lacks prostatic fluid that can protect her from urinary tract infections. In addition, the anatomical proximity of the urethra to the vagina and rectum predisposes the female to migration of bacteria from those orifices. Since *Escherichia coli* is the most frequent source of UTI infection, it underscores the necessity for good hygiene practices. Tissue trauma during sexual intercourse may also predispose the female to higher incidence of urinary tract infections.

Page 242: Solution—Many medical conditions and diseases can cause hematuria or blood in the urine. What the client describes in this case is gross hematuria. Blood may also be present in the urine without the individual noticing it and may be observed with microscopic analysis. Any client with hematuria should seek evaluation from a healthcare provider. Since hematuria is the most frequent sign of renal cancer and tumors of the urinary tract, early diagnosis and intervention is vital.

Page 244: Solution—Since fluid retention is common in glomerulonephritis, sodium restriction should be included in the teaching plan. The client should be taught to check labels on food products to ascertain the amount of sodium in them. A low-protein diet is also instituted particularly when there is elevation of BUN and creatinine levels. A high-carbohydrate, high-calorie diet is necessary to prevent utilization and breakdown of protein stores. Collaboration with the dietician for detailed meal planning should also be sought.

Chapter 7

Page 264: Solution—The client should be instructed to keep the temperature of the room air cool (68 to 70°F) with the humidity maintained at 30 to 40 percent. Itching may be relieved by taking a cool or tepid bath containing colloidal substances such as oatmeal, cornstarch, or soybean powder. Emollient lotions should be used rather than lotions containing alcohol, which can dry the skin.

Page 272: Solution—There are several types of viral hepatitis. Transmission for hepatitis A is through the fecal-oral route. For example, people who have hepatitis A may transmit it to others if they do not wash their hands well after using the toilet and then handle food. Hepatitis A is also transmitted in seafood harvested from contaminated water or food eaten raw that has been washed in contaminated water. It may be transmitted sexually by oral contact with the rectum of a contaminated individual. Hepatitis B, C, and D are transmitted through contact with blood and blood products of individuals with the disease. It is also transmitted sexually, and the hepatitis B virus has been found in saliva, semen, urine, feces, and other body fluids. Hepatitis C is found in blood and semen, but most people with hepatitis C have no known risk factors.

Page 279: Solution—The client's vital signs are taken every 15 minutes for an hour, every 30 minutes for an hour, every hour for 2 hours, every 4 hours four times and then every 6 hours thereafter. The nurse should observe the dressing for oozing on the same schedule as the vital signs. Direct pressure should be applied to the biopsy site directly after the procedure, and the client is positioned on the right side. The client is usually kept on bedrest for 24 hours and can resume fluids 2 hours after the procedure. Anything that increases intra-abdominal pressure should be avoided for 1 to 2 weeks (coughing, lifting, straining).

Page 282: Solution—The purpose of lactulose is ultimately to reduce the ammonia level. It is a disaccharide laxative that is not absorbed by the GI tract and pulls water into the bowel, causing diarrhea and preventing the absorption of ammonia.

Page 287: Solution—The client with cholelithiasis should be instructed to eat small, frequent, low-fat meals. The obese client should be encouraged to lose weight, but the client should be cautioned against very rapid weight loss with an extreme calorie restriction since this increases the risk for developing gallstones.

Page 289: Solution—The client should be monitored for the level of pain, and pain should be treated before it becomes too intense. Vital signs should be taken at least every 4 hours and the client should be monitored for signs of peritonitis. The incision should be kept clean and dry and monitored for bleeding and drainage. To prevent pulmonary infection the client should be encouraged to use the incentive spirometer every hour and cough and deep-breathe at least every 2 hours.

Chapter 8

Page 306: Solution—Because there is radiation involved in this diagnostic test, all women of childbearing age should be asked if they are or could be pregnant. During the procedure, the client is placed in the CAT scan machine, which is just slightly larger than the body; therefore, anyone with claustrophobia may have difficulty completing this test. All clients should be asked if they have claustrophobia before the test. Some CAT scans are performed using a contrast medium containing iodine so the client should be questioned about allergy to shellfish or iodine.

Page 308: Solution—Each step of the procedure should be explained to the client so that the level of anxiety can be minimized. The client is placed in a high-Fowler's position. The tube is measured from the tip of the nose to the ear and down to the xyphoid process and marked at this place. The tube is inserted through the nose with the client's head bent slightly forward, which helps to close the epiglottis and promotes movement of the tube into the esophagus rather than the trachea. The client is asked to swallow or sip water during insertion for this reason as well. Once the predetermined mark is reached, the tube is taped to the nose. Placement is checked by instilling 10 to 20 mL of air into the tube and auscultating for the flow of air "burp" in the left upper quadrant.

Page 312: Solution—Initial assessment of the postoperative colostomy client includes vital signs, lung sounds, bowel sounds, intake and output, level of consciousness, level of pain, and drainage from any tubes and drains. The incision should be assessed for drainage, wound approximation, and signs of infection. Of particular importance is a thorough assessment of the stoma. The stoma should be red or pinkish red and shiny. A stoma that appears dark, purplish red, or blue may be ischemic and should be reported to the surgeon immediately. Drainage from the stoma is typically bloody and scant immediately post-op. The drainage will increase as the client begins to take fluids, but should not contain blood.

Page 320: Solution—Barrett's epithelium is the body's way of compensating for chronic exposure of the esophagus to gastric juice. The normal squamous epithelium in the distal portion of the esophagus is replaced with columnar epithelium, also called Barrett's epithelium. This columnar epithelium is more resistant to gastric acid and actually supports healing of the chronic inflammation. The one disadvantage is that this type of cell is a premalignant tissue and the client with Barrett's epithelium has an increased risk of developing cancer of the esophagus, and therefore, needs periodic follow-up and testing.

Page 323: Solution—Peptic ulcer is a generic term for ulceration of tissue in the GI tract that comes in contact with gastric juice. The most common locations are the stomach and duodenum. Gastric ulcers are not necessarily caused by increased gastric acid secretion as are duodenal ulcers, but rather, are caused from a disruption of the normal gastric mucosal protective barrier, which prevents the diffusion of acid back across the membrane. Gastric ulcers also involve an area of gastritis surrounding the ulcer crater, and duodenal ulcers do not have this feature. Prostaglandins produced in the gastric mucosa increase the resistance of the mucosa to the effects of acid. Drugs that inhibit prostaglandins, such as aspirin and NSAIDs, contribute to gastric ulcer formation.

Chapter 9

Page 341: Solution—The client should be told that he will be in a cylinder-like tube and that he will need to be still for the procedure to be completed. There is a possibility that a contrast medium might be used. If so, the physician will inform him and will ask him about allergies.

Page 341: Solution—MRI is contraindicated in any client who has a metal implant of any type such as a pacemaker, prosthetic, or surgical clip. Clients with a history of claustrophobia might

have difficulty in some MRI machines that enclose them in the diagnostic imaging machine. Clients who are unstable, or who require intravenous pumps, are not good candidates for an MRI procedure.

Page 351: Solution—The risk factors associated with osteoporosis that are appropriate to include in teaching this client are inadequate dietary intake of calcium, sedentary lifestyle, smoking, and excessive alcohol intake. All these factors involve lifestyle modifications that can prevent the disease.

Page 359: Solution—Priority interventions include:

1. Immobilize the fracture by the application of a splint.
2. Assess neurovascular status. Check for the pulse distal to the injury. Evaluate for the presence of paresthesia, inability to move the toes, coolness of the distale extremity, or delayed capillary refill. The tibial artery and/or the peroneal nerve may have been damaged by the injury and can cause neurovascular deficits.
3. Cover the skin opening with a sterile dressing.
4. Assess for signs of hemorrhage and shock.

Page 364: Solution—Gout is characterized by elevated serum uric acid level. When serum uric acid levels increase, monosodium urate crystals form in tissues of the body. This initiates the inflammatory response that causes the pain of gout. Probenecid (Benemid) is a uricosuric drug. This drug acts by blocking the tubular reabsorption of urate and promotes elimination of uric acid through the kidneys.

Chapter 10

Page 384: Solution—Evaluation of the mole should include the ABCD (Assymetry, Border, Color, Diameter) method of evaluation. Encourage monthly evaluation of the skin, especially new moles that may be changing. If concerned about any changes in moles, the client should consult the healthcare provider for further evaluation.

Page 385: Solution—Encourage skin protection with the use of sunscreen with an SPF 15 or greater when outdoors. Using clothing for skin protection along with a hat is recommended. Also avoid peak sun hours when the rays are strongest between the hours of 10:00 A.M. and 2:00 P.M. Encourage clients to monitor the skin monthly with skin checks, using the ABCD method to evaluate any moles or skin lesions.

Page 386: Solution—Methods used to prevent spreading impetigo include good handwashing, keeping hands away from the lesions, not sharing drinks or straws, no kissing or allowing anyone to touch the lesions. Inform contacts regarding the infection to encourage all children to use good preventive measures from contacting impetigo.

Page 389: Solution—Discuss with the client that herpes virus remains in the body for life. The virus may lay dormant for long periods of time. The fact that she has not had any lesions for several years does not mean that the virus has disappeared. She still has the virus and the lesion she has today could possibly be a genital herpes lesion. The virus can be reactivated at any time and then present with active lesions. Things that cause reactivation of the virus include illness and stress. However, she needs to have the lesion evaluated today.

Page 390: Solution—Warts are caused by a virus that remains in the body for life, and the virus can be reactivated at any time. Even removal of the wart with treatments such as over-the-counter products and cryotherapy is not a guarantee that the wart will not reappear at a later date. Recommend to the client that there are options for removal, such as cryotherapy, however the wart may still reappear at a later time or place. Even if no treatment is applied to the wart, the likelihood of the wart resolving on its own within 6 to 12 months is likely.

Chapter 11

Page 423: Solution—Immunizations provide a client with artificial natural immunity that offers protection against specific diseases. The antigen is introduced to the client through vaccination (injection) and then the client develops antibodies to the specific antigens to afford protection. If a client is "up to date" on the immunization schedule, the body will have enough serum antibody levels to maintain protection against specific disease processes.

Page 426: Solution—It is important to assess and monitor the client for a potential allergic reaction (Type 1 hypersensitivity). The basic concepts of ABC (airway, breathing, and circulation) are of critical importance. It is also important to determine whether the client has a history of having this type of reaction before, other allergic reactions associated with food and medication, and any other pertinent medical conditions that might affect the individual. If there is a positive client history, the client may already have an EpiPen in his or her possession and may have to utilize the device as directed by the prescribing physician. Removal of the offending agent is required and the client should not be allowed to eat further strawberries even if the breathing pattern returns to normal.

Page 440: Solution—The concept of autoimmune disease involves a chronic condition with acute exacerbations and remissions. Autoimmunity involves the body's inability to maintain normal lines of defense and reaction by not recognizing one's "self." This can lead to an overactive immune response where the body develops autoantibodies that can lead to organ and system damage.

Page 441: Solution—Genetic counseling can provide a framework to identify specific etiologies for primary immunodeficiency disorders. This can be helpful to clients in the childbearing years and for family members to become aware of potential genetic traits that can be passed on to family members. This allows the client to be informed and promotes client advocacy.

Page 443: Solution—An ANC of 500 indicates that the client is severely immunosuppressed and neutropenic precautions should be instituted. The client should be placed on reverse isolation and the ANC level should be monitored to see if immune system function returns. Medication therapy such as colony-stimulating factors may be used to boost the immune response. A neutropenic diet

should be instituted for the client. Client, staff, and family members must be made aware of and educated regarding these precautions and they should be maintained until the ANC count raises to an acceptable level as determined by the physician.

Page 445: Solution—Megace is being prescribed for its effect to be an appetite stimulant and to promote weight gain. Even though it is considered a female hormone, it does provide this effect and is used in many disease states where weight loss and decreased appetite has become a problem.

Page 447: Solution—The vast number of medications used to control this disease can certainly cause one to feel like "there is no way to comply," but each prescribed medication provides a specific function. The medications are aimed at working together to provide the best therapeutic response in the hopes of decreasing symptoms, decreasing viral load, and promoting the immune response.

Page 448: Solution—Contact precautions relate to the prevention of spread of diseases through direct contact. Bodily fluids such as emesis, drainage, and diarrhea may spread these diseases. Measures include basic handwashing, use of gloves when providing client contact, and proper handling and disposal of bodily fluids in separate identified biohazard containers. A sign should be placed on the client's door indicating to staff and visitors that certain precautions will be instituted when entering the client's room. Additional teaching may be required for visitors who are not familiar with these types of precautions. Cultures of body specimens may be required to identify specific infection and help establish therapeutic management.

Chapter 12

Page 467: Solution—First, recognize that cancer causes fear and anxiety in the client and psychosocial support should be ongoing. Acknowledge the client's fears and concerns and encourage expression of concerns. He may be responding to misconceptions told to him by others ("My mother had radiation and no one could get closer than 6 feet to her."). Teach the client about external radiation, and tell him that there is no risk of harm or exposure to radiation to his son or others coming in contact with him.

Page 473: Solution—Recall that the client with a decreased platelet count (thrombocytopenia) is at risk for bleeding. Precautions to prevent bleeding include avoiding intramuscular injections and monitoring intravenous site at least every 2 hours. Other interventions include monitoring stool, urine, and vomitus for blood, posting a bleeding precaution sign on the door to the client's room, and teaching client measures to prevent bleeding. The decreased leukocyte count places the client at high risk for infection. Interventions include placing client in private room, instituting protective isolation, maintaining strict aseptic technique, screening visitors for infection, avoiding raw fruits and vegetables, and teaching the client measures to prevent infection.

Page 474: Solution—The client is experiencing stomatitis, a common side effect of chemotherapy and radiation. Interventions include teaching client proper oral care, using a soft toothbrush, avoiding mouthwashes, and rinsing mouth with water or saline frequently. Because the ulcerations are painful and interfering with nutritional intake, the client may benefit from viscous lidocaine to rinse mouth with; teach client not to swallow xylocaine. To manage nausea, round-the-clock antiemetics may be necessary. Teach client dietary habits to help reduce diarrhea. Encourage client to eat small, frequent meals, as these may be tolerated easier. Since the client is at risk for inadequate nutrition, suggest maintaining a food diary to record daily intake of food and fluid.

Page 475: Solution—Severe pain at the infusion site can indicate of infiltration. Discontinue the infusion immediately. If the chemotherapeutic agent is a vesicant, proceed with the protocol for infiltration of that agent and inform the oncologist for specific actions to be taken. Assess the intravenous site, document the infiltration, actions taken, appearance of the site, and provide written and oral instructions to client.

Page 478: Solution—Early symptoms of spinal cord compression include progressive back and leg pain and numbness. Because of the potential for irreversible paraplegia, spinal cord compression is considered an oncological emergency. Assessment includes a thorough investigation of all complaints of back pain and neurological changes. The physician should be notified immediately if spinal cord compression is suspected.

Chapter 13

Page 493: Solution—The treatment goal in a client with SIADH is to restore normal fluid volume and serum osmolality. The client should be taught that excess ADH causes volume expansion and dilutional hyponatremia. The ingestion of too much fluid will therefore aggravate the serum hypo-osmolality and hyponatremia. Limiting fluids to 1000 mL per day will aid in the normalization of serum sodium. The client can be taught to decrease thirst by using of ice chips and hard candy to blunt the thirst sensation.

Page 498: Solution—The treatment of Graves' disease does not reverse the changes associated with exophthalmos. Thus the client needs to know how to protect the eyes from injury, prevent infection and promote comfort and visual acuity.

Page 501: Solution—Low levels of thyroid hormone associated with hypothyroidism cause altered lipid metabolism, leading to elevated serum triglyceride and cholesterol levels, and thereby increasing the risk for atherosclerosis and cardiovascular disease. In hypothyroidism constipation results from decreased gastrointestinal motility, peristalsis, and the reduced physical activity associated with low thyroid hormone induced fatigue.

Page 505: Solution—The body needs a therapeutic level of glucocorticoids to maintain fluid and electrolyte balance. If the medication is going to be stopped or dose decreased it need to be done gradually. A sudden decrease in the amount or sudden stopping of the medication does not allow the adrenal gland to begin functioning to produce glucocorticoid. When people take additional glucocorticoid medication to treat a condition, the adrenal

gland slows down or may stop its own production of the glucocorticoid as a negative feedback mechanism.

Page 512: Solution—Insulin availability at the beginning of exercise affects the body's response. During exercise the muscles get energy from the breakdown of muscle glycogen and liver production of glucose. During prolonged exercise fatty acids are broken down for energy. If there is an insufficient amount of insulin during exercise, the glucose produced by the body cannot be used by the muscles. The glucose accumulates in the body, causing hyperglycemia, and forces the muscles to use fatty acids for energy, causing ketosis. Hypoglycemia can occur 6 to 15 hours up to 24 hours after sustained high intensity exercise. Hyperglycemia can occur and last for several hours following exercise. Regular moderate exercise improves glucose control for the patient with diabetes, improves glucose clearance, lowers insulin requirements, and promotes weight loss. Prior to exercise the client should check his fasting blood glucose level, and if it is greater than 250 mg/dL he should check his urine for ketones. Ketones in the urine are a contraindication for exercise indicating that fatty acids are currently broken down for energy and there is insufficient insulin present.

Chapter 14

Page 529: Solution—The nurse should make sure that a signed consent has been completed. The nurse explains to the client about the procedure. Instructions should be given about not moving during the procedure. After the bone marrow biopsy has been completed, the nurse should apply a sterile pressure dressing on the puncture site. Direct pressure should be applied for at least 5 minutes. The direct pressure required might be longer in cases where the client has thrombocytopenia. Periodic checks to monitor for evidence of bleeding should be continued up to 4 hours after the procedure.

Page 530: Solution—If an immediate IV access cannot be established within 20 minutes, then the unit of blood should be returned to the blood bank. Unused blood may not be refrigerated in other areas except in the blood bank.

Page 531: Solution—The chills may be a sign of a transfusion reaction and therefore the nurse has to implement the specific protocol of the agency or setting in which this occurred. The blood transfusion should be discontinued immediately. The blood product and the IV tubing are disconnected from the IV access site. New IV tubing and normal saline will be initiated to keep the IV line open. The client will be assessed for other signs of reactions and to evaluate vital signs. The physician and the blood bank will be notified of this reaction and established protocol will be followed. Throughout this process the nurse establishes intensive monitoring of the client, and emergency interventions are provided as they arise.

Page 537: Solution—Folic acid anemia is most likely to occur in individuals who are undernourished. This group includes the elderly, alcoholics, and those with substance abuse. Alcoholics usually develop this type of anemia because alcohol interferes with the metabolism of folic acid. In addition to this group, other individuals who might be susceptible to folic acid deficiency anemia are those with high metabolic requirements, including those who are pregnant, infants, and teenagers. Additional factors to the development of this anemia are certain medications, hemodialysis, and total parenteral nutrition supplementation.

Page 541: Solution—An individual with sickle cell trait is heterozygous, with one-fourth of the hemoglobin in the S form. Sickle cell anemia is an autosomal recessive genetic disorder that results from the inheritance of the sickle cell hemoglobin gene. If an individual who has sickle cell trait has a child with another with the trait, there is 25 percent likelihood that a child may inherit two abnormal genes and thus will develop the disease.

Chapter 15

Page 576: Solution—The client receiving continuous bladder irrigation (CBI) who develops bladder spasms should be assessed to determine the cause. One of the most common causes of spasms is urinary drainage tubing that is kinked or blocked (by the client's leg, position, etc.), and this should be checked first. Another cause is the size of the balloon at the tip of the catheter. The pressure exerted by the balloon on the bladder and the straining to attempt to void "against" the catheter causes the spasms. In addition, blood clots and bleeding can cause the spasms. If the discomfort is due to the pressure of the balloon and straining, then pain medication, including antispasmodics, should be given as prescribed. The client should also be instructed to avoid straining. If the spasms are caused by blood clot formation and urinary catheter obstruction, then increasing the instillation flow of the CBI or manual irrigations of the bladder should be performed.

Page 582: Solution—Mumps could lead to orchitis, which results in a reduced sperm count in about half of the men affected. Many organisms can cause orchitis including viruses, bacteria, parasites, and fungi.

Page 584: Solution—The client should be instructed to use condoms in the future and to avoid sexual intercourse until all sexual partners have been examined and treated. Sexually transmitted disease is the most common factor in causing the disorder in younger men. In older men, the most common etiology is urinary tract infection or prostatitis.

Page 586: Solution—Males between the ages of 15 and 40 are more likely to develop a varicocele. The major complication in this disorder is that varicocele could cause testicular atrophy, resulting in infertility, or it could cause diminished sperm count (the major complication).

Page 588: Solution—Testicular torsion or twisting of the testes and spermatic cord is a potential medical emergency because compromised blood flow may lead to testicular ischemia and necrosis. Detorsion of the testicle and fixation to the scrotum is performed immediately to prevent the necrosis from occurring.

Page 590: Solution—Testicular cancer, the most common cancer in men between the ages of 15 and 35, has a cure rate of 90% to date.

Page 592: Solution—The classic symptoms of an enlarged prostate gland include difficulty starting and stopping urinary stream, overflow dribbling, and urinary frequency. Narrowing of the prostatic urethra cause all these symptoms.

Page 599: Solution—Client education is very important in treating clients with syphilis to prevent recurrence of the disease and to prevent infection of the client's sexual partner. Sexually transmitted diseases, including syphilis, are common in individuals who lack motivation for seeking early treatment, which underscores the importance of education to help in arresting the spread of the disease.

Page 601: Solution—The client should be informed that there is no cure for herpes. This disease has a latency period however, which is characterized by the virus laying dormant into nerve fibers until its recurrence. During this stage, there may be no symptoms but is not an indication that the condition has been cured.

Page 603: Solution—Genital warts are caused by human papilloma virus (HPV) and are transmitted by all types of sexual contact.

Page 605: Solution—Chlamydia, which is the most common sexually transmitted disease in the United States, is difficult to diagnose based on physical examination alone because most clients are asymptomatic. Female clients seek consultation when the infection has invaded the uterus and uterine tubes causing acute symptoms. Nearly a third of men with the infection remain asymptomatic.

Chapter 16

Page 637: Solution—There are no symptoms in the early stages of glaucoma. This disorder is characterized by a loss of peripheral vision that is so gradual it is virtually unnoticeable to the person affected. The vision that is lost, however, cannot be regained. The condition can lead eventually to blindness unless eye medications are taken daily for life, and periodic eye exams are done to monitor intraocular pressure and disease progression.

Page 644: Solution—The client's reported symptom is a classic finding with detached retina. The nurse should question the client about other manifestations, such as the presence of floating spots (floaters), flashing lights, blurring of vision, visual field deficits, and presence of pain (detached retina is painless). Immediate interventions are to:

- Protect the eye from further damage (bedrest, cover both eyes with eye patches)
- Instruct the client not to bend forward or make sudden or jerking head movements
- Position the client with detached area dependent/inferior as ordered
- Protect the client from injury by keeping the bed low, side rails up, call bell within reach, and assisting with care
- Reinforce explanations about surgical repair
- Provide psychological support to alleviate anxiety

Page 648: Solution—Use the bed as a reference point to orient the client to the room and the bedside area. Using the face of a clock as an analogy, describe the location of different parts of the room in terms of where they are located on the clock face, such as "When you are lying in bed, the bathroom is at 3 o'clock in reference to you." Point out and demonstrate the use of the call bell for the client, and have the client practice to ensure it can be used when needed. Also point out controls for radio and TV to provide diversion. Encourage the client to call for assistance before getting out of bed to prevent injury, and check on the client often.

Page 654: Solution—Instruct the client to:

- Keep the outer ear dressing clean and dry
- Avoid activities that increase middle ear pressure, such as blowing nose, sneezing, coughing, straining; if necessary, cough or sneeze with mouth open; blow nose one nostril at a time with mouth open
- Avoid drinking through a straw for 2 to 3 weeks and avoid air travel until allowed by surgeon
- Prevent constipation by increasing fluids and fiber and maintain mobility
- Do not shower or shampoo hair until allowed by surgeon, and no swimming or diving until fully healed
- Take medications as ordered and report persistent postoperative headache, increased drainage or bleeding from site, fever, new or increased ear pain or dizziness, or decreasing hearing to the surgeon.

Page 655: Solution—Otosclerosis leads to conductive hearing loss. It is a hereditary disorder of the labyrinthine capsule, in which abnormal bone growth occurs around the ossicles and causes stiffening or fixation of the stapes bone. Surgical correction may be needed. To enhance communication, the following should be done:

- Approach the client from within the client's line of vision or tap the client lightly on the shoulder to get attention before beginning to speak

- Reduce background noise, such as radio or TV, before beginning to speak
- Avoid covering mouth with hands or other objects while speaking
- Face the client and speak slowly and clearly—pronounce words clearly without over-articulating them; speak using low-pitch and normal loudness
- Use nonverbal cues and written messages to enhance communication
- Repeat sentences using different words if client has difficulty understanding
- Ask client to repeat directions or teaching that was done to ensure the client's understanding

Chapter 17

Page 673: Solution—The goals for the care of the client with multiple contiguous fractured ribs would be to:

1. Ensure ABCs.
2. Maintain an effective breathing pattern; mechanical ventilation may be necessary.
3. Achieve pain control.
4. Maintain hemodynamic stability.

Page 698: Solution—The preferred placement for an arterial line would be the radial artery. Other sites that can be used would be the femoral and brachial arteries.

Page 711: Solution—The primary areas of concern for shock are maintenance of adequate oxygenation, adequate cardiac output and tissue perfusion, and resolution of underlying cause.

Page 715: Solution—No spontaneous respirations and/or no palpable pulse are indications for cardiopulmonary circulation.

Page 719: Solution—Immediate, definitive care would be defibrillation (for a total of three shocks if needed at joules of 200, 300, and 360 shocks). If no defibrillator is available, call for assistance and begin CPR until a defibrillator is available.

➤ *Case Study Suggested Answers*

Chapter 1

1. The questions should be directed to obtain the following information:
   - When did the abdominal pain, nausea and vomiting start (time, setting)?
   - What were you doing at the time? what had you been eating or drinking?
   - Is there pain associated with the nausea or does it occur without nausea at times?
   - If there is pain, where is the pain located and does it radiate anywhere?
   - Are there any foods, medications, or activities that aggravate or alleviate the pain, nausea, or vomiting?

   - How disruptive is this to your normal activities?

2. Tests would likely include:
   - Serum amylase: indicates pancreatic tissue damage
   - Serum lipase: usually elevated with acute pancreatitis
   - Serum glucose: may be elevated because of pancreatic cell damage
   - WBC: indicates inflammation or infection

3. Diagnostic procedures may include the following:
   - Ultrasound to assess for the presence of gallstones or pancreatic mass
   - CT of the abdomen to assess for pancreatic size, fluid, or necrosis

- Abdominal x-ray to assess for the presence of stones or fluid accumulation in the area of the pancreas

4. Client teaching related to these procedures would include the following:
   - The client will require no special preparation for the abdominal x-rays, however, ultrasound and CT procedures require special preparation.
   - Ultrasound of the abdomen will require that the client have a relatively clean bowel and be NPO for a period of time prior to procedure. Stool, gas, and air can alter the transmission of the sound waves and cause altered recorded images.
   - The CT of the abdomen will require that the client drink approximately 42 ounces of contrast media prior to the test. The client will also need to have IV access for administration of additional contrast material as needed.

5. Three possible nursing diagnoses that would be appropriate for this client are Pain; Risk for altered nutrition: less than body requirements; and Risk for fluid volume deficit. Other possible nursing diagnoses based upon the particular client assessment may include: Ineffective breathing pattern related to pulmonary effusion or pain, Risk for activity intolerance, Altered health maintenance related to knowledge deficit of disease process, and Sleep pattern disturbance related to pain.

Chapter 2

1. Impaired gas exchange. Maintaining adequate gas exchange is the physiological priority for the client with acute exacerbation of COPD and acute lung infection of pneumonia. Activity intolerance and self-care deficit are also reasonable nursing diagnoses for this client who has been hospitalized.

2. Debris produced by dead bacteria accounts for purulent secretions in the client with a bacterial origin of pneumonia. This finding is a classic sign that helps to distinguish bacterial pneumonia from other etiologies of pneumonia. With viral pneumonia, the client typically has a nonproductive cough.

3. Clients with COPD are often underweight because of the fatigue associated with eating. This client has acutely increased energy needs because of the hypermetabolism associated with acute infection of pneumonia. Providing small quantities of calorie-dense foods will help to achieve needed calorie and protein intake while perhaps avoiding increased fatigue associated with eating.

4. Ventilation and perfusion are gravity-dependent, so when the client is lying on his/her side, gravity accounts for greater ventilation and perfusion to that dependent lung. Since pneumonia produces excess secretions and possible obstructed airways, ventilation and perfusion will be optimized when the client is placed in a position with the good lung in a dependent position.

5. Carbon dioxide level in the blood is a major stimulus for breathing. Clients with COPD retain carbon dioxide and typically have higher than normal blood levels of carbon dioxide and develop a hypoxic respiratory drive. Lowering carbon dioxide levels by administration of high concentration of oxygen lowers or removes this stimulus for breathing. Initial oxygen supplementation for clients with suspected or known COPD should be low concentration, 1 to 2 L/min via nasal cannula to avoid respiratory depression or arrest.

Chapter 3

1. Instruct client in routine preoperative teaching, turning and deep-breathing (vigorous coughing is discouraged because it may increase intrathoracic pressure and cause instability in the sternal area), incentive spirometry to prevent respiratory complications, and leg exercises to prevent emboli formation. Explain expected client status immediately postoperatively including respiratory support on a ventilator with an endotracheal tube; suctioning; surgical incisions, chest tubes, multiple intravenous lines, tubes, drains, and monitors with alarms and noises; pain management, communication techniques, visiting policies, and expected length of hospitalization and recovery period. Include family members in preoperative teaching and explanations. Ensure that all consents are signed. Evaluate the client's understanding of the preoperative teaching. Ensure that all preoperative orders are complete.

2. In the preoperative phase, the nurse monitors the hemodynamic status of the client, and carefully monitors for signs of ischemia or decreased cardiac output. This includes continuous ECG monitoring, vital signs, and careful assessment and monitoring of any chest pain or dyspnea.

3. Nursing diagnoses that are appropriate for a client in the postoperative period are Pain, Ineffective breathing pattern, Risk for decreased cardiac output, Risk for dysrhythmia, Risk for infection, Anxiety, Fear.

4. In the period after critical care, the nurse monitors the client for potential complications. These include decreased cardiac output, ineffective breathing and fluid accumulation in lungs, infection in surgical wounds, activity intolerance, or dysrhythmias.

5. When the client is ready to go home after surgery, the nurse will instruct client about new medication regime, symptoms to report to MD upon discharge including chest pain, shortness of breath, decrease in activity tolerance, fever, redness, swelling or drainage from surgical incisions, activity plan for home, cardiac rehabilitation, and resumption of sexual activity. The client may resume sexual activity when he or she can walk up two full flights of stairs without shortness of breath or chest pain. The client should be rested when resuming sexual activity. Sexual activity should be avoided after a heavy meal or after the intake of alcohol. Instruct client that clinical depression occurs in about 20 percent of clients up to 6 months after cardiac surgery, and client should notify physician because antidepressants are every effective. Include family in teaching and planning for discharge.

Chapter 4

1. The most likely cause of Mr. B.'s foot ulcer is venous insufficiency. Venous ulcers usually develop around the ankles, especially in the area of the medial malleoli.

2. Venous insufficiency may present with edema of the lower extremities, ulcerations that are moist around the ankles, complaints of aching or heaviness in the calf or thigh, cyanosis of the extremity when dependent, and a leathery or brawny appearance to the skin of the lower extremities. Pulses and normal hair distribution are usually present and the skin is warm to touch.

3. Nursing diagnoses include: Impaired skin integrity, Risk for infection related to decreased peripheral circulation and skin ulcers; Altered tissue perfusion; Altered health maintenance related to lack of knowledge of venous insufficiency

4. Primary nursing interventions include:
   Education on improving venous return
   - Keep legs elevated above heart level as much as possible
   - Avoid prolonged standing/sitting or flexing legs
   - Wear support hose when ambulatory
   - Do not wear tight or restrictive clothing or shoes
   - Avoid injury or trauma to legs and feet
   Treating venous stasis ulcer
   - Open sores treated with hydrocolloid or wet dressings of boric acid, Burrow's solution, or normal saline QID
   - Unna boot may be applied and changed every 1 to 2 weeks
   - Teach client proper hand washing and infection control measures
   - Assess for infection
   Education on high-protein, low-sodium diet and proper weight control

5. Outcomes of nursing care include:
   - No infection and healing of venous ulcers
   - Decreased peripheral edema
   - Verbalization of knowledge of wound care, improved venous return, and diet

Chapter 5

1. The focal neurological assessment should include the client's level of consciousness, Glasgow Coma Scale score, mental status assessment, motor and sensory evaluation, and possibly cranial nerve testing. It is important to assess pupil reaction to light, hand grasps, and foot pushes for strength and equality. A full neurological exam can proceed when the client is stabilized.

2. Intracranial hemorrhage can be diagnosed by CT scan or MRI.

3. Increased ICP is indicated by a deteriorating level of consciousness, focal neurological deficits, and by the classic signs of increasing systolic blood pressure, widening pulse pressure, and bradycardia.

4. A quiet peaceful environment that minimizes environmental stimuli will help prevent rises in intracranial pressure. Keep lights low, provide physical care to client, maintain bedrest, minimize stimulants such as radio, TV, newspaper, and others. Ingested stimulants should also be avoided, including coffee, tea, cola drinks, cigarette smoke, and others.

5. No specific medication is indicated to treat hematomas; medication such as anticonvulsants and steroids could be used as indicated to treat seizures and increased ICP if they occur as complications.

Chapter 6

1. Aminoglycoside antibiotics are known to be nephrotoxic and should be used with extreme care for clients with decreased renal function.

2. The client's blood glucose level should decrease as waste products are removed from his blood. Monitor his glucose levels and observe for signs of hypoglycemia.

3. The client's lungs are already compromised by pneumonia. Missing his dialysis treatment may lead to fluid overload, which places him at risk for congestive heart failure and pulmonary edema.

4. Metabolic acidosis may lead to a fruity odor on the breath. Other signs of metabolic acidosis include general malaise, headache, nausea and vomiting, and abdominal pain.

5. Atrophy of the sweat glands and metabolic wastes not eliminated by the kidneys can lead to dry, itching skin. To help with the client's pruritus, avoid harsh soaps; instead use mild soap or a cleansing cream and bath oils. If soap is used, rinse well. Use a humidifier to add moisture to the air. Apply unscented lotion when the skin is slightly damp after bathing. Teach him that it isn't necessary to bathe every day.

Chapter 7

1. Lab values will reflect liver injury and decreased liver function and include: elevated ALT and AST, low serum albumin, prolonged prothrombin time, elevated total bilirubin, hyponatremia, possible elevated serum ammonia level, anemia, thrombocytopenia, and leukopenia.

2. Since the liver is such a vascular organ, the priority of care is to monitor for bleeding. Vital signs are taken q 15 min × 4; q 30 min × 2; q 1 hr × 2; q 4 hr × 4; then every 6 hr. The dressing should be monitored for bleeding and the client should be positioned on the right side, which helps apply pressure to the biopsy site. The client is usually maintained on bed rest for 24 hr to reduce the risk of bleeding.

3. Complications of hepatitis B include the development of chronic hepatitis, which destroys the liver and leads to cirrhosis and liver failure. The complications of cirrhosis are portal hypertension leading to esophageal varices, right-sided heart failure, and varicose veins. Ascites, hepatic encephalopathy, and hepatorenal syndrome are also complications of cirrhosis.

4. The client with cirrhosis is usually on a protein, sodium, and fluid-restricted diet. Foods to avoid would be canned and processed foods (high in sodium), chicken, meat, eggs, and dairy products (high in protein), and fluids are usually limited.

5. The long-term outcome of cirrhosis is death. If the complications of cirrhosis can be controlled the prognosis is better. Liver transplant is an effective treatment for end-stage liver disease for those individuals who meet certain criteria.

Chapter 8

1. An upper-GI series will probably be ordered and can show lower esophageal sphincter (LES) function as well as ulceration. An esophagogastroduodenoscopy can be more diagnostic because it is a direct visualization of the tissue of the esophagus and can show inflammation. The gastric and duodenal mucosa are also visualized directly and ulcerations are evident. The advantage of endoscopy over an upper-GI series is that tissue samples can be obtained for determining the presence of cancer, Barrett's epithelium, or *H. pylori*. Gastric analysis may also be used to determine the pH and acid output of the stomach.

2. An upper-GI series usually involves the ingestion of barium, which is constipating. The client should be encouraged to drink fluids and ambulate. Aspiration of barium during the procedure is a possibility, so the nurse should assess lung sounds and monitor for signs of aspiration such as fever, cough, and dyspnea. For the client after esophagogastroduodenoscopy, it is extremely important to assess for the return of swallowing and the gag reflex since the throat is anesthetized for the procedure. The client is sedated for the procedure, therefore general safety measures should be instituted (side rails up, bed in low position).

3. Lifestyle and diet modifications are key to controlling GERD. The client should be instructed to avoid eating within 2 hours of bedtime and should remain in an upright position after eating. Tight clothing (belts, tight waistbands), straining (weight lifting, bending over, lifting heavy objects), and vigorous physical activity increase intra-abdominal pressure aggravate GERD and should be avoided. A reduction in dietary fat and an increase in complex carbohydrates encourage more rapid gastric emptying and reduction in symptoms of GERD. The client should be instructed to avoid substances that decrease LES tone such as caffeinated beverages, chocolate, peppermint, spearmint, smoking, and fried foods. The client should be encouraged to elevate the head of the bed about 12 inches to prevent reflux at night.

4. The complications of GERD are limited to the development of Barrett's epithelium, cancer, and esophageal stricture. Symptoms include dysphagia, pain, and more systemic symptoms such as fatigue, dyspnea, and activity intolerance. Complications of PUD are perforation, hemorrhage, gastric cancer (gastric ulcer), and pyloric obstruction. The client should be instructed to report any of the following symptoms: vomiting, hematemesis, black tarry stools, pain, rapid heart rate, abdominal rigidity, and fever as they may indicate a complication.

5. Clients with GERD may develop Barrett's epithelium and be at a greater risk for cancer if GERD remains untreated, so it is important that the client follow the treatment regimen. If the client has a duodenal ulcer, the risk for developing cancer as a result are minimal; however, there is an increased incidence of gastric cancer in people with gastric ulcers. Continued follow-up is therefore important in this population.

Chapter 9

1. The nurse should perform a neurovascular assessment, which includes assessing the right lower extremity for pulses, capillary refill, temperature, movement, and paresthesias. The dressing should also be inspected for bleeding. The respiratory status should be assessed since the client is on a PCA pump for the management of pain. The client's level of pain should also be assessed to evaluate the effectiveness of the PCA dosing.

2. The client should be turned alternately on the back or the non-operative side. Avoid positioning the client on the operative side. When the client is turned, abduction pillows or abduction splints should be used between the knees. The nurse can also support the client's right ankle and right thigh to maintain abduction of the hip during turning. Sandbags can also be used to prevent external rotation of the hip. When the head of the bed is raised, remember that the hip should not be flexed beyond 90 degrees.

3. The pillow (or an abduction splint) prevents external rotation, supports the legs and prevents adduction. Adduction of the right leg past the midline can cause the right hip to dislocate.

4. Any activity that forces the hip into more than 90 degrees of flexion puts this client at risk for hip dislocation. These activities include using a low chair or a low commode, stooping, and bending. Any activity that causes the leg on the operated side to cross the midline, such as leg crossing, can cause dislocation of the affected hip.

5. It is important that activities are normalized as early as possible to lessen the complications of bedrest. Specifically, complications such as skin pressure ulcers, venous thrombosis, atelectasis, pneumonia, and contractures are prevented with early mobility.

Chapter 10

1. Questions to ask the client regarding the rash include:
   - Is there a family history of psoriasis?
   - Are you on any current or new medications?
   - Has here been any local trauma or irritation to the skin recently?
   - Have you had any recent infections?

- Have you ever been tested or diagnosed with HIV?
- When did the rash begin?

Ask the client to describe the course of the rash.
- Does the rash itch or is it painful?
- Have you used any new soaps, detergents, or lotions?
- Have you had any exposure to any toxic substances?
- Have you ever noticed what time of year you usually experience the rash?

2. Psoriasis is a chronic skin condition that affects approximately 3 percent of the population. It usually peaks during adolescence and young adulthood, and then reoccurs in the later adult years. The cause of the skin disorder is unknown. Some evidence indicates the condition can be familial and can be exacerbated by stress and cold climates. The plaques are thought to be produced from an overactive production of the skin cells, along with inflammation of the dermis and epidermis.

2. Psoriasis is a chronic skin condition that may require long-term treatment. The goal of treatment for psoriasis is to control the skin condition. To maintain control of the disorder and/or to prevent psoriasis the client will need to be compliant with recommended therapies.

4. Over-the-counter products that are useful for controlling psoriasis include emollients such as Eucerin™ cream, Lubriderm Moisture Plus™, or Moisturel™. For scalp involvement, the coal tar shampoos are recommended. Encourage daily use of these products and stress the importance of daily routines.

5. Outdoor environments are safe as long as the client wears sunscreen with an sun protection factor (SPF) of 15 or greater to protect the skin from burning. Sunlight exposure may help this chronic skin condition. However, a few clients will react differently to the sun, and it may even cause the psoriasis to worsen. Therefore initial exposure to the sun should be limited to determine how the skin will react to the sunlight exposure.

Chapter 11

1. Background information that would demonstrate how the client is "reacting" to the diagnosis would include identification of social support systems, religious and cultural beliefs, and discussion of coping strategies that the client has utilized in the past to deal with life's dynamic changes.

2. A multisystem disease is one that eventually can affect every body organ. The progression of a multisystem disease can lead to changes in how each of the body's organ systems handles everyday immune responses.

3. Diagnostic tests that would serve to provide a baseline include antinuclear antibody (ANA), complement assay, ESR, CBC, and urinalysis. Depending on client's status at time of diagnosis, specific symptom complaints and results from baseline labs may require further testing to determine organ involvement.

4. Discharge planning should include measures aimed at minimizing stress, and establishing rest periods. Symptom management may require the use of medications such as NSAIDs to provide relief from arthritic manifestations. Skin protection along with proper skin care should be promoted to prevent possible exacerbation of disease. Client should be instructed to avoid potential infection exposure as this can cause exacerbation of problems in a client who already has an altered immune response. Adequate nutrition should be stressed to help the client remain well hydrated and maintain ideal body weight. Since the client is of childbearing age, birth control selection should be discussed since certain methods may be contraindicated for clients with this disease. While pregnancy is not contraindicated, discussion can be directed towards the concept of a "planned" pregnancy at a time when the disease has been in a stable state. Additionally, since the effects of this disease are multi-system in nature, the client may have to deal with concepts of altered body image and altered coping. Counseling and available support systems should be in place to help the client and family members live with this disease process.

Chapter 12

1. The client with cancer may experience anxiety, for example, as a response to the specific disease, fear of the unknown, and fear of pain, disfigurement, or death. Nursing interventions include allowing the client to express feelings, establishing a therapeutic relationship with client, and assessing the client's level of anxiety. Additionally, informing the client about the disease, expected treatments and outcomes will allow the client a sense of control. Provide the client with resources to assist with coping, such as the American Cancer Society's "I Can Cope" program, which provides counseling, education, and support for clients with cancer.

2. Begin by asking her what information has been provided to her. Even though clients have been provided information, they may not have understood the specific details. Knowing what the client has been told and her level of understanding will assist you in explaining or clarifying information to her. From this point, you will teach her about chemotherapy, radiation, and other treatments that are included in the treatment plan.

3. You will provide the client with information regarding the chemotherapeutic agent, which includes expected side effects, signs of reaction or infiltration, and interventions before chemotherapy, such as taking anti-emetics. Side effects should be specific, for example, nausea, alopecia, xerostomia, bone marrow suppression. To reduce potential complications, you should continually evaluate the client's understanding of the teaching you provide.

4. You should administer an anti-emetic before beginning the chemotherapy. Suggest that the client consume small, frequent meals and drink cool liquids. Provide an atmosphere that is calm and quiet and free from odors. The client may require anti-emetics around-the-clock to reduce the nausea and vomiting.

5. The client with hair loss may experience a body image disturbance. Interventions should include allowing the client to

express feelings and concerns about the change in body appearance. Also, encourage active participation in the management of hair loss, such as purchasing a hairpiece or wig, hats, or scarves. Suggest support programs such as "Look Good…Feel Better." Instruct the client that hair will begin to grow back after the chemotherapy is completed, though the texture and color may be different.

Chapter 13

1. Oral tracheal suction supplies, emergency tracheostomy tray with tracheostomy kit, two sand bags, thermometer, sphygmomanometer, ice collar, and a pole for the IV infusion should be placed in the client's room.
2. Respiratory distress and hemorrhage are most likely to occur during the first 24 hours postsurgery.
3. The client should keep the head neutral while lying in semi-Fowler's position with an ice collar over the incision area when in bed. The client should support her head and neck with her hands behind the neck when turning in bed. The client should turn to her side, then move to sitting at the bedside, and then walk to the bedside chair.
4. You should monitor the dressing for amount and frequency of drainage and degree of tightness around the neck. Assess the lower neck, back of neck, and below the dressing for bleeding. Auscultate the neck for stridor and stertor. Assess the client for numbness or tingling of extremities, lips, or mouth, and for Trousseau's and Chvostek's signs. Assess vital signs, breathing effort, skin color and ask the client about a sensation of tightness around the neck. Assess the client's voice for weakness and tone indicating laryngeal nerve damage.
5. The medication should be taken daily for life, in the morning 1 hour before food or 2 hours after food. The client should not change the brand without consulting the physician.

Chapter 14

1. The predisposition to develop disseminated intravascular coagulopathy in this client may be due to septic shock. Both septicemia and shock are conditions which predisposes an individual to the development of DIC. Endotoxins from Gram-negative bacteria activates several steps in the coagulation cascade and therefore increase the likelihood of the development of DIC.
2. The nurse has to perform a thorough assessment of the client for other signs and symptoms of this syndrome to be able to do appropriate planning and intervention. In DIC, there are both thrombotic and bleeding manifestations. The assesment finding relating to the left lower extremity points to the possibility that this client has a thrombotic phenomenon occuring in that area. Other areas should be explored to assess the extent of this thrombotic possibility. In addition, measures to assess and control bleeding should be instituted, particularly in areas where direct pressure could be applied. The physician should be notified of these observations so that appropriate interventions could be instituted.

3. Clients who have DIC will have screening tests which includes prothrombin time (PT), partial thromboplastin time (PTT), thrombin time, fibrinogen, platelets, fibrin split products, antithrombin III, and D-dimers. These laboratory tests attempt to evaluate the degree of firinolysis that is occuring. In DIC, the normal coagulation mechanisms are enhanced initially. However, excessive clotting activates the fibrinolytic system eventually, which in turn lysis the newly formed clots. This process increases the fibrin split products which inhibits normal clotting because of its anticoagulant properties. These mechanisms can be deduced by examining the results of these laboratory tests.
4. The typical DIC presentation will show the following laboratory results: prothrombin time—prolonged; PTT—prolonged; thrombin time—prolonged; fibrinogen—reduced; platelets—reduced; fibrin split products—elevated; antithrombin III—reduced, and D-dimers—elevated.
5. Ineffective tissue perfusion; Decreased cardiac output; Pain

Chapter 15

1. The procedure is usually done under local anesthesia. A piece of tissue will be surgically removed from the breast, using a small incision. The section of removed tissue will be sent to the laboratory for histologic examination.
2. The client who undergoes a breast biopsy and is later informed that she has a malignancy will have the following possible nursing diagnoses included in her care plan: Anxiety, Decisional conflict, Anticipatory grieving, Risk for Body Image Disturbance.
3. A mastectomy causes changes in the client's body image. The client and her husband may have anxiety and fear about the diagnosis and the resulting body changes that may occur with treatment and interventions.
4. The nurse should provide up-to-date written material and assist the client understand the options she has for treatment. The nurse should answer all questions posed by the client. For those questions she is unable to answer, the nurse should assist the client in writing them down so that the physician may clarify them. Attentive listening and therapeutic communication techniques should be employed throughout the discussion with the client. The nurse should also share information about the American Cancer Society's programs for the woman with breast cancer, making a referral as soon as the diagnosis is made.
5. Modified radical mastectomy is the removal of breast tissue and lymph nodes under the arm, leaving the chest wall muscles intact.

Chapter 16

1. This procedure is typically done on an outpatient basis and generally requires less intensive nursing care than with some other types of surgery. Questions to ask this client include the questions typically asked of a preoperative client as well as a few particular to this procedure:

- The time of the last intake of food or fluids (includes smoking and gum chewing)?
- What medications, if any, were taken on the morning of surgery?
- Any there any remaining questions about the procedure?
- Who is available to drive the client home after surgery?
- Does the client have someone to help at home as needed after the procedure?
- Does the client have dark glasses available to use following surgery?

2. Assessments will those typically done in the preoperative period: baseline vital signs, general physical assessment, and results of preoperative laboratory or diagnostic tests.
3. Postoperative care includes the following:
   - Baseline assessments as for all postoperative clients: vital signs, level of consciousness, status of dressing
   - Maintain eye patch or eye shield in place to prevent injury to eye, and instruct client not to rub or touch the area
   - Elevate head to 30 to 45 degrees and have client lie on back or unaffected side (to reduce intraocular pressure); use small pillows at sides of head to immobilize head when lying on back
   - Instruct and assist the client to avoid activities that increase IOP, such as coughing or sneezing, if these are necessary, client should do so with mouth open
   - Maintain client safety: orient to environment, keep articles and call bell on unaffected side, use side rails with stretcher/bed/chair in low position, and assist with ambulation
   - Give antibiotic, antiinflammatory, and other prescribed topical (eye) or systemic medications
   - Give analgesics as ordered, avoiding or using caution with opioids to prevent postoperative nausea, vomiting, and constipation; discomfort may be described as achy or scratching; avoid morphine, which can cause miosis
   - Assess for possible surgical complications that should be reported immediately to preserve sight: sudden sharp eye pain (possibly indicating hemorrhage, sudden rise in IOP or other ocular emergency), hemorrhage, retinal detachment (client sensations of flashes of light, floaters, or a curtain being drawn over the eye), corneal edema—noted by a cloudy appearance to cornea (may not be visible if dressing in place)

4. The following points are included in discharge teaching:
   - Leave eye shield in place until the surgeon's office visit; then use eye shield at night during sleep for eye protection
   - Avoid rubbing, scratching, touching, squeezing, or putting pressure on surgical eye
   - Avoid activities that increase intraocular pressure, (sneezing, coughing, vomiting, straining, moving rapidly, bending, or lifting more than 5 pounds)
   - Maintain sedentary lifestyle for approximately 2 weeks or as prescribed by surgeon

- Avoid reading until allowed by surgeon, and then read in moderation during healing
- Use measures to prevent constipation (adequate fiber and fluid intake, maintain mobility, use stool softener P.R.N.)
- Wear sunglasses with side shields when out of doors (photophobia)
- Proper techniques for use of eye patch or shield and/or instillation of eye drops
- Medication names, dose, schedule, side effects, purpose, and anticipated duration of use
- Symptoms to report to physician: new, increased or severe eye pain or pressure, decreased vision, redness, cloudiness, drainage, floaters or light flashes, halos around brightly lit objects

5. The client's vision may take several weeks to stabilize as healing occurs. A final prescription for corrective lenses will be given once vision has stabilized. In the meantime, it is very important to keep all follow-up appointments.

Chapter 17

1. The triage category would be "emergent" based upon potential for extensive organ system damage.
2. The priorities in treating this client are:
   - Stabilization of ABCs
   - Supplemental oxygen
   - IV access
   - Determination of medication serum level at present and serial levels
   - Prevention of further absorption and enhanced elimination of medication
   - If acetylcysteine (Mucomyst) is used do not give charcoal to prevent binding of the antidote to the drug
3. The methods that could be utilized to decrease absorption of this medication are:
   - Emesis with syrup of ipecac
   - Gastric lavage
   - Administration of activated charcoal
   - Enhanced elimination may be of some use for medications primarily absorbed in the lower GI tract
   - Hemoperfusion

   Remember that an alteration in mental status may preclude the use of any or all of these methods unless the airway has been protected by endotracheal intubation.

4. Suggestions for the three priority nursing diagnoses for this client would be:
   - Fluid volume deficit related to detoxification and elimination treatments
   - Risk for impaired tissue perfusion
   - Risk for injury

5. Three evaluation criteria indicating successful treatment of this client could include any of the following:
   - Absorption is minimized and toxic by-products are reduced

- Tissue integrity is maintained
- Fluid volume deficit is corrected
- Tissue and organ perfusion is adequate
- No further organ damage occurs

Credits

Chapter 1

Figure 01–01 Art, © Prentice Hall Health, Upper Saddle River, New Jersey.

Figure 01–02 From Health Assessment in Nursing, by Lina K. Sims, Donita D. D'Amico, Johanna K. Stiesmeyer, Judith A. Webster, " 1995 by Addison-Wesley Publishing Company, Inc., Redwood City, CA; Page 30, Figure 02–05.

Chapter 2

Figure 02–01 Art, From Medical Surgical Nursing: Critical Thinking in Client Care, by Priscilla LeMone, Karen M. Burke, Edition 3, © 2004 by Prentice-Hall, Inc., Upper Saddle River, New Jersey; Page 1116, Fig. 36–12; Artist: Kristin N. Mount

Figure 02–02 Art, From Medical Surgical Nursing: Critical Thinking in Client Care, by Priscilla LeMone, Karen M. Burke, Edition 2, © 2000 by Prentice-Hall, Inc., Upper Saddle River, New Jersey; Page 1474, Fig. 34–21; Artist: Nea Hanscomb.

Chapter 3

Figure 03–01 Art, From Recognizing and Interpreting Arrhythmias by Ginger Ochs, Melvin A. Ochs, Edition 3, © 1997 by Prentice-Hall, Inc., Upper Saddle River, New Jersey; Page 02, Fig. 01–01.

Figure 03–02 Art, From Recognizing and Interpreting Arrhythmias by Ginger Ochs, Melvin A. Ochs, Edition 3, © 1997 by Prentice-Hall, Inc., Upper Saddle River, New Jersey; Page 04, Fig. 01–03.

Table 03–01 Art, From Medical Surgical Nursing: Critical Thinking in Client Care, by Priscilla LeMone, Karen M. Burke, Edition 3, © 2004 by Prentice-Hall, Inc., Upper Saddle River, New Jersey; Page 845–847, Table 29–6. Artists: GTS Graphics and Kristin N. Mount.

Chapter 4

Figure 04–01 Art, From Medical Surgical Nursing: Critical Thinking in Client Care, by Priscilla LeMone, Karen M. Burke, Edition 3, © 2004 by Prentice-Hall, Inc., Upper Saddle River, New Jersey; Page 920, Fig. 31–01.

Figure 04–02 Art, From Medical Surgical Nursing: Critical Thinking in Client Care, by Priscilla LeMone, Karen M. Burke, Edition 3, © 2004 by Prentice-Hall, Inc., Upper Saddle River, New Jersey; Page 921, Fig. 31–2.

Chapter 5

Figure 05–01 Art, From Medical Surgical Nursing: Critical Thinking in Client Care, by Priscilla LeMone, Karen M. Burke, Edition 3, © 2004 by Prentice-Hall, Inc., Upper Saddle River, New Jersey; Page 1304, Fig. 40–18 & 40–19; Artist: Precision Graphics.

Fig. 05–02 Art, From Medical Surgical Nursing: Critical Thinking in Client Care, by Priscilla LeMone, Karen M. Burke, Edition 3, © 2004 by Prentice-Hall, Inc., Upper Saddle River, New Jersey; Page 1324, Fig. 41–05, Artist: Kristin N. Mount.

Figure 05–03 Art, From Medical Surgical Nursing: Critical Thinking in Client Care, by Priscilla LeMone, Karen M. Burke, Edition 3, © 2004 by Prentice-Hall, Inc., Upper Saddle River, New Jersey; Page 1367, Fig. 42–04; Artist: Precision Graphics.

Chapter 6

Figure 06–01 Art, From Medical Surgical Nursing: Critical Thinking in Client Care, by Priscilla LeMone, Karen M. Burke, Edition 3, © 2004 by Prentice-Hall, Inc., Upper Saddle River, New Jersey; Page 695, Fig. 25–01 "A"; Artist: Wendy Hiller Gee/Kristin N. Mount/ Nea Hanscomb.

Figure 06–02 Art, From Medical Surgical Nursing: Critical Thinking in Client Care, by Priscilla LeMone, Karen M. Burke, Edition 3, © 2004 by Prentice-Hall, Inc., Upper Saddle River, New Jersey; Page 715, Fig. 26–02; Artist: Kristin N. Mount

Figure 06–03 Art, From Medical Surgical Nursing: Critical Thinking in Client Care, by Priscilla LeMone, Karen M. Burke, Edition 3, © 2004 by Prentice-Hall, Inc., Upper Saddle River, New Jersey; Page 725, Fig. 26–06 "B"; Artist: Kristin N. Mount

Chapter 7

Figure 07–01 Art, © Prentice Hall Health, Upper Saddle River, New Jersey.

Figure 07–02 Art, From Medical Surgical Nursing: Critical Thinking in Client Care, by Priscilla LeMone, Karen M. Burke, Edition 3, © 2004 by Prentice-Hall, Inc., Upper Saddle River, New Jersey; Page 587, Multisystem Effects of Cirrhosis; Artist: Wendy Hiller Gee/Kristin N. Mount.

Figure 07–03 Art, From Medical Surgical Nursing: Critical Thinking in Client Care, by Priscilla LeMone, Karen M. Burke, Edition 3, © 2004 by Prentice-Hall, Inc., Upper Saddle River, New Jersey; Page 590, Fig. 22–3; Artist: Kristin N. Mount

Chapter 8

Figure 08–01 Art, © Prentice Hall Health, Upper Saddle River, New Jersey.

Figure 08–02 Art, From Medical Surgical Nursing: Critical Thinking in Client Care, by Priscilla LeMone, Karen M. Burke, Edition 3, © 2004 by Prentice-Hall, Inc., Upper Saddle River, New Jersey; Page 592, Fig. 22–05; Artist: Kristin N. Mount

Figure 08–03 Art, From Medical Surgical Nursing: Critical Thinking in Client Care, by Priscilla LeMone, Karen M. Burke, Edition 3, © 2004 by Prentice-Hall, Inc., Upper Saddle River, New Jersey; Page 567, Fig. 21–13 "A&B"; Artist: Kristin N. Mount

Figure 08–04 Art, From Medical Surgical Nursing: Critical Thinking in Client Care, by Priscilla LeMone, Karen M. Burke, Edition 3, © 2004 by Prentice-Hall, Inc., Upper Saddle River, New Jersey; Page 551, Fig. 21–05 "A&B"; Artist: Kristin N. Mount

Chapter 9

Figure 09–01 Art, From Medical Surgical Nursing: Critical Thinking in Client Care, by Priscilla LeMone, Karen M. Burke, Edition 3, © 2004 by Prentice-Hall, Inc., Upper Saddle River, New Jersey; Page 1199, Fig. 38–5; Artist: Precision Graphics.

Figure 09–02 Art, From Medical Surgical Nursing: Critical Thinking in Client Care, by Priscilla LeMone, Karen M. Burke, Edition 3, © 2004 by Prentice-Hall, Inc., Upper Saddle River, New Jersey; Page 1268, Fig. 39–09; Artist: Christopher Burke

Figure 09–03 Art, From Medical Surgical Nursing: Critical Thinking in Client Care, by Priscilla LeMone, Karen M. Burke, Edition 3, © 2004 by Prentice-Hall, Inc., Upper Saddle River, New Jersey; Page 1206, Fig. 38–09; Artist: Kristin N. Mount

Chapter 10

Figure 10–01 From Health Assessment in Nursing, by Lina K. Sims, Donita D. D'Amico, Johanna K. Stiesmeyer, Judith A. Webster, " 1995 by Addison-Wesley Publishing Company, Inc., Redwood City, CA; Page 126, Figure 8–2.

Figure 10–02 From Medical Surgical Nursing: Critical Thinking in Client Care, by Priscilla LeMone, Karen M. Burke, Edition 3, © 2004 by Prentice-Hall, Inc., Upper Saddle River, New Jersey; Page 355, Table 13–2; Artist: Kristin N. Mount

Figure 10–3 Art, From Medical Surgical Nursing: Critical Thinking in Client Care, by Priscilla LeMone, Karen M. Burke, Edition 3, © 2004 by Prentice-Hall, Inc., Upper Saddle River, New Jersey; Page 415, Fig. 15–4; Artist: Precision Graphics.

Chapter 11

Figure 11–01 Art, From Medical Surgical Nursing: Critical Thinking in Client Care, by Priscilla LeMone, Karen M. Burke, Edition 3, © 2004 by Prentice-Hall, Inc., Upper Saddle River, New Jersey; Page 196, Fig.08–03; Artist: Christopher Burke.

Figure 11–02 Art, From Medical Surgical Nursing: Critical Thinking in Client Care, by Priscilla LeMone, Karen M. Burke, Edition 3, © 2004 by Prentice-Hall, Inc., Upper Saddle River, New Jersey; Page 196, Fig. 08–02; Artist: Christopher Burke.

Figure 11–03 Art, © Prentice Hall Health, Upper Saddle River, New Jersey.

Chapter 12

Figure 12–01 Art, © Prentice Hall Health, Upper Saddle River, New Jersey.

Figure 12–02 Art, © Prentice Hall Health, Upper Saddle River, New Jersey.

Chapter 13

Figure 13–01 Art, From Medical Surgical Nursing: Critical Thinking in Client Care, by Priscilla LeMone, Karen M. Burke, Edition 3, © 2004 by Prentice-Hall, Inc., Upper Saddle River, New Jersey; Page 85, Multisystem Effects of Fluid Volume Deficit (FVD); Artist: Wendy Hiller Gee/Kristin N. Mount.

Figure 13–02 Art, From Medical Surgical Nursing: Critical Thinking in Client Care, by Priscilla LeMone, Karen M. Burke, Edition 3, © 2004 by Prentice-Hall, Inc., Upper Saddle River, New Jersey; Page 446, Multisystem Effects of Hyperthyroidism; Artist: Wendy Hiller Gee/Kristin N. Mount.

Figure 13–03 Art, From Medical Surgical Nursing: Critical Thinking in Client Care, by Priscilla LeMone, Karen M. Burke, Edition 3, © 2004 by Prentice-Hall, Inc., Upper Saddle River, New Jersey; Page 479, Multisystem Effects of Diabetes Mellitus; Artist: Wendy Hiller Gee/Kristin N. Mount.

Chapter 14

Figure 14–01 Art, From Medical Surgical Nursing: Critical Thinking in Client Care, by Priscilla LeMone, Karen M. Burke, Edition 3, © 2004 by Prentice-Hall, Inc., Upper Saddle River, New Jersey; Page 934, Fig. 32–04; Artist: Christopher Burke.

Figure 14–02 Art, From Medical Surgical Nursing: Critical Thinking in Client Care, by Priscilla LeMone, Karen M. Burke, Edition 2, © 2000 by Prentice-Hall, Inc., Upper Saddle River, New Jersey; Page 1290, Fig. 31–9; Artist: Nea Hanscomb.

Chapter 15

Figure 15–01 Art, From Medical Surgical Nursing: Critical Thinking in Client Care, by Priscilla LeMone, Karen M. Burke, Edition 3, © 2004 by Prentice-Hall, Inc., Upper Saddle River, New Jersey; Page 1513, Fig. 46–01; Artist: Barbara Cousins/Nea Hanscomb.

Figure 15–02 Art, From Medical Surgical Nursing: Critical Thinking in Client Care, by Priscilla LeMone, Karen M. Burke, Edition 3, © 2004 by Prentice-Hall, Inc., Upper Saddle River, New Jersey; Page 1516, Fig. 46–02; Artist. Wendy Hiller Gee/Nea Hanscomb.

Figure 15–03 Art, From Medical Surgical Nursing: Critical Thinking in Client Care, by Priscilla LeMone, Karen M. Burke, Edition 3, © 2004 by Prentice-Hall, Inc., Upper Saddle River, New Jersey; Page 1589, Fig. 48–13; Artist: Precision Graphics.

Figure 15–04 Art, From Medical Surgical Nursing: Critical Thinking in Client Care, by Priscilla LeMone, Karen M. Burke, Edition 3, © 2004 by Prentice-Hall, Inc., Upper Saddle River, New Jersey; Page 1557, Multisystem Effects of Premenstrual Syndrome; Artist: Wendy Hiller Gee/Kristin N. Mount.

Chapter 16

Figure 16–01 Art, From Medical Surgical Nursing: Critical Thinking in Client Care, by Priscilla LeMone, Karen M. Burke, Edition 3, © 2004 by Prentice-Hall, Inc., Upper Saddle River, New Jersey; Page 1475, Fig. 45–05; Artist: Kristin N. Mount.

Figure 16–02 Art, From Medical Surgical Nursing: Critical Thinking in Client Care, by Priscilla LeMone, Karen M. Burke, Edition 3, © 2004 by Prentice-Hall, Inc., Upper Saddle River, New Jersey; Page 1504, Fig. 45–16; Artist: Kristin N. Mount.

Chapter 17

Figure 17–01 Art, From Medical Surgical Nursing: Critical Thinking in Client Care, by Priscilla LeMone, Karen M. Burke, Edition 3, © 2004 by Prentice-Hall, Inc., Upper Saddle River, New Jersey; Page 877, Fig. 30–03; Artist: Precision Graphics.

Figure 17–02 Art, From Medical Surgical Nursing: Critical Thinking in Client Care, by Priscilla LeMone, Karen M. Burke, Edition 3, © 2004 by Prentice-Hall, Inc., Upper Saddle River, New Jersey; Page 1169, Fig. 36–24; Artist: Nea Hanscomb.

Index